Articular Cartilage Lesions

Springer Science+Business Media, LLC

Brian J. Cole, MD, MBA
*Associate Professor, Departments of Orthopaedics and Anatomy,
Director, Rush Cartilage Restoration Center,
Rush University Medical Center, Chicago, Illinois*

M. Mike Malek, MD
Washington Orthopaedic and Knee Clinic, Inc., Fairfax, Virginia

Articular Cartilage Lesions
A Practical Guide to Assessment and Treatment

With 302 Illustrations in 547 Parts, 301 in Full Color

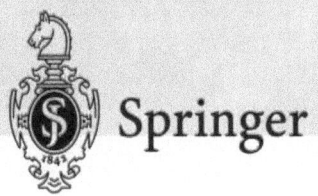

Springer

Brian J. Cole, MD, MBA
Associate Professor
Departments of Orthopaedics and Anatomy
Director, Rush Cartilage Restoration Center
Rush University Medical Center
Chicago, IL 60612
USA

M. Mike Malek, MD
Washington Orthopaedic and Knee
  Clinic, Inc.
Fairfax, VA 22031
USA

.

Library of Congress Cataloging-in-Publication Data

Cole, Brian J.
   Articular cartilage lesions : a practical guide to assessment and treatment / Brian J. Cole,
M. Mike Malek
       p.   cm.
   Includes bibliographical references and index.
    ISBN 978-1-4757-9289-8   ISBN 978-0-387-21553-2 (eBook)
    DOI 10.1007/978-0-387-21553-2

    1. Articular cartilage—Wounds and injuries. 2. Articular cartilage—Surgery. I. Malek,
M. Mike, II. Title.

RD560.C64 2004
617.4'72044—dc22   2003063338

ISBN 978-1-4757-9289-8   Printed on acid-free paper.

© 2004 Springer Science+Business Media New York
Originally published by Springer-Verlag New York, Inc. in 2004
Softcover reprint of the hardcover 1st edition 2004

9 8 7 6 5 4 3 2 1   SPIN 10885672

www.springer-ny.com

springeronline.com

Foreword

For more than 250 years, surgeons have been trying to find ways to restore articular cartilage surfaces, efforts that for most of the last quarter of a millennium yielded little progress. In the last few decades, however, advances in understanding of articular cartilage biology and biomechanics have led to new approaches to restoring articular cartilage, including stimulating cartilage repair from marrow and synovial cells, chondrocyte transplantation, osteochondral autografts and allografts, and alterations of joint loading, including joint distraction. These new approaches to the treatment of articular cartilage injuries have created considerable public interest and led patients and orthopaedic surgeons to believe that restoration of articular cartilage structure and function is possible.

Yet, many questions concerning the treatment of articular cartilage injuries remain, leaving patients and surgeons uncertain about the current best treatment for a specific injury, or if surgical treatment should be attempted. Some of this uncertainty results from the difficulties in performing well-designed prospective studies of different approaches to restoring articular surfaces. Does chondrocyte transplantation produce better results than microfracture repair for specific types of articular cartilage injury? Or, do fresh osteochondral allografts produce better results than chondrocyte transplantation? Answers to questions like these will require expensive and time-consuming prospective clinical research and the cooperation of large numbers of patients.

In addition, the natural history of many types of articular cartilage injuries has not been defined, so it is not clear which injuries should be treated surgically. Understandably, most patients with articular cartilage injuries turn to their orthopaedic surgeons to provide them with clear treatment recommendations. Yet, many knowledgeable surgeons have limited experience with the spectrum of current treatments for articular cartilage injuries.

For these reasons, there is a clear need to critically analyze the available information to help patients and surgeons make treatment decisions concerning articular cartilage injuries. This book will help orthopaedic surgeons evaluate the massive and often confusing information about articular cartilage injuries and their treatment to help make the best possible decisions. The book takes the refreshing approach of examining the various approaches to treatment of articular cartilage and then uses case studies that help illustrate and explain the decision-making process and the treatment of patients. The next decades will bring substantial new information about chondral injuries and new treatments, but this book fills a clear and important present need, and the authors and editors deserve great credit for this effort to improve the care of patients with articular cartilage injuries.

Joseph A. Buckwalter, MD
Professor and Chair
Department of Orthopaedic Surgery
University of Iowa Hospitals and Clinics
Iowa City, IA

Preface

In the last 20 years, the subspecialty of cartilage repair has gradually emerged in the field of orthopaedics. It offers options where none previously existed. In the early 1990s, not uncommonly, knee arthroscopies were performed on young patients who were unable to remain active because of joint pain, swelling, and mechanical symptoms that resulted from their articular cartilage disease. As residents, we remember feeling helpless when postoperatively these patients were told to live with their disease because no reliable treatments were available. The only option—besides the eventual knee arthroplasty that many of these patients would predictably undergo in the future—was debridement and lavage or marrow stimulation. The situation was even more complex because patients experienced a combination of pathology including articular cartilage defects, meniscal deficiency, ligament disruption, and malalignment. Thus, any biologic solution used as an alternative to arthroplasty would, by necessity, be multifactorial. This complimentary approach would seek to maximize the treatment outcome.

Articular cartilage defects are unlike traditional orthopaedic pathology, in which surgeons are accustomed to evaluating, treating, and predicting a likely outcome. In the case of articular cartilage disease, very little is known about its cause and incidence—and even less about the natural history of the incidental defect in an otherwise healthy knee. But because articular cartilage defects can and do cause pain and disability in some patients, many of us remain committed to critical investigation of the basic science and clinical results of the existing and emerging technology. Unlike solutions used to treat traditional orthopaedic pathology, the solutions for treating articular cartilage disease and meniscal deficiency have a relatively short track record, are resource intense, and may require a prolonged period of time before the patient actually has demonstrable relief of pain and increased function. These factors create an especially difficult, but warranted, approach to the management of articular cartilage disease and meniscal deficiency.

Few subspecialties are held to the standards that are intrinsic to the field of cartilage repair. Clearly, the concerted efforts of the basic scientists and clinicians who cross multiple disciplines will lead to an evidence-based approach to the decision making required to manage this patient population. Although successful clinical outcomes can be anticipated in the majority of patients who are appropriately indicated for cartilage repair procedures, we must continue to indicate our patients wisely. Remembering that not all articular cartilage defects will become symptomatic and that not all meniscectomized knees will become arthritic is of primary importance. Furthermore, those who are appropriately indicated may only be provided a greater number of pain-free years, and the natural history of the underlying disease process and inevitable outcome may not always be avoidable. Thus, because our success is primarily predicated upon a reduction in the patient's symptoms and increases in function, we should avoid treating solely for the purpose of eliminating the need for knee arthroplasty in the future. It is critical to avoid choosing treatment options early in the disease process that can potentially burn bridges for the implementation of future options, or even worse, create new problems for patients who were otherwise minimally symptomatic. At this juncture, our judgment is guided by our experience and emerging peer-reviewed clinical outcomes.

René Descartes taught that "our eyes do not see what our minds do not know." I think that this is especially true of articular cartilage and meniscal pathology. Although we have become comfortable attributing a patient's symptoms to specific pathoanatomy, it is imperative that we avoid the temptation to think linearly about a patient's problem. In other words, the mere existence of an articular defect or a post-meniscectomized state is not always synonymous with a symptomatic state. Knee pain has many causes, both known and unknown. Ascribing a patient's symptoms to an incidentally discovered defect that may have no clinical relevance can lead to the eventual implementation of an inappropriate treatment option. We often tell patients that articular cartilage defects are a bit like real estate—location counts. For example, an 18-year-old woman without swelling or mechanical symptoms who has a known defect of the posterior medial femoral condyle but who only complains of anterior knee pain going up and down stairs has patellofemoral pain treatable with appropriate physical therapy until proven otherwise. Because the available technology used to treat these patients is perceptively seductive to patients and physicians alike, we have an unprecedented obligation to implement these technologies both responsibly and ethically.

As orthopaedic surgeons, we traditionally focus on techniques and the "how to" rather than when to implement a solution that is likely to match or exceed our patient's expectations. Despite volumes of clinical and basic science research literature, more questions than answers remain. Adoption of a single technique is based upon the composite influence of what we know, what we think we know, and what we have little knowledge about. How do we fill these voids? How do we make the best decisions with our patients? With so much technology and so much difficulty arriving at a consensus regarding the indications for these procedures, it is imperative that an up-to-date composite body of work be available as a practical guide to manage these lesions.

Articular Cartilage Lesions: A Practical Guide to Assessment and Treatment reflects our commitment to fill the current void in the management of articular cartilage disease and meniscal deficiency. We have asked experts to contribute to this book with a very specific mission in mind: to help you develop an evidence-based decision-making framework to be used as a practical guide for the assessment and management of patients with articular cartilage lesions and meniscal deficiency. Because clinical outcomes are rapidly appearing in the literature, and new technology is emerging at a feverish pace, we mandated that this project be completed in an expedited manner. To maximize the quality and accuracy of the contents herein, the entire project was completed within eighteen months.

The book is divided into three logical parts. Part I, Background and Patient Assessment, provides a framework to understand the underlying pathoanatomy, evaluate the prospective patient, consider nonoperative or palliative management, and offer a potential treatment algorithm. Part II, Surgical Techniques, includes a concise compendium of every available treatment option with a step-by-step approach to each technique ranging from arthroscopy and debridement through unicondylar arthroplasty. Part III, Case Studies, highlights the decision-making process through case-based learning. Nearly 40 illustrated cases have been completely prepared with preoperative planning and postoperative outcomes. They include virtually every permutation and combination of cartilage repair currently in clinical use.

Articular Cartilage Lesions: A Practical Guide to Assessment and Treatment is timely, comprehensive, and up to date. We would like to thank the contributing authors who have put forth enormous effort to help create what we believe will remain a primary reference for orthopaedic surgeons, fellows, residents, basic scientists and any clinician committed to implementing sound judgment, excellence in surgical technique and perioperative management of the patient with articular cartilage disease and meniscal deficiency. We would also like to thank Rob Albano, Peter Bak, and Barbara Chernow for helping to assure that this project was completed on time and with excellence from the time the cover is opened until the final case is presented.

Brian J. Cole, MD, MBA
M. Mike Malek, MD

Genzyme Biosurgery is proud to have collaborated with Springer-Verlag to support the publication of this book. We are committed to improving patient care through education, research and advancing the field of cartilage repair. We applaud the efforts of the books' contributors and believe this text will be a valuable reference for clinicians seeking expert guidance in this emerging field.

Genzyme Biosurgery
A division of Genzyme Corporation
Cambridge, MA

Contents

Contributors

Mats Brittberg, MD, PhD
Department of Orthopaedics, Cartilage Research Unit, Göteborg University, Kungsbacka Hospital, S-434 80 Kungsbacka, Sweden

Tim Bryant, RN
Cartilage Repair Center, Brigham and Women's Hospital, Chestnut Hill, MA 02467, USA

William D. Bugbee, MD
Department of Orthopaedic Surgery, University of California, San Diego, La Jolla, CA 92037 USA

Richard D. Coutts, MD
Department of Orthopaedic Surgery, University of California, San Diego, La Jolla, CA 92093, and Department of Orthopedic Surgery, Sharp Memorial Hospital, San Diego, CA 92123, USA

Brian J. Cole, MD, MBA
Associate Professor, Departments of Orthopaedics and Anatomy, Director, Rush Cartilage Restoration Center, Rush University Medical Center, Chicago, IL 60612, USA

Michael G. Dennis, MD
Attending Physician, Orthopaedic Care Center, Aventura Hospital and Medical Center, Aventura, FL 33180, USA

Jeffrey R. Dugas, MD
Department of Orthopaedic Sports Medicine, American Sports Medicine Institute, Healthsouth Medical Center, Birmingham, AL 35255, USA

Gregory C. Fanelli, MD
Sports Injury Clinic, Department of Orthopaedic Surgery, Geisinger Clinic Medical Center, Danville, PA 17822, USA

Jack Farr, MD
Department of Orthopedic Surgery, Indiana University School of Medicine, Indianapolis, IN 46202, and Cartilage Restoration Center, OrthoIndy Knee Care Institute, Indianapolis, IN 46237, USA

Peter J. Fowler, MD, FRCS (C)
Department of Orthopaedic Surgery, Fowler Kennedy Sport Medicine Clinic, University of Western Ontario, London, Ontario N6A 3K7, Canada

Wayne K. Gersoff, MD
Department of Orthopedics, Sky Ridge Medical Center, Denver, CO 80220, USA

Thomas J. Gill, MD
Department of Orthopedic Surgery, Massachusetts General Hospital, Harvard Medical School, Boston, MA 02114, USA

Scott D. Gillogly, MD
Atlanta Sports Medicine and Orthopaedic Center, Atlanta, GA 30327, USA

Daniel A. Grande, PhD
Department of Orthopaedic Surgery, North Shore/Long Island Jewish Health System, Manhasset, NY 11030, USA

Laurence D. Higgins, MD
Division of Orthopaedic Surgery, Duke University Medical Center, Durham, NC 27708, USA

Michael J. Langworthy, MD
Department of Orthopaedics, Naval Medical Center, San Diego, Chula Vista, CA 91910, USA

Andrew S. Levy, MD
Department of Orthopedics, New Jersey Medical School, Newark, NJ 07103, and Center for Advanced Sports Medicine, Knee and Shoulder, Medical Arts Center, Summit, NJ 07901, USA

Yan Lu, MD
Department of Medical Sciences, University of Wisconsin-Madison, Madison, WI 53706, USA

Bert R. Mandelbaum, MD
Santa Monica Orthopaedic and Sports Medicine Research Foundation, Santa Monica, CA 90404, USA

Mark D. Markel, DVM, PhD
Department of Medical Sciences, School of Veterinary Medicine, University of Wisconsin, Madison, WI 53706, USA

L. Pearce McCarty, III, MD
Harvard Combined Orthopaedic Residency, Boston, MA 02114, USA

Steven W. Meier, MD
Department of Orthopedic Surgery, Overlook Hospital, Summit, NJ 07902, USA

R. Michael Meneghini, MD
Department of Orthopaedic Surgery, Rush University Medical Center, Chicago, IL 60612, USA

Lyle J. Micheli, MD
Department of Orthopaedic Surgery/Sports Medicine, Children's Hospital, Harvard Medical School, Boston, MA 02115, USA

Tom Minas, MD, MS
Department of Orthopedics, Cartilage Repair Center, Brigham and Women's Hospital Harvard Medical School, Chestnut Hill, MA 02467, USA

Steve A. Mora, MD
725 LaVeta, Orange, CA 92868, USA

Fred R.T. Nelson, MD
Department of Orthopaedics, Henry Ford Hospital, Detroit, MI 48170, USA

Daniel R. Orcutt, MD, MS
Department of Orthopaedic Surgery, Geisinger Medical Center, Danville, PA 17822, USA

Justin P. Roe, MB, BS, BSc(Med), FRACS
Department of Orthopaedic Surgery, North Sydney Orthopaedic and Sport Medicine Centre, Sydney, New South Wales 2065, Australia

Giles R. Scuderi, MD
Department of Orthopaedic Surgery, Beth Israel Medical Center, New York, NY 10128, USA

Mitchell B. Sheinkop, MD
Adult Reconstruction Program, Department of Orthopaedic Surgery, Rush University Medical Center, Chicago, IL 60612, USA

J. Richard Steadman, MD
Steadman Hawkins Clinic, Vail, CO 81657, USA

Kenneth R. Zaslav, MD
Department of Orthopedic Surgery, Virginia Commonwealth University, Richmond, VA 23284, and The Sports Medicine Center, Advanced Orthopedic Centers, Richmond, VA 23294, USA

PART I

Background and Patient Assessment

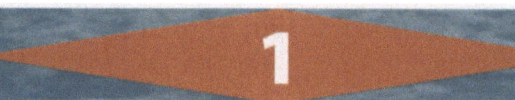

Basic Science

Michael J. Langworthy, Fred R.T. Nelson, and Richard D. Coutts

Articular cartilage is the specialized organ covering the ends of diarthrodial joints. It is tough, resilient, and structured to undergo years of cyclic loading without breaking down. This endurance is achieved by a highly stable collagen architecture that contains the high swelling pressure of the water, which is attracted by the predominant proteoglycan, aggrecan. This living tissue is immunoprivileged, aneural, and appears to rely on mechanical forces for biologic regulation. Current research is focused on the embryonic and fetal development of the articular cartilage end organ, the mechanical and biochemical accelerators of degradation, and the mechanisms of degradation and repair, including potential disease-modifying agents.

It is remarkable that in most joints, cartilage is only 2 to 3 mm thick, has a relatively stable collagen architecture, and at some locations supports 1 to 4 megapascals (Mpa) (150 to 600 pounds per square inch) of force[1-3] an average of 2 million times each year.[4] It is even more remarkable that it can remain attached to bone without separation for a lifetime. In addition, the structure and chemistry vary from location to location within one joint[5] and from one joint to another.[6] There is no comparison in the industrial world.

FORMATION AND STRUCTURE

Cells that are destined to form articular cartilage begin their development before 8 weeks of gestation.[7] Homeobox and other genes transcribe the mRNA of the cells based on the orientation of the cells in a three-plane axis. By 8 weeks of gestation, the articular cartilage is heterogeneous, with distinct chondrocyte populations for surface growth and others for the eventual epiphysis. Precise cytokine expression directs the development of the variously shaped diarthrodial joints.[8,9] After the development of the epiphyseal center of ossification, there is a relatively small growth plate that develops on the bony surface with chonodrocyte division leading away from the ossifying front. This growth plate allows for the expansion in size and shape of the eventual adult bone architecture. It has recently been determined that the cells near the articular surface of joints have the residual growth-regulating protein that is an intracellular signaling molecule seen in early articular cartilage development.[8] Other intracellular signaling proteins are responsible for the events that lead to the segregation of the chondrocytes into specialized layers.[10]

Adult articular cartilage is layered into superficial, transitional, deep, and calcified zones (Figure 1.1). Each of these zones has a specific chondrocyte orientation, biology, structural organization, and physiologic response to force (Figure 1.2). The biomechanical responses of articular cartilage vary with depth, location, and age.[11-14] Matrix composition and structural orientation allow articular cartilage to convert shear and compression forces into tensile forces at the bone surface.[15] Per volume of tissue, articular cartilage has a relatively sparse number of chondrocytes distributed throughout an extracellular matrix of proteoglycans, collagen, proteins, and water. The structure and density composition varies not only throughout the depth of the extracellular matrix, but also about the territorial regions of the individual chondrocytes. From the articular surface to the subchondral bone there are distinct histologic areas that can be demonstrated with specific stains (see Figure 1.2).

The superficial zone is composed of chondrocytes that are elongated and oriented along with thin collagen fibrils parallel to the joint surface (Figure 1.3). The high tensile integrity of articular cartilage is produced by the horizontally directed fibers as well as a thin surface collagen structure called the lamina splendens. Hydration is high in this zone, and proteoglycan content is lower than in the other zones. The transitional (middle) zone contains chondrocytes that are rounder in appearance. Collagen fibrils are larger and organized in a crossing pattern. The proteoglycan concentration is the highest, with a corresponding decrease in the hydration of this zone. The chondrocytes in the deep zone are also round but are arranged in a columnar pattern. The collagen is likewise oriented in a columnar pattern and is perpendicular to the underlying subchondral bone. The zone of calcified cartilage contains some chondrocytes. The matrix has apatitic salts and an orientation that unites directly with the underlying bone. The deep zone and calcified zone are separated by the tidemark, which is thought to act as a barrier to vascular penetration.

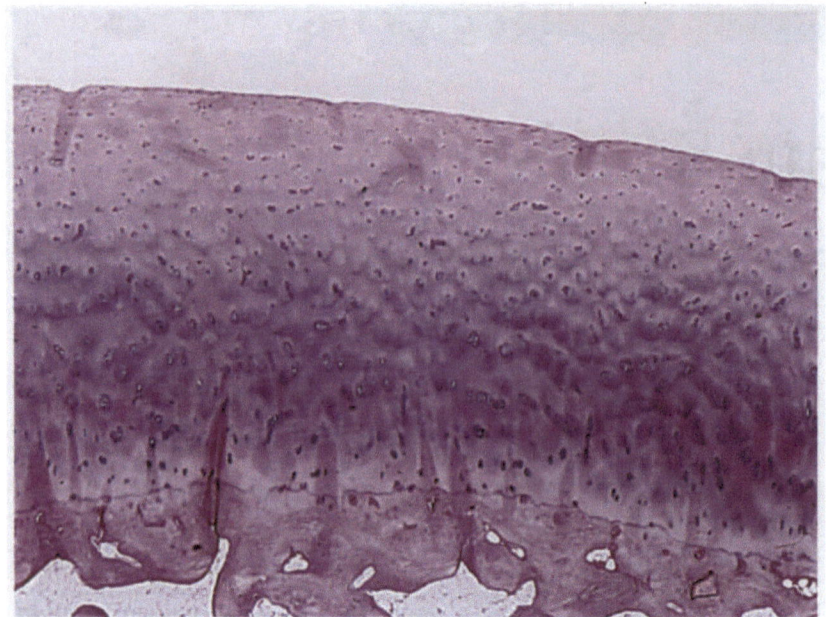

FIGURE 1.1 Stained section of normal adult articular cartilage shows typical horizontal orientation of chondrocytes, relative decreased number of chondrocytes per volume in deeper layer, intact tidemark without vascular ingrowth, and absence of cellular cloning.

CHONDROCYTES AND MATRIX

The matrix surrounding the widely spaced chondrocytes is composed of three zones (Figure 1.2). The pericellular matrix closest to the cell is high in type VI collagen and has a relatively high metabolic turnover. The territorial matrix immediately adjacent to the pericellular matrix, although exhibiting less metabolic activity, is the first to have increased matrix turnover in osteoarthrosis. The interterritorial matrix is more stable and the last to show response to osteoarthrosis.

Electron microscopy demonstrates considerable variation in chondrocyte intracellular structure. This anatomic speci-ficity has been correlated with the position of the chondrocyte as related to depth within the articular cartilage.[16] Depending on their zonal location, chondrocytes make up less than 10% of the volume of articular cartilage. All components of the matrix are synthesized by the chondrocyte. Oxygen utilization has been shown to be lower in cartilage than in other tissues, despite the presence of a well-defined glycolytic pathway, and the cells appear to rely on energy production from an anaerobic pathway.[17] Transient changes in metabolic activity can occur with minor injury and may result in full recovery of the structure and function of the matrix, provided the chondrocyte continues to remain viable.

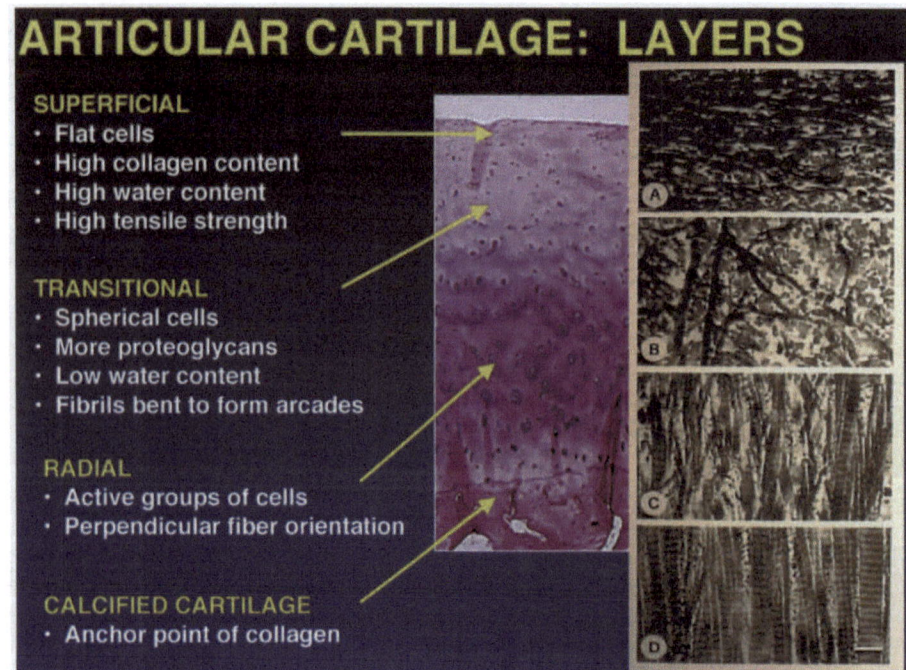

FIGURE 1.2 Specific layers show different morphology by histology and electron microscopy.

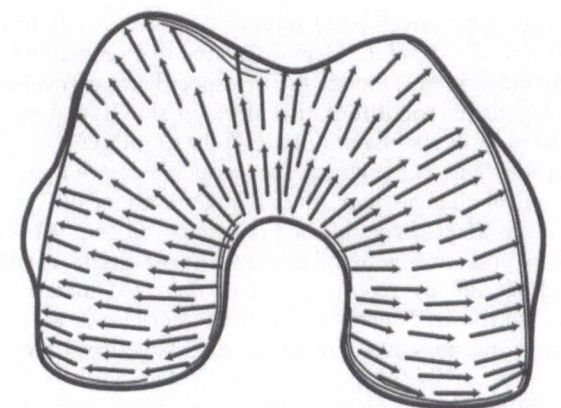

FIGURE 1.3 Split lines demonstrate specific parallel orientation of superficial collagen fibers.

Despite intensive investigation, it is not exactly clear how the chondrocyte obtains its nutrition to fuel its anaerobic and aerobic metabolism. Interruption of contact between cartilage and vascularized subchondral bone appears to result in degradation of cartilage in an animal model.[18] Uninjured adult articular cartilage has no vascular supply. Perfusion of the matrix and chondrocytes occurs from movement of the synovial fluid that occurs with the loading that accompanies joint motion. Because of the small pore size in the superficial zone (around 50 Å), it may take 10 s to several hours for molecular diffusion into the cartilage to occur, depending on the structure, size, charge, and weight of the molecule.[19,20] Some growth factors (interleukin-1) appear to move freely through the cartilaginous matrix. Fragmented and degraded portions of proteoglycans that are generated during normal turnover are able to passively leave the matrix.[20]

MATRIX COMPOSITION

Between 65% and 80% of the wet weight of normal articular cartilage is water.[21] More than 70% of the dry weight of cartilage is collagen. Type II collagen makes up more than 95% of the total collagen content of hyaline cartilage.[22,23] Type II collagen is composed of three identical collagen fibers that form a triple helix and is assembled outside the cell in a staggered fashion. Normally, there is very little turnover of collagen in the adult.[24–26] Collagen fibrils create a mesh that entraps aggrecan and provides the tensile strength of cartilage[13,27] (Figure 1.4). The passage of strongly charged ions through the soluble, fixed, and charged molecular surface of articular cartilage produces physiologically important effects.[28] Collagen types V, VI, IX, and XI also participate in matrix structure and function.[21] Types V, IX, and XI associate with type II collagen fibrils, whereas type VI is a nonfibrillar pericellular collagen. Because the hydroxylation of proline to hydroxyproline is a posttranslational event in collagen formation, tritiated proline is often used as a method for determining collagen synthesis, whereas hydroxyproline is used to measure the amount of total collagen.[29]

Aggrecan constitutes 80% to 90% of all the proteoglycans in articular cartilage. It is composed of extremely hydrophilic glycosaminoglycan chains that branch out from a 220-kDa protein core. More than 100 chondroitin sulfate and keratin sulfate chains are covalently bonded to a protein core. The core protein is attached to hyaluronic acid by a link protein. Hyaluronic acid is a disaccharide repeat of *N*-acetyl glucosamine and glucuronic acid. Up to 100 aggrecan molecules can associate with a single hyaluronic acid chain. The repeating carboxyl or sulfate groups of chondroitin sulfate and keratan sulfate are responsible for a high avidity for water because they impart a strong negative charge that attracts the positive charge of water. In cartilage degradation, the relative water content of cartilage increases as a result of collagen loss or proteoglycan depletion with increased hydration (Figure 1.5). [35]S is used as an indicator of proteoglycan synthesis because of its high concentration in aggrecan. Two other important proteoglycans are biglycan and decorin. Decorin is thought to participate in posttranslational collagen fibril modification; biglycan also plays a role in collagen organization.[30] Despite the small molecular weight of these proteoglycans, they numerically equal the content of the larger aggrecan in total matrix content.

BIOMECHANICS

Adult articular cartilage on average experiences about 2 MPa of force in the hip, knee, and ankle.[1,2,31,32] Meniscal or anterior cruciate injury can increase articular forces to well over 8 MPa, which is well beyond the normal loads of 1 to 4 MPa;

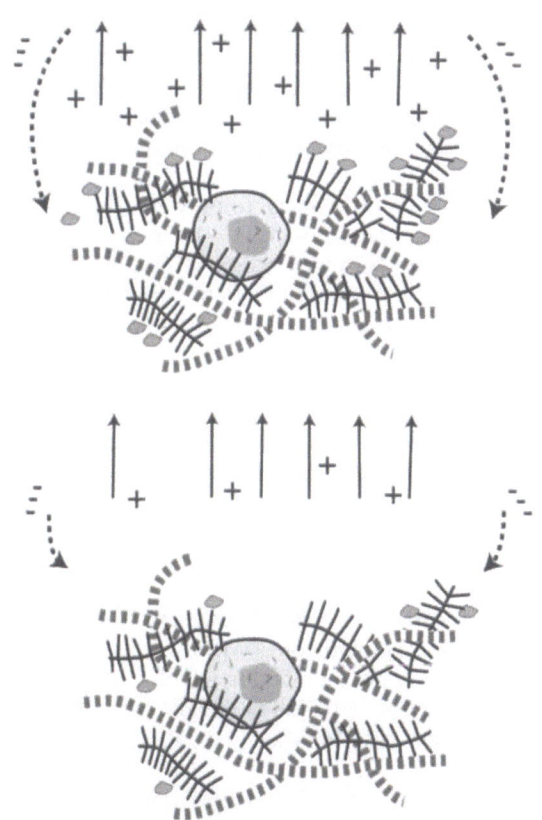

FIGURE 1.4 Relationship of collagen to proteoglycan results in charge density with development of physiologically important charge.

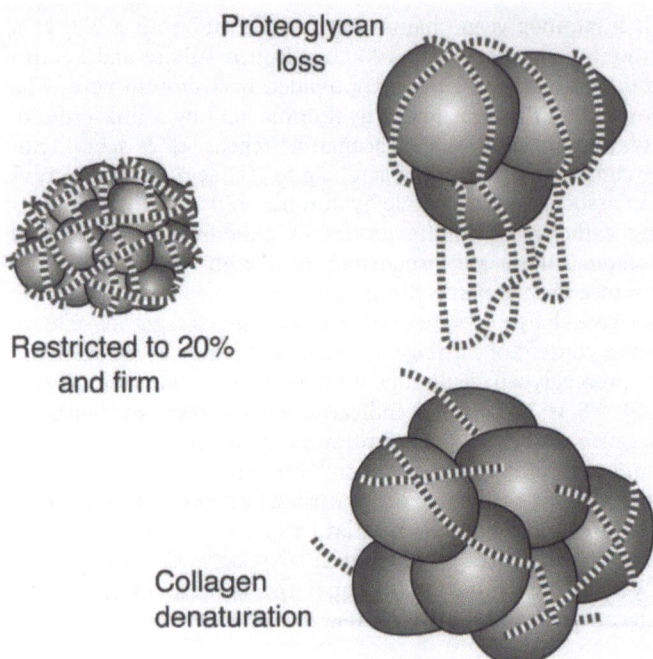

Proteoglycan loss

Restricted to 20% and firm

Collagen denaturation

FIGURE 1.5 Restriction of swelling of proteoglycan and effect of either collagen or collagen loss on tensile property of cartilage.

this might explain subsequent arthritic degeneration over months and years.[33] Articular cartilage is viscoelastic, which in biology means a property of tissue that exhibits both viscous and elastic behavior (creep and stress relaxation); the material's stress strain behavior depends on strain rate.[34] Articular cartilage is anisotropic, which means that the intrinsic material properties depend on the matrix orientation and composition, as well as the direction in which the cartilage is loaded. This anisotropic orientation has been demonstrated with India ink staining. Collagen restricts the swelling pressure of aggrecan to only 20% of its capacity to associate with water, which is 50 times its weight.[35] The internal pressure within cartilage is 0.5 MPa (75 pounds/in²).

The four zones of cartilage behave somewhat differently with statically applied strains.[12] The highest axial strain measurements have been found in the transitional zone. However, this was significant only with respect to the upper and lower radial zones. It is thought that this relatively low axial strain pattern in the lower radial zone is most likely related to the high proteoglycan content of this zone and its attachment to the underlying subchondral bone.[36] A constant force will produce creep and the deformation from the stress will increase with time, so long as the force is maintained.

On the surface of articular cartilage, the collagen fibers have a tensile strength of 30 MPa in the young adult. To understand the relevance of this figure, compare aluminum, which has a tensile strength of 70 MPa, with nylon, having a tensile strength of 80 MPa.[37]

Isolated Chondral Injury Versus Osteoarthrosis

The concept of the relationship between duration, intensity, and frequency of an applied force on articular cartilage is

described as an envelope of injury.[38] Single-event traumatic episodes tend to produce lesions isolated to a geographic area and are most often associated with a specific injury event. On the other hand, conditions that develop slowly and are not associated with trauma are more likely to influence a wider area of the joint. These changes are associated with long-term biochemical changes that affect a larger amount of cartilage around the affected site, leading to osteoarthrosis.[39] Articular chondrocytes are generally able to maintain cartilage throughout life by replacing lost or damaged matrix with freshly synthesized material. Synthetic activity is very well regulated and increases rapidly to well above basal levels in response to cartilage injury, suggesting that synthesis activity is linked to matrix loss through some damage control mechanism. A major stimulator of matrix synthesis is insulin-like growth factor I (IGF-I). Its availability in cartilage is controlled by IGF-binding proteins (IGFBPs) that are secreted by the chondrocytes. IGFBPs are part of a complex system, termed the IGF-I axis, that tightly regulates IGF-I activity. The IGFBPs block IGF-I activity by sequestering IGF-I from its cell receptor. The binding protein IGFBP-3 has recently been studied and found to increase with chondrocyte age, paralleling an age-related decline in matrix synthesis activity. IGFBP-3 is actually overexpressed in osteoarthritic cartilage with resultant disturbances in metabolic activity and subsequent matrix degeneration. These observations may indicate that IGFBP-3 plays a crucial role in regulating matrix synthesis in cartilage. Cartilage damage control mechanisms may fail due to age-related changes in IGFBP-3 expression or distribution. It is likely that the chondrocyte and the area of the territorial matrix play important roles in the cartilage damage control by interfering with the chondrocyte's ability to respond to IGF-1.[40]

Basic Research and Current Methods of Treatment for Cartilage Damage

NATURAL COURSE OF CARTILAGE INJURY

Shetland ponies were used to compare 3-mm, 9-mm, 15-mm, and 21-mm defects in the knee over a course of 6 months. The 3-mm defects completely filled. Both the 9- and 15-mm defects were still apparent at 6 months, with a softening of surrounding cartilage in the 15- and 21-mm defects.[41] In the other study, although immature rabbits (3–4 months) were used, 2-mm diameter superficial surfaces were shaved off with a sharp knife blade. The shaved surfaces smoothed over, but there was no filling of these very small and thin defects. The surrounding chondrocytes reacted with matrix changes, particularly in the pericellular area, but there was no matrix expansion or new cells.[42]

MARROW STIMULATION

Early research has been directed at filling articular defects with tissue that approximates articular cartilage by stimulating a repair tissue from the marrow. Stem cells are capable of developing into a multitude of tissues. Bone, muscle, fat, tendon, and cartilage have all been obtained from these multipotential cells. A stem cell population capable of differentiating into cells that can produce cartilage is obtainable from the bone marrow. In human studies, the fraction of stem cells that retain the ability to develop various types of tissue has been found to decline radically from 1 in 20,000 cells in juvenile humans to only 1 in 4,000,000 during late adult life.[43]

Microfracture of the subchondral bone is believed to deliver stem cells from the bone to the articular surface, resulting in nechondrogenesis. The majority of studies are based on human clinical results from microfracture.[44,45] Based on studies in rabbits, protection of the joint and the use of continuous passive motion (CPM) appear to have a positive effect on cartilage development.[46]

The origin and differentiation of cells in the repair of 3-mm-diameter cylindrical, full-thickness articular cartilage and bone defects were studied by Shapiro et al. in New Zealand white rabbits.[47] In the first few days, fibrinous arcades were established in the defects within a clot from surface edge to surface edge. At 10 days, safranin O staining revealed evidence of a glycosaminoglycan (GAG) containing extracellular matrix. By 14 days, a type of cartilage-like tissue was present immediately beneath the surface of the fibrinous arcade. This substance was densely populated with flattened fibrocartilaginous cells. By 3 weeks, the sites of almost all the defects had a well-demarcated layer of cartilage-like tissue. Autoradiography, after labeling with ^{3}H-thymidine and ^{3}H-cytidine, demonstrated that chondrocytes from the adjacent native cartilage did not participate in the repopulation of the defect. The cartilaginous repair appeared to be mediated by the proliferation and differentiation of mesenchymal cells from the bone marrow. Interestingly, the radioisotope label taken up by undifferentiated mesenchymal cells appeared not only in the new chondrocytes but also in fibroblasts and osteoblasts. Early traces of degeneration of the new cartilage matrix were seen in many of the defects by 12 weeks, with the prevalence and severity of the degeneration increasing at 24 to 48 weeks. Polarized light microscopy demonstrated that the newly synthesized matrix had failed to integrate with the native cartilage adjacent to the drilled hole. It was hypothesized that the lack of integration allowed motion of the repair substance with resultant early degeneration.

It has been demonstrated that periosteal and bone marrow-derived cells can produce a similar pattern of differentiation into articular cartilage in New Zealand white rabbits.[48] Trypsin was used to digest free periosteal and bone marrow-derived cells, which were then injected into a type I collagen gel implanted into the site. Defects filled with carrier gel and defects left empty did not have the same repair of cartilage and subchondral bone fill within the 3-mm defects as the cell-impregnated gel defects. The cell-impregnated gels had good reparative tissue that resembled hyaline cartilage. This hyaline-like cartilage thinned out over a period of 24 weeks.

OSTEOCHONDRAL GRAFTS

The successful transplantation of articular cartilage that is capable of restoring joint function, providing pain relief, and giving long-term, reproducible, and excellent outcomes has been the holy grail of cartilage repair. Lexer attempted substitution of whole joints as far back as 1908.[49,50] By 1925, it was noted that even though whole joint transplantation had an initial good clinical result, the ones that did not fail due to infection developed frank degenerative changes in the cartilage. It was not until the early 1950s that a canine animal model was used to study morphologic and histologic differences between autografts and allografts following transplantation.[51] An extensive subsequent literature in this area has recorded variable results and outcomes. Several critical factors have been identified that contribute to the success of cartilage transplantation. The chondrocytes must survive the transplantation, and they must remain viable and capable of continued production of normal matrix. The matrix must remain mechanically competent without degeneration or substitution to a fibrocartilage. The bony portion of the graft must integrate and form a mechanically sound union with the host recipient site. Mechanical instability may to indicate the development of an immune response.[52]

In the late 1970s and early 1980s, a number of studies examined various aspects of cartilage transplantation in animals to delineate the optimal conditions of transplantation. Autograft and allograft osteochondral transplantation were studied using gross observation, radiology, histology, histochemistry, and biochemistry. Lane and Brighton[53] examined joint resurfacing in the New Zealand white rabbit utilizing autologous transplanted femoral condyles. The lateral femoral condyle was completely excised and then fixed back into its original position with a straight Keith needle. Subsequent examination revealed that the cartilage surface appeared normal in 80% of these cases. At 1 year, histologic examination demonstrated that the thickness of the cartilage had been preserved, with the exception of a few areas of localized thinning of the cartilage. Biochemical analysis of the harvested implants revealed that DNA, hydroxyproline content, and SO_4 incorporation were equal to those of the non-harvested portions of the joint and also to sham-operated intact condyles.[53]

Lipton et al.[54] utilized a similar protocol to study allotransplantation of osteochondral grafts. Osteochondral femoral allografts were performed in male adult New Zealand white rabbits, paired arthrotomies being performed simultaneously in different rabbits. The left lateral femoral condyles were osteotomized and an osteochondral graft was harvested with 5 mm of subchondral bone. Care was taken to avoid transplanting any soft tissue. The grafts were then switched, transplanted from one rabbit to the other, and fixed with small K-wires. The rabbits were allowed full weight bearing without immobilization. The condyles were then harvested at 3, 6, and 18 months. Physical examination of the joints before harvest revealed no swelling, inflammation, or instability of any of the knee joints. However, gross inspection of the joints at necropsy revealed that one third of the joints had sustained advanced cartilaginous degeneration, with fraying and even loss of articular cartilage leading to eburnation of the bone, although two thirds of the joints appeared normal. The arthritic degeneration was noted to correlate with the joints that had not maintained an anatomic reduction following allograft transfer. Histologic analysis of the allografts that had maintained anatomic reduction revealed no differences when compared to cartilage from the undisturbed contralateral joint.

Biochemical testing performed on the anatomically reduced allografts at 3, 6, and 18 months following transplantation showed no statistical difference with respect to protein, collagen, hexosamine, or hydroxyproline content. The incorporation of SO_4 was studied in both in vivo and in vitro, and no statistically significant differences were noted between the experimental and control condyles, indicating active metabolism was occurring. Biomechanical testing of the harvested specimens that had retained anatomic reduction revealed that there was no statistically significant difference in percent of creep, instantaneous shear modulus, or relaxed shear modulus between allograft and control cartilage. The allografts that failed appeared to do so because of mechanical problems of fixation, and not graft rejection.[54]

In 1980, De Nubile et al.[55] published data on allotransplantation of preserved and fresh articular cartilage utilizing an osteochondral plug model. It was thought that the plug geometry would be a mechanically stable construct and that the grafts would not undergo premature degeneration. Osteochondral plugs measuring 3 to 5 mm in diameter were obtained from New Zealand white rabbits, with a remnant thickness of 1 mm of subchondral bone. A recipient rabbit was prepared and the donor plug was press-fit into place. No additional fixation besides the press-fit was utilized for graft stabilization. The allografts transplanted in this manner were examined at 3, 6, and 18 months. Gross examination revealed that there was almost complete preservation of cartilage thickness, and in the majority of the specimens, the edges were well united with no clefts. Safranin O staining revealed that the proteoglycan content of the allograft was preserved. A few of the plugs failed to unite to the recipient host bone, and there was a proliferation of fibrous material around the plug. Some of the plugs also appeared to have subsided or were left protruding. The cases in which there was evidence of mechanical instability, subsidence, or protrusion, showed poor preservation of the cartilage matrix. Of special note, a few of the specimen samples appeared to have developed an immunologic reaction that was interpreted as rejection. There were areas around these plugs that contained large numbers of monocytic and plasma inflammatory cells. The authors thought that overall good to excellent results had been achieved in 60% of the specimens.[55] Those plugs that were mechanically unstable appeared to manifest this inflammatory response.

AUTOGRAFT MOSAICPLASTY

In 1991, Lazlo Hangody[56] conceived of a method to use small cylindrical autologous osteochondral plugs for the treatment of focal chondral and osteochondral defects of the femoral condyles in the knee. He tested the concept of mosaicplasty osteochondral transplant on a breed of working dogs. The graft sizes ranged from 2.7 to 4.5 mm. The peripheral margin of the distal femoral supracondylar ridge was selected as the donor site because of its thick cartilage morphology and nonweight-bearing location. At 4 weeks, the cancellous bone between the donor plugs and recipient graft site had united. At 8 weeks, there was a seal between the recipient and donor surface that was interpreted to be a fibrocartilage that produced matrix integration. The original donor sites filled in with cancellous bone and fibrocartilage. This fibrocartilage was also firmly adhered to the surrounding cartilage. Histologic examination of the grafts revealed that the hyaline morphology of both the chondrocytes and cartilage matrix was maintained.[56] In another study, the grafts were all 4.5 mm; 18 were on the nonweight-bearing lateral side and 18 were on the weight-bearing medial side. The lateral side fared better over a year's time, and there was sustained good inter-

plug fibrocartilage fill.[57] Based on these results, the technique was then taken to the clinic and used on humans.

ALLOGRAFT

It is useful to compare organ allografts from other parts of the body to understand the considerations for osteochondral allograft surgery.[58] In the case of a heart transplant, the cells must remain alive for function, and there is no tissue replacement from the recipient. The matrix is not replaced and is maintained by the original organ cells. Tissue donor-to-host compatibility is important. In the case of osteoarticular transplantation, the attached fresh or frozen bone is usually dead on transplantation, unless there is a grafted vascular supply. Over time, dead bone is replaced by living bone. In the case of cortical bone, this process is slow and may only involve a few millimeters of depth. Tissue donor-to-host compatibility is a minor issue unless marrow elements are present. Unfrozen articular cartilage has chondrocyte survival, no rejection, and no host-to-graft cell repopulation (chimerism). Although the graft articular cartilage matrix appears to be maintained over many years, there are studies of cartilage metabolism in allogeneic osteochondral grafts that show a lower cell count and reduced metabolism. The bone is eventually replaced by host bone, but the bone of the cartilage–bone interface does not participate in this process.

Brighton et al.[59] examined methods of articular cartilage storage with the application of tissue culture techniques. Mechanical and histologic examination of the stored constructs was normal when compared to controls. Brighton performed another study in which osteoarticular constructs were stored for 30 days, and it was again found that the biomechanical properties of the constructs were essentially normal when compared to controls. Histologic examination demonstrated that there was only minor swelling of the chondrocytes and that the histochemistry appeared to be normal. Incorporation of SO_4 appeared to be increased when compared to fresh control samples, but there appeared to be normal amounts of hydroxyproline and hexosamine.[59]

Animal studies were then undertaken with transplantation of the stored osteoarticular allograft plugs into New Zealand white rabbits. The results were evaluated at 12 months after transplantation with gross examination as well as mechanical and biochemical testing. More than 70% of the transplanted osteoarticular grafts demonstrated loss of cartilage thickness, irregularity, and fibrillation. Histologically, several of the grafts demonstrated evidence of an immune reaction with large numbers of inflammatory cells and apparent graft necrosis. There was only 50% retention of proteoglycan content, but hydroxyproline content was not significantly different from control values. Only 20% of the grafts appeared to have preserved matrix integrity. Gel filtration chromatography of sulfate-labeled macromolecules in guanidine HCl was utilized to index the quality of the proteoglycans synthesized by fresh and stored osteoarticular allograft plugs. A characterization of the proteoglycans eluted from the grafts revealed that the stored grafts had partially degraded molecules despite a normal staining with Safranin O and normal SO_4 content.[59] This qualitative degradation of cartilage proteoglycan was thought to result in susceptibility to mechanical and immunologic failure. Oates et al.[60] evaluated 12-week postimplanted osteochondral allograft transplants, comparing allografts stored for 14 days in media with 8.8% fetal calf serum at 4°C with fresh allografts. The authors found no significant difference in histology, glycosaminoglycan content, collagen content, permeability, or modulus in the two groups.[60]

Osteochondral allografts can be of three types: shell allograft, mosaicplasty, and large-fragment osteochondral allograft. Fresh allograft replacement surgery has been performed for primary osteoarthritis, osteonecrosis, osteochondritis dissecans, and posttraumatic defects. Procedures for procurement of fresh allograft material have been established by the American Association of Tissue Banks. Donors are typically under 30 years of age, which is thought to maximize cartilage quality. The grafts are harvested under strict aseptic conditions and usually within 24 hours after death. The entire joint is harvested with joint capsule, ligaments, cartilage and metaphyseal bone being excised en bloc. Cultures are taken after harvest, and the entire joint is immersed in lactated Ringer's solution with cefazolin and bacitracin antibiotics being included in the solution. After the container is sealed off, it is stored at 4°C. Histocompatibility markers are not obtained. Donor and recipient are matched for size, and transplantation must take place in less than 1 week.

A biomechanical and biochemical study conducted by Jimenez and Brighton[52] studied fresh-frozen osteochondral allografts in rabbits. The graft was stored for 30 days in tissue culture conditions. They found that 70% to 75% of the sample did not appear normal and manifested early degenerative changes, including fibrillation and loss of proteoglycan.[52] By comparing cryopreservation techniques with fresh osteochondral allografts, it was found that cryopreservation resulted in less immunologic antigenicity, but also marked degeneration of the cartilaginous matrix and chondrocyte viability.[61] A 1985 study by Czitrom et al.[62] found that chondrocyte viability in fresh osteochondral allografts ranged from 69% to 99% when assessed in culture media from biopsy specimens by SO_4 and ^{3}H-cytidine autoradiography in grafts 1 to 6 years after implantation.[62] One six-year graft had only 37% chondrocyte viability, but they were actively producing proteoglycans. Human chondrocytes in the cartilage of a fresh osteochondral allograft can apparently survive for long periods of time. Oakeshott et al.[63] analyzed 18 cases of failed fresh allografts and found that the grafted bone had indeed died; 12 of 18 grafts had viable cells at 13 to 92 months. Convery et al.[64] have also found allograft chondrocyte survival 8 years after implantation. There appears to be a cell-mediated immune response that is responsible for the allografted bone graft rejection.

Langer et al.[65] have demonstrated a positive lymphocytic migration test following graft transplantation. The allograft may actually soften, with subsequent creeping substitution from the host tissue taking place over several years. Graft subsidence has actually been observed at 2 to 3 years after the index surgery, likely because of a delay in early revascularization as a result of the immune response and softened subchondral bone. Basic animal research has demonstrated the importance of isolation of allogeneic chondrocytes from host subchondral bone. Mahomed et al.[66] followed 92 patients with posttraumatic knee injuries who received fresh allograft reconstruction of small osteochondral lesions of either the tibia or femur. Failure was defined as less than 20 points of improvement on the Knee Assessment Scoring System from

the Hospital for Special Surgery (HSS), any revision procedure, or subjective patient assessment that the knee was worse. There was clinical success in 75% at 5 years, 64% at 10 years, and 63% at 14 years after implantation.

Currently, various tissue processing organizations are using culture environments that allegedly maintain chondrocyte viability. These organizations offer "prolonged-fresh" osteoarticular grafts available from 14 days to 45 days postharvest in some instances. The benefits include overcoming the logistics and timing required for clearing these grafts for serology and virus testing which can take upwards of 14 days in some settings before final cultures are obtained. Unfortunately, basic science evaluating cell viability and activity remains limited at this time.

AUTOGENOUS CHONDROCYTE IMPLANTATION

Human chondrocytes have been cultured for autologous chondrocyte implantation in humans since 1987. Peterson et al.[67] reported on successful treatment of focal patellar defects in a rabbit model with the use of transplanted cultured autologous chondrocytes. The cultured chondrocytes were injected under a periosteal flap, which was sutured over the patellar defect. Examination one year after transplantation revealed that a cartilage-like tissue covered about 70 percent of the defects. In 1994, Brittberg et al.[28] reported on the results of 23 patients treated with ACI, with a 16 to 66 month follow-up. Second-look arthroscopy allowed clinical examination at 3 months. These examinations revealed that the transplants were level with the surrounding tissue and somewhat spongy when probed. A second arthroscopic examination was performed on a subset of these patients at 12 to 46 months, and clinical examination revealed that the transplant had progressed through a maturation process and had firmed up. During the second arthroscopic procedure, biopsy specimens extending to the subchondral bone were taken from the central portion of the transplant. Histologic examination and biochemical staining of the transplant biopsies revealed that the transplant had an abundance of type II collagen, similar to normal articular cartilage. Bovine articular chondrocytes in agarose culture produce a matrix capable of developing physiologically important potentials under mechanical stress.[28]

It has been theorized that, because chondrocytes are encased by matrix, they lack the ability to migrate to the site of chondral injury and actively participate in a repair process.[68,69] Animal studies have demonstrated that partial-thickness chondral injuries can sometimes undergo repair by stem cell migration from adjacent synovial tissues.[70] Full-thickness chondral lesions in adult humans have not demonstrated the capacity to heal. Stem cell migration from the underlying subchondral bone with defect filling by fibrocartilage has been studied extensively and has produced variable results as to its effectiveness. The resulting fibrocartilage repair tissue is predominantly fibrous in nature, with variable numbers of chondrocytes present. The tissue, at a microscopic level, appears unorganized and lacks the biomechanical and viscoelastic characteristics of normal hyaline cartilage.[71] Rabbit studies with ACI have shown superior filling of a 3 mm articular cartilage defect. Defects with transplanted cells have more hyaline-like cartilage than untreated defects when analyzed with quantitative stereology. The implanted chondrocytes, when studied with radioisotope labeling, appear to physically adhere to the wound bed and significantly contribute to the repair tissue.[72] Breinan et al.[73] created 4-mm defects in the trochlear groove in three randomized groups of dogs. One group had an empty defect, one group had periosteum sewn over the defect, and the third group had autogenous chondrocyte transplantation with periosteum. Histomorphometric analyses at 12 and 18 months revealed the defect fill was 36% to 76%, hyaline-like cartilage was 10% to 23%, and integration with surrounding cartilage was 16% to 32%, with no significant difference between the three groups.

Peterson et al.[74] performed arthroscopic second looks on 65 patients who had undergone ACI during a 2 to 9-year outcome study. Quality of the repair tissue was assessed as to defect fill, integration with the surrounding cartilage, and surface mechanical characteristics. Biopsy specimens from the central portion of the grafted site were also obtained. Macroscopic assessment of the repair tissue revealed that the implant slowly matured over the course of a year. Arthroscopy done in the first 2 to 3 months demonstrated a repair construct that was typically soft and had a wavelike pattern of graft movement when probed. By 12 months, the repair tissue was almost as firm as the adjacent cartilage. Histopathologic analysis was performed on 37 biopsy specimens. Three pathologists who had been blinded to treatment outcomes were asked to evaluate the tissue samples. The majority of the specimens were thought to have a homogeneous matrix with low cellularity, with rounded chondrocytes encased in typical lacunae. The size, shape, and cell features were characteristic of hyaline cartilage. Immunohistochemical staining was positive for type II cartilage and normal proteoglycan content in all specimens that had a hyaline-like appearance. There was a positive correlation between hyaline-like reconstitution of the defect and clinical outcome. Differences on histologic examination demonstrated a greater number of chondrocytes with more random distribution of cell colonies and absence of columnar organization. Because a periosteal envelope was created to facilitate the construct application, it should be noted that in some biopsy specimen the most superficial layer was composed of remnant fibrocytes which were likely incorporated from the periosteum.

The periosteum appears to incorporate into the repair tissue via metaplasia and is mechanically debrided from the surface of the construct during the first 3 to 5 months. Contaminating cells may not come only from just the periosteal envelope. Cells from the synovium and bone may also contribute biologically to the chondrocyte culture medium. Lövstedt et al.[75] found that by utilizing a combination of primers for osteocalcin and collagen types 2A+B they were able to positively identify chondrocytes before cell culturing. The culturing of chondrocytes for ACI is time dependent. Cell culture methods usually require that cell isolation take place within 6 hours after surgery, followed by augmentation and implantation in 14 to 21 days. Leela and Bentley[76] examined the capability of chondrocytes from damaged articular cartilage to function in ACI. In an effort to avoid iatrogenic damage to the knee, the debrided cartilage in the perilesional area was collected and enzymatially digested and processed according to standard protocol. Histologic and immunohistochemical analysis was carried out as well as assays for DNA and GAGs. The chondrocytes obtained from the debrided cartilage lesion were equivalent to those obtained from harvested healthy cartilage areas. Sufficient cell numbers for implantation were achieved for all patients. The only difference was that significantly longer times in culture were required to attain the required number of cells in patients who had cartilage scavenged from large degenerative lesions.

CONCLUSIONS

Orthopaedic surgeons involved in cartilage replacement and preservation surgery must be aware of the many outstanding basic biologic issues they face. Articular cartilage and its adjoining bony surface is a remarkable organ that demands respect for its biology and requires attention to the many mechanical and biochemical details that should be considered for surgical planning. It is also incumbent on the surgeon to keep abreast of changes in the biologic literature and evidence-based clinical literature that will continually alter their practice. Cartilage has a highly stable component to its matrix, and it is capable of recovery and prolonged life given the proper environment.

References

1. Genda E, Li G, Barrance PJ, MacWilliams BA, Chao EYS. Functional analysis of hip joint contact pressure. Trans Orthop Res Soc 1996;21:416.
2. Kitaoka HB, Kura H, Luo ZP, An KN. Contact features of the ankle joint. Trans Orthop Res Soc 1996;21:396.
3. Bendjaballah MZ, Shirazi-Adl A, Zukor DJ. Biomechanics of the human knee joint in compression: reconstruction mesh generation and finite element analysis. Knee 1995;2:69–79.
4. Silva M, Shepherd EF, Jackson WO, Dorey FJ, Schmalzriede TP. Average patient walking activity approaches 2 million cycles per year: pedometers under-record walking activity. J Arthroplasty 2002;17:693–697.
5. Akizuki S, Mow VC, Muller F, et al. Tensile properties of human knee joint cartilage. II. Correlations between weight bearing and tissue pathology and the kinetics of swelling. J Orthop Res 1987;5:173–186.
6. Kempson GE. Age-related changes in the tensile properties of human articular cartilage: a comparative study between the femoral head of the hip joint and the talus of the ankle joint. Biochim Biophys Acta 1991;1075:223–230.
7. Zaleski DJ. Cartilage and bone development. Instr Course Lect 1998;47:461–468.
8. Archer CW, Redman S, Bowyer S, Bishop S, Dowthwaite GP. The identification and characterization of articular cartilage progenitor cells. Trans Orthop Res Soc 2002;48:9.
9. Archer CW, Morrison H, Pitsillides AA. Cellular aspects of the development of diarthrodial joints and articular cartilage. J Anat 1994;184:447–456.
10. Noskina Y, Cole A. Presence of proliferation markers in human articular chondrocytes. Trans Orthop Res Soc 2002;27:375.
11. Akizuki S, Mow VC, Muller F, Pita JC, Howell D, Manicourt DH. Tensile properties of human knee joint cartilage: I. Influence of ionic conditions, weight bearing, and fibrillation on the tensile modulus. J Orthop Res 1986;4:379–372.
12. Schinagl RM, Gurskis D, Chen AC, Sah RL. Depth-dependent confined compression modulus of full-thickness bovine articular cartilage. J Orthop Res 1997;15:499–506.

13. Kempson GE, Muir H, Pollard C, Tuke M. The tensile properties of the cartilage of human femoral condyles related to the content of collagen and glycosaminoglycans. Biochim Biophys Acta 1973;297:456–472.

14. Kempson GE. Relationship between the tensile properties of articular cartilage from the human knee and age. Ann Rheum Dis 1982;41:508–511.

15. O'Connor JJ, Johnston J. Transmission of rapidly applied load through articular cartilage: the mechanics of osteoarthrosis. In: Turner-Smith AR (ed) Micromovement in Orthopaedics. Oxford: Clarendon Press, 1993:244–268.

16. Buckwalter JA, Hunziker EB. Articular cartilage biology and morphology. In: Mow VC, Ratcliff A (eds) Biomechanics of Diarthrodial Joints. New York: Springer-Verlag; 1993.

17. Guilak F, Sah R, Sutton LA. Physical regulation of cartilage metabolism. In: Mow VC, Hayes WC (eds) Basic Orthopaedic Biomechanics. Philadelphia: Lippincott Raven; 1997:197–207.

18. Malinin T, Ouellette EA. Articular cartilage nutrition is mediated by subchondral bone: a long term study in baboons. Osteoarthritis Cartilage 2000;8:483–491.

19. Wallis WJ, Simlin PA, Nelp WB. Protein traffic in human synovial effusions. Arthritis Rheum 1987;30:57–63.

20. Maroudas A, Bullough P, Swanson SAV, Freeman MAR. The permeability of articular cartilage. J Bone Joint Surg 1968;50B:166–177.

21. Poole AR. Cartilage in health and disease. In: McCarthy DJ, Koopman WJ (eds) Arthritis and Allied Conditions. A Textbook in Rheumatology, 12th edn. Philadelphia: Lea & Febiger, 1993:279–333.

22. Mayne R. Cartilage collagens: what is their function, and are they involved in articular disease. Arthritis Rheum 1989;32:241–246.

23. Hollander AP, Heathfield TF, Webber C, et al. Increased damage to type II collagen in osteoarthritic cartilage detected by a new immunoassay. J Clin Invest 1994;93:1722–1732.

24. Verzijl N, DeGroot J, Bank RA, Bijlsma JWJ, Lafeber FPJG, TeKoppele JM. Increased collagen turnover during cartilage degeneration is not restricted to focal lesions. Trans Orthop Res Soc 2002;48:166.

25. Verzijl N, DeGroot J, Thorpe SR, et al. Effect of collagen turnover in the accumulation of advanced glycation end products. J Biol Chem 2000;275:39027–39031.

26. Nelson F, Dahlberg L, Laverty S, et al. Evidence for altered synthesis of type II collagen in patients with osteoarthritis. J Clin Invest 1998;102:2115–2125.

27. Mow VC, Setton LA, Ratcliffe A, Howell DS, Buckwalter JA. Structure–function relationships of articular cartilage and the effects of joint instability and trauma on cartilage function. In: Brandt KD (ed) Cartilage Changes in Osteoarthritis. Indiana School of Medicine: Ciba-Geigy, 1990:22–42.

28. Buschmann MD, Gluzband YA, Grodzinsky AJ, Hunziker EB. Chondrocytes in agarose culture synthesize a mechanically functional extracellular matrix. J Orthop Res 1992;10:745–758.

29. Burton-Wurster N, Hui-Chou CS, Greisen HA, Lust G. Reduced deposition of collagen in the degenerated articular cartilage of dogs with degenerative joint disease. Biochim Biophys Acta 1982;718:74–84.

30. Ameye L, Young, MF. Mice deficient in small leucine-rich proteoglycans: novel in vivo models for osteoporosis, osteoarthritis, Ehlers-Danlos syndrome, muscular dystrophy, and corneal diseases. Glycobiology 2002;12:107R–116R.

31. Tsumura H, Miura H, Iwamoto Y. Three-dimensional pressure distribution of the human hip joint—comparison between normal hips and dysplastic hips. Fukuoka Igaku Zasshi 1998;89:109–118.

32. Walker PS, Erkman MJ. The role of the menisci in force transmission across the knee. Clin Orthop 1975;109:184–192.

33. Brown TD, Shaw DT. In vitro contact stress distribution on the femoral condyles. J Orthop Res 1984;2:190–199.

34. Buckwalter JA, Einhorn TA, Simon SR. Orthopaedic Basic Science. Chicago: American Academy Orthopaedic Surgeons, 2000.

35. Hascall VC, Sajdera SW. Physical properties and polydispersity of proteoglycan from bovine nasal cartilage. J Biol Chem 1970;245:4920–4930.

36. Wong M, Wuethrich P, Buschmann MD, Eggli P, Hunziker E. Chondrocyte biosynthesis correlates with local tissue strain in statically compressed adult articular cartilage. J Orthop Res 1997;15(2):189–196.

37. Cochran GVB. A Primer of Orthopaedic Biomechanics. New York: Churchill Livingstone, 1982:413.

38. Dye SF. The knee as a biologic transmission with an envelope of function: a theory. Clin Orthop 1996;325:10–18.

39. Goldberg VM, Kuettner KE. Osteoarthritic Disorders. Chicago: American Academy Orthopaedic Surgeons, 1995:xxii–xxiii.

40. Martin JA, Scherb MB, Lembke LA, Buckwalter JA. Damage control mechanisms in articular cartilage: the role of the insulin-like growth factor I axis. Iowa Orthop J 2000;20:1–10.

41. Convery FR, Akeson WH, Keown GH. The repair of large osteochondral defects. Clin Orthop 1972;82:253–262.

42. Fuller JA, Ghadially FN. Ultrastructural observations on surgically produced partial-thickness defects in articular cartilage. Clin Orthop 1972;86:193–205.

43. Caplan AI. Mesenchymal stem cells. J Orthop Res 1991;9:641–650.

44. Rodrigo JJ, Steadman JR, Sillman JF, Fulstone HA. Improvement of full-thickness chondral defect healing in the human knee after debridement and microfracture using continuous passive motion. Am J Knee Surg 1994;7:109–116.

45. Steadman JR, Rodkey WG, Singleton SB, Briggs KK. Microfracture technique for full-thickness chondral defects: technique and clinical results. Oper Tech Orthop 1997;7:300–304.

46. Salter RB, Simmonds DF, Malcolm BW, Rumble EJ, MacMichael D, Clement ND. The biological effect of continuous passive motion on the healing of full-thickness defects in articular cartilage. J Bone Joint Surg 1980;62A:1232–1251.

47. Shapiro F, Koide S, Glimcher MJ. Cell origin and differentiation in the repair of full-thickness defects of articular cartilage. J Bone Joint Surg 1993;75A:532–553.

48. Wakitani S, Goto T, Pineda SJ, et al. Mesenchymal cell-based repair of larger, full-thickness defects of articular cartilage. J Bone Joint Surg 1994;76A:579–592.

49. Lexer EL. Joint transplantations and arthroplasty. Surg Gynecol Obstet 1925;40:782.

50. Lexer EL. Substitution of whole or half joints from freshly amputated extremities by free plastic operation. Surg Gynecol Obstet 1908;6:601.

51. Herndon CH, Chase SW. The fate of autogenous and massive homogenous bone grafts including articular surfaces. Surg Gynecol Obstet 1954;98:273–290.

52. Jimenez SA, Brighton CT. Experimental studies on the fate of transplanted articular cartilage. In: Friedlaender GE, Mankin HJ, Sell KW (eds) Osteochondral Allografts, Banking and Clinical Applications. Boston: Brown, 1983:73–79.

53. Lane JM, Brighton CT. Joint resurfacing in the rabbit using an autologous osteochondral graft: a biochemical and metabolic study of cartilage viability. J Bone Joint Surg 1977;59A:218.

54. Lipton MA, et al. Allotransplantation: a histological, biochemical, and biomechanical study. Trans Orthop Res Soc 1978;3:12.

55. De Nubile NA, et al. Allotransplantation of preserved and fresh articular cartilage in an osteochondral plug model. Trans Orthop Res Soc 1980;5:74.

56. Hangody L, Kish G, Karpati Z, Eberhardt R. Autogenous osteochondral graft technique for replacing knee cartilage defects in dogs. Int Orthop 1992;5:175–181.

57. Hangody L, Kisk G, Karpati Z, et al. Autogenous osteochondral graft technique for replacing knee cartilage defects in dogs. Int Orthop 1997;5:175–181.
58. Nelson FR. Chondrocyte engineering: in search of articular cartilage. MUSC Orthop J 1999;2:26–31.
59. Brighton CT, Shadle CA, Jimenez SA, Irwin JT, Lane JM, Lipton M. Articular cartilage preservation and storage I. Application of tissue culture techniques to the storage of viable articular cartilage. Arthritis Rheum 1979;22:1093–1101.
60. Oates KM, Chen AC, Young EP, Kwan MK, Amiel D, Convery FR. Effect of tissue storage on the in vivo survival of canine osteochondral allografts. J Orthop Res 1995;13:562–569.
61. Stevenson S, Dannucci GA, Sharkey NA, Pool RR. The fate of articular cartilage after transplantation of fresh and cryopreserved tissue-antigen-matched and mismatched osteochondral allografts in dogs. J Bone Joint Surg 1989;71A:1297–1307.
62. Czitrom AA, Keating S, Gross A. The viability of articular cartilage in fresh osteochondrl allografts after clinical transplantation. J Bone Joint Surg 1990;72A:574–581.
63. Oakeshott RD, Farine I, Pritzker KPH, Langer F, Fross AE. A clinical and histologic analysis of failed fresh osteochondral allografts. Clin Orthop 1988;233:283–294.
64. Convery FR, Akeson WH, Amiel D, Meyers MH, Monosov A. Long-term survival of chondrocytes in osteochondral articular cartilage allograft. J Bone Joint Surg 1996;78A:1082–1088.
65. Moskalewski S, Hyc A, Osiecka-Iwan A. Immune response by host after allogeneic chondrocyte transplantation to the cartilage. Microsc Res Tech 2002;58:3–13.
66. Mahomed MN, Beaver RJ, Gross AE. The long-term success of fresh, small fragment osteochondral allografts used for intra-articular post-traumatic defects in the knee joint. Orthopaedics 1992;15:1191–1199.
67. Peterson L, Menche D, Grande D, et al. Chondrocyte transplantation: an experimental model in the rabbit. Tran Orthop Res Soc 1984;18:218.
68. Hirotani H, Ito T. Chondrocyte mitosis in the articular cartilage of femoral heads with various diseases. Acta Orthop Scand 1975; 46:979–986.
69. Rothwell AG, Bentley G. Chondrocyte multiplication in osteoarthritic articular cartilage. J Bone Joint Surg 1973;55B: 588–594.
70. Hunziker EB, Rosenberg LC. Repair of partial-thickness defects in articular cartilage: cell recruitment from the synovial membrane. J Bone Joint Surg 1996;78A:721–733.
71. Johnson LL. Arthroscopic abrasion arthroplasty historical and pathologic perspective: Present status. Arthroscopy 1986;2: 54–69.
72. Grande DA, Pitman MI, Peterson L, Menche D. Klein M. The repair of experimentally produced defects in rabbit articular cartilage by autologous chondrocyte transplantation. J Orthop Res 1989;7:208–218.
73. Breinan HA, Minas T, Hsu H-P, Nehrer S, Sledge CB, Spector M. Effect of cultured autologous chondrocytes on repair of chondral defects in a canine model. J Bone Joint Surg 1997;79A: 1439–1451.
74. Peterson L, Minas T, Brittberg M, Nilsson A, Sjogren-Jansson E, Lindahl A. Two- to 9-year outcome after autologous chondrocyte transplantation of the knee. Clin Orthop 1999;374:212–234.
75. Lövstedt K, Thornemo M, Lindahl A. Identification of Contaminating Cells from Biopsies Used for Articular Cartilage Repair. Toronto: International Cartilage Repair Society. 2002:73.
76. Leela CB, Bentley G. A Novel Source of Cells for Autologous Chondrocyte Transplantation in the Adult Knee. Toronto: International Cartilage Repair Society. 2002:54.

2

Patient Evaluation

Laurence D. Higgins

Symptomatic chondral injuries of the knee in the young, athletic individual remain among the most challenging orthopaedic conditions to treat. Treatment of these disorders is further complicated by the magnitude of the problem, uncertainty of the natural history of chondral injuries, and the lack of adequate clinical research to create a reliable, clinically sound treatment algorithm. These injuries are at times problematic both to diagnose and to treat because the etiology, presentation, and associated maladies create endless variety in their clinical presentation. With the advent of new techniques to address chondral injuries, renewed interest in their treatment has sparked both much-needed debate and research on virtually every aspect of articular cartilage injury and restoration. The purpose of this chapter is to review the incidence and natural history of chondral lesions; to review the common clinical presentations and the standard evaluation process (with appropriate diagnostic tools), and to discuss the use of diagnostic arthroscopy and classification of chondral lesions.

INCIDENCE

New chondral lesions are reported to affect nearly 1 million individuals annually, accounting for an estimated 5% to 10% of all hemarthrosis.[1,2] High-grade lesions account for more than 200,000 surgical procedures annually and may be encountered in almost two thirds of all knee arthroscopies.[1] Curl and associates[3] reviewed 31,516 knee arthroscopies maintained in a regional database to quantify the prevalence of chondral injuries, location, grade, and associated pathologic changes encountered. Sixty percent of patients had high-grade chondral lesion (Outerbridge grade III or IV). Curl further analyzed the data to delineate what is believed to be a subset of patients who most likely would benefit from newer restorative chondral techniques. In those patients under 40 years of age, grade IV monopolar lesions on the medial femoral condyle were found in 4% of all cases studied, representing what may be the "ideal" candidate for intervention. Although the medial femoral condyle represented the most common location to encounter a grade IV lesion (32%), the lateral femoral condyle and patellofemoral joint were also common sites. Most patients with multifocal lesions were over 40 years of age.[3]

NATURAL HISTORY

It is widely believed and often stated that chondral lesions progress and, anecdotally, it is commonplace to hear that they progress to osteoarthritis. Although some studies have demonstrated that some chondral lesions progress radiographically, to date no well-designed and controlled study has documented that this is invariably the case. This lack in part results from the difficulty in accurate classification of lesions with noninvasive means, and the complexity associated with following these patients longitudinally over time. Following clinically symptomatic lesions may become practical with continued advancement in magnetic resonance imaging (MRI); however, it is not practical, but it is far more difficult to study asymptomatic lesions. Currently, there are no data to support the conjecture that asymptomatic lesions will become symptomatic, and clinical recommendations must take this into consideration.

There have been several long-term studies on the radiographic progression of chondral lesions and a plethora of anecdotal reports of progression of lesions with a wide spectrum of treatment. The former reports add to our continued belief that lesions likely progress; the latter serve to remind us that our treatments to date have not succeeded in restoring functional, durable hyaline articular cartilage in most cases.

Sahlström and associates[4] reported on a large Swedish cohort study with 20-year follow-up for osteoarthritis. In patients with subchondral sclerosis or osteophytes with preserved joint space (Ahlback stage 0), 57% demonstrated radiographic progression. In patients with Ahlback stage 1 osteoarthritis (50% joint space narrowing), 61% showed progression. For those patients with more advanced disease as determined by radiographs (Ahlback stage 2 or higher), 100% demonstrated progression. In summary, those with early disease exhibited variable radiographic progression, whereas those with significant radiographic changes demonstrated advanced radiographic osteoarthritis.

Messner and Maletius[5] reported on 28 patients with isolated chondral lesions followed for 14 years after diagnosis. Although most of these patients demonstrated progressive radiographic abnormalities consistent with osteoarthritis, 22 of the 28 had good or excellent clinical results without treatment. The same authors also reported on a minimum 12-year follow-up on 42 patients who were treated with or without meniscectomy in the presence of a chondral lesion. By matching patients, those individuals with meniscectomy and chondral lesions had a more rapid progression of radiographic abnormalities than those without meniscectomy. It should be noted the nonmeniscectomy group did demonstrate some progression of radiographic changes consistent with osteoarthritis on weight-bearing X-rays.

The natural history of chondral lesions, in the absence of any plain radiographic abnormality, is unknown. There are currently no well-controlled treatment matched studies for chondral injury that may shed light on the progression of these injuries. What is clear, however, is that animal studies do confirm that articular incongruity alone will lead to progressive chondral loss and histologic changes in the subchondral bone with cyst formation mimicking osteoarthritis.[6–10]

Posttraumatic changes and chondral injuries sustained with concomitant anterior cruciate ligament (ACL) rupture have been investigated. It is clear that a wide spectrum of injury exists with impaction injuries of the lateral femoral condyle at the time of ACL rupture. In fact, Indelicato and Bittar[11] reported a 23% prevalence of osteochondral injuries with operative ACL reconstructions in their series. While the prevalence of bone bruises may exceed 75% acutely, all disappeared on repeat MRI at 16 weeks (Figure 2.1).

CLINICAL PRESENTATION

The clinical presentation of chondral injuries encompasses the gamut from incidentally noted, asymptomatic lesions to dramatic, disabling arthritic symptoms. A thorough history is essential, and the patient should be queried regarding any previous treatment. A history of ligament injury (often the ACL), patellar dislocation, or a traumatic "dashboard" injury to the knee may be elicited. Hemarthroses are encountered in virtually all acute injuries that create a full thickness chondral injury.

Other common scenarios include loose-body symptoms that often connote a full-thickness articular injury. Pain is frequently worse with activity, and swelling is often intermittent and activity related in chronic cases. Pain with prolonged sitting, stair climbing, and kneeling may localize the pain to the patella or femoral trochlea. Activities that provoke pain should be specifically queried. To assess disability, work requirements should be noted and what, if any, limitations the patient is currently experiencing. Athletic participation and patient expectations regarding return to sports or activity are critical to note, as they are often unrealistic.[12] Previous treatments, including both surgical and nonsurgical interventions must be discussed as well as the patients' clinical responses. Medications, including viscosupplementation and chondrosupplementation with glucosamine or chondroitin or both, are important interventions that must be recorded.

The presence of pain is a result of the loss of the cushioning function of the articular cartilage. As such, the subchon-

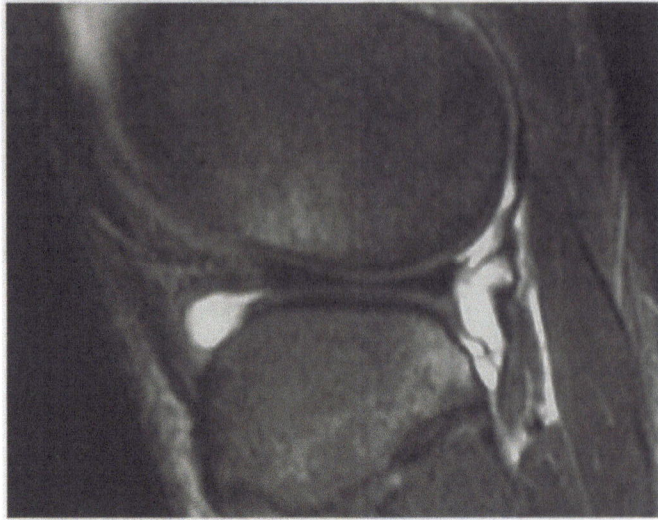

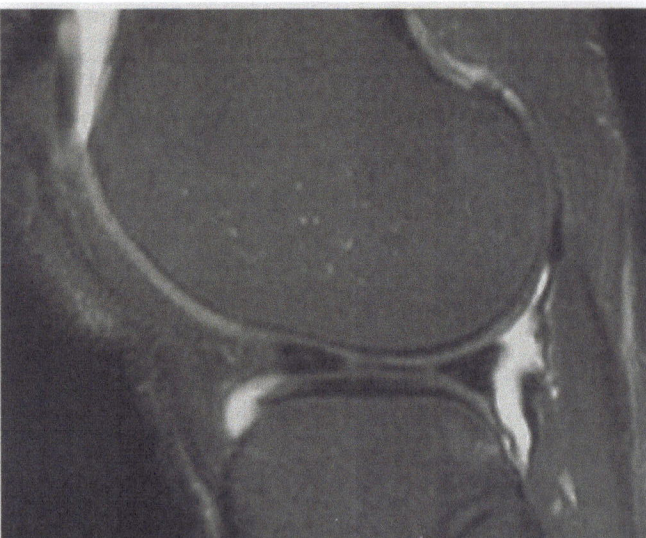

FIGURE 2.1 A. T_2-weighted fast spin echo (FSE) fat saturation (sagittal) image of bone bruises to lateral femoral condyle one week after ACL injury. **B.** T_2-weighted FSE fat saturation image of resolved bone bruise.

dral bone is exposed to increased pressure, and pain fibers in this region are stimulated. Increased venous flow accompanies bony sclerosis and congestion of the cancellous bone occurs (Figure 2.2). With this, a vicious cycle ensues, only exacerbated by further mechanical trauma to the joint, often in the form of sporting activity. The presence of an effusion caused by enzymatic breakdown of articular cartilage can lead to capsular distension and synovitis, worsening symptoms. These pathologic changes create a feeling of achiness deep in the joint.

After a thorough history, several key points on the physical examination should be specifically noted. While the palpation of a loose body may confirm the presence of an articular cartilage injury, other reproducible and consistent findings are lacking. Pain may be poorly localized, and crepitus may be present. The audible nature of crepitus may be alarming to patients, but asymptomatic crepitus should not be alarming and the patient should be reassured. However, painful crepitus and other mechanical symptoms should be carefully noted and, if possible, localized. The overall align-

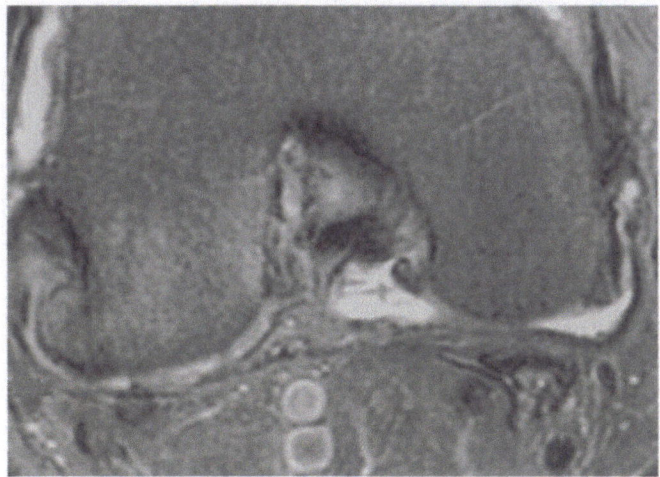

FIGURE 2.2 Subacromial edema (bone bruise) secondary to degenerative joint disease (DJD). Note loss of overlying articular cartilage.

ment should be clinically assessed, with the understanding that precise analysis requires radiographs. Quadriceps atrophy and nonarticular patellofemoral pain are potentially reversible causes of knee pain and must be sought.

RADIOGRAPHIC EVALUATION

Standard radiographs of the knee, comprising anteroposterior (AP), lateral, and an axial view of the patella have served as the standard X-ray series for the knee (Figure 2.3A–C). Furthermore, radiographic changes have served as the de facto outcome measure for many orthopaedic procedures, particularly osteoarthritis and its surgical treatment. Fairbanks[13] described three classic radiographic findings of osteoarthritis of the knee: narrowing of the joint space, flattening of the femoral condyles and formation of marginal osteophytes. Ahlbäck[14] stressed the importance of obtaining weight-bearing radiographs to illustrate these important findings, using posteroanterior (PA) views.

The presence of articular cartilage lesions in the knee has been noted to occur more commonly between 30° and 60° of knee flexion. To confirm these suspicions, Rosenberg et al.[15] performed radiographs on a consecutive series of patients obtaining 45° PA weight-bearing views. By using a 2-mm decrease in joint space compared to the contralateral side as indicative of "major degeneration" (grade III or IV chondral lesion), comparisons were made to conventional extension weight-bearing AP radiographs. The 45° PA views (Figure

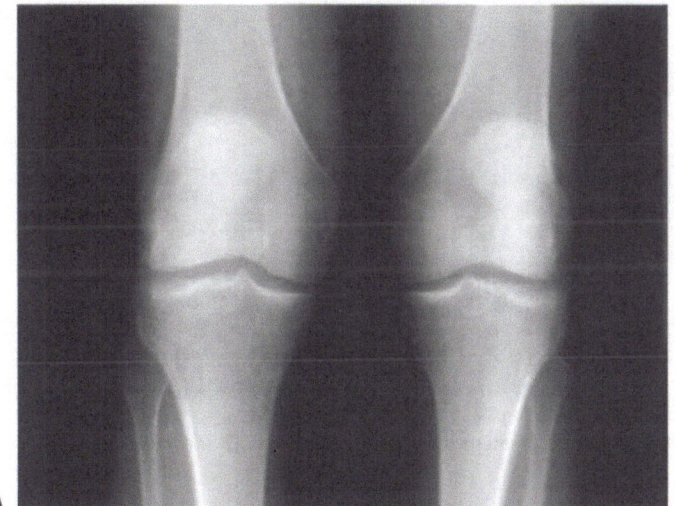

A

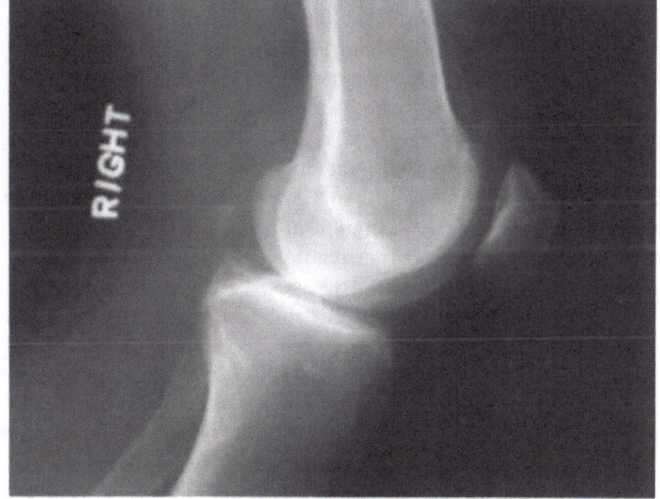

B

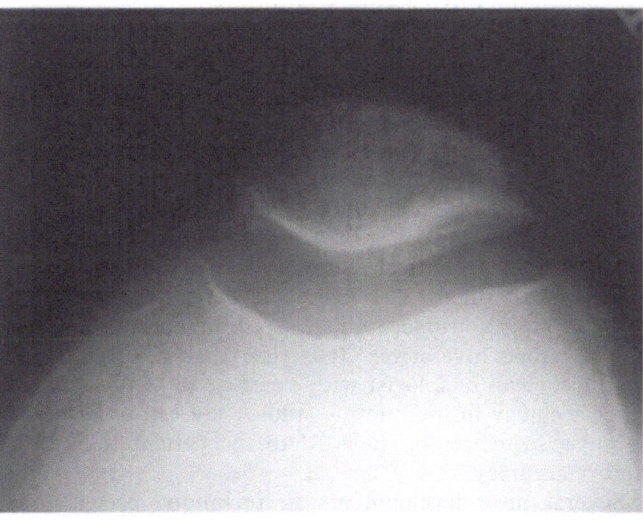

C

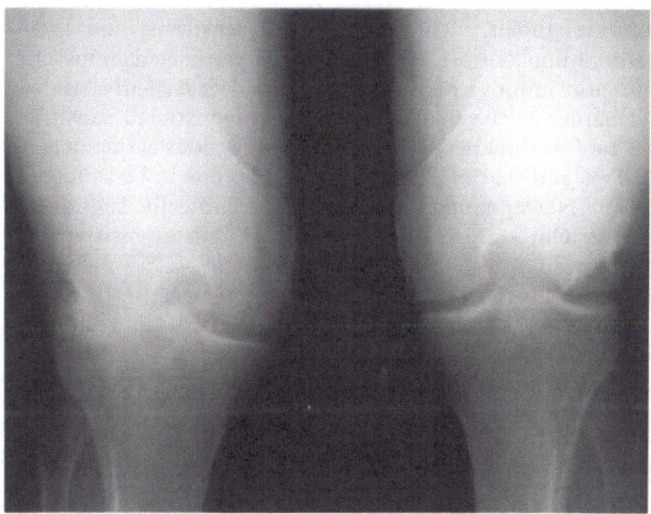

D

FIGURE 2.3 A. Standing anterior-posterior (AP) radiograph of the knee. **B.** Lateral radiograph of the knee. **C.** Axial view of the patella. **D.** Rosenberg view of the knee of the same patient. Note the complete loss of the joint space demonstrated by this radiographic view.

2.3D) were statistically more accurate, more specific (no false positives), and more sensitive in detecting "significant chondral lesions" using arthroscopy as the gold standard.[15] While plain radiographs may be helpful to delineate osteochondral lesions, they may fail to reveal chondral lesions, particularly if the lesion is small. In this setting, the use of MRI may be more helpful.

Although several imaging techniques have been proposed to serve as the standard technique for articular cartilage imaging, MRI has emerged as the imaging method of choice. The contrast that MRI is able to produce in the soft tissues and its multiplanar capability are superior to other imaging modalities. Additionally, MRI provides information about the subchondral cancellous bone. However, MRI still demonstrates significant limitations in sensitivity and specificity despite marked improvements in image acquisition.[16] Certain protocols for imaging have emerged as standard sequences for articular cartilage, and newer protocols continually emerge. Furthermore, the higher field strength magnets and local gradient coils have demonstrated enhanced imaging due to higher signal-to-noise ratios and stronger local gradient fields.[17]

There is no standard appearance of articular cartilage on MR imaging, with the final appearance very technique dependent. With the complex architecture of articular cartilage and zonal biochemical differences, even adjacent areas may demonstrate significantly different signal characteristics. Standard pulse sequences for articular cartilage frequently include a T_2-weighted image with or without fat suppression (Figure 2.4A) and a T_1-weighted fat-suppressed three-dimensional spoiled gradient-echo technique (Figure 2.44B). These protocols benefit from the arthrogram-producing effect of the differential signal intensity on the joint fluid, which highlights irregularity or defects of the joint surface. On the T_1-weighted images, cartilage is higher in signal intensity than joint fluid; the reverse is true for the T_2-weighted images.[16,18-23]

The addition of contrast material to the joint does not necessary improve the accuracy of MRI for articular cartilage injuries. There is ample evidence, however, that the addition of a contrast agent may enhance the ability to detect loose bodies[24] as well as to grade and detect unstable osteochondral injuries with improved sensitivity and specificity over noncontrast studies.[25] The results of the sensitivity and specificity of noncontrast MRI on articular cartilage demonstrate dramatic improvement over the past decade. Early studies evaluating MRI versus arthroscopy demonstrated sensitivities for full-thickness articular cartilage lesions of the knee to be 41% and that of partial-thickness lesions to be as low as 15%.[27] Newer studies have detected clinically significant lesions (Outerbridge grade 2, 3, and 4) with a sensitivity of 87%, specificities of 94%, and accuracy of 92%.[28,29] As would be expected, the thickness of the articular cartilage of the patellofemoral joint provides enhanced diagnostic results in this region. No studies have demonstrated that MRI can accurately grade cartilage lesions, which to date are still recorded on the basis of direct arthroscopic visualization.

The field strength of the magnet is critical to obtaining valid results. Currently 1.5 T magnets have been validated for efficacy in evaluating chondral lesions[28,29] whereas the lower field strength studies have not been validated. In fact, direct comparison between 0.2 T and 1.5 T field strength magnets

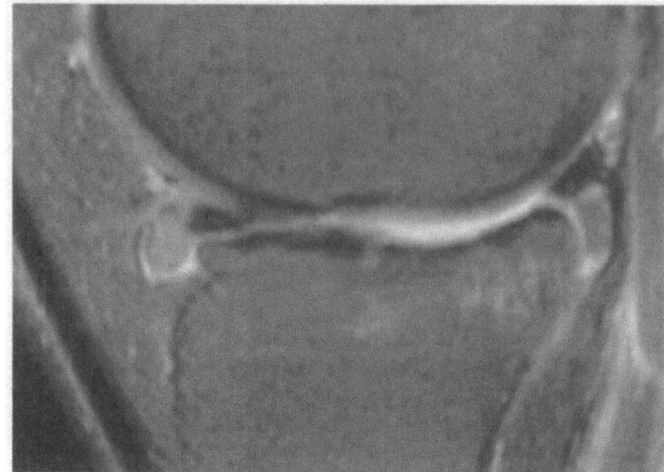

A

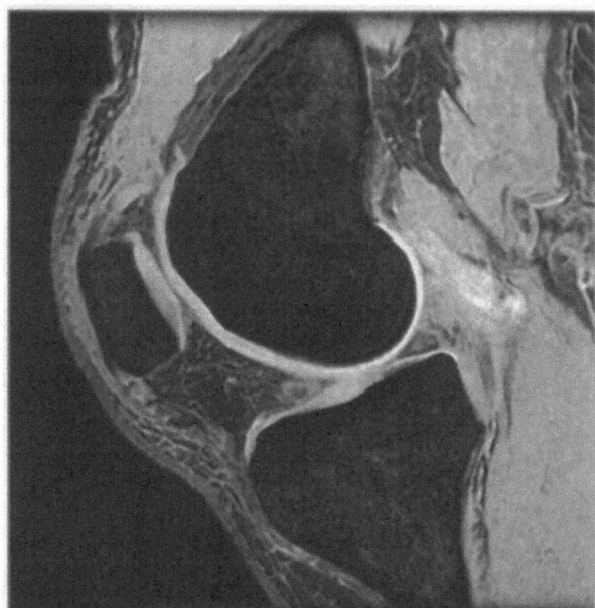

B

FIGURE 2.4 A. T_2-weighted fat saturation view of the condyle. **B.** 3-D spoiled gradient recalled acquisition with fat saturation.

have shown improved accuracy of the 1.5 T magnet.[30] While the use of local coils is widely encouraged to enhance the signal-to-noise ratio and improve contrast in all knee MRIs at suppression remains superior with higher field strength magnets and, as such, may improve their ability to detect injury.[31]

The current recommended sequences have dramatically improved detection of chondral lesions of the knee, but sizing of such lesions is still problematic. There are no current studies documenting accuracy in determining the area of the chondral defect, a critical factor in determining treatment options. Furthermore, T_1-weighted sequences are very susceptible to metal artifacts which may limit their usefulness in the postoperative state.[31] It is clear that an experienced musculoskeletal radiologist with expertise in MRI will have higher accuracy in interpreting studies and can often tailor the pulse sequences of the MRI to the patient to further improve accuracy.

Several new developments in technique can further enhance MR accuracy for cartilage lesions. The current techniques do little to evaluate the structure of the cartilage itself and rely on chondral defects to identify areas of injury. The use of ionic gadolinium appears to show promise in its ability to detect injured cartilage. When ionic gadolinium is injected into the joint, healthy cartilage rich in negatively charged proteoglycans repels the contrast. Injured cartilage, which demonstrates a predictable loss of proteoglycans, will demonstrate signal enhancement with contrast because it does not repel the contrast.[32] The use of ultrashort echo times has been investigated by Brossmann et al.[26] to detect early chondral changes. Such sequences, which have long acquisition times, demonstrated statistically higher accuracy than those obtained with T_1-weighted fat-suppressed three-dimensional spoiled gradient-echo images. Furthermore, these sequences may be useful to obtain proton spectra in articular cartilage, which may connote early biochemical degradation.[20] Finally, the multiplanar ability of MRI may allow the creation of surface models of articular cartilage. The ability of MR to calculate cartilage volume is inherent in the technique and has been demonstrated to be highly accurate.[33] Thus, this technique may allow more precise determination of the area involved. Although this is an established technique, early reports are mixed on the usefulness of chondral surface maps in osteoarthritis.[34]

Imaging of the articular cartilage after surgical treatment is, as expected, complex. The noninvasive nature of MR makes this technique the most appealing, but interpretation of these studies is difficult. Further studies into the normal appearance of repair tissue are needed to differentiate pathologic progression. As MR field strength and the ability to routinely assess the biochemical nature of the cartilage repair with contrast agents and new sequences improves, great strides will be made in patient treatment.

DIAGNOSTIC ARTHROSCOPY AND CLASSIFICATION

Arthroscopy of articular cartilage lesions is accepted as the most accurate and reliable mechanism to assess chondral lesion size, depth, surface appearance, and precise location. It is universally believed that each of these characteristics is critical to determining the appropriate therapeutic options for the patient with a symptomatic chondral lesion and to document the current disease extent.[3,35–41] Despite the critical nature of these findings, there is little consensus regarding the optimal system to document chondral injuries. Many classification systems exist with widely different rationales and there is no consensus scoring system for documenting such injuries. Early systems did not specify whether measurements of cartilage injury should be recorded in the pre- or postdebridement state. Most surgeons with expertise now believe that the postdebridement measurements are more clinically relevant, although no data have been published to support this contention[42–50] (Figure 2.5).

Two new classification systems that have recently been proposed to precisely record the size, depth, and location of the lesions will greatly facilitate research into etiology, prognosis, and the outcomes of both operative and nonoperative treatment. Each of these systems uses postdebridement measurements, with the International Cartilage Research Society (ICRS) system also recording predebridement measurements.[45,51] What is still inadequately conveyed in current sys-

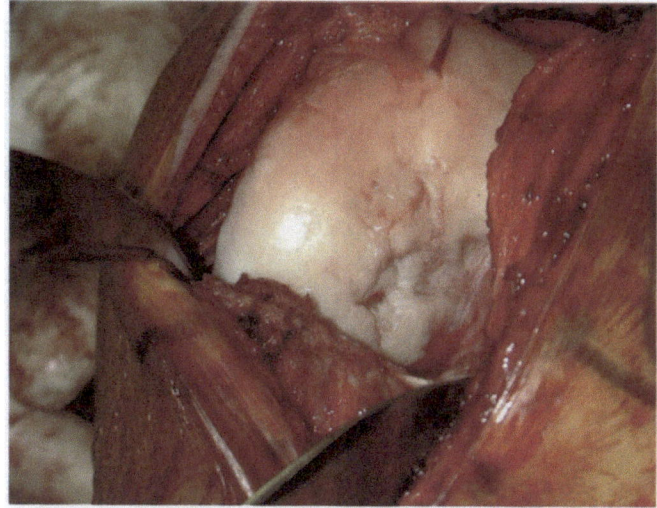

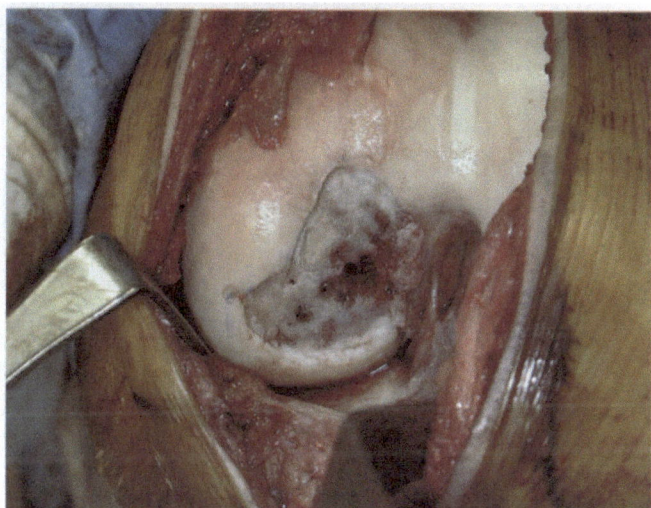

FIGURE 2.5 Predebridement **A.** and postdebridement **B.** images of an articular cartilage lesion. Note the substantial change in the size of the lesion after debridement.

tems is the status of the subchondral bone and a mechanism to connote the state of the opposing articulating surface for the lesion in question.

Many of the early classification systems used both appearance and size of the lesions to assign a grade within a classification system.[49] Table 2.1 lists the current systems, showing the vast differences between scales. Although not exhaustive, this table provides an overview of the most commonly used systems and the specifics for their classification of chondral lesions. The first true grading system for articular cartilage was advanced by Outerbridge[52] to describe the incidence of chondromalacia patella at the time of meniscectomy. Outerbridge carefully documented the extent of the chondral lesions of the patella and proposed a four-grade system for such lesions, based upon size and depth of the lesion (see Table 2.1). What is most evident is that the only difference between grade II and III lesions is size alone, and depth of penetration is not considered. Lesions that are less than 0.5 inches in diameter are grade II and those larger are grade III. In fact, Outerbridge's initial descriptions of chondral lesions of the patella were subsequently adapted as the Outerbridge classification for all chondral surfaces.

TABLE 2.1 Compilation of available articular cartilage grading systems.

Author	Year	Grade	Description	Defect Size
Outerbridge[52]	1961	I	Softening and swelling	
		II	Fragmentation/fissuring	<1/2 inch
		III	Fragmentation/fissuring	>1/2 inch
		IV	Erosion with exposed of subchondral bone	
Insall[57]	1976	I	Softening	
		II	Fissuring to subchondral bone	
		III	Fibrillation	
		IV	Erosion with exposure of subchondral bone	
Ficat et al.[58]	1977	I	Closed chondromalacia, surface intact, softening	
		II	Open chondromalacia (surface not intact)	
		IIA	Fissuring to subchondral bone	
		IIB	Erosion with exposure of subchondral bone	
Casscells[59]	1982	I	Superficial erosion	1 cm
		II	Deeper layers of cartilage involved	1–2 cm
		III	Eroded cartilage, exposed subchondral bone	2–4 cm
		IV	Articular cartilage completely destroyed	"wide area"
Beguin and Locker[53]	1983	I	Softening and swelling	
		II	Superficial chondral fissuring	
		III	Deep chondral fissuring	
		IV	Erosion with exposed subchondral bone	
Bentley and Dowd[60]	1984	I	Fibrillation/fissuring	<0.5 cm
		II	Fibrillation/fissuring	0.5–1 cm
		III	Fibrillation/fissuring	1–2 cm
		IV	Fibrillation with/without exposed subchondral bone	>2 cm
Noyes and Stabler[50]	1989	I	Intact cartilage	
		IA	Softening	<1 cm
		IB	Softening with deformation	1.5 cm
		II	Fibrillation/fissuring	
		IIA	Fibrillation/fissuring	$<^1/_2$ thickness
		IIB	Fibrillation/fissuring	$>^1/_2$ thickness
		III	Exposure of subchondral bone	
		IIIA	Exposure of subchondral bone, intact	
		IIIB	Exposure of subchondral bone, with bony excavation	
French Society of Arthroscopy grading system (Dougados et al.[47])	1994	0	Grade 0 = 100%	NOTE: Uses Beguin and Locker(6) grades in description
		I	Grade IV = 0% and grade 0 ≥ or = 80%	
		II	Grade IV = 0% and grade 0 < 80% and grade III < 15%	
		III	(Grade IV = 0% and grade 0 < 80% and grade III ≥ or = 15%) OR (grade IV ≥ or = 1% and grade 0 ≥ or = 65%)	
		IV	Grade IV ≥ or = 1% and grade 0 < 65%	
Lewandrowski et al.[49]	1996	No grades purely descriptive	Appearance (six categories) Depth ($<^1/_2$ or $>^1/_2$ thickness) Area (< or = 1 cm², 1–4 cm², >4 cm²) Clinical Stage (acute, subacute, chronic) Location (Patellofemoral, Femorotibial) Severity (3 stages, depth and size dependant)	
ICRS[45]	1998	0 (normal)		NOTE: Exact dimensions and chondral mapping noted separately
		I (nearly normal)	Superficial with soft indentation or cracks	
		II (abnormal)	$<^1/_2$ thickness	
		III (severely abnormal)	≥ or = $^1/_2$ thickness, but bone intact	
		IV (severely abnormal)	osteochondral lesion	
Hunt et al.[48]	2001	I	Same as Outerbridge	NOTE: Exact dimensions and chondral mapping noted separately
		II	Same as Outerbridge	
		III	Same as Outerbridge	
		IV	Same as Outerbridge	

The classification system of Beguin and Locker[53] proposed four stages of depth, completely removing size as a component. Grades I and IV were similar to the Outerbridge classification, whereas grade II described superficial chondral fissuring and grade III deep fissuring. Only in grade III may the fissuring reach the subchondral surface, and thus the use of a probe was encouraged. Grade III also was used to define deep cartilage ulcerations, regardless of diameter.[47,53] This system is frequently used and mistakenly attributed to Outerbridge, with the size of the lesion separately noted.

To address some of the deficiencies of the existing classification systems, the International Cartilage Research Society (ICRS) developed a clinical cartilage injury evaluation system in 1998 and revised the system in 2000.[45,51] This system addressed the deficiencies of precise mapping of the lesion by creating a grid on the articular cartilage of the knee (Figure 2.6). By dividing the articular surface into 21 femoral zones, 18 tibial zones, and 3 trochlear zones, precise mapping of the site of the lesion is possible. Direct measurement of the lesion is also performed, and finally, the depth of the lesion by

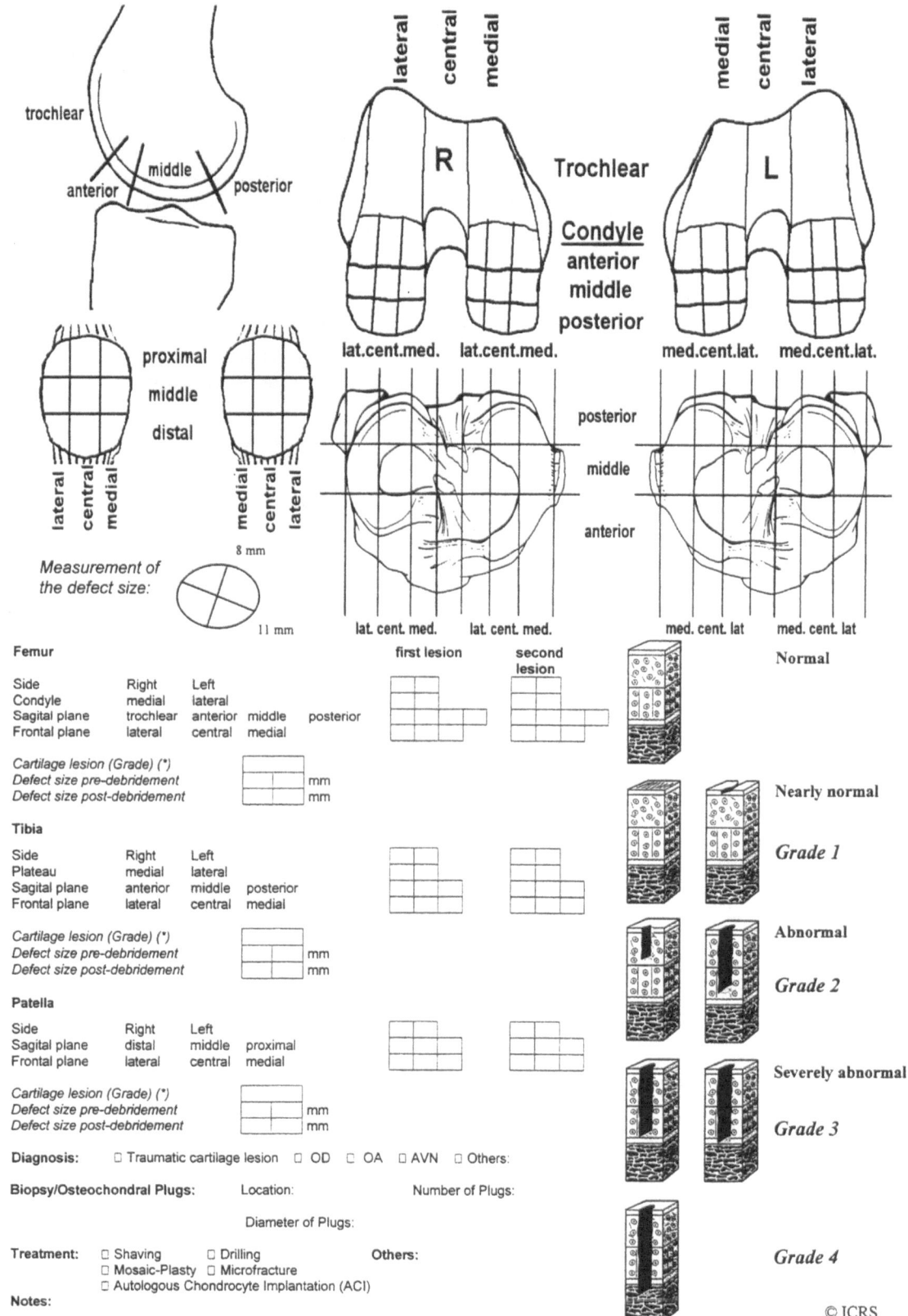

FIGURE 2.6 International Cartilage Repair Society (ICRS) chondral map to document articular cartilage lesions of the knee. (With permission from ICRS, February, 2003.)

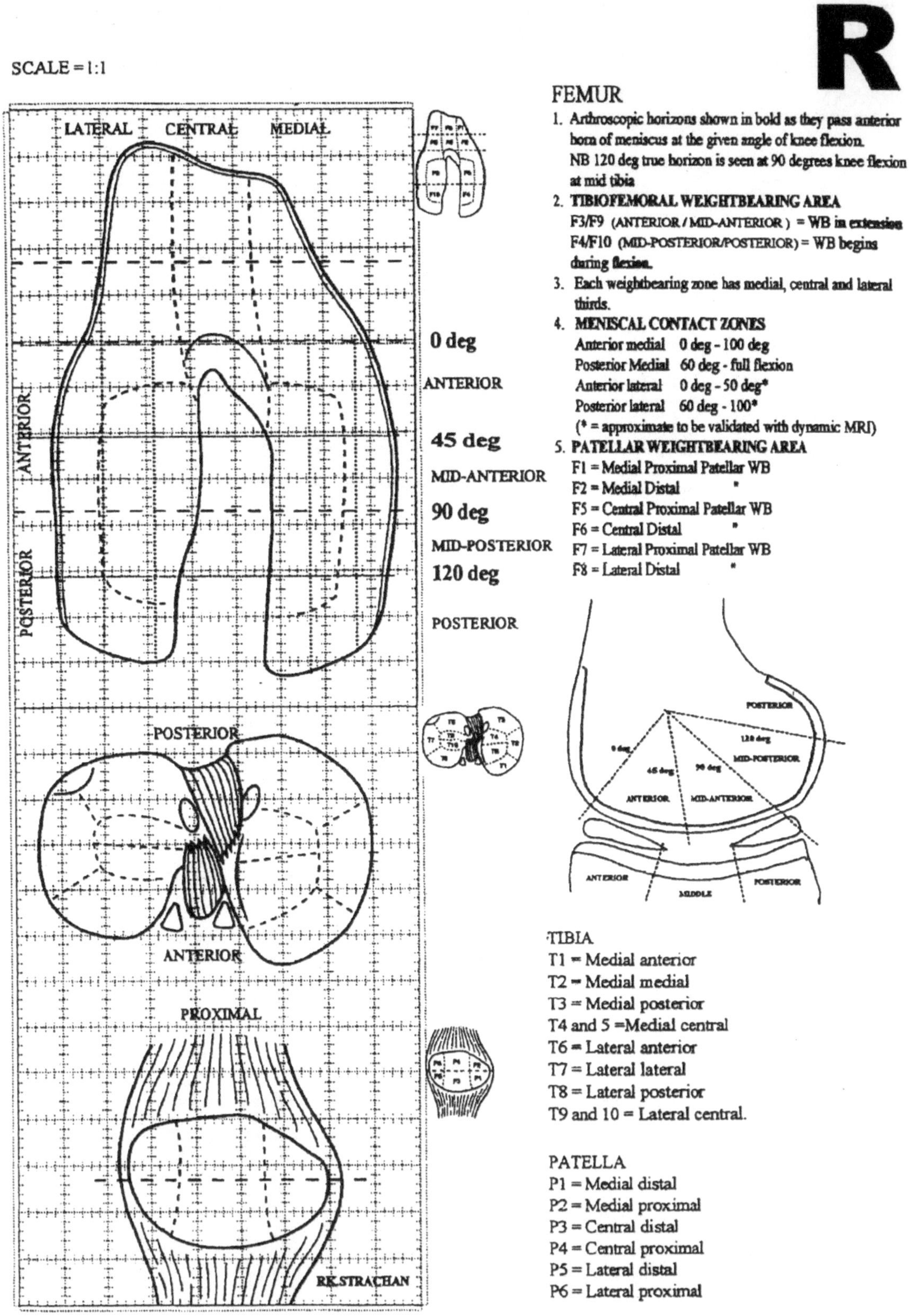

R

SCALE = 1:1

LATERAL   CENTRAL   MEDIAL

ANTERIOR

POSTERIOR

0 deg

ANTERIOR

45 deg

MID-ANTERIOR

90 deg

MID-POSTERIOR

120 deg

POSTERIOR

POSTERIOR

ANTERIOR

PROXIMAL

R.K.STRACHAN

FEMUR

1. Arthroscopic horizons shown in bold as they pass anterior horn of meniscus at the given angle of knee flexion. NB 120 deg true horizon is seen at 90 degrees knee flexion at mid tibia

2. **TIBIOFEMORAL WEIGHTBEARING AREA**
   F3/F9 (ANTERIOR / MID-ANTERIOR) = WB in extension
   F4/F10 (MID-POSTERIOR/POSTERIOR) = WB begins during flexion.

3. Each weightbearing zone has medial, central and lateral thirds.

4. **MENISCAL CONTACT ZONES**
   Anterior medial   0 deg – 100 deg
   Posterior Medial   60 deg - full flexion
   Anterior lateral   0 deg – 50 deg*
   Posterior lateral 60 deg – 100*
   (* = approximate to be validated with dynamic MRI)

5. **PATELLAR WEIGHTBEARING AREA**
   F1 = Medial Proximal Patellar WB
   F2 = Medial Distal   "
   F5 = Central Proximal Patellar WB
   F6 = Central Distal   "
   F7 = Lateral Proximal Patellar WB
   F8 = Lateral Distal   "

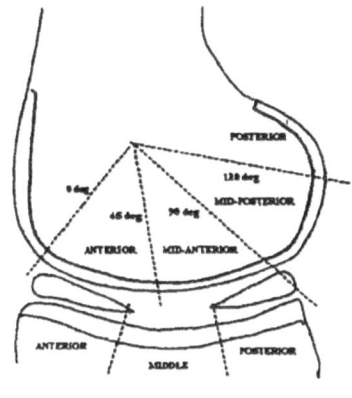

TIBIA
T1 = Medial anterior
T2 = Medial medial
T3 = Medial posterior
T4 and 5 = Medial central
T6 = Lateral anterior
T7 = Lateral lateral
T8 = Lateral posterior
T9 and 10 = Lateral central.

PATELLA
P1 = Medial distal
P2 = Medial proximal
P3 = Central distal
P4 = Central proximal
P5 = Lateral distal
P6 = Lateral proximal

FIGURE 2.7 Cartilage map proposed by Hunt et al. Notice that this map geographically represents the articular cartilage lesion in reference to the meniscus. (Reprinted from Arthroscopy, Vol. 17, Hunt N, Sanchez-Ballester J, Pandit R, Thomas R, Strachan R. Chondral lesions of the knee: a new localization method and correlation with associated pathology, 481–490, copyright 2001, with permission from Elsevier.)

the ICRS standards in recorded. This system is very thorough and is particularly well suited for focal chondral defects. Unfortunately, there is no formal assessment of the meniscus in this system.

Hunt et al.[48] have proposed a similar scoring system, although the authors have departed from the rectangular grids of the ICRS system to employ more anatomic and functional referencing. Femoral and tibial zones were determined by their meniscal relations and, while not representing equal surface areas as advocated by the ICRS, the grids represent the articular contact zones with respect to the meniscus and central ridge of the patella (Figure 2.7). Femoral condyle zones are further divided by flexion/extension zones (with 0°, 45°, 90°, and 120° horizons) on the basis of tibiofemoral weight-bearing. The size of the lesion is directly measured and then drawn on the chondral map of the knee. Of note, the areas of the particular lesions are measured by using an overlying grid system to determine what percentage of the condyle is involved. The status of the meniscus is included in Hunt's grading system, with the meniscal lesion drawn directly on a specific map to correlate with the area of chondral injury. Any meniscal surgery, including repair or resection, may be recorded on this meniscal map.

Both of the recently developed grading systems have certain deficiencies, but they represent the most complete and practical way to gather information on chondral injuries. Few orthopaedic surgeons take the effort to specifically document the size, depth, and specific location of cartilage lesions.[3,48,51] These two systems serve as simple ways to prospectively document the nature of the pathology and allow better tracking of the lesion over time. As few surgeons utilize strict criteria for describing chondral lesions in operative findings, accurately relaying information to specialists in articular cartilage restoration remains challenging. One of the key features of any scoring system is a high degree of inter- and intraobserver reliability. If a scoring system has poor reliability, it cannot have accurate prognostic and therapeutic value. Both the Outerbridge and French Society of Arthroscopy (SFA) grading system have been evaluated with kappa statistics to evaluate reliability. The reliability of a variety of scoring systems have been analyzed in several recent studies.[43–46,48,51,54–56] Results show the importance of training sessions in the analysis and classification for any scoring system.[41]

The SFA grading and Hunt scoring systems have been validated with kappa statistics only for interobserver reliability,[43,44,46,48,54] whereas the Outerbridge classification has been evaluated for both inter- and intraobserver reliability.[46] Although the Outerbridge system has demonstrated high intraobserver reliability, interobserver reliability was fair. In fact, interobserver reliability was enhanced when physicians with more than 5 years of clinical expertise in knee arthroscopy assigned the grade. The SFA grading system has demonstrated good interobserver reliability; it is a semiquantitative variable assigning a category to the severity of chondropathy in each compartment. What is common in each of these reliability studies is the use of video to determine reliability. A recent study (LD Higgins, unpublished data) demonstrated that arthroscopic photos had poor interobserver and intraobserver reliability and that kappa statistics were markedly improved with the use of video for chondral assessment.

To date, no scoring system has become the standard. However, both the ICRS[45,51] and the scoring system proposed by Hunt[48] have obvious advantages over other methods. The use of chondral maps and clear documentation of the size and depth of the lesion are critical features to note accurately and will allow meaningful comparison between treatment groups. Only when the prospective assessment of chondral lesions is documented can the orthopaedic community assess the impact of both nonoperative and operative management of articular cartilage injuries.

References

1. Cole BJ, Frederick R, Levy A. Management of a 37 year old man with recurrent knee pain. J Clin Outcomes Management 2002; 6:46–57.
2. Noyes FR, Bassett RW, Grood ES, Butler DL. Arthroscopy in acute traumatic hemarthrosis of the knee. Incidence of anterior cruciate tears and other injuries. J Bone Joint Surg Am 1980;62:687–695, 757.
3. Curl WW, Krome J, Gordon ES, Rushing J, Smith BP, Poehling CG. Cartilage injuries: a review of 31,516 knee arthroscopies. Arthroscopy 1997;13:456–460.
4. Sahlstrom A, Johnell O, Redlund-Johnell I. The natural course of arthrosis of the knee. Clin Orthop1997;340:152–157.
5. Maletius W, Messner K. The effect of partial meniscectomy on the long-term prognosis of knees with localized, severe chondral damage. A twelve- to fifteen-year followup. Am J Sports Med 1996;24:258–262.
6. Atkinson PJ, Haut RC. Subfracture insult to the human cadaver patellofemoral joint produces occult injury. J Orthop Res 1995; 13:936–944.
7. Messner K, Fahlgren A, Persliden J, Andersson BM. Radiographic joint space narrowing and histologic changes in a rabbit meniscectomy model of early knee osteoarthrosis. Am J Sports Med 2001;29:151–160.
8. Newberry WN, Garcia JJ, Mackenzie CD, Decamp CE, Haut RC. Analysis of acute mechanical insult in an animal model of post-traumatic osteoarthrosis. J Biomech Eng 1998;120:704–709.
9. Newberry WN, Mackenzie CD, Haut RC. Blunt impact causes changes in bone and cartilage in a regularly exercised animal model. J Orthop Res 1998;16:348–354.
10. Newberry WN, Zukosky DK, Haut RC. Subfracture insult to a knee joint causes alterations in the bone and in the functional stiffness of overlying cartilage. J Orthop Res 1997;15:450–455.
11. Indelicato PA, Bittar ES. A perspective of lesions associated with ACL insufficiency of the knee. A review of 100 cases. Clin Orthop 1985;198:77–80.
12. Messner K, Maletius W. The long-term prognosis for severe damage to weight-bearing cartilage in the knee: a 14-year clinical and radiographic follow-up in 28 young athletes. Acta Orthop Scand 1996;67:165–168.
13. Fairbank, TJ. Knee joint changes after meniscectomy. J Bone Joint Surg, 30-B:664–670, 1948.
14. Ahlbäck S. Osteoarthritis of the knee: a radiographic investigation. Acta Radiol Suppl 1968;277:7–72.
15. Rosenberg TD, Paulos LE, Parker RD, Coward DB, Scott SM. The forty-five-degree posteroanterior flexion weight-bearing radiograph of the knee. J Bone Joint Surg Am 1988;70: 1479–1483.
16. Chung CB, Frank LR, Resnick D. Cartilage imaging techniques: current clinical applications and state of the art imaging. Clin Orthop 2001;(391 Suppl):S370–S378.
17. Karantanas AH, Zibis AH, Kitsoulis P. Fat-suppressed 3D-T_1-weighted-echo planar imaging: comparison with fat-suppressed 3D-T_1-weighted-gradient echo in imaging the cartilage of the knee. Comput Med Imaging Graph 2002;6:159–165.

18. Gold GE, Beaulieu CF. Future of MR imaging of articular cartilage. Semin Musculoskelet Radiol 2001;5:313–327.

19. Matsui N, Kobayashi M. Application of MR imaging for internal derangement of the knee (orthopedic surgeon view). Semin Musculoskel Radiol 2001;5:139–141.

20. McCauley TR, Recht MP, Disler DG. Clinical imaging of articular cartilage in the knee. Semin Musculoskel Radiol 2001; 5:293–304.

21. Recht M, Bobic V, Burstein D, et al. Magnetic resonance imaging of articular cartilage. Clin Orthop 2001;391(suppl):S379–S396.

22. Sonin AH, Pensy RA, Mulligan ME, Hatem S. Grading articular cartilage of the knee using fast spin-echo proton density-weighted MR imaging without fat suppression. AJR Am J Roentgenol 2002;179:1159–1166.

23. Uetani M. MR imaging of cartilage lesions of the knee: what is the clinical indication? (radiologist's view). Semin Musculoskel Radiol 2001;5:147–149.

24. Chandnani VP, Ho C, Chu P, Trudell D, Resnick D. Knee hyaline cartilage evaluated with MR imaging: a cadaveric study involving multiple imaging sequences and intraarticular injection of gadolinium and saline solution. Radiology 1991; 178:557–561.

25. Kramer J, Recht MP, Imhof H, Stiglbauer R, Engel A. Postcontrast MR arthrography in assessment of cartilage lesions. J Comput Assist Tomogr 1994;18:218–224.

26. Brossmann J, Preidler KW, Daenen B, et al. Imaging of osseous and cartilaginous intraarticular bodies in the knee: comparison of MR imaging and MR arthrography with CT and CT arthrography in cadavers. Radiology 1996;200:509–517.

27. Speer KP, Spritzer CE, Goldner JL, Garrett WE. Magnetic resonance imaging of traumatic knee articular cartilage injuries. Am J Sports Med 1991;19:396–402.

28. Bredella MA, Tirman PF, Peterfy CG, et al. Accuracy of T_2-weighted fast spin-echo MR imaging with fat saturation in detecting cartilage defects in the knee: comparison with arthroscopy in 130 patients. Am J Roentgenol 1999;172: 1073–1080.

29. Potter HG, Linklater JM, Allen AA, Hannafin JA, Haas S. Magnetic resonance imaging of articular cartilage in the knee. An evaluation with use of fast-spin-echo imaging. J Bone Joint Surg Am 1998;80:1276–1284.

30. Disler DG, McCauley, TR, Kelman CG, et al. Fat-suppressed three-dimensional spoiled gradient-echo MR imaging of hyaline cartilage defects in the knee: comparison with standard MR imaging and arthroscopy. AJR Am J Roentgenol 1996;167: 127–132.

31. McCauley TR, Disler DG. Magnetic resonance imaging of articular cartilage of the knee. J Am Acad Orthop Surg 2001;9: 2–8.

32. Mlynarik V, Trattnig S, Huber M, Zembsch A, Imhof H. The role of relaxation times in monitoring proteoglycan depletion in articular cartilage. J Magn Reson Imaging 1999;10:497–502.

33. Piplani MA, Disler DG, McCauley TR, Holmes TJ, Cousins JP. Articular cartilage volume in the knee: semiautomated determination from three-dimensional reformations of MR images. Radiology 1996;198:855–859.

34. Gandy SJ, Dieppe PA, Keen MC, Maciewicz RA, Watt I, Waterton JC. No loss of cartilage volume over three years in patients with knee osteoarthritis as assessed by magnetic resonance imaging. Osteoarthritis Cartilage. 2002;10:929–937.

35. Brittberg M, Tallheden T, Sjogren-Jansson B, Lindahl A, Peterson L. Autologous chondrocytes used for articular cartilage repair: an update. Clin Orthop 2001;391(suppl):S337–S348.

36. Browne JE, Branch TP. Surgical alternatives for treatment of articular cartilage lesions. J Am Acad Orthop Surg 2000;8: 180–189.

37. Cain, EL, Clancy WG. Treatment algorithm for osteochondral injuries of the knee. Clin Sports Med 2001;20:321–342.

38. Minas T. The role of cartilage repair techniques, including chondrocyte transplantation, in focal chondral knee damage. Instr Course Lect 1999;48:629–643.

39. O'Driscoll SW. The healing and regeneration of articular cartilage. J Bone Joint Surg Am 1998;80:1795–1812.

40. Peterson L, Brittberg M, Kiviranta I, Akerlund EL, Lindahl A. Autologous chondrocyte transplantation. Biomechanics and long-term durability. Am J Sports Med 2002;30:2–12.

41. Sellards RA, Nho SJ, Cole BJ. Chondral injuries. Curr Opin Rheumatol 2002;14:134–141.

42. Ayral X. Diagnostic and quantitative arthroscopy: quantitative arthroscopy. Baillieres Clin Rheumatol 1996;10:477–494.

43. Ayral X., Gueguen A., Ike RW, et al. Inter-observer reliability of the arthroscopic quantification of chondropathy of the knee. Osteoarthritis. Cartilage. 1998;6:160–166.

44. Brismar BH, Wredmark T, Movin T, Leandersson J, Svensson O. Observer reliability in the arthroscopic classification of osteoarthritis of the knee. J Bone Joint Surg Br 2002;84:42–47.

45. Brittberg M, Peterson L. Introduction to an articular cartilage classification. ICRS Newsl 1998;1:5–8.

46. Cameron ML, Briggs KK, Steadman JR. Reproducibility and reliability of the Outerbridge classification for grading chondral lesions of the knee arthroscopically. Am J Sports Med 2003;31:83–86.

47. Dougados M, Ayral X, Listrat V, et al. The SFA system for assessing articular cartilage lesions at arthroscopy of the knee. Arthroscopy 1994;10:69–77.

48. Hunt N, Sanchez-Ballester J, Pandit R, Thomas R, Strachan R. Chondral lesions of the knee: a new localization method and correlation with associated pathology. Arthroscopy 2001;17: 481–490.

49. Lewandrowski KU, Ekkernkamp A, David A, Muhr G, Schollmeier G. Classification of articular cartilage lesions of the knee at arthroscopy. Am J Knee Surg 1996;9:121–128.

50. Noyes FR, Stabler CL. A system for grading articular cartilage lesions at arthroscopy. Am J Sports Med 1989;17:505–513.

51. Brittberg M. Evaluation of cartilage injuries and cartilage repair. Osteologie 2000;9:17–25.

52. Outerbridge RE. The etiology of chondromalacia patella. J Bone Joint Surg Br 1961;43:752–757.

53. Beguin J, Locker B. Chondropathie rotulienne. 2ème Journee d'Arthroscopie du Genou 1983;1:89–90.

54. Ayral X, Dougados M, Listra V, Bonvarlet JP, Simonnet J, Amor B. Arthroscopic evaluation of chondropathy in osteoarthritis of the knee. J Rheumatol 1996;23:698–706.

55. Brooks S, Morgan M. Accuracy of clinical diagnosis in knee arthroscopy. Ann R Coll Surg Engl 2002;84:265–268.

56. van Kampen A, Waal Malefijt MC, Jerosch J, Castro W, Busch M, Pape M. Interobserver variance in diagnostic arthroscopy of the knee. Knee Surg Sports Traumatol Arthrosc 1998;6:16–20.

57. Insall J. Disorders of the patella. In: Insall J (ed) Surgery of the Knee. New York: Churchill Livingston 1984:191–260.

58. Ficat RP, Philippe J, Hungerford DS. Chondromalacia patellae: a system of classification. Clin Orthop 1979;144:55–62.

59. Casscells SW. Gross pathological changes in the knee joint of the aged individual: a study of 300 cases. Clin Orthop 1978;132: 225–232.

60. Bentley G, Dowd G. Current concepts of etiology and treatment of chondromalacia patellae. Clin Orthop 1984;189:209–228.

3

Nonoperative Treatment

Kenneth R. Zaslav and Jeffrey R. Dugas

Primary osteoarthritis is the most common disorder affecting the musculoskeletal system. Prevalence nears ubiquity over the age of 65 and therefore it has been considered a degenerative disease of the elderly[1] Prevalence rates however, approximate 200–250/1000 population in patients 40 to 60 years of age. Many of these patients still desire an active athletic lifestyle.[2] In patients with ligament or meniscal injury, as well as those patients with acute chondral injury, the curve representing the onset of secondary arthritis over time slopes upward earlier and steeper. Acute chondral injury has been reported by one study to occur in at least 5% of all arthroscopies performed on patients younger than 40, and it has been estimated that 900,000 Americans suffer acute articular cartilage injuries each year.[3] Replacement of joint surfaces in younger, more active patients is fraught with danger and therefore many of these patients need more effective palliative treatments. Recent years have seen advances in the nonsurgical management options for painful arthritis and articular surface loss.

Hyaline cartilage is a three-dimensional construct composed of water, type II collagen, and cells. The cellular percentage of the total volume is minimal, only 2%. The second most important structural element, after water, is type II collagen. It is arranged in three layers, with the middle layer called "the netting." The netting is composed of aggregates of proteoglycans called glycosaminoglycans (GAGs). This layer gives the hyaline cartilage its hydrophilic character, enabling it to act as low friction substrate for motion.[2] The joint fluid itself is composed largely of hyaluronic acid, a high molecular weight substance that also adds to the low friction environment. The rheologic environment is completed by the healthy exchange of wear by-products and diffusion of nutrients across the cell membranes provided by motion through this joint fluid.

In arthritis GAGs are altered and found in lower volumes, allowing water to flow more freely through the netting as its structural support is broken down. Hyaluronic acid is decreased in diseased joints as well, promoting more wear and tear on these injured surfaces. Theoretically, effective nonoperative therapies would address the loss of GAGs and hyaluronan plus attempt to maintain the normal rheology of the joint. A mechanical shift in alignment could also help to avoid high stress across areas of injured articular cartilage. The last decade has seen a plethora of literature addressing potential supplements, injectables, orthotic manipulation, and exercise to address these specific factors. Each intervention in its own way can contribute to decreasing symptoms and increasing lifestyle choices in patients with these injured joints. This chapter focuses on the research behind the more traditional conservative approaches as well as these newer advances.

TRADITIONAL MEDICATIONS

Oral administration of countless over-the-counter and prescription medications has long been the most frequently utilized modality for addressing pain related to arthritis and cartilage injury. Although several classes of medications are prescribed, the simple analgesics, narcotics, and nonsteroidal antiinflammatory drugs (NSAIDs) are currently the most common.

Simple analgesics include medications such as aspirin and acetaminophen. In a placebo controlled study, 4 g/day of acetaminophen was shown to significantly reduce pain and increase function in patients with osteoarthritis.[4] Narcotic pain medications have the advantage of effective pain blockade; however, addiction, allergic reaction, constipation, and altered mentation are among the common detrimental effects of this class of drugs. Several dozen NSAIDs are currently available in both prescription and non-prescription strengths. Although several comparative studies exist, no single NSAID has been shown to be significantly more effective than the others in relieving the symptoms of arthritis. Comparative trials of NSAIDs versus simple analgesics found that acetaminophen alone is enough to control pain in many patients with osteoarthritis, and that in patients requiring NSAID therapy, the addition of acetaminophen may reduce the necessary dosage of NSAIDs.[5–7]

Traditional NSAIDs are effective at relieving pain associated with arthritis by reversibly and nonspecifically blocking the cyclooxygenase (COX) side of the arachidonic acid metabolism pathway. This blockade effectively decreases the production of inflammatory agents such as prostaglandins.

Although the beneficial effects of pain relief and decreased inflammation are common, so also are the side effects of blocking the protective effects of prostaglandins. These negative effects are manifested in the form of dyspepsia (most common side effect), gastrointestinal (GI) ulceration, hepatotoxicity, renal toxicity, and cardiac failure. Unlike aspirin, which has a permanent antiplatelet effect that lasts the life of the platelet, NSAIDs have only a short-term effect on coagulation, which usually resolves within 12 to 24 hours. Most side effects are directly related to dosage and are most frequently seen in the elderly population. Contraindications to oral NSAID therapy include concurrent anticoagulation therapy, active hepatic or renal dysfunction, or a history of GI disease.[8]

Although NSAID therapy can control symptoms, studies indicate no evidence of chondroprotection and no diminution in the rate of disease progression.[9] In fact, there is evidence that shows that NSAIDs have an antimetabolite function because they inhibit GAG synthesis by articular cartilage in vitro, thereby inhibiting attempts at matrix repair.[8] COX-2 inhibitors have been shown to provide equally effective pain relief from the symptoms of osteoarthritis with significantly lower GI toxicity and less platelet effect than traditional non-steroidal anti-inflammatory medications.[10,11] Despite the decrease in COX-1 blockade, dyspepsia remains the most frequently reported side effect of the COX-2 inhibitors.[12] However a significant decrease in POBs (perforations, obstructions, and bleeding ulcers) has been demonstrated.[13,14] Other side effects, similar to those of standard NSAIDs, include potential liver and renal toxicity and effects on hypertension. These drugs are not, however, strictly contraindicated with anticoagulation therapy and have no significant effect on platelet function, thereby offering some benefits for preoperative and postoperative care.[15] COX-2 drugs with even more specific COX-2 inhibition are coming to market at this time and may offer future advantages.

CORTICOSTEROID INJECTION

Intraarticular injection of corticosteroid is an effective means of decreasing pain and localized inflammation. Osteoarthritics with acute symptomatic flare or significant effusion are good candidates for injection of corticosteroid because of the powerful antiinflammatory effect of these types of medications. Two broad categories of corticosteroid preparations are available, including the soluble variety (e.g., betamethasone) and the crystalline variety (e.g., triamcinolone). The soluble types rarely induce any inflammatory reaction but tend to be short acting, whereas the crystalline types tend to have slower absorption and longer effect but a higher potential for synovitis or poststeroid flare. Although not mandated at the time of corticosteroid injection, joint aspiration may serve to decrease local inflammation and effusion.

Several small randomized placebo-controlled trials have been performed that demonstrate the positive pain-relieving effect of corticosteroid injection, although the beneficial effects tend to be short lived.[16,17] In another review of three clinical trials, results were noted to be short lived with no permanent beneficial effect noted at 12-month follow-up.[18] No evidence for chondroprotection exists in animal or human studies. Although long-term detrimental effect is difficult to quantify, several review articles on the subject of medical management of osteoarthritis have suggested that a patient should not receive more than three or four injections of corticosteroid per year into a single joint because corticosteroid may have a catabolic effect on joint GAGs.[19,20] Other common side effects of corticosteroid injection include subcutaneous fat atrophy, changes in skin pigmentation, and elevation of serum glucose levels in diabetics.

ACTIVITY MODIFICATION: EXERCISE AND WEIGHT LOSS

An association between obesity and osteoarthritis has been demonstrated in longitudinal studies of men and women, although obesity seems to be a greater risk factor in women.[21] Weight gain tends to occur as physical activity decreases. Messier et al.[22] demonstrated that weight loss can be achieved and maintained over a 6-month period, and that weight loss and exercise or exercise alone can lead to improvements in pain, disability, and performance. Obviously aerobic exercise and good cardiovascular fitness will aid in maintaining appropriate weight status, but in the context of the arthritic patient one has to be concerned with the detrimental effects of load bearing on these injured joints.[2] Animal and human studies have shown that inactivity and sedentary lifestyle contribute to the loss of proteoglycan and matrix seen naturally with arthritis.[23-25] The reversibility of these changes in response to running and load bearing has been demonstrated in animal models.[26] Penninx et al. have demonstrated that aerobic and resistance exercise can reduce the incidence of daily disability in older persons with knee arthritis.[27] Last, the psychologic effects of inactivity on well-being measures in our population of injured ex-athletes with early osteoarthritis (OA) should not be underemphasized.[28,29] In the face of these contradictory needs for the patient with chondral injury and arthritis, an effective exercise regimen needs to be based on sound science and goals that are feasible to achieve.

Minor et al.[30] performed a prospective study on 120 volunteers with OA and rheumatoid arthritis with three exercise protocols: aerobic walking, aerobics with an aquatics program, and a control of formal customized range of motion (ROM) only. All three groups showed improvements in flexibility, well-being assessments and health status questionnaires. No increase in morning stiffness was noted, no adverse effects were recorded, and retention over a 9-month period remained high at over 85%.

Other studies have consistently shown that breaking the cycle of immobility and disuse that often accompanies chondral injury or arthritis offers both physiologic and psychological benefits in all stages of osteoarthritis.[31-34] Hoffman[35] suggested that to keep compliance high, programs should be instituted slowly and in a specific sequence to prepare inflamed joints for new stresses. Effective programs begin with gentle stretching, add isometric and isotonic passive resisting exercise (PRE), and finally aerobic exercise. For patients with earlier stages of injury and disease, modified recreational athletics can then be instituted with appropriate precautions and bracing. Counseling patients to obtain their aerobic high and socialized recreation with low-impact activities is important. Bicycling, skating, walking, or swimming is suggested over running and cutting sports that cause high shear stress across the joints. Cycling activities have been shown to cause little elongation of the anterior cruciate ligament (ACL) and lower joint stresses than running and yet yield four times higher activity in the quadriceps mechanism.[36]

Strength adds important benefits to these patients in several ways. Increased muscle acts to eccentrically decrease shear stresses across abnormal joint surfaces and allows the patient to move more efficiently during activities. It also improves gait in the elderly and decreases falls. To increase muscle mass, the muscle must be stressed by more weight than it normally sustains, and therefore the use of exercise tubing and ankle weights is helpful.[37] Studies have shown that even in the ninth decade of life patients can gain muscle mass from isometric exercise and that strength gain therefore is not age dependent.[38,39]

Careful monitoring of reactive joint inflammation in response to exercise with adjunctive antiinflammatory and activity modification is important for the long-term success of any of these programs.

NEUTRACEUTICAL ORAL SUPPLEMENTS FOR OSTEOARTHRITIS

Because of the adverse effects of long-term NSAID use as well as the detrimental effects of repeated steroid injections, interest has recently been focused on a newly recognized class of compounds that can give pain relief and may offer an additional cartilage-sparing or chondroprotective effect. Anecdotal reports abound for many herbal compounds, but this chapter concentrates on the compounds substantiated by peer-reviewed, published clinical studies and evaluates those studies along with in vitro research to substantiate these claims. Chondroprotective agents have been defined by Ghosh as those that do the following:

1. Stimulate proteoglycan and collagen synthesis.
2. Exert an inhibiting effect on cartilage degradation.
3. Inhibit thrombus formation in the subchondral blood vessels.[40]

Glucosamine and chondroitin sulfate are two compounds that are produced endogenously and have proven effective in orally administered forms to meet one or more of these criteria. They are also the most widely distributed supplements for this purpose. More recent terminology refers to these agents as symptomatic structure-modifying osteoarthritic drugs (SMOADs). They are not, however, regulated by the U.S. Food and Drug Administration (F.D.A.). Therefore, the buyer must beware that all products marketed as glucosamine and chondroitin sulfate may not actually contain what the label purports. One study done at the University of Maryland found that the actual content of glucosamine in a group of products found in a pharmacy contained variably 25% to 115% of the label claim in the tested samples.[41]

In Vitro Studies

The role of inflammation in the pathophysiology of early chondral wear and OA is supported by observations that C-reactive protein levels are elevated in early OA and that high values predict those patients whose disease will progress.[42] Tissue destruction and disease progression associated with joint inflammation are mediated by the action of proteases and inflammatory cytokines. Typically, elevated levels of interleukin (IL)-1, IL-6, and tumor necrosis factor found within the synovial fluid indicate catabolic activity in articular cartilage or matrix breakdown in both early inflammatory arthritis and early OA.[43] The potential therapeutic value of glucosamine and chondroitin sulfate in arthrosis relies on their involvement in effecting articular cartilage biosynthesis and synovial metabolism.[44]

Glucosamine is an amino acid precursor to GAGs endogenously synthesized from glucose and an amine group from glutamine. It is the structural base unit from which all the monosaccharides that make up the GAGs are created. Its theoretical actions include synoviocyte stimulation to synthesize hyaluronic acid, chondrocyte stimulation to produce type II collagen though GAG synthesis, and a direct antiinflammatory action through its ability to decrease proteolytic enzyme activity. All three of these actions were seen in dog serum cultured with calf cartilage and glucosamine in a study by McNamara et al.[45] Glucosamine has also been shown more recently to reverse the decrease in proteoglycan synthesis and UDP (uridine diphosphate)-transferase I mRNA expression induced by IL-1β and also to interfere with IL-1 activation of nuclear factor NF-kappaB.[46] It, as well as chondroitin sulfate, has been shown to inhibit cytokine activity responsible for the generation of proinflammatory prostaglandins and metalloproteases, substances that degrade cartilage matrix in OA.[47-49]

Chondroitin sulfate is the most abundant GAG in articular cartilage. It is found in other human organs including intervertebral disks, cornea, and heart valves. It is composed of linear strands of disaccharide units of galactosamine sulfate and glucuronic acid, which, as mentioned earlier, are derived from the glucosamine molecule. The biologic activity of GAGs such as chondroitin sulfate have been described as early as 1972 by Dorfman et al.[50,51] at the University of Chicago. In vitro cultured chondrocytes were stimulated to synthesize new GAGs when exposed to chondroitin sulfate. Further studies confirmed the anabolic activity of chondroitin as well as glucosamine on articular cartilage and synoviocytes.[52-55] Chondroitin sulfate has also been found to have a strong anticatabolic (inhibitory) effect on enzymes that degrade articular cartilage. These studies showed vast differences in enzyme mRNA activity after exposure to chondroitin sulfate and glucosamine.[56-58]

More recently, two in vitro and in vivo studies have revealed two unique phenomena concerning the effects of glucosamine and chondroitin sulfate on articular cartilage. Interestingly, the response of young healthy articular cartilage to either agent is minimal in terms of biosynthetic pathway activity. However, aged or injured tissues respond with greater intensity,[55,59] which may mean that chondrocytes and synoviocytes in injured or stressed cartilage are more sensitive once activated by a pathologic process. Clinically, this finding may suggest that there is a greater capacity for repair in these injured or stressed tissues. The second phenomenon is that mRNA synthesis is stimulated in chondrocytes by a combination of glucosamine and chondroitin sulfate to an extent greater than the additive value of either agent alone, suggesting a synergistic effect.[54,60]

Clinical Studies

Commercially available glucosamine is produced in various grades of purity and is derived from the processing of crustacean shells such as those of crab and shrimp to obtain the chitin component. Through hydrolysis, this water-insoluble polymer is cleaved into glucosamine subunits that are also insoluble. Further processing is required to produce a water-soluble ionized form: either glucosamine hydrochloride or glucosamine sulfate. Both these salt forms are absorbed in the GI tract at approximately 87% and are equally efficacious. However, a higher dose of the sulfate form is needed to provide an equal amount of glucosamine to the subject compared with the hydrochloride form (40% more glucosamine sulfate is needed to match the amount of glucosamine provided by the hydrochloride form).[61–64] This fact should be taken into account by the various dosing regimens indicated in over-the-counter preparations.

Once administered either orally or parenterally, glucosamine is distributed in the articular cartilage, kidney, and liver and is excreted primarily in the urine.[64,65] Randomized placebo-controlled studies now exist that document efficacy of glucosamine in reducing pain and swelling in arthritic joints.[63,66] Studies also exist comparing its use with NSAIDs (specifically Ibuprofen), indicating equal yet longer-lasting effect.[67] When taken at doses of 1500 mg/day, its antiinflammatory and pain-blocking action is slow, requiring nearly 2 months for maximum onset; however, no toxicity or abnormal biochemical, hematologic, or other side effects have been reported with the use of either of these glucosamine salts in these prospective studies. These supplements have been used extensively in Europe and in veterinary treatment for more than 20 years, and no detrimental effects have been reported in other retrospective studies in the literature during the past 20 years that belie its high safety profile.[45,63,66,68–70]

Although the theoretic basis for chondroprotection with the use of glucosamine has been known for years from in vitro studies,[45,52,58] animal studies have now shown an anti-reactive effect in those animals treated with glucosamine in arthritis models such as meniscectomized rabbits.[54] Most recently its chondroprotective effect was also demonstrated in a placebo-controlled double-blind human study published in *Lancet*. In a study of 212 osteoarthritic patients with grade II or III radiographic change, radiographs were followed for 3 years. A statistically significant loss of joint space was seen (average, 4 mm) in the placebo group whereas no statistical loss was seen in the group taking glucosamine for the 3 years. Increases in WOMAC (Western Ontario and McMaster Universities Arthritis Index) scores were also noted in the glucosamine sulfate group whereas symptoms worsened in all patients in the placebo group.[66]

Chondroitin sulfate is synthesized in cartilage intracellularly by chondrocytes and assembled on protein backbones forming proteoglycan units that are attached to hyaluronan at the cell membrane. These components are then extruded into the cartilage matrix. Commercially available chondroitin sulfate varies widely in purity, quality, and molecular weight, which can range up to 50,000 daltons. All published randomized controlled studies in the United States and Europe that have demonstrated effectiveness of chondroitin sulfate in humans have used a specific 95% pure low molecular weight chondroitin sulfate derived from bovine trachea that is fractioned to approximately 14,000 to 18,000 daltons.[71] The same chemical (manufactured and provided by Bioiberica Pharmaceuticals, SA, Barcelona, Spain) has been selected for a large ongoing multi-center clinical trial by the U.S. National Institutes of Health (NIH).

In human and animal pharmacokinetic studies, only 12% to 15% of orally administered chondroitin sulfate is absorbed by the GI tract.[71] An affinity of chondroitin sulfate for synovial fluid and cartilage has been shown, as well as bioaccumulation of chondroitin in the plasma following continuous dosing.[72] Chondroitin sulfate is metabolized in the liver and excreted in the urine. Unfortunately, incorporation of orally or parenteral administered chondroitin into cartilage matrix has never been demonstrated. Its activity appears to be as a competitive inhibitor to degradative enzymes such as metalloproteinases that break down cartilage matrix and synovial fluid in progressive OA.[58,73] It also acts as a signaling molecule to stimulate proteoglycan synthesis by chondrocytes[74] and to inhibit thrombus formation in subchondral and synovial vasculature, which occurs in the osteoarthritic process.[20]

As has glucosamine, chondroitin sulfate has demonstrated exceptional safety and no toxicity with long-term use, and it is generally well tolerated with minimal to no side effects.[45,69,75–78] Published randomized, placebo-controlled clinical studies of chondroitin sulfate using a dose of 1200 mg/day have demonstrated effectiveness in treating OA as measured by reduction in pain and increase in patient mobility.[76,78–80] Studies to determine a chondroprotective effect with chondroitin sulfate have also been performed. Although one small study with only six subjects showed no statistical difference, two other larger prospective studies, one on the finger joint and one on knees, did show a statistically significant difference in osteoarthritic changes and joint space height in the groups taking chondroitin sulfate versus those on placebo.[79,80]

Synergistic Activity in Clinical Studies

In the United States, a combination of 99% pure glucosamine hydrochloride and 95% pure chondroitin sulfate has been available as an over-the-counter supplement since 1992. All randomized prospective studies published to date on combination drugs have been with this trademarked material. (Cosamine DS). Lipiello et al.[81,82] have shown synergy in both in vitro and in vivo animal studies in slowing cartilage damage when using the combination drug versus either chemical alone. In vitro, collagenase and aggrecanase activity was inhibited most when exposed to both glucosamine and chondroitin. In menisectomized rabbits (a model for arthritis) followed for 4 months, no severe lesions were seen in the articular cartilage, and a statistically significant decrease in moderate lesions was seen in the combination group versus the group with glucosamine or chondroitin alone.[54]

In conclusion, both glucosamine as well as chondrotin sulfate and the combination compounds have been shown to be safe, well-tolerated treatments that can decrease pain, increase activity, and offer some potential chondroprotection in many patients with arthritis. Patients should look for those preparations that have been studied to check their purity to assure effective dosing as the FDA does not control these supplements.

VISCOSUPPLEMENTATION

Viscosupplementation is a newer intraarticular modality that is now approved by numerous regulatory bodies internationally. The research underpinning its development has spanned several decades, however. The discovery that the synovial fluid of the osteoarthritic joint has hyaluronan of a smaller molecular size and in lower concentrations with consequently reduced elastoviscous protective effects spurred research to explore its augmentation by an exogenous hyaluronan with improved elastic and viscous properties.[83–86] In osteoarthritic synovial fluid, the molecular weight and concentration of hyaluronan are decreased by dilutional effects, abnormalities in synthesis, and free radical degradation.[83] Consequently, the biologic and mechanical properties normally provided to synovial fluid by hyaluronan are compromised in OA.

The concept of viscosupplementation thus originated in an attempt to restore the normal rheologic environment to an osteoarthritic joint. In the 1970s, a noninflammatory fraction of hyaluronan (Healon) with an average molecular weight of about 2 million was used in arthritic racehorse and human knees. In the 1980s, purified hyaluronan preparations with molecular weights of 0.5 to 0.75 million, generally given in courses of five or more injections, were approved for treating human knee OA in Italy and Japan. Hylans, cross-linked forms of a noninflammatory fraction of hyaluronan, were then developed to increase the molecular weight, elastoviscous properties, and intraarticular residence time of viscosupplements.

In the United States, three hyaluronan-based preparations are currently marketed for intraarticular injection in human knee OA. They were approved for marketing as medical devices because their primary mode of action was considered to be mechanical; hence, they have been called synovial prostheses. These products include lower molecular weight hyaluronan preparations with molecular weights ranging from 0.5 to 1.7 million (Hyalgan, Fidia, Italy; Supartz, Seikagaku, Japan), and one higher molecular weight hylan product (Synvisc, Genzyme, United States) with an average molecular weight of 6 million. In addition to the differences in molecular weight, the devices have different injection schedules: hylan G-F 20 requires three weekly injections, whereas the hyaluronan products require five weekly injections.

Properties of Hyaluronan

Hyaluronan is the suggested International Union of Pure and Applied Chemistry (IUPAC) nomenclature for the polysaccharide previously referred to as hyaluronic acid or sodium hyaluronate.[85] It is a simple, linear polysaccharide (glycosaminoglycan), composed of the repeating disaccharide unit N-acetylglucosamine and glucuronic acid, linked by alternating β_{1-4} and β_{1-3} glycosidic bonds. The identical molecule occurs in species ranging from bacteria to primates, and is ubiquitous in human tissues.[87] In diarthrodial joints, it is continually synthesized and released into synovial fluid by specialized synoviocytes. The linear hyaluronan molecule adopts a coiled configuration; because of this and its large size, it forms an entangled network even at low concentra-

tions in solution.[88] This configuration gives synovial fluid the elasticity and viscosity responsible for shock absorption under rapid, high-impact or shear conditions, and lubrication in slow-impact, lower-load conditions. Synovial fluid in healthy adults contains a high concentration of hyaluronan molecules of high molecular weight, its average molecular weight is 4 to 5 million and its concentration ranges from 2.5 to 4 mg/mL.[83,89,90]

In addition to its contributions to the rheologic environment, hyaluronan appears to affect inflammatory cell migration and concentrations of some inflammatory mediators.[83,91] Additional molecular weight-dependent roles include antinociception,[92,93] and feedback effects that improve the quality of endogenous hyaluronan synthesis.[94] The latter may explain in part the persistence of clinical benefits well beyond the residence time of the viscosupplements in the joint. There is also accumulating evidence for anticatabolic effects and roles in chondrocyte metabolism.[95]

Clinical Trials of Efficacy of Viscosupplements in Knee Osteoarthritis

Overall, in clinical trials and in practice, viscosupplements have effectively modified osteoarthritic pain and functional disability. Clinical trials have demonstrated significantly greater pain relief for both low molecular weight hyaluronan and high molecular weight hylan preparations compared with an intraarticular saline control.[96–98] Multicenter, prospective, comparative trials have demonstrated that viscosupplementation is at least as effective as NSAIDs.[96,99,100] Some of the results of these trials are reviewed next.

Hyaluronan Viscosupplements

Hyalgan and Supartz are the two lower molecular weight hyaluronan preparations that are marketed in the United States. A number of the studies of Hyalgan were not double blind or controlled.[26,101–103] Of the seven studies that were, two demonstrated efficacy at their 60-day endpoints,[104,105] one demonstrated short-term differences that were no longer evident at the 6-month follow up,[106] and one demonstrated efficacy through the 6-month endpoint.[96] One 6-month study also demonstrated efficacy similar to naproxen.[96] The remainder of the studies did not demonstrate significant differences with the control treatment.[16,107,108]

The results of clinical comparisons of corticosteroids with Hyalgan have been inconsistent, demonstrating either some degree of superiority for hyaluronan or similar responses to both treatments. One 6-month study compared Hyalgan with triamcinolone hexacetonide in knees with effusions; the study had a high rate of discontinuation and did not demonstrate differences by intent-to-treat analysis.[76] However, in completed patients at the study endpoint, the hyaluronan group had significantly less pain. A comparison of Hyalgan with methylprednisolone 40 mg, each administered in three weekly intraarticular doses in inflammatory knee OA, demonstrated significant differences favoring Hyalgan at 60 days after the first injection.[109] Another study compared methylprednisolone 40 mg with Hyalgan, each in three weekly intraarticular doses, and demonstrated similar improvement with both treatments over a 1-year follow-up period.[110]

Supartz was developed in Japan, so many studies were published in Japanese and are not reviewed here. Published large-scale double-blind studies of Supartz have either demonstrated no difference from control[111,112] or efficacy only in a subset of patients.[63]

Viscosupplemetation with Hylan G-F 20

To date, there have been seven controlled, double-blind clinical trials of hylan G-F 20. In four, the control was arthrocentesis or intraarticular saline injections; in two, the comparison was with oral NSAIDs; and in one, the comparison was with a lower molecular weight hyaluronan. The first two trials were studies comparing two injections or three injections over a 2-week period versus control regimens of intraarticular saline.[97] Both hylan G-F 20 regimens were statistically superior to saline, and three injections were superior to two at a 6-month telephone follow-up. Following this, a larger-scale study was performed with a saline control in which hylan G-F 20 was superior to control through a telephone follow-up at 26 weeks.[113] In another study, hylan G-F 20 was effective in a subset of patients whose OA flared on withdrawal of their conventional (primarily NSAID) therapy.[114] In a comparative trial with a 6-month follow-up, hylan G-F 20 was compared with continuous oral NSAIDs or hylan plus NSAIDs.[99] The groups treated with hylan G-F 20 had significantly better improvement than did patients treated with NSAIDs alone. A 3-month comparison of hylan G-F 20 with diclofenac also demonstrated superiority for hylan G-F 20.[100]

Only one clinical study has directly examined the relationship of molecular weight to analgesic effect. This study was a double-blind, randomized, multicenter, 12-week study comparing three weekly 2-mL injections of a lower molecular weight hyaluronan (Artz, Seikagaku, Japan, 0.75 million molecular weight) with the same regimen of higher molecular weight hylan G-F 20 (6 million molecular weight).[115] At the 12-week endpoint, knees treated with hylan G-F 20 were significantly better in all primary outcome measures, including weight-bearing pain, overall treatment response, and improvement in knee movement, than those treated with Artz.

Four open-label studies of hylan G-F 20, one retrospective and three prospective, examined clinical experience. One retrospective survey of hylan G-F 20 as used among Canadian rheumatology practices in a 2.5-year period found more than 75% of the knees improved after a first course of treatment.[116] A Canadian prospective study[117] compared the effectiveness, cost-effectiveness, and cost utility of appropriate care (as defined by the American College of Rheumatology guidelines[118]) for knee OA including hylan G-F 20 with appropriate care exclusive of hylan G-F 20. At 12 months, improvement in the WOMAC A (pain) was significantly greater in the hylan G-F 20 group. Quality-of-life assessments were also significantly better when hylan G-F 20 was included. Results of a related cost-utility analysis were favorable regarding the benefit of treatment with hylan G-F 20 gained in return for its societal costs.[119] In a second prospective, open-label study, the effectiveness of hylan G-F 20 on quality of life 6 months after treatment was demonstrated in several categories of the SF-36, indicating a measurable improvement in overall functioning in these patients.[120] An open-label safety study substantiated the tolerance and effectiveness observed in earlier, blinded clinical trials.[98]

It should be noted that the controlled clinical trials usually excluded radiographic grade 4 OA. As is the case with other symptom-modifying OA therapies, viscosupplementation is more effective in earlier radiographic grades of OA.[116]

Response Duration and Repeat Treatment

In a chronic arthropathy such as OA, long-term duration of symptomatic relief should be one important factor in decisions regarding therapeutic management. Many of the earlier viscosupplementation trials were modeled on NSAID trials and were 3 months or less in duration. There are only a few longer trials, not always controlled or double blinded, on which to base projections of duration of benefits. Although repeat treatment with viscosupplementation is a common occurrence, no prospective, controlled, double-blind studies of repeat treatment have been published, so the open studies must provide guidance.

Controlled, prospective, blinded studies of hylan G-F 20 in osteoarthritic knees demonstrated significant symptomatic improvements that were sustained through follow-up evaluations at 6months after a single course of hylan G-F 20.[99,113] A Canadian open-label, retrospective study revealed that only 12.2% of patients treated initially with a single three-injection course required repeat administration at a mean time of 8.2 months after the first course, suggesting a longer duration of effect than the 6-month studies were designed to detect.[116] The response to the second course was at least strong as that to the first, with more than 80% of patients reporting improvement. The prospective open-label study that compared appropriate care without hylan G-F versus appropriate care plus hylan G-F 20 allowed repeat treatments.[117] Sixty-nine percent of hylan G-F 20-treated knees were improved in pain at 12 months, significantly more than the 40% improved in the appropriate care without hylan G-F 20 group. Although repeat courses were permitted, 62% of knees did not require additional courses during the 12-month follow-up, and among knees that did, the mean time interval between courses was 7 months.

An open-label study of Hyalgan included data on patients who had repeat treatment, in that the design permitted a second injection course 4 to 8 months after the initial five-injection course.[121] For the 55% of patients who were observed for 12 months after the first treatment cycle, significant improvements from baseline pain lasted 12 months. Patients who had a second treatment course were reported to have further amelioration of symptoms.

In the absence of well-designed clinical trial results from which to establish evidence-based guidelines on repeat treatment, clinicians can bear in mind that repeat treatment seems to be effective in some patients. There is considerable "between-patient" variability in duration of effect (from 2.4 to 18.6 months in one study in the knee[116]), and predictors of the duration of response to initial or repeat treatments have not yet been identified. An individual patient's response to their initial course of viscosupplementation is probably the key deciding factor. Some clinicians have established criteria of an improvement from pretreatment knee pain sustained for at least 3 months with a subsequent return to the pretreatment pain levels before administering a repeat course.[122]

Safety

Overall, viscosupplementation is relatively well tolerated in comparison to the adverse event profile of other agents and surgical options for knee OA. The systemic adverse events considered possibly treatment related in clinical trials of viscosupplements were infrequent, did not have serious sequelae, and did not recur after second injections. Local reactions after viscosupplementation consisting of pain or swelling in the knee joint occur in approximately 6% to 7% of knees and 2% to 3% of injections.[97,99,113,115] Reactions have ranged from mild to severe, but they are typically transient and have resolved within 1 to 2 days with or without symptomatic treatment with oral analgesics, NSAIDs, ice, elevation, rest, and occasionally corticosteroid injection and arthrocentesis.

More severe local reactions, accompanied by large effusions with extremely high white blood cell counts ($>10^5$ cells/mm^3) have been reported.[98] Clinical resolution occurs after arthrocentesis, intramuscular corticosteroid injections, ice to the knee, and rest. Infection, although rare, is a risk that accompanies any intraarticular injection and that risk increases with the number of injections. Therefore, injections must always be performed under strict aseptic conditions. A knee with severe reaction should be aspirated; the aspirate must be Gram stained and cultured for aerobic and anaerobic bacteria in an effort to either treat an actual infection or avoid unnecessary treatment of a joint that only appears to be septic.

The mechanism of these reactions may be characterized on further study, but it is not necessarily allergic. Unilateral reactions have occurred in bilaterally treated patients and, furthermore, reactions do not necessarily recur in the same patients on subsequent injections.[98,116]

Some percentage of the side effects in the knee that occur with viscosupplementation treatment are likely caused by inaccurate injection technique. Even experienced injectors miss the intraarticular space, as documented in a study of injection accuracy among rheumatologists, where injection accuracy was uncertain 19% of the time and extraarticular 29% of the time.[123] Viscosupplement is then injected into the soft tissues surrounding the joint space, the physical and physiologic effects on the synovial fluid cannot be delivered, and a painful reaction may occur. Accurate placement of the viscosupplement is critical to realize its beneficial effects and will eliminate a potential source of local reactions.

Thorough joint aspiration before viscosupplementation injection is important and can also contribute to good clinical outcomes, not only because intraarticular placement of the needle is confirmed, but also because one avoids the dilutional effects of osteoarthritic synovial fluid on the injected viscosupplement, which would reduce its elastoviscosity.

Even in "dry" joints, the orthopedist can confirm accurate needle placement by several means. Waddell et al.[124] have described a method using fluoroscopic guidance. Injection techniques using mini air-arthrography or ultrasound guidance to confirm intraarticular placement have been reported.[38,77] Our experience is that these techniques are rarely needed by an experienced arthroscopist.

FUTURE DIRECTIONS

Viscosupplementation

Although viscosupplements are currently indicated for use in the knee, they may prove useful therapy in any diarthrodial joint diagnosed with OA. Preliminary findings indicate possible utility in treatment of OA of the hip, shoulder, and other joints.[125–129] Initial synergies with NSAIDs, intraarticular corticosteroids, or surgery are also areas for research. Applications in intraarticular drug delivery for OA and other arthritic diseases may be developed, and therapeutic roles in cartilage injury may emerge. A chondroprotective effect seen in vivo in meniscetomized animals, as well as improved meniscal repair healing seen in animal models, may offer future hope for chondroprotection of injured human joints.[130] Chondroprotection has not yet been reported in humans with viscosupplementation.

Braces and Orthotics

Malalignment of the lower extremity may be both the cause and the result of arthritic changes in the knee. If the medial joint space experiences increased stress because of varus alignment, early degeneration may take place. By the same token, if the medial compartment experiences some early wear or injury, this loss of articular surface height may lead to progressive varus deformity and more rapid deterioration. Mechanical devices such as braces and orthotics may by useful in decreasing the stress of weight bearing in the affected compartment. Lateral heel wedge orthotics inclined at approximately 5° have been shown to significantly reduce knee varus torque during walking in patients with medial compartment OA.[131] Despite these findings, clinical studies have variably reported reliable pain relief with the use of these types of shoe inserts. In one study, although no significant pain relief could reliably be predicted on the basis of clinical outcome scores, patient compliance was improved and medication (NSAID) usage decreased with the use of orthotics.[132] Several other studies have demonstrated reliable pain relief with the use of lateral wedge orthotics along with significant improvement in subjective functional scores.[133–135] In one study, more than 75% of patients experienced statistically significant improvements in Hospital for Special Surgery pain scores at an average of 12-month follow up.[133]

Soft knee braces provide only compressive forces without altering mechanical alignment. Even so, some patients report decreased pain with the use of compressive type wraps or braces, possibly due to alterations in proprioceptive feedback. Until the advent of newer unloading braces, mechanical nonoperative unloading of abnormal joint surfaces had not been demonstrated with conventional bracing. These unloader braces apply a three-point bending moment to the knee to create an alteration in the joint reactive force. Pain relief is related to actual condylar separation, which has been demonstrated at heel strike and during the midstance phases of gait with the use of unloader braces.[136–138]

Lindenfeld et al.[139] have shown that unloading braces can achieve a statistically significant shift in the mean adduction moment greater than 10% with a custom orthotic unloader.

These gait studies were augmented by clinical and Visual Analogue Scale (VAS) evaluation in 11 patients with varus arthritis of the knee versus age-matched controls. These studies indicated a analgesic pain scale improvement of 48% and 79% improvement in functional activity scale performance with valgus bracing. Matsuno et al.[138] in Japan studied 20 patients with OA over the age of 55. All patients were followed for 12 months and wore G-II custom unloading braces (G II Medical); 19 of 20 patients indicated pain relief and all showed significant strength gains in quadriceps dynamometer testing. A mean shift of 2° was seen in the tibial-femoral angle measured on X-ray at 12 months on 12 of these patients.

Although some patients find the braces cumbersome and uncomfortable, one study reported a 50% decrease in patient complaints when using the brace for 7 hours per day, 5 days per week.[140] A recent study by Pollo et al.[141] demonstrated a 13% average decrease in net varus moment about the knee and an average decrease in medial compartment load of 11% with the use of a calibrated 4° valgus brace. This same study also demonstrated that increasing the degree of valgus alignment had a greater effect on joint forces than did increasing strap tension. Another recent study demonstrated significant decreases in resting pain, night pain, and activity-related pain with the use of unloader bracing, but no difference was noted in bone scans before and after 3 months of bracing.[142]

In the most comprehensive study to date, a Canadian group performed a prospective randomized clinical trial comparing unloading braces (G-II Medical) with use of a neoprene sleeve alone and with NSAID use alone in 119 patients. Patients were concomitantly stratified by age, degree of deformity, and presence or absence of ACL. Quality of life scales, functional testing, and mechanical gait analysis were evaluated at baseline and 6 months. Mechanical axis was shifted with unloading braces effectively and a statistically significant improvement was noted in quality of life scales and functional testing when comparing unloading bracing to either NSAID or neoprene brace use alone. Few adverse effects were noted, and compliance remained high for the 6 months.[138] Although no data exist to suggest that mechanical bracing or orthotics alter the composition or structure of the diseased and deteriorated articular surface, clinical evidence is strongly in favor of these devices in the management of unicompartmental osteoarthritis. Both off-the-shelf and custom braces may be effective.[143]

Recent experience has shown that unloading braces can be used effectively to supplement other invasive procedures discussed in this volume. They can be used to predict the potential pain-reducing benefits of osteotomy before undergoing the procedure. They offer a predictable and convenient way to unload injured or chondroplastied surfaces for 3 to 6 months while repair tissue matures, thereby allowing weight bearing to stimulate proper joint nutrition and avoid muscle atrophy and disuse osteoporosis. These braces could act similarly after articular cartilage implants of osteoarticular autografts or allografts to allow protection to these newly formed surfaces postoperatively or on resumption of sports activity. Randomized prospective studies of these potential uses have not been published to date.

CONCLUSION

Although operative treatment may be necessary for chondral injury and early osteoarthritis it should be coupled with appropriate nonoperative care to offer the most comprehensive program to our patients.

References

1. Felson DT, Zhang Y. An update on the epidemiology of knee and hip osteoarthritis with a view to prevention. Arthritis Rheum 1998;41:1343–1355.
2. Buckwalter JA. Aging sports and osteoarthritis. Sports Med Arthritis Rev 1996;4(2):276–287.
3. Cole BJ, Frederick RW, Levy AS, et al. Management of a 37-year-old man with recurrent knee pain: case study and commentary. JCOM 1999;6(6):46–57.
4. Amadio P, Cummings DM. Evaluation of acetaminophen in the management of osteoarthritis of the knee. Curr Ther Res 1983;34:59–66.
5. Bradley JD, Brandt KD, Katz BP, et al. Comparison of an anti-inflammatory dose of ibuprofen, an analgesic dose of ibuprofen, and acetaminophen in the treatment of patients with osteoarthritis of the knee. N Engl J Med 1991;325:87–91.
6. March L, Irwig L, Schwarz J, et al. Trials comparing a non-steroidal anti-inflammatory drug with paracetamol in osteoarthritis. Br Med J 1994;309:1041–1045.
7. Williams HJ, Ward JR, Egger MJ, et al. Comparison of naproxen and acetaminophen in a two year study of treatment of osteoarthritis of the knee. Arthritis Rheum 1993;36:1196–2006.
8. Abraham, Weissman, et al. Mechanics and action of NSAIDS. Arthritis Rheum 1989.
9. Brandt, KD. Should osteoarthritis be treated with non-steroidal anti-inflammatory drugs. Rheum Dis Clin North Am 1993; 19:697–712.
10. Ehrich EW, Schnitzer TJ, McIlwain H, et al. Effect of specific COX-2 inhibition in osteoarthritis of the knee: a 6 week double blind, placebo controlled pilot study of rofocoxib. J Rheumatol 1999;26:2438–2447.
11. Scott LJ, Lamb HM. Rofocoxib. Drugs 1999;58:499–505.
12. Langman MJ, Jensen DM, Watson DJ, et al. Adverse upper gastrointestinal effects of rofecoxib compared with NSAIDs. JAMA 1999;282:1929–1933.
13. Reicin A, et al. Comparison of upper gastrointestinal toxicity of rofecoxib and naproxen in patients with rheumatoid arthritis. N Engl J Med 2000;343:1520–1528.
14. Lane NE. Pain management in osteoarthritis: the role of COX-2 inhibitors. J Rheumatol 1997;24(suppl 49):20–24.
15. Reuben SS, Connelly NR. Postoperative analgesic effects of celecoxib or rofecoxib after spinal fusion surgery. Anesth Analg 2000;91:1221–1225.
16. Creamer P, Sharif M, George E, et al. Intra-articular hyaluronic acid in osteoarthritis of the knee: an investigation into mechanisms of action. Osteoarthritis Cartilage 1994;2:133–140.
17. Jones A, Doherty M. Intra-articular corticosteroids are effective in osteoarthritis but there are no clinical predictors of response. Ann Rheum Dis 1996;55:829–832.
18. Towheed TE, Hochberg MC. A systematic review of randomized controlled trials of pharmacological therapy in osteoarthritis of the knee with an emphasis on trial methodology. Semin Arthritis Rheum 1997;26:755–770.
19. Marshall KW, Waddell DD. Nonoperative management of osteoarthritis of the knee. Phys Sports Med 2000; (special report):14–19.
20. Manek NJ, Lane NE. Osteoarthritis: current concepts in diagnosis and management. Am Fam Physician 2000:1–13.

21. Felson DT, Anderson JJ, Naimark A, et al. Obesity and knee osteoarthritis. The Framingham study. Ann Inern Med 1988; 109:18–24.
22. Messier SP, Loeser RF, Mitchell MN, et al. Exercise and weight loss in obese older adults with knee osteoarthritis: a preliminary study. J Am Geriatr Soc 2000;48:1062–1072.
23. Jurvelin J, Helminen HJ, Lauritsalo S, et al. Influences of joint immobilization and running exercise on articular cartilage surfaces of young rabbits. Acta Anat (Basel). 1985;122:62–68.
24. Palmoski MJ, Brandt KD. Running inhibits the reversal of atrophic changes in canine knee cartilage after removal of a leg cast. Arthritis Rheum 1981;24:1329–1337.
25. Pita J, Muller FJ, Manicourt DH, et al. Early matrix changes in experimental osteoarthritis and joint disuse atrophy. In: Kuettner KE, Schleyerbach R, Peyron JG, Hascall VC (eds) Articular Cartilage and Osteoarthritis. New York: Raven Press. 1992, pp. 455–467.
26. Jurvelin J, Kiviranta I, Saamanen A-M, et al. Partial restoration of joint immobilization-induced softening of canine articular cartilage after remobilization of the knee (stifle) joint. J Orthop Res 1989;7:352–358.
27. Penninx BW, Messier SP, Rejeski WJ, et al. Physical exercise and the prevention of disability in activities of daily living in older persons with osteoarthritis. Arch Intern Med 2001;161(19): 2309–2316.
28. Rosenbaum M. Learned resourcefulness, stress, and self regulation. In: Learned Resourcefulness: Coping Skill, Self Control, and Adaptive Behavior. New York Springer, 1990, pp. 3–30.
29. Scheir MF, Carver CS. Dispositional optimism and physical well being: Influence of generalized outcome expectancies and health. J Personality 1987;155:169–210.
30. Minor MA, Hewett JE, Webel RR, Anderson SK, Kay DR. Efficacy of physical conditioning exercise in patients with rheumatoid arthritis and osteoarthritis. Arthritis Rheum 1989;32(11):1396–1405.
31. Bunning RD, Materson RS. A rational program of exercise for patients with osteoarthritis. Semin Arthritis Rheum 1991; 21(suppl 2):33–43.
32. Ettinger WH Jr, Afable RF. Physical disability from knee osteoarthritis: the role of exercise as an intervention. J Am Coll Sports Med 1994;26(12)1435–1440.
33. Pothier B, Allen M. Kinesiology and the degenerative joint. Rheum Dis Clin North Am 1990;16(4):989–2002.
34. Ytterberg SR, Mahowald ML, Krug HE. Exercise for arthritis. Baillieres Clin Rheumatol 1994;8(1):161–189.
35. Hoffman DF. Arthritis and exercise. Arthritis 1993;20(4):895–909.
36. Henning CE, Lynch MA, Glick KR. An in vitro study of elongation of the ACL. Am J Sports Med 1985;11:303–307.
37. Semble E, Loeser RF, Wise CM. Therapeutic exercise for rheumatoid arthritis and osteoarthritis. Semin Arthritis Rheum 1990;20(1):32–40.
38. Fiatarone MA, Marks EL, Ryan ND, et al. High intensity strength training in nonagenarians: Effect on skeletal muscle. JAMA 1990;263(22):3029–3039.
39. McCubbin JA. Resistance exercise training for persons with arthritis. Rheum Dis Clin North Am 1900;16(4):1990.
40. Ghosh P. Second-line agents in osteoarthritis. In: Second-Line Agents in the Treatment of Rheumatic Diseases. New York: Dekker, 1992, pp. 363–427.
41. Adebowale AO, Cox DS, Liang Z, et al. Analysis of glucosamine and chondroitin sulfate in marketed products. J Am Neutraceutical Assoc 2000;3(1):32–38.
42. Chikanza I, Fernandes L. Novel strategies for the treatment of osteoarthritis. Expert Opin Investig Drugs. 2000;9:1499–1510.
43. Amin AR, Abramson SB. The role of nitric oxide in articular cartilage breakdown in osteoarthritis. Curr Opin Rheumatol 1998; 10:263–268.
44. Bali JP, Cousse H, Neuzil E. Biochemical basis of the pharmacologic action of chondroitin sulfates on the osteoarticular system. Semin Arthritis Rheum 2000;31:58–68.
45. McNamara PS, Barr SC, Erb HN. Hematologic, hemostatic, and biochemical effects in dogs receiving an oral chondroprotective agent for thirty days. Am J Vet Res 1996;57(9):1390–1394.
46. Schaible HG, Schmidt RF. Effects of an experimented arthritis on sensory properties of the afferent units. J Neurophysiol 1985; 54:1109–1112.
47. Conrozier T. Death of articular chondrocytes. Mechanisms and protection. Presse Med 1998;27:1859–1861.
48. Gouze JN, Bordji K, Gulberti S, et al. Interleukin-beta down regulates the expression of glucuronosyltransferase I, a key enzyme priming glycosaminoglycan biosynthesis: influence of glucosamine on interleukin-1-beta mediated effects in rat chondrocytes. Arthritis Rheum 2000;44:351–360.
49. Stove J, Huch K, Gunther KP, et al. Interleukin-1 beta induces different gene expression of stromelysin, aggrecan, tumor necrosis factor-stimulated gene 6 in human OA chondrocytes in vitro. Pathobiology 2000;68:144–149.
50. Nevo Z, Dorfman A. Stimulation of chondromucoprotein synthesis in chondrocytes by extracellular chondromucoprotein. Proc Natl Acad Sci USA 1972;69:2069–2072.
51. Schwartz NB, Dorfman A. Stimulation of chondroitin sulfate proteoglycan production by chondrocytes in monolayer. Connect Tissue Res 1975:115–122.
52. Bassleer C, Rovati L, Franchimont P. Stimulation of proteoglycan production by glucosamine sulfate in chondrocytes isolated from human osteoarthritic articular cartilage in vitro. Osteoarthritis Cartilage 1998;6:427–434.
53. Fenton JI, Chlebek-Brown KA, Peters TL, Caron JP, Orth MW. The effects of glucosamine derivatives on equine articular cartilage degradation in explant culture. Osteoarthritis Cartilage 2000;8:444–451.
54. Lippiello L, Woodward J, Karpman R, Hammad TA. In vivo chondroprotection and metabolic synergy of glucosamine and chondroitin sulfate. Clin Ortho Res 2000;381:229–240.
55. Nerucci F, Fioravanti A, Cicero MR, et al. Effects of chondroitin sulfate and interleukin-1 beta on human chondrocyte cultures exposed to pressurization: a biochemical and morphological study. Osteoarthritis Cartilage 2000;8:279–287.
56. Bobacz K, Erlacher L, Graninger WB. The effect of chondrosulf (sodium chondroitin sulfate) on proteoglycan synthesis by human osteoarthritic and bovine juvenile articular cartilage chondrocytes: an in vitro study. Acta Med Aust 2000;29:20–25.
57. Gouze JN, Bianchi A, Becuwe P, et al. Glucosamine modulates IL-1 activation of rat chondrocytes at a receptor level, and by inhibiting the NF-kappa B pathway. FEBS Lett 2000;510: 166–170.
58. Mims TT, O'Grady C, Marwin S, et al. Effects of dietary supplements on cartilage metabolism and its potential role in osteoarthritis. Presented at the 46th Annual Meeting of the Orthopaedic Research Society, Session 39, Orlando FL, March 14, 2000 (Abstract).
59. Lippiello L, Han MS. Articular cartilage response to glucosamine HCl and chondroitin sulfate under simulated conditions of joint stress. Abstract 15, Presented at the 28th Annual Meeting of the American Orthopaedic Society for Sports Medicine Orlando, FL, 2002.
60. McCarty MF, Russell AL, Seed MP. Sulfated glycosaminoglycans and glucosamine may synergize in promoting synovial hyaluronic acid synthesis. Med Hypotheses 2000;54:798–802.
61. Deal CL, Moskowitz RW. Nutraceuticals as therapeutic agents in osteoarthritis. Rheum Dis Clin North Am 1999;25:379.
62. Fenton JI, et al. The effects of glucosamine derivatives on equine arthicular cartilage degradation in explant culture. Osteoarthritis Cartilage 2000;8(6):444–451.

63. Pujalte JM, et al. Double-blind clinical efficacy and safety of intramuscular glucosamine sulfate in osteoarthritis of the knee. Arzneim Forsch (Drug Res) 1980:30(I).

64. Setnikar I, Palumbo R. Pharmacokinetics of glucosamine in man. Arzneim Forsch (Drug Res) 1993;43(II):1109–1113.

65. Setnikar I, Giacchetti C, Zanolo G: Pharmacokinetics of glucosamine in dog and in man. Arzneim Forsch (Drug Res) 1986;36(4):729–734.

66. Reginster JY, DeroistR, Rovati LC, et al. Long term effects of glucosamine sulfate on osteoarthritis progression: a randomized placebo controlled clinical trial. Lancet 2001;357(9252):251–256.

67. Muller-Fassbender H, et al. Glucosamine sulfate compared to ibuprofen in osteoarthritis of the knee. Osteoarthritis Cartilage 1994;2:61–69.

68. Anderson MA, Slater MR, Hammad TA. Results of a survey of small-animal practitioners on the perceived clinical efficacy and safety of an oral nutraceutical. Prev Vet Med 1999;38:65–73.

69. McNamara PS, Barr SC, Erb HN, et al. Hematological, hemostatic, and biochemical effects in cats receiving an oral chondroprotective agent for thirty days. Am J Vet Res 2000;1(2):108–117.

70. O'Driscoll SW. Current concepts review the healing and regeneration of articular cartilage. J Bone Joint Surg 1998;80(12):1795–1812.

71. Ronca G, et al. Antiinflammatory activity of chondroitin sulfate. Singapore: The Third International Congress of the Osteoarthritis Research Society, 1997:6.

72. Du J, et al. Bioavailability and disposition of the dietary Supplements, FCHG49TM Glucosamine and TRH122TM chondroitin sulfate in dogs after single and multiple dosing. Poster presentation of the American Association of Pharmaceutical Scientists, October 21–25, 2001.

73. Conte A, et al. Biochemical and pharmacokinetic aspects of oral treatment with chondroitin sulfate. Arzneimittelforschung 1995;45:918–925.

74. Grande D, O'Grady C, Garone E, et al. Chondroprotective and gene expression effects of nutritional supplements on articular cartilage. Osteoarthritis Cartil 2000;8(suppl):S34–S35.

75. Beals CA, Lampman RM, Banwell BF, et al. Measurement of exercise tolerance in patients with rheumatoid arthritis and osteoarthritis. J Rheumatol 1985;12:458–461.

76. Das AK, Hammad TA. Efficacy of a combination of FCHG49 glucosamine hydrochloride, TRHI22 low molecular weight sodium chondroitin sulfate and manganese ascorbate in the management of knee osteoarthritis. Osteoarthritis Cartil 2000;8(5):343–350.

77. Fioravanti A, et al. Clinical efficacy and tolerance of galactosaminoglycuronoglycan sulfate in the treatment of osteoarthritis. Drugs Exp Clin Res 1991;17(1):41–44.

78. Leffler CT, Philippi AF, Leffler SG, Mosure IC, et al. Glucosamine, chondroitin and manganese ascorbate for degenerative joint disease of the knee or low back: a randomized, double-blind, placebocontrolled pilot study. Mil Med 1999;164(2):85–91.

79. Conrozier T, et al. Prospective randomized study of the effect of chondroitin sulfate on tibial-femoral osteoarthritis. Presse Med 1998;27:1862–1865.

80. Verbruggen G, et al. Chondroitin Sulfate in the treatment of finger joint OA Osteoarthritis Cartilage. 1998;6(suppl):37–38.

81. Lippiello L, Hammad T. Dose response and synergistic effect of glucosamine HCL and chondroitin sulfate on in vitro proteoglycan synthesis by bovine and human chondrocytes. Proceedings of the 67th Meeting of the American Academy of Orthopaedic Surgeons, Orlando, FL 2000.

82. Lohmander LS, Dalén N, Englund G, et al. Intra-articular hyaluronan injections in the treatment of osteoarthritis of the knee: a randomised, double blind, placebo controlled multicentre trial. Ann Rheum Dis 1996;55:424–431.

83. Balazs EA, Briller SO, Denlinger JL: Na-hyaluronate molecular size variations in equine and human arthritic synovial fluids and the effects on phagocytic cells. In: Talbott JH (ed) Seminars in Arthritis and Rheumatism. New York: Grune & Stratton, 1981:141–143.

84. Balazs EA, Denlinger JL. Sodium hyaluronate and joint function. J Equine Vet Sci 1985;5:217–228.

85. Balazs EA, Laurent TC, Jeanloz RW. Nomenclature of hyaluronic acid. J Biochem 1986;235:903.

86. Balazs EA, Watson D, Duff IF, et al. Hyaluronic acid in synovial fluid. I. Molecular parameters of hyaluronic acid in normal and arthritic human fluids. Arthritis Rheum 1967;10:357–376.

87. Laurent TC, Fraser JRE. Hyaluronan. FASEB J 1992;6:2397–2404.

88. Laurent TC. Structure of hyaluronic acid. In: Balazs EA (ed) Chemistry and Molecular Biology of the Intercellular Matrix. New York: Academic Press, 1970:703–732.

89. Balazs EA. The physical properties of synovial fluid and the special role of hyaluronic acid. In: Helfet A (ed) Disorders of the Knee. 2nd ed. Philadelphia: Lippincott; 1982:61–74.

90. Balazs EA. Viscoelastic properties of hyaluronic acid and biological lubrication (Proceedings of Symposium: Prognosis for Arthritis: Rheumatology Research Today and Prospects for Tomorrow, 1967). Univ Mich Med Cent J (Suppl) 1968;9:255–259.

91. Balazs EA, Darzynkiewicz Z. The effect of hyaluronic acid on fibroblasts, mononuclear phagocytes and lymphocytes. In: Kulonen E, Pikkarainen J (eds) Biology of the Fibroblast (papers of a symposium held in Turku, Finland, 1972.) London: Academic Press, 1973:237–252.

92. Belmonte C, Pozo MA, Balazs EA. Modulation by hyaluronan and its derivatives (hylans) of sensory nerve activity signalling articular pain. In: Laurent TC (ed) The Chemistry, Biology, and Medical Applications of Hyaluronan and its Derivatives (Proceedings of the Wenner-Gren Foundation International Symposium, Sept 18–21, 1996, Stockholm, Sweden, vol. 72). London: Portland Press, 1997:205–217.

93. Pozo MA, Balazs EA, Belmonte C. Reduction of sensory responses to passive movements of inflamed knee joints by hylan, a hyaluronan derivative. Exp Brain Res 1997;116:3–9.

94. Smith MM, Ghosh P. The synthesis of hyaluronic acid by human synovial fibroblasts is influenced by the nature of the hyaluronate in the extracellular environment. Rheumatol Int 1987;7:113–122.

95. Marshall KW. Intra-articular hyaluronan therapy. Curr Opin Rheumatol 2000;12:648–674.

96. Altman RD, Moskowitz R, Hyalgan Study Group. Intraarticular sodium hyaluronate (Hyalgan®) in the treatment of patients with osteoarthritis of the knee: a randomized clinical trial. J Rheumatol 1998;25:2203–2212.

97. Scale D, Wobig M, Wolpert W. Viscosupplementation of osteoarthritic knees with hylan: a treatment schedule study. Curr Ther Res 1994;55:220–232.

98. Wobig M, Beks P, Dickhut A, et al. Open-label multicenter trial of the safety and efficacy of viscosupplementation with hylan G-F 20 (Synvisc) in primary osteoarthritis of the knee. J Clin Rheumatol 1999;5(suppl):S24–S31.

99. Adams ME, Atkinson MH, Lussier AJ, et al. The role of viscosupplementation with hylan G-F 20 (Synvisc®) in the treatment of osteoarthritis of the knee: A Canadian multicenter trial comparing hylan G-F 20 alone, hylan G-F 20 with non-steroidal anti-inflammatory drugs (NSAIDs) and NSAIDs alone. Osteoarthritis Cartilage 1995;3:213–225.

100. Dickson DJ, Hosie G, English JR, the Primary Care Rheumatology Society OA Knee Study Group. A double-blind, placebo-controlled comparison of hylan G-F 20 against diclofenac in knee osteoarthritis. Clin Res 2001;4:41–52.

101. Bragantini A, Cassini M, De Bastiani G, et al. Controlled single-blind trial of intra-articularly injected hyaluronic acid (Hyalgan®) in osteoarthritis of the knee. Clin Trials J 1987;24:333–340.

102. Dougados M, Nguyen M, Listrat V, et al. High molecular weight sodium hyaluronate (hyalectin) in osteoarthritis of the knee: a 1 year placebo-controlled trial. Osteoarthritis Cartilage 1993;1:97–103.

103. Huskisson EC, Donnelly S. Hyaluronic acid in the treatment of osteoarthritis of the knee. Rheumatology 1999;38:602–607.

104. Corrado EM, Peluso GF, Gigliotti S, et al. The effects of intra-articular administration of hyaluronic acid in osteoarthritis of the knee: a clinical study with immunological and biochemical evaluations. Eur J Rheumatol Inflamm 1995;15:47–56.

105. Grecomoro G, Martorana C, Di Marco C. Intra-articular treatment with sodium hyaluronate in gonarthrosis: a controlled clinical trial versus placebo. Pharmatherapeutica 1987;5:137–141.

106. Carrabba M, Paresce E, Angelini M, et al. The safety and efficacy of different dose schedules of hyaluronic acid in the treatment of painful osteoarthritis of the knee with joint effusion. Eur J Rheumatol Inflamm 1995;15:25–31.

107. Dixon ASJ, Jacoby RK, Berry H, et al. Clinical trial of intra-articular injection of sodium hyaluronate in patients with osteoarthritis of the knee. Curr Med Res Opin 1988;11:205–213.

108. Henderson EB, Smith EC, Pegley F, et al. Intra-articular injections of 750 kD hyaluronan in the treatment of OA: a randomised, double-blind placebo-controlled trial of 91 patients demonstrating lack of efficacy. Ann Rheum Dis 1994;53(8):529–534.

109. Leardini G, Mattara L, Franceschini M, et al. Intra-articular treatment of knee osteoarthritis. A comparative study between hyaluronic acid and 6-methyl prednisolone acetate. Clin Exp Rheumatol 1991;9:375–381.

110. Leardini G, Franceschini M, Mattara L, et al. Intra-articular sodium hyaluronate (Hyalgan®) in gonarthrosis. Clin Trials J 1987;24:341–350.

111. Dahlberg L, Lohmander LS, Ryd L. Intraarticular injections of hyaluronan in patients with cartilage abnormalities and knee pain. A one-year double-blind, placebo-controlled study. Arthritis Rheum 1994;37:521–528.

112. Lohmander LS. A controlled, randomized, double-blind multi-center trial of intra-articular hyaluronan treatment in osteoarthrosis of the knee. Acta Orthop Scand 1995;66(suppl 265):35–36.

113. Wobig M, Dickhut A, Maier R, et al. Viscosupplementation with hylan G-F 20: a 26-week controlled trial of efficacy and safety in the osteoarthritic knee. Clin Ther 1998;20:410–423.

114. Moreland L, Arnold W, Saway A, et al. Efficacy and safety of intra-articular hylan G-F 20 (Synvisc), a viscoelastic derivative of hyaluronan, in patients with osteoarthritis of the knee. Am Coll Rheumatol, San Antonio, TX, Nov. 7–11, 1993(Abstract 165).

115. Wobig M, Bach G, Beks P, et al. The role of elastoviscosity in the efficacy of viscosupplementation for osteoarthritis of the knee: a comparison of hylan G-F 20 and a lower-molecular-weight hyaluronan. Clin Ther 1999;21:1549–1562.

116. Lussier A, Cividino AA, McFarlane CA, et al. Viscosupplementation with hylan for the treatment of osteoarthritis: findings from clinical practice. Can J Rheumatol 1996;23:1579–1585.

117. Raynauld JP, Torrance GW, Band PA, et al. A prospective, randomized, pragmatic, health outcomes trial evaluating the incorporation of hylan G-F 20 into the treatment paradigm for patients with knee osteoarthritis (part 1 of 2): clinical results. Osteoarthritis Cartil 2002;10(7):506–517.

118. American College of Rheumatology Subcommittee on Osteoarthritis Guidelines. Recommendations for the medical management of osteoarthritis of the hip and knee. 2000 update. Arthritis Rheum 2000;43:1905–1915.

119. Torrance GW, Raynauld JP, Walker V, et al. A prospective, randomized, health outcomes trial evaluating the incorporation of hylan G-F 20 into the treatment paradigm for patients with knee osteoarthritis: Osteoarthritis Cartilage. 2002;10(7):518–527.

120. Goorman SD, Watanabe TK, Miller EH, et al. Functional outcome in knee osteoarthritis after treatment with hylan G-F 20. Arch Phys Med Rehabil 2000;81:479–483.

121. Kotz R, Kolarz G. Intra-articular hyaluronic acid: duration of effects and results of repeated treatment cycles. Am J Orthop 1999;28 (suppl 11):5–7.

122. Waddell D, Estey D, Bricker DC. Viscosupplementation under fluoroscopic control. Am J Sports Med 2001;3:237–241, 249.

123. Jones A, Regan M, Ledingham J, et al. Importance of placement of intraarticular steroid injections. Br Med J 1993;307:1329–1330.

124. Waddell D, Estey D, Bricker DC. Viscosupplementation under fluoroscopic control. Am J Sports Med 2001;3:237–241, 249.

125. Chevalier X, Conrozier T, Bertin P, et al. Treatment of patients with symptomatic hop OA—a pilot study with intra-articular hylan G-F 20 (Synvisc) Presented at the American College of Rheumatology, 64th Annual Scientific Meeting. Oct. 30–Nov. 3, 2000, Philadelphia, PA [abstract].

126. Jones AC, Pattrick M, Doherty S, et al. Intra-articular hyaluronic acid compared to intra-articular triamcinolone hexacetonide in inflammatory knee osteoarthritis. Osteoarthritis Cartilage 1995;3:269–273.

127. Masuda K, Masuko T, Ito M. Evaluation of hyaluronate preparations for the treatment of peri-arthritis of the shoulder. J Asahikawa Kosei General Hospital 1997;113:19–21.

128. Srejic U, Calvillo O, Kabakibou K. Viscosupplementation: a new concept in the treatment of sacroiliac joint syndrome: a preliminary report of 4 cases. Reg Anesth 1999;24:84–88.

129. Justin D, Kryshtalskyj B, Galea A. Use of hylan G-F 20 for viscosupplementation of the temporomandibular joint for the management of osteoarthritis: a case report. J Orofac Pain 1995;9:375–379.

130. Vangsness CT Jr, Soma C, Marshall GJ, et al. The effects of hyaluronic acid on the injured meniscus: An in vivo analysis of healing response: Presented at the American Orthopaedic Society for Sports Medicine Specialty Day, Anaheim, CA, 1999.

131. Kerrigan DC, Lelas JL, Goggins J, et al. Effectiveness of a lateral wedge insole on knee varus torque in patients with knee osteoarthritis. Arch Phys Med Rehabil 2002;93:889–893.

132. Maillefert JF, Hudry C, Baron G, et al. Laterally elevated wedged insoles in the treatment of medial knee osteoarthritis: a prospective randomized control study. Osteoarthritis Cartil 2001;9(8):738–745.

133. Keating EM, Faris PM, Ritter MA, et al. Use of lateral heel and sole wedges in the treatment of medial osteoarthritis of the knee. Orthop Rev 1993;22:921–924.

134. Sasaki T, Yasuda K. Clinical evaluation of the treatment of osteoarthritic knees using a newly designed wedged insole. Clin Orthop 1987;221:181–187.

135. Yasuda K, Sasaki T. The mechanics of treatment of the osteoarthritic knee with a wedged insole. Clin Orthop 1987;215:162–172.

136. Kirkley A, Webster-Bogaert S, Litchfield R, et al. The effect of bracing on varus gonarthrosis. J Bone Joint Surg 1999;81A:539–548.

137. Komistek RD, Dennis DA, Northcut EJ, et al. An in vivo analysis of the effectiveness of osteoarthritis knee brace during heel strike gait. J Arthroplasty 1999;14:738–742.

138. Matsuno H, Kadowaki KM, Tsuji H. Generation II knee bracing for severe medial compartment osteoarthritis of the knee. Arch Phys Med Rehabil 1997;78:745–749.

139. Lindenfeld TN, Hewett TE, Andriacchi TP. Joint loading with valgus bracing in patients with varus gonarthrosis. Clin Orthop Relat Res 1997;344:290–297.

140. Hewitt TE, Noyes FR, Barber-Westin SD, Heckmann TP. Decrease in knee joint pain and increase in function in patients with medial compartment arthrosis: a prospective analysis of valgus bracing. Orthopedics 1998;21:131–138.

141. Pollo FE, Otis JC, Backus MA, et al. Reduction of medial compartment loads with valgus bracing of the osteoarthritic knee. Am J Sports Med 2002;30:414–421.

142. Finger S, Paulos LE. Clinical and biomechanical evaluation of the unloading brace. J Knee Surg 2002;15:155–159.

143. Otis JC, Backus MA, Warren RF, et al. Valgus bracing for the osteoarthritic knee. Presented at the American Orthopaedic Society for Sports Medicine Specialty Day Meeting, San Francisco, CA, 1997.

4

Cartilage Injury: Overview and Treatment Algorithm

Bert R. Mandelbaum and Steve A. Mora

The athlete's knee is exposed to various degrees of sporting activity, injury, and chronologic aging effects, which frequently result in a spectrum of meniscal, ligamentous, and articular cartilage disorders. Participation in routine and competitive sports may result in a higher incidence of acute and chronic injury, chronic overuse syndromes, and osteoarthritis. One of the goals of this chapter is to introduce a new concept, *chondropenia*, the earliest degenerative cartilage lesion, and highlight and highlight its pathogenesis leading to the end-stage articular cartilage lesion, *osteoarthritis*. The "chondropenia curve," a working concept, is also introduced. A treatment algorithm for knee articular cartilage injuries, based on the current understanding of the natural history of cartilage injuries and the current state-of-the-art treatments, is covered in detail. The emphasis of this algorithm is on preservation of long-term joint function.

THE LOSS OF FORM AND FUNCTION: CHONDROPENIA, THE EARLIEST ARTICULAR CARTILAGE LESION

Articular cartilage is a viscoelastic material that allows variable load bearing during daily functional and athletic activities. Functionally, stress reduction on the subchondral bone and minimization of friction are essential in fulfilling this role. The characteristics of articular cartilage are dependent on its specific structural composition and organization.[1] Normal articular hyaline cartilage is composed of an extracellular matrix, chondrocytes, and water. The range of water concentration varies from 65% to 85% depending on the load status and the presence or absence of degenerative changes. This structure is contiguous with and overlies the subchondral bone of the joint. The extracellular matrix is primarily made up of type II collagen fibers. Sulfated proteoglycans are linked to hyaluronate proteins that facilitate the creation of a hydrophilic latticework and are responsible for tensile strength and resiliency of articular cartilage. The functional organizational unit of articular cartilage is composed of four layers, including the tangential zone, intermediate zone, calcified cartilage, the tidemark, and the subchondral bone. The subchondral bone and the calcified cartilage are crucial sup-

portive structures that become thickened and abnormal in the process of arthrosis. The complexities of composition, organization and morphology dictate the material and structural properties of articular cartilage.

It is the resilience of the functional load-bearing unit that is essential for functional success. The elite athlete is able to consistently perform at the highest levels of activity (dose) and perform (response) without any symptoms elicited from the knee joint. It is only loss of articular integrity, through injury, pathologic loading, and aging, that results in chondropenic and degenerative changes over time. These changes initially include loss of cartilage volume, then later articular cartilage defects with subsequent elevation of joint contact pressures develop. The clinical results of these changes amount to a conceptual drop on the dose–repose curve, or "*chondropenia curve*" (Figure 4.1). Clinically, as the articular cartilage integrity fails and with each step down the curve, the athlete finds he is unable to reach the same levels of performance (response) with an executed activity (dose).

The concept of the chondropenia curve defines a strategy aimed at maintaining the knee and its cartilage functional through the application of therapeutic interventions. Without intervention, the injured joint is destined to fail and succumb to dysfunction and further degeneration. In summary, the loss of cartilage integrity falls within a continuum, with chondropenia and osteoarthritis on the opposite poles of the spectrum. Therefore, the goal of the sports medicine physician is to optimize performance by maintaining articular cartilage integrity and preventing a downward slide on this chondropenia curve.

PATHOGENESIS OF CHONDROPENIA AND OSTEOARTHRITIS

A New Dilemma: Identifying Chondropenia

One of the principal challenges for the benchtop scientist and clinician comes from a lack of accurate measurement tools to objectively identify chondropenia and the pathologic progression of articular cartilage failure. For osteoporosis, the early osseous lesion, osteopenia, that predisposes patients to patho-

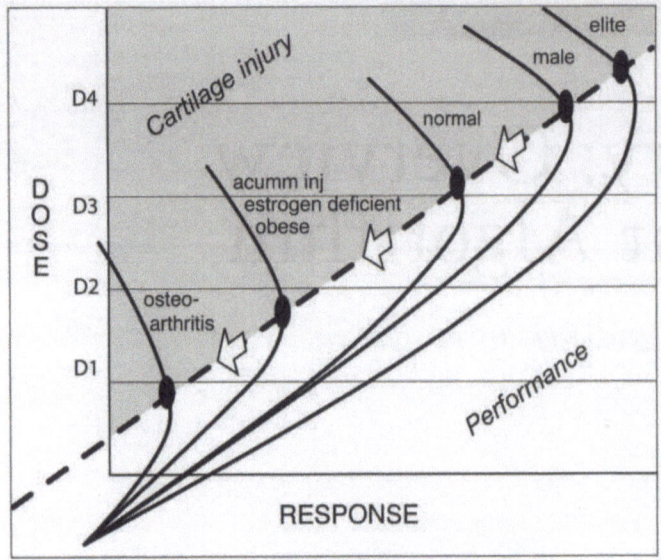

FIGURE 4.1 The chondropenia curve.

logic fractures can be reliably identified with dual-energy X-ray absorptiometry (DEXA). A DEXA-type scan for osteopenia does not yet exist for articular cartilage. To a limited degree, magnetic resonance imaging (MRI) with T_1 fat suppression and fast spin echo offers increased sensitivity for assessing cartilage volume and proteoglycan content. At this time, MRI with the proper sequencing selection and the introduction of intraarticular contrast is effective mainly for identifying deep, full-thickness defects. Stronger MRI magnets will improve the sensitivity in the future.

Alternative methods, such as molecular markers, which sensitively measure cartilage turnover, may also prove to be effective for quantitatively, reliably, and sensitively detecting osteoarthritic changes in the joints at an early stage of the disease.[2] In addition, these markers may be important for the development of new disease-modifying therapies. The use of pressure and biologically sensitive cartilage probes that can measure and profile biomechanical and biochemical properties is also on the horizon. The future goal is to have a tool, or combination of methods, that will allow clinicians not only to diagnose chondropenia and osteoarthritis early but also use it for prognosis, monitoring the disease progression, and for measuring treatment efficacy.

The Increased Incidence of Injury

The female athlete has a greater incidence of knee injuries and as a consequence is at greater risk for chondropenia and osteoarthritis. In a National Collegiate Athletic Association (NCAA) study on knee injury, Arendt and Dick in 1995[3] found a female rate of 1.6 per 1,000 exposures as compared to a 1.3 in the age-matched male. In addition, the age of anterior cruciate ligament (ACL) injury in females is younger (19 versus 23 years) and has an incidence in the 15- to 20-year-old female fourfold greater than in males. In fact, if all studies are taken simultaneously, the incidence of female ACL injuries is two to six times as common as that for males.[3-8] Several risk factors have been examined to determine the etiology of ACL

tears. These risk factors are multiple and are classified as anatomic, hormonal, environmental, and biomechanical. Griffin et al.[5] concluded that the biomechanical variables are the major risk factor, causing a pathokinetic chain that results in the noncontact ACL tears.

Acute Injury and Biochemical Response

In the athlete, symptomatic articular cartilage injuries lead to a reduction in performance levels and chronically to further articular cartilage degeneration. We now know that an acute knee injury in the athlete, such as an ACL rupture or a meniscus tear, is likely to have long-term chronologic effects resonating beyond the index injury and possibly leading to degenerative joint disease. The degenerative process arises from an insidious biochemical response that begins with the intraarticular release of interleukins and other preinflammatory cytokines after the acute injury. The adverse milieu is amplified by variables such as instability, meniscus tissue deficiencies, and limb malalignment. The impact of sports knee injuries and the subsequent production of the harmful intraarticular biochemical response was defined by Lohmander and others, who observed the synovial fluid of ACL and/or meniscus injured knees had higher concentrations of aggrecan fragments and higher concentration of enzymes that cleave articular cartilage.[9-11] In addition the observation of increased cartilage oligomeric matrix protein (COMP), C-propeptide of type II collagen (CPII), bone sialoprotein, matrix metalloproteinases (MMP) 1 and 3, stromelysin, and tissue inhibitor of metalloproteinases 1 adds more direct evidence of cartilage catabolism by degradative factors after an ACL injury of the knee. These changes are the initial biochemical effects after a knee injury that are thought to lead to progressive chondropenia and then osteoarthritis. A future goal is to counteract this inflammatory effect that follows a knee injury with agents which halt the destructive process and therefore change the long-term outcome.

It is also important to point out mechanical and anatomic factors associated with ACL injuries. The role of chronology, including age of the patient and time elapsed since knee injury, is critical to the pathogenesis of cartilage degeneration.[12] The accumulation of time after an ACL injury equates to higher likely hood of degenerative problems.[12] This knowledge is the foundation for programs aimed at ACL injury prevention and overuse injury avoidance in young athletes. ACL injuries are rarely an isolated problem. This fact is important and should influence the way that patients are educated about knee injury. Subchondral bones bruises are present in up to 80% of the ACL injuries.[13-16] This complex of injuries is more commonly encountered in soccer and basketball.[17-19] These studies collectively highlight the biochemical and mechanical complexities of articular cartilage injury and its potential for degeneration. Bringing these concepts to surface is a 9-year data registry study by Johnson et al.,[20] which demonstrated an acute articular cartilage defect incidence of 1.9%, but an overall long-term incidence of 19% in the ACL-injured population. Others have also found significant loss of articular cartilage and meniscus injuries after ACL tears.[12,21]

A study by Murrell et al.[12] found that patients whose injuries had occurred more than 2 years before the examination had more than sixfold greater cartilage loss and damage compared with those whose injuries had occurred within the past 2 months. Meniscal loss was associated with a threefold increase in cartilage damage or loss. The group of patients with meniscal loss, whose initial ACL injury had occurred more than 2 years before examination, exhibited 18 times the amount of cartilage loss or damage as did the group that had no meniscal loss and whose injury occurred less than 1 month before examination. The presence of an articular cartilage lesion in and of itself can result in chondropenia and osteoarthritis.[22] Guertller et al.[23] demonstrated, in athletes under the age of 14 years, that the presence of an articular cartilage defect resulted in osteoarthritis. This study found a significant increase in contact pressure and load with presence of a significant 10-mm cartilage lesion that is exponentially exacerbated with varus alignment. These findings and other studies suggest that an acute ACL injury with disruption of the osteochondral functional unit, in combination with an unstable knee, unleashes a destructive biochemical process that results in progressive deterioration of the articular cartilage over time.

Anterior cruciate ligament reconstruction may not alter the natural history of osteoarthritis, but it does improve the patient's ability to return to the preinjury activity level within a relatively short period of time. There is no consensus that ACL reconstruction lessens the risk for developing osteoarthritis.[24] To date, there is no controlled study demonstrating a difference in development of osteoarthritis after non-surgical versus surgical interventions. Andersson et al.[24] found that after ACL reconstruction there was a decreased risk of meniscal injury.[24] Interestingly, Daniel et al.,[25] in a prospective, nonrandomized outcome study, found that after ACL reconstruction there was a higher incidence of radiographic osteoarthritis The criticism of this study is the selection bias that resulted in the surgical selection of patients with severe injuries. An additional explanation for the higher rate of osteoarthritis in ACL-reconstructed patients is the fact that these patients were able to return to their preinjury levels of activity without dropping down the dose–response slope; therefore, they continued to "abuse" their knees. Patients who were not reconstructed were incapable of participating in pivoting/cutting sports, which decreased the hours per year of sports participation and therefore decreased their exposure to the level and intensity of damaging athletic activities.

The risk of developing osteoarthritis after suffering a meniscus tear has also been investigated. Several studies have shown that after meniscal surgery, partial or total meniscectomy, there is a significant risk of developing future osteoarthritis.[26–31] Ferretti et al.[32] performed a radiographic and clinical study on 114 knees after ACL reconstruction with a mean 5-year follow-up and observed that there was a significant correlation between the magnitude of the meniscectomy and radiographic degenerative changes. In ACL-deficient knees with irreparable meniscal tears, or in which meniscectomy had been undertaken, the development of osteoarthritis seemed independent of the degree of stability, but in such knees with no meniscal tear or meniscal repair, reconstruction appeared to save the menisci and preserve the joint. The time period before developing degenerative changes after meniscectomy is not clear. Kellgren and Lawrence[33] found that 75% of the patients

studied had radiologic changes 21 years after a total meniscectomy.

Studies have found that meniscus repair in stable knees decreases the potential for osteoarthritis.[34–36] This finding adds support to the known concept that meniscus preservation or repair has significant joint-preserving benefits. Patients with a meniscus tear and a concomitant ACL injury have a greater risk of developing osteoarthritis than those with isolated meniscus tears.[37] Neyret et al.[37] compared two groups of soccer players that underwent a meniscus-preserving partial meniscectomy, one group with and one without an ACL-deficient knee. The subjects with unstable knees had greater radiologic evidence of osteoarthritis and required an increased number of surgeries for arthritis. Roos et al. demonstrated that 50% of ACL injuries have radiographic changes 10 to 15 years after the ACL tear.[38,39] Because the presence of a meniscal injury with an ACL injury is between 70% and 80%, the risk of osteoarthritis is much greater in a patient with this constellation of injuries.

In conclusion, there is no definitive evidence that meniscal surgery or ACL reconstruction diminishes the risk for developing osteoarthritis. Patients who suffer from these injuries may find themselves on a path leading toward the development of degenerative changes. The likelihood of degeneration increases with the coexistence of other intraarticular pathology. Therefore, the current literature reports that knee injuries with ACL ruptures, meniscus tears, and articular or subchondral injury are at risk of developing early osteoarthritis with or without surgical intervention.[40]

The Biomechanical Response

In recent years, through collaboration with basic scientists and engineers, exact relationships between biomechanical and biochemical variables have been defined. To study the effects of injurious compression on the degradation and repair of cartilage in vitro, studies have evaluated the effects of strain and strain loading on cartilage specimens. Grodzinsky et al.[41] have demonstrated in calf cartilage disks that injurious compression and immobilization result in glycosaminoglycan (GAG) loss and matrix metalloproteinase (MMP)-3 elevation. They concluded that cartilage injuriously compressed at high strain rates can lose its characteristic anabolic response to low-amplitude cyclic mechanical loading. Sah et al.[42] also found that cyclic oscillatory compression results in greater prostaglandin (PG) synthesis and content. Nitric oxide (NO) production and NO synthase (NOS) expression are increased in osteoarthritis and rheumatoid arthritis, suggesting that NO may play a role in the destruction of articular cartilage.

Chowdhury et al.[43] concluded that dynamic compression counteracts the negative effects of interleukin-1 by suppressing NO and postaglandin E_2 (PGE_2) synthesis. Last, Fermor et al.[44] revealed that compressive forces inhibit cyclooxygenase 2 (COX-2) inhibitors, the production of PGE_2, and NO. These findings indicate that NO production by chondrocytes is influenced by mechanical compression in vitro and suggest that biomechanical factors may in part regulate NO production in vivo. Therefore, the specific consequences of mechanical loads have significant impact on the biochemical and cellular integrity of articular cartilage.

Repetitive Trauma

Another important variable common in high-level sports participation and adding to the degenerative risk is pathologic high rate repetitive loading of the joint. Repetitive pathologic loading of damaged articular cartilage accelerates its destruction. For the healthy athlete, the dose of activity (duration, intensity, frequency) has a positive linear correlation with athletic performance until a threshold is reached. The important question therefore surrounds the details of the "dose" threshold, that is, how much exercise or athletic performance is excessive or deleterious to the joint? Athletes who "abuse" their knees, such as soccer players, are at greater risk because of the likelihood of ligamentous and cartilage injuries in combination with their repetitive joint loading. A number of studies have evaluated the effects of cumulative trauma and its influence on the manifestation of osteoarthritis.[45–51] In an animal study, Kirivanta[52–54] found that moderate running, 4 km/day, increased knee articular cartilage stiffness and matrix content of proteoglycan in normal female beagle dogs whereas 20 km/day decreased proteoglycan content. In another dog model, Arokoski et al.[45] documented the detrimental effects of long-term running. An adaptive response leading to loss of proteoglycan and softening of articular cartilage was observed. Researchers have also been able to correlate similar results in human studies.[55–59] Felson et al.[40,55,56] and others[58,60–62] have demonstrated that the increased loading in occupations such as firefighters, coal miners, laborers, farmers, and construction workers and in athletes has a greater risk of osteoarthitis of the knee. Felson found that, in the group of high-demand participants, any increase in activity and loading beyond the articular cartilage threshold for injury results in a clinical overuse response with the potential negative consequences of chondropenia and an increased risk of developing osteoarthritis. In summary, the literature is not conclusive but does suggest that recurrent overuse trauma foreshadows late degenerative changes.

Intraarticular Modulators

Damage to the joint and cartilage can also be attributed to various potent proinflammatory mediators known as cytokines that include interleukin-1 (IL-1), tumor necrosis factor-α (TNF-α), and several others. The local inflammatory response is modulated by the intraarticular IL-1 and TNF release in response to injury. The direct effect of these proinflammatory cytokines is to upregulate metalloproteinases, aggrecanases, and collagenases. These enzymes cleave extracellular matrix products and stimulate NO and PGE$_2$, both of which exert negative effects on all chondrocyte function. Additionally, IL-1 is an endogenous pyrogen, regulates the immune system systemically and locally, augments activation of T and B lymphocytes, causes macrophages to release proteolytic enzymes and chemotactic factors, and also stimulates osteoclasts to resorb bone.

Systemically, estrogen deficiencies have direct consequences on cartilage thickness resulting in chondropenia. Claassen et al.[63] found alpha- and beta-receptors in articular cartilage and noted that estrogen and calcium deficiency states resulted in a loss of extracellular cartilage matrix and volume. Richmond et al.[64] observed that estrogen replacement produces insulin-like growth factor-binding protein 2

and proteoglycan synthesis locally, and increases cartilage volume by 7.7% as demonstrated by MRI T$_1$ fat suppression images. Interestingly, a subset of females with osteoarthritis of the knee had greater bone mineral density than those without osteoarthritis. Dennison et al.,[65] studying female subjects scheduled for hip replacement, found a significant higher risk of osteoarthritis after oophorectomy. This risk could be decreased by 40% after hormonal replacement therapy. Therefore, estrogen has direct effects on cartilage and its deficiency is associated with chondropenia and osteoarthritis.

Nutritional disorders and respective interventions are proving to have significant impact on articular cartilage integrity. Well-known consequences of normal aging include loss of muscle mass (sarcopenia), loss of bone mass (osteopenia), the escalation of body fat percent, and the development of obesity. There is also progressive cartilage loss (chondropenia) and osteoarthritis as an independent variable. The latter changes have been documented by Manninen et al.[66] who evaluated Finnish farmers over a 10-year period and found that obese women have a strong risk factor for disabling knee osteoarthritis. Supporting this idea is a study by other researchers who demonstrated that obesity and aging are risk factors for development of osteoarthritis.[58,67,68]

In recent years, oral glucosamine sulfate and chondroitin sulfate have been popularized as a treatment for osteoarthritis. However, the mechanism of the antiarthritic activities is still poorly understood. Studies have attempted, with some success, to prove the antiinflammatory effects of N-acetylglucosamine. Several studies indicate beneficial effects of supplementation on inflammatory variables and cartilage volume. Shikhman et al.[69] demonstrated inhibition of IL-1β, TNF-α, and other inflammatory cytokines known to be adverse toward articular cartilage integrity and chondrocyte viability. Gouze et al.[70] studied the influence of glucosamine sulfate on the proinflammatory agent IL-1β in an in vitro rat chondrocyte model. They first confirmed that IL-1β inhibited proteoglycan synthesis. Glucosamine was able to prevent, in a dose-dependent manner, the inhibitory effects of IL-1β. In the same way, glucosamine reduced NO$_2^-$ and PGE$_2$ production induced by IL-1β. Glucosamine also completely prevented the upregulation of stromelysin-1 mRNA expression by IL-1β. Although the mechanisms of glucosamine and chondroitin are not completely clear, benchtop research is helping us better define these complex biomechanical mechanisms.

The rationale for hyaluronic acid or viscosupplementation is predicated on the ability of proteoglycan and GAG to bind to a collagen mesh and aid in hydration and biomechanical function for shock absorption and lubrication. With normal aging, there is a decrease in concentration and molecular weight, resulting in decreased articular cartilage viscoelastic resiliency. Viscosupplementation decreases the inflammatory response and improves viscoelastic properties.[71] In addition, this results in a greater chondrocyte density with a greater territorial matrix and metabolism.[72] Clinical outcome in several studies has demonstrated that hyaluronic acid is effective in diminishing knee pain and improving function associated with osteoarthitis.[73,74]

Aging

Over time, the chronology of age results in biochemical, biomechanical, and cellular changes in cartilage. Biochemically, there is an accumulation of advanced glycosylation end products and pentosides, resulting in a stiffer and brittle cartilage.[75] Moreover, there is less aggregan synthesis and less capability to make large molecular size aggregates. The cellular response in human chondrocytes more than 45 years of age is senescence. There is decreased beta-galactosidase and mitotic activity, resulting in the inability of chondrocytes to maintain and support articular cartilage integrity.[75] In time, this change results in the loss of articular cartilage volume and subchondral bone.[76] Finally, transitions consistent with osteoarthritis in the superficial zones, including fibrillations, chondrocyte clusters and degenerative matrix changes occur. In addition, the degenerative cartilage contains interleukin-1β, TNF-α, and six different MMPs.[77]

MANAGEMENT OF ARTICULAR CARTILAGE DISORDERS

Hunter in 1743 stated that "...once violated...articular cartilage defects are a troublesome thing...they don't heal."[78] Therefore the goals of the sports medicine physician are injury care, injury prevention, and performance maximization. To accomplish these goals the practitioner must be proactive, collaborative, interactive, and counteractive.

Proactive

ACL PREVENTION

Despite recent positive strides in treating damaged articular cartilage, treatment of these injuries remains a formidable challenge. Because the impact of articular cartilage injuries is functionally and financially costly, greater emphasis is being placed on knee injury prevention strategies. These programs include multicomponent physical training regimens and athlete–trainer counseling approaches to curb pathologic repetitive joint loading. The goal is to ultimately influence the trend toward degenerative arthritis by eliminating the index knee lesion through prevention and education. To increase the success of such programs, the populations that are at the highest risk, that is, female athletes, need to be targeted. Numerous studies have found that female athletes who participate in jumping and pivoting sports are four to six times more likely to sustain a knee ligament injury, such as ACL injury, than male athletes participating in the same sports.[3–8] The reasons are numerous; however, biomechanical and neuromuscular deficits have been documented as central factors contributing to higher ACL injuries in women. Additionally, there has been a surge in athletic participation by young female athletes in the past two decades. Most ACL injuries in women occur by noncontact mechanisms, often during landing from a jump or making a lateral pivot while running.

Ferretti et al.,[32] in considering ACL injuries in national-caliber volleyball players, found that women, who accounted for 61% of the players studied, sustained 81% of the ACL injuries over a 10 year period. Shelbourne and Gray[79] followed basketball related injuries seen in their clinic over a 2.5 year period and noted 19 ACL ruptures per 76 female basketball players seen versus only 4 ACL ruptures in 151 male basketball players injured during the same time period. Arendt and

Dick[3] used data compiled by the NCAA over a 5-year period from 1989 to 1992 to compare ACL injury rates between men and women in collegiate basketball and soccer. The ACL injury rate in women's soccer was more than double than that of the men, while the rate in women's basketball was more than four times higher. In soccer, 63% of the women's ACL injuries were due to a noncontact mechanism versus 48% for the men; in basketball, 80% of the female ACL injuries were noncontact versus 65% for the men.

Current ACL prevention programs focus on improvements in strength, flexibility, agility, proprioception avoidance of at-risk situations, and pliometrics. Early results from these programs have shown statistical impact on ACL tear rates.[3,5,7,80,81,84–87] In conclusion, it is essential to make an effort to minimize the potential for injury in populations at high risk for ACL ruptures by using preventative programs that include proprioception, strengthening, flexibility, agility, and avoidance of at-risk playing positions and situations.

Collaborative

The goal of the collaborative approach is to employ innovative strategies involving mainstream orthopaedic concepts in conjunction with new biotechnologies such as nutritional intervention, rehabilitative protocols, viscosupplementation and hormonal therapies that contribute to chondroprotection and chondropreservation.

NUTRITIONAL INTERVENTION

Patients who are overweight should be strongly encouraged and guided toward an achieving ideal body weight, reducing body fat, and enhancing their muscle mass with resistance training and conditioning therapies.

REHABILITATIVE PHYSICAL AND CONDITIONING THERAPY

The goal for the patient and the physical therapist is to maximize quadriceps strength thereby diminishing knee pain. O'Reilly et al.[88] demonstrated that quadriceps strength is strongly associated with knee pain and disability. Rogind et al.[89] found that a daily home program including general fitness, coordination, balance, and stretching appears to be beneficial to patients with osteoarthritis of the knee. Bautch et al.[90] demonstrated that a daily exercise program decreased knee pain without accelerating disease progression. The study design attempted to assess the role of the biologic markers keratin sulfate and hydroxyproline, and found that the markers showed neither improvement nor exacerbation of cartilage status with exercise. Rehabilitation programs must focus more on the details of training progressions and crosstraining including swimming, Stairmaster, elliptical trainers, and flexibility training such as yoga.

VISCOSUPPLEMENTATION

Usage of hyaluronic acid viscosupplementation will improve resiliency and therefore increase the threshold of activities by 10% to 20% with improvements in 70% of patients.[72–74]

HORMONAL THERAPY

The benefits of estrogen replacement treatment on articular cartilage must be considered and balanced with the potential risks such as breast cancer and cardiovascular disease.

Interactive

The goal of the interactive approach is to effectively execute contemporary treatment principles and procedures that maintain meniscus integrity, ligamentous integrity, and limb alignment in conjunction with state-of-the-art articular cartilage repair techniques. In the situation of an ACL-deficient knee and associated internal derangement, the future goal will be to restore stability and athletic performance as well as to minimize the probability of further joint degeneration. Benchtop researchers are defining the biochemical mechanisms responsible for the chronologic destruction of articular cartilage after injury. The therapeutic goal is to curtail these destructive events with novel therapies such as intraarticular injectable drugs given at the time of the initial injury which can lessen or prevent the adverse intra articular joint environment.

It is also imperative to identify and correct limb malalignment. Normal alignment is crucial for successful management of articular and meniscal abnormalities and for prevention of future degeneration. Uncorrected malalignment can result in significant increases in contact pressure and can lead to deleterious biochemical alterations and cellular apoptosis and death.[79] Sharma et al.[40] in an epidemiological study demonstrated incidences of osteoarthritis four- to fivefold greater in those individuals with malalignment. Research in this area has shown that alterations on the axial alignment of the knee allow cartilage regeneration by removing excessive loads on the articular surface; this concept is the basis for high tibial osteotomies.[91,92]

Meniscus repairs up to 90% to 100% are successful when associated with concomitant ACL reconstruction.[93] In contrast, a success rate of 30% to 70% has been reported in unstable knees.[93,94] In ACL-intact knees with isolated meniscus tears, healing rates are less than in ACL-reconstructed knees with meniscus tears. Although older patients have been shown to heal as well as younger patients in selected ACL tears, there is a higher complication rate and the long-term benefit of preserving the meniscus is less in the older population. Human meniscus allograft transplantation is currently becoming more popular for restoration of native meniscus tissue. The long-term follow-up is limited and therefore requires further investigation to assess its effectiveness in restoring normal meniscal function, prevention of malalignment, and preventing osteoarthritis.[95,96]

In recent years, there has been rapid evolution and progress in articular cartilage repair techniques. The challenge to restore damaged articular cartilage has generated an enormous interest from researchers, clinicians, and industry. The procedural details of these techniques are thoroughly discussed in other chapters of this volume. The ideal repair technique should be cost effective, durable, easily available, minimally invasive, safe, and effective. Historically, the first-generation articular cartilage repair techniques were based on the concept of mesenchymal stem cell stimulation. These techniques employed procedures including lavage, debridement, abrasion, drilling, and microfracture.[97–99] The principle behind these early techniques was based on the attraction of mesenchymal stem cells into the cartilage defect from deep subchondral bone and the subsequent creation of reparative tissue. These techniques fill the defect with fibrocartilage repair tissue, principally type I collagen and rarely type II, VI, and IX, which are found in hyaline cartilage. These techniques are limited by the availability of chondrocytes and the inferior biomechanical properties of fibrocartilage. More recently, cartilage substitution replacement techniques utilizing fresh allografts[100] and autografts[101] have been successfully applied to large articular cartilage defects. More recently, biologic articular cartilage replacement techniques have been introduced utilizing autologous chondrocyte implantation (ACI).[38,102] It is premature at this time to make concrete conclusions regarding the effectiveness of these techniques for recreating a durable articular cartilage surface; however, midterm follow-up studies using these new resurfacing techniques have been encouraging.[102,103] Newer techniques on the horizon include the use of bioabsorbable extracellular scaffolds; use of genetically modified chondrocytes, and in vitro construction of a transplantable articular cartilage functional unit.[104] The clinician, therefore, must scrutinize potential surgical options with respect to efficacy, safety, and the long-term impact on joint chondropenia and osteoarthritis risk reduction.

ALGORITHM FOR THE TREATMENT OF ARTICULAR CARTILAGE DEFECTS

A comprehensive algorithm has been developed for the management of articular cartilage defects (Figure 4.2). The algorithm defines 10 patient-directed situations based on lesion size, depth, and associative issues such as alignment, ligament, and meniscal integrity. Each situation considers categorically the problem, the therapeutic options, and the unresolved issues at this moment.

SITUATION 1

Problem: meniscus tears and partial-thickness articular cartilage defect, a common problem that the orthopaedist sees in practice.

- Treatment options: arthroscopic debridement and partial meniscectomy followed by rehabilitation and physical and conditioning therapy.
- Unresolved issues:
  - Role of radiofrequency probes; do they cause chondrocyte death or decrease regenerative and more degenerative or avascular consequences? Which device (bipolar versus monopolar) is more effective and safe?
  - When to use glucosamine and chrondroitin sulfate and viscosupplementation?

SITUATION 2

Problem: femoral articular cartilage defects less than 1 cm².

- Treatment options:
  - Debridement
  - Microfracture
  - Osteochondral grafting (OCG)
  - Unresolved Issues: do small defects heal sufficiently well with mesenchymal stem cell stimulation techniques such as microfracture?

SITUATION 3

Problem: femoral articular cartilage defects including osteochondritis dissecans (OCD) of 1 to 2 cm².

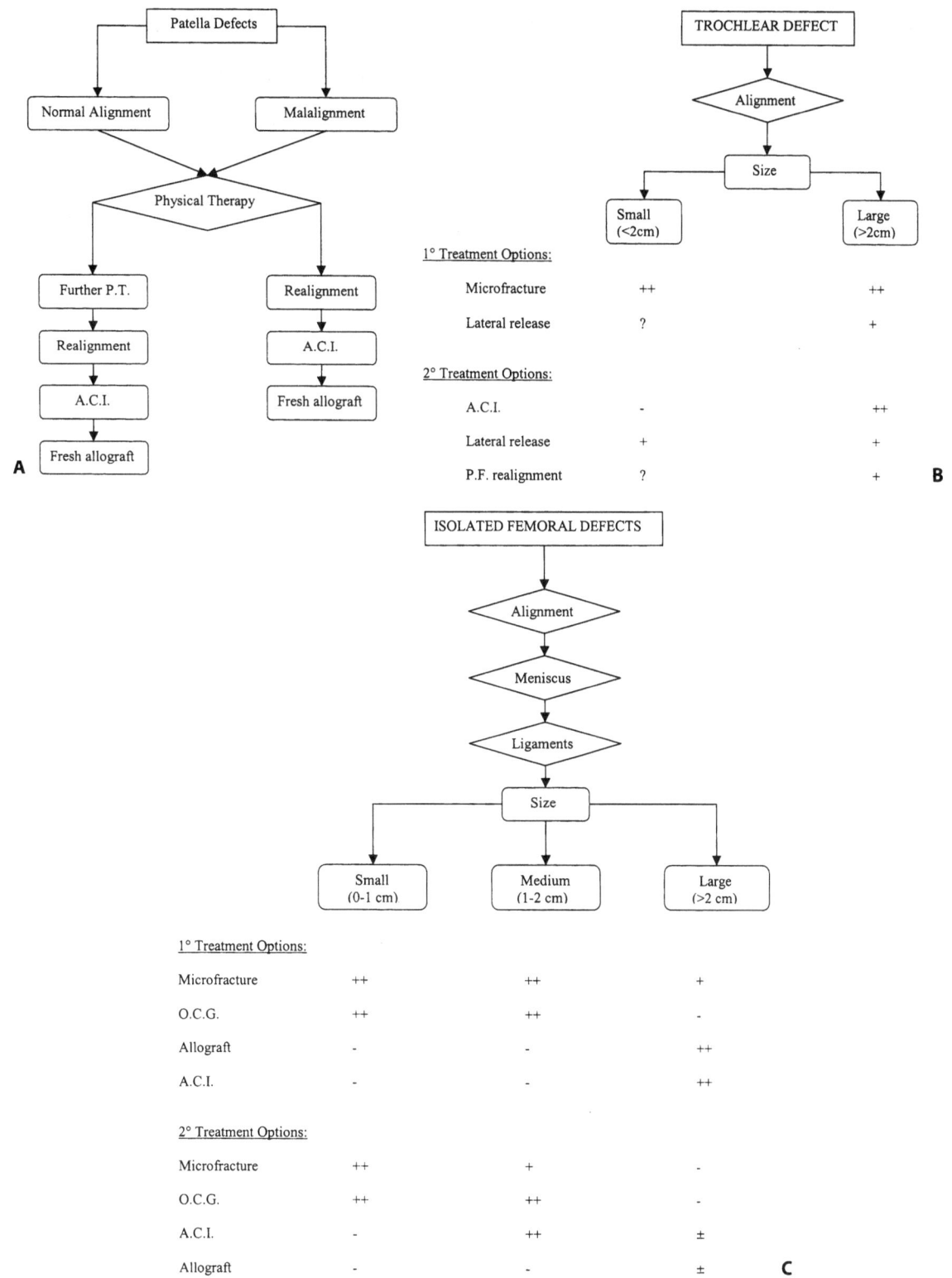

FIGURE 4.2 Treatment algorithm for **A.** femoral, **B.** trochlear and **C.** patellar defects that considers defect size and associated comorbidites as part of the decision process.

- Therapeutic primary options:
  - Debridement
  - Microfracture
  - OCG
  - ACI
- Therapeutic secondary options:
  - OCG
  - ACI
  - Unresolved Issues: Is a mesenchymal stem cell stimulation technique an acceptable primary option?

SITUATION 4

Problem: femoral articular cartilage defects including OCD greater than $2\,cm^2$.

- Therapeutic Primary options:
  - ACI
  - Fresh allograft
- Therapeutic secondary options:
  - ACI
  - Fresh allograft
  - Unresolved Issues: What is the optimal and maximal size of lesion to which autograft OCG can be applied?

SITUATION 5

Problem: complex femoral articular defects with malalignment and ligament and/or meniscal deficiency.

- Therapeutic Primary options:
  - Osteotomy
  - Meniscal repair or allograft
  - Cruciate reconstruction(s)
  - ACI, fresh allograft, or OCG autograft depending on size.
- Unresolved Issues:
  - How to optimally stage procedures so that index postoperative protocol does not compromise integrity of secondary or tertiary procedure?
  - Which meniscus allograft, osteotomy, or ligament reconstruction procedure to utilize?

SITUATION 6

Problem: patella and/or trochlear articular cartilage defects with no malignment or instability.

- Therapeutic primary options:
  - Physical and conditioning therapy including taping, bracing and pelvic stabilization
- Therapeutic secondary options:
  - Arthroscopy and lateral release
- Therapeutic tertiary options:
  - ACI+ Anteromedialization or patellofemoral realignment osteotomy
- Unresolved issues:
  - What are the definitive indications for arthroscopic lateral release?
  - Does viscosupplementation have a role early in management of patellofemoral chondromalacia syndrome?

SITUATION 7

Problem: patella and trochlear articular cartilage defects; significant malalignment or instability.

- Therapeutic primary options:
  - Physical and conditioning therapy including taping, bracing, and pelvic stabilization
- Therapeutic secondary options:
  - ACI+ anteromedialization or patellofemoral realignment osteotomy
- Unresolved issues:
  - Is the role of osteotomy beneficial at an early stage such that it will prevent osteoarthitis of the patellofemoral joint?

SITUATION 8

Problem: tibial articular cartilage defects; no significant malignment or instability.

- Therapeutic options:
  - Osteotomy as required in relation to the degree of malalignment in combination with microfracture or ACI depending on size of lesion
- Unresolved Issues:
  - Successful access may require release of collateral ligaments and detach meniscus insertions
  - Potentially conflicting postoperative rehabilitative protocol.

SITUATION 9

Problem: significant chondropenia and early osteoarthritis (OA) (global grade III/IV articular cartilage defects) in 30- to 60-year-olds with degenerative meniscal tears

- Therapeutic options:
  - NSAID/COX-2 inhibitors
  - Hyaluronic ACID
  - Glucosamine/chondroitin sulfate
  - Bike for exercise
  - Unloading braces
  - Arthroscopy for mechanical symptoms, loose bodies, and meniscal tears
  - Osteotomy selectively as required in relation to the degree of malalignment or joint space narrowing
- Unresolved issues:
  - Is there a role for concomitant biologic resurfacing with realignment procedures?

SITUATION 10

Problem: degenerative meniscal tears and global grade IV articular cartilage defect (late OA).

- Therapeutic options:
  - NSAID/COX-2 inhibitors
  - Hyaluronic acid
  - Glucosamine/chondroitin sulfate
  - Bike for exercise
  - Unloading braces
  - Arthroscopy for mechanical symptoms, loose bodies and meniscal tears

- Osteotomy selectively as required in relation to the degree of malalignment or joint space narrowing
- Total knee arthroplasty
- Unresolved Issues:
  - What is the role of arthroscopy in late OA other than alleviation of mechanical symptoms?

Counteractive

Athletes who have sustained a significant ACL, meniscal, or articular injury at a young age while involved in team sports such as soccer and basketball are at risk for accelerating their OA. The group that returns to high level sports after injury and recovery may be at greatest risk. The pathogenesis of OA is a multivariable phenomenon, such that there are negative and positive modulators. Important negative modulators of this maladaptive response include pathologic repetitive joint loading, repetitive injuries, chronic ligamentous instability, malalignment, hormonal deficiencies, and obesity. Roos et al.[39] have stated that the longer the duration of time after ACL rupture, the higher the risk of radiologic signs of OA. An ACL injury places the 20 to 40-year-old athlete at greatest risk for early OA by the age of 50. It is also becoming clearer that female athletes have a higher rate of OA of the knee in comparison to their male counterparts. Therefore, the goals are to develop new technologies and disease-modifying interventions that protect and preserve the knee joint over time by maintaining biochemical, biomechanical, and cellular integrity. Potential interventions include disease-modifying osteoarthritis drugs including:

- Anti-TNF or TNF-α antagonists,
- Anti-IL-1 factors and IL-1Ra (receptor antagonist),
- Bone morphogenetic protein 2 (BMP-2) (local),
- BMP-16 (systemic),
- Estrogen,
- Osteopontin inherent inhibitor of IL-1, NO, and PGE_2,
- Cyclosporin, and
- Calcium pentosan polysulfate (CaPPS) agents.

CONCLUSIONS

Taking care of the athlete requires a multilevel approach that includes injury prevention, acute injury management, and the long-term need to preserve joint function and athletic performance. Articular cartilage disorders in athletes continue to be an ongoing challenge for the clinician, researcher, and the injured athlete. As our patients seek to push new physical and competitive boundaries, clinicians and researchers are challenged to maintain them at their highest possible level of performance and function. The degeneration of articular cartilage is a complex multivariable process that occurs along an uncertain line of chronology and is initiated by injury, biologic modulators, and the aging process. A spectrum of articular injury exists. Chondropenia defines the early loss of normal articular cartilage integrity. The goals for the future include injury prevention, further development and refinement of articular cartilage resurfacing procedures, growth factor science, genetic engineering, tissue engineering, innovative technologies, and disease-modifying interventions that protect and preserve the joint by preserving its biochemical, biomechanical, and cellular integrity.

As a consequence, the sports medicine orthopaedic surgeon can no longer be reactive toward acute knee injuries but should also be proactive, collaborative, interactive and counteractive in the comprehensive management of the athlete.

References

1. Burks RT. Arthroscopy and degenerative arthritis of the knee: a review of the literature. Artroscopy 1990;6:43–47.
2. Verzijl N, DeGroot J, Bank RA, et al. Age-related accumulation of the advanced glycation endproduct pentosidine in human articular cartilage aggrecan: the use of pentosidine levels as a quantitative measure of protein turnover. Matrix Biol 2001; 20:409–417.
3. Arendt E, Dick R. Knee injury patterns among men and women in collegiate basketball and soccer: NCAA data and review of literature. Am J Sport Med 1995;23:694–701.
4. Buhl Nielsen A. The epidemiologic aspects of anterior cruciate ligament injuries in atheletes. Acta Orthop Scand 1991; 62(suppl)243:13.
5. Griffin LY, Agel J, Albohm MJ, et al. Noncontact anterior cruciate ligament Iinjuries: risk factors and prevention strategies. J Amer Acad Orthop Surg 2000;8:141–150.
6. Harmon KG, Ireland ML. Gender differences in noncontact anterior cruciate ligament injuries. Clin Sports Med 2000;19: 287–302.
7. Heidt RS, Sweeterman LM, Carlonas RL, et al. Avoidance of soccer injuries with preseason conditioning. Am J Sports Med 2000;28:659–662.
8. Engström B, Johansson C, Törnkvist H. Soccer injuries among elite female players. Am J Sports Med 1991;4:372–375.
9. Lohmander LS, Roos H, Dahlberg L, Hoerrner LA, Lark MW. Temporal patterns of stromelysin, tissue inhibitor and proteoglycan fragments in synovial fluid after injury to knee cruciate ligament or meniscus. J Orthop Res 1994;12:21–28.
10. Lohmander LS, Roos H. Knee ligament injury, surgery and osteoarthrosis. Truth or consequences? Acta Orthop Scand 1994;65:605–609.
11. Cameron M, Buchgraber A, Passler H, et al. The natural history of the anterior cruciate ligament-deficient knee. Changes in synovial fluid cytokine and keratan sulfate concentrations. Am J Sports Med 1997;25:751–754.
12. Murrell GA, Maddali S, Horovitz L, et al. The effects of time course after anterior cruciate ligament injury in correlation with meniscal and cartilage loss. Am J Sports Med 2001;29(1): 9–14.
13. Johnson DL, Urban WP, Caborn NM, et al. Articular cartilage pathology associated with MRI detected "bone bruises" after ACL rupture. Presented at the American Academy of Orthopedic Surgeons Society for Sports Medicine Specialty Day, Atlanta, GA, 1996.
14. Mink JH, Deutsch AL. Occult cartilage and bone injuries of the knee: detection, classification and assessment with MR imaging. Radiology 1989;170:823–829.
15. Speer KP, Spritzer CE, Goldner JL, et al. Magnetic resonance imaging of traumatic knee articular cartilage injuires. Am J Sports Med 1991;19:396–402.
16. Spindler KP, Schils JP, Bergfeld JA, et al. Prospective study of osseous, articular and meniscal lesions in recent anterior cruciate ligament tears by magnetic resonance imaging and arthroscopy. I 1993;21:551–557.

17. Luthje P, Nurmi I, Kataja M, et al. Epidemiology and traumatology of injuries in elite soccer: a prospective study in Finland. Scand J Med Sci Sports 1996;6:180–185.

18. Malone TR, Hardaker WT, Garrett WE, et al. Relationship of gender to anterior cruciate ligament injuries in intercollegiate basketball players. J South Orthop Assoc 1993;2:36–39.

19. Maehlum S, Daljord OA. Football injuries in Oslo: a one year study. Br J Sports Med 1984;18:186–190.

20. Johnson DL, Urban WP, Caborn NM, Carlson C, Van Arthos W. Articular cartilage pathology associated with MRI detected "bone bruises" after ACL rupture. Presented at the American Academy of Orthopedic Surgeons Society for Sports Medicine Specialty Day, Atlanta, GA, 1996.

21. Faber KJ, Dill JR, Amendola A, Thain L, Spoiuge A, Fowler PJ. Occult osteochondral lesions after anterior cruciate ligament rupture. Six-year magnetic resonance imaging follow-up study. Am J Sports Med 1999;27(4):489–494.

22. Mandelbaum B, Browne JE, Fu F, et al. Articular cartilage lesions of the knee. Am J Sports Med 1998;26:853–861.

23. Guettler JH, Glisson RR, Stubbs AJ, et al. The triad of varus malalignment, meniscectomy and chondral damage: a biomechanical explanation for joint degeneration based on pressure and force distribution within the medial knee compartment. Presented at the American Orthopaedic Society for Sports Medicine Annual Meeting, Orlando, FL, 2002.

24. Andersson C, Odensten M, Good L, et al. Surgical or non-surgical treatment of acute rupture of the anterior cruciate ligament. A randomized study with long-term follow-up. J Bone Joint Surg Am 1989;71A:965–974.

25. Daniel DM, Stone ML, Dobson BE, et al. Fate of the ACL injured patient. A prospective outcome study. Am J Sports Med 1996; 22:632–644.

26. Bolano LE, Grana WA. Isolated arthroscopic partial meniscectomy. Functional radiographic evaluation at five years. Am J Sports Med 1993;21:432–437.

27. Allen PR, Denham RA, Swan AV. Late degenerative changes after meniscectomy. Factors affecting the knee after operation. J Bone Joint Surg Br 1984;66:666–671.

28. DeHaven KE, Black KP, Griffiths HJ. Open meniscus repair. Technique and two to nine year results. Am J of Sports Med 1989;17:788–795.

29. Faunø P, Buhl-Nielsen A. Arthroscopic partial meniscectomy: a long-term follow-up. Arthroscopy 1992;8:345–348.

30. Gillquist J, Messner K. Long-term results of meniscal repair. Sports Med 1993;1:159–163.

31. Hede A, Larsen E, Sandberg H. Partial versus total meniscectomy. A prospective, randomized study with long-term follow-up. J Bone Joint Surg 1992;74B:118–121.

32. Ferretti A, Conteduca F, De Carli A, Fontana M, Mariani PP. Osteoarthritis of the knee after ACL reconstruction. Int Orthop 1991;15:367–371.

33. Kellgren JH, Lawrence JS. Radiological assessment of osteoarthrosis. Ann Rheum Dis 1957;16:494–502.

34. Rockborn P, Gillquist J. Outcome of arthroscopic meniscectomy. A 13-year physical and radiographic follow-up of 43 patients under 23 years of age. Acta Orthop Scand 1995; 66(2):113–117.

35. Rockborn P, Gillquist J. Results of open meniscus repair. Long-term follow-up study with a matched uninjured control group. J Bone Joint Surg Br 2000;82(4):494–498.

36. Sommerlath KG. Results of meniscal repair and partial meniscectomy in stable knees. Int Orthop 1991;15:347–350.

37. Neyret P, Donell ST, DeJour D, DeJour H. Partial meniscectomy and anterior cruciate ligament rupture in soccer players. A study with a minimum 20-year followup. Am J Sports Med 1993; 21:455–460.

38. Roos EM, Ostenberg A, Roos H, et al. Long-term outcome of meniscectomy: symptoms, function, and performance tests in patients with or without radiographic osteoarthritis compared to matched controls. Osteoarthritis Cartilage 2001;9(4): 316–324.

39. Roos H, Adalberth T, Dahlberg L, et al. Osteoarthrosis of the knee after injury to the anterior cruciate ligament or meniscus. The influence of time and age. Osteoarthitis Cartilage 1995;3:261–267.

40. Sharma L, Song J, Felson DT, Cahue S, Shamiyeh E, Dunlop DD. The role of knee alignment in disease progression and functional decline in knee osteoarthritis. JAMA 2001;286:188–195.

41. Kurz B, Jin M, Patwari P, Lark MW, Grodzinsky AJ. Biosynthetic response and mechanical properties of articular cartilage after injurious compression. J Orthop Res 2001;19:1140–1146.

42. Sah RL, Kim YJ, Doong JY, et al. Biosynthetic response of cartilage explants to dynamic compression. J Orthop Res 1989; 7:619–636.

43. Chowdhury TT, Bader DL, Lee DA. Dynamic compression inhibits the synthesis of nitric oxide and PGE(2) by IL-1beta-stimulated chondrocytes cultured in agarose constructs. Biochem Biophys Res Commun 2001;285:1168–1174.

44. Fermor B, Weinberg JB, Pisetsky DS, Misukonis MA, Banes AJ, Guilak F. The effects of static and intermittent compression on nitric oxide production in articular cartilage explants. J Orthop Res 2001;19:729–737.

45. Arokoski J, Kiviranta I, Jurvelin J, et al. Long-distance running causes site-dependent decrease of cartilage glycosaminoglycan content in the knee joints of beagle dogs. Arthritis Rheum 1993;36:1451–1459.

46. Kellgren JH, Lawrence JS. Rheumatism in miners. X-ray study. Br Med J 1952;9:197–207.

47. Kirkeskov Jensen L, Eenberg W. Occupation as a risk factor for knee disorders. Scand J Work Environ Health 1996;22:165–175.

48. Klünder K, Rud B, Hansen J. Osteoarthritis of the hip and knee joint in retired football players. Acta Orthop Scand 1980; 51:925–927.

49. Lindberg H, Roos H, Gärdsell P. Prevalence of coxarthrosis in former soccer players: 286 players compared with matched controls. Acta Orthop Scand 1993;64:165–167.

50. Marti B, Knobloch M, Tschopp A, Jucker A, Howald H. Is excessive running predictive of degenerative hip disease? Controlled study in former elite athletes. Br Med J 1989;299:91–93.

51. McAlindon TE, Cooper C, Kirwan JR, et al. Determinants of disability in osteoarthritis of the knee. Ann Rheum Dis 1993;52:258–262.

52. Jurvelin J, Kiviranta I, Säämänen A-M, et al. Indentation stiffness of young canine knee articular cartilage–influence of strenuous joint loading. J Biomech 1990;23:1239–1246.

53. Kiviranta I, Tammi M, Säämänen A-M, et al. Moderate running exercise augments glycosaminoglycans and thickness of articular cartilage in the knee joint of young beagle dogs. J Orthop Res 1988;6:188–195.

54. Kiviranta I, Tammi M, Jurvelin J, et al. Articular cartilage thickness and glycosaminoglycan distribution in the canine knee joint after strenuous (20 km/day) running exercise. Clin Orthop 1992;283:302–308.

55. Felson D. The course of osteoarthritis and factors that affect it. Rheum Dis North Am 1993;19:607–615.

56. Felson DT, Hannan MT, Naimark A, et al. Occupational physical demands, knee bending, and knee osteoarthritis: results from the Framingham study. J Rheumatol 1991;18:1587–1592.

57. Konradsen L, Berg Hansen E-M, Söndergaard L. Long distance running and osteoarthrosis. Am J Sports Med 1990;18:379–381.

58. Kohatsu ND, Schurman DJ. Risk factors for the development of osteoarthrosis of the knee. Clin Orthop 1990;261:242–246.

59. Lane NE, Michel B, Bjorkengren A, et al. The risk of osteoarthritis with running and aging: a five year longitudinal study. J Rheumatol 1993;20:461–468.

60. Lequesne MG, Dang N, Lane NE. Sport practice and osteoarthritis of the limbs. Osteoarthritis Cartilage 1997;5:75–86.

61. Spector TD, Dacre JE, Harris PA, et al. Radiological progression of osteoarthritis; an 11 year follow up study of the knee. Ann Rheum Dis 1992;51:1107–1110.

62. Spector TD, Harris PA, Hart DJ, et al. Risk of osteoarthritis associated with long term weight-bearing sports: a radiologic survey of the hips and knees in female ex-athletes and population controls. Arthritis Rheum 1996;39:988–995.

63. Claassen H, Hassenpflug J, Schunke M, Sierralta W, Thole H, Kurz B. Immunohistochemical detection of estrogen receptor alpha in articular chondrocytes from cows, pigs and humans: in situ and in vitro results. Ann Anat 2001;183:2237.

64. Richmond RS, Carlson CS, Register TC, Shanker G, Loeser RF. Functional estrogen receptors in adult articular cartilage: estrogen replacement therapy increases chondrocyte synthesis of proteoglycans and insulin-like growth factor binding protein 2. Arthritis Rheum 2000;43:2081–2090.

65. Dennison EM, Arden NK, Kellingray S, Croft P, Coggon D, Cooper C. Hormone replacement therapy, other reproductive variables and symptomatic hip osteoarthritis in elderly white women: a case-control study. Br J Rheumatol 1998;37:1198–1202.

66. Manninen P, Heliovaara M, Riihimaki H. et al. Int J Obes Relat Metab Disord 1996;20:595–597.

67. Leach RE, Baumgard S, Broom J. Obesity: its relation to osteoarthritis of the knee. Clin Orthop 1973;93:271–273.

68. Kannus P, Järvinen M: Age, overweight, sex, and knee instability: their relationship to the posttraumatic osteoarthrosis of the knee joint. Injury 1998;19:105–108.

69. Shikhman AR, Kuhn K, Alaaeddine N, Lotz M. N-Acetylglucosamine prevents IL-1 beta-mediated activation of human chondrocytes. J Immunol 2001;15;166(8):5155–5160.

70. Gouze JN, Bordji K, Gulberti S, et al. Interleukin-1beta down-regulates the expression of glucuronosyltransferase I, a key enzyme priming glycosaminoglycan biosynthesis: influence of glucosamine on interleukin-1beta-mediated effects in rat chondrocytes. Arthritis Rheum 2001;44:351–360.

71. Abatangelo G, Botti P, Del Bue M, et al. Intra-articular sodium hyaluronate injections in the Pond-Nuki experimental model of osteoarthritis in dogs. II. Morphological findings. Clin Orthop 1989;241:278–299.

72. Guidolin DD, Ronchetti IP, Lini E, Guerra D, Frizziero L. Morphological analysis of articular cartilage biopsies from a randomized, clinical study comparing the effects of 500–730 kDa sodium hyaluronate (Hyalgan) and methylprednisolone acetate on primary osteoarthritis of the knee. Osteoarthritis Cartilage 2001;9:371–381.

73. Lussier A, Cividino AA, McFarlane CA, et al. Viscosupplementation with hylan for the treatment of osteoarthritis: findings from clinical practice in Canada. J Rheumatol 1996;23:1579–1585.

74. Wobig M, Dickhut A, Maier R, Vetter G. Viscosupplementation with Hylan G-F 20: a 26-week controlled trial of efficacy and safety in the osteoarthritic knee. Clin Ther 1998;20:410–423.

75. Verbruggen G, Cornelissen M, Almqvist KF, et al. Influence of aging on the synthesis and morphology of the aggrecans synthesized by differentiated human articular chondrocytes. Osteoarthritis Cartilage 2000;8:170–179.

76. Yamada K, Healey R, Amiel D, Lotz M, Coutts R. Subchondral bone of the human knee joint in aging and osteoarthritis. Osteoarthritis Cartilage. 2002;10:360–369.

77. van den Berg WB. Lessons from animal models of osteoarthritis [review].Curr Opin Rheumatol 2001;13:452–456.

78. Hunter W. Of the structure and diseases of articulating cartilages. Clin Orthop 1743;470:514.

79. Shelbourne KD, Gray T. Results of anterior cruciate ligament reconstruction based on meniscus and articular cartilage status at the time of surgery. Am. J Sports Med 2000;28:446–453.

80. Hewett TE, Lindenfeld TN, Piccobene JV, et al. The effect of neuromuscular training on the incidence of knee injury in female athletes. Am J Sports Med 1999;27:699–705.

81. Hewett TE, Stroupe AL, Nance TA, et al. Plyometric training in female athletes: decreased impact forces and increased hamstring torques. Am J Sports Med 1996;24:765–773.

82. Ettlinger CF, Johnson RJ, Shealy JE. A method to help reduce the risk of serious knee sprains incurred in Alpine skiing. Am J Sports Med 1995;23:531–537.

83. Ekstrand J, Gillquist J, Möller M, et al. Incidence of soccer injuries and their relation to training and team success. Am J Sports Med 1983;11:63–67.

84. Heidt RS, Sweeterman LM, Carlonas RL, et al. Avoidance of soccer injuries with preseason conditioning. Am J Sports Med 2000;28:659–662.

85. Henning CE, Griffis ND. Injury prevention of the anterior cruciate ligament (videotape). Mid-America Center for Sports Medicine, 1990.

86. Caraffa A, Cerulli G, Projetti M, et al. Prevention of anterior cruciate ligament injuries in soccer: A prospective controlled study of proprioceptive training. Knee Surg Sports Traumatol Arthrosc 1996;4:19–21.

87. Cerulli G, Benoit DB, Caraffa A, et al. Proprioceptive training and prevention of anterior cruciate ligament injuries in soccer. J Orthop Sports Phys Ther 2001;31:655–660.

88. O'Reilly SC, Muir KR, Doherty M. Effectiveness of home exercise on pain and disability from osteoarthritis of the knee: a randomised controlled trial. Ann Rheum Dis 1999;58:15–19.

89. Rogind H, Bibow-Nielsen B, Jensen B, Moller HC, Frimodt-Moller H, Bliddal H. The effects of a physical training program on patients with osteoarthritis of the knees. Arch Phys Med Rehabil 1998;79:1421–1427.

90. Bautch JC, Malone DG, Vailas AC. Effects of exercise on knee joints with osteoarthritis: a pilot study of biologic markers. Arthritis Care Res 1997;10:48–55.

91. Li KW, Williamson AK, Wang AS, Sah R. Modulators of cartilage. Growth responses to cartilage to static and dynamic compression. Clin Orthop 2001;391:34–38.

92. Coventry M. The effects of axial alignment of the lower extremity on articular cartilage of the knee. In: Ewing J (ed) Articular Cartilage and Knee Joint Function. New York: Raven Press, 1990.

93. Cannon WD, Vittori JM. The incidence of healing in arthroscopic meniscal repair in anterior cruciate ligament reconstructed knees versus unstable knees. Am J of Sports Med 1992;20:176–181.

94. DeHaven KE. Decision making factors in the treatment of meniscus lesions. Clin Orthop 1990;252:49–54.

95. Cole BJ, Carter TR, Rodeo SA. Allograft meniscal transplantation: background, techniques, and results. J Bone Joint Surg Am 2002;84A:1236–1250.

96. Garrett JC, Stevensen RW. Meniscal transplantation in the human knee: a preliminary report. Arthroscopy 1991;7:57–62.

97. Johnson LL. Arthroscopic abrasion arthroplasty historical and pathologic perspective: present status. Arthroscopy 1986;2:54–69.

98. Pridie KW. A method of resurfacing osteoarthritic joints. J Bone Joint Surg 1959;41B:618–619.

99. Steadman JR, Rodkey WG, Rodrigo JJ. Microfracture: surgical technique and rehabilitation to treat chondral defects. Clin Orthop 2001;391(suppl):S362–S369.

100. Bugbee WD. Fresh osteochondral allografts. J Knee Surg 2002;15:191–195.

101. Hangody L, Feczko P, Bartha L, Bodo G, Kish G. Mosaicplasty for the treatment of articular defects of the knee and ankle. Clin Orthop 2001;391(suppl):S328–S336.

102. Peterson L, Minas T, Brittberg M, Nilsson A, Sjogren-Jansson E, Lindahl A. Two- to 9-year outcome after autologous chondrocyte transplantation of the knee. Clin Orthop 2000;374:212–234.

103. Micheli LJ, Browne JE, Erggelet C, et al. Autologous chondrocyte implantation of the knee: multicenter experience and minimum 3-year follow-up. Clin J Sport Med 2001;11:223–228.

104. Brittberg M, Tallheden T, Sjogren-Jansson B, Lindahl A, Peterson L. Autologous chondrocytes used for articular cartilage repair: an update. Clin Orthop 2001;391(suppl):337–348.

Radiofrequency Energy for Cartilage Treatment

Yan Lu and Mark D. Markel

Treatment methods for articular cartilage lesions are controversial. Some lesions progress to osteoarthritis and joint dysfunction without proper treatment whereas others remain relatively stable. The traditional treatment options for injured or diseased articular cartilage include the removal and debridement of loose or chondromalacic cartilage with the purpose of creating a smooth surface. This surgical procedure is typically accomplished with a mechanical shaver and hand instruments. Unfortunately, mechanical shavers cannot produce a smooth surface and often remove an excessive amount of adjacent healthy articular cartilage. Hand instruments are most applicable for eradication of thickened cartilaginous fronds and flaps; they are ineffective at smoothing chondromalacic cartilage with fine fronds.

In 1989, Miller et al.[1] compared the effects of the Nd:YAG laser with electrocautery and mechanical debridement on articular cartilage lesions and concluded that the laser had biologic advantages over mechanical resurfacing and electrocautery in arthroscopic procedures. In 1990, Raunset and Lohnert[2] reported the results of the excimer laser for chondromalacic cartilage of Outerbridge grades 2 and 3. The results of this study demonstrated significant pain relief and reduction of reactive synovitis in treated patients. In 1994, Grifka et al.[3] also reported that the use of the excimer laser on chondromalacic cartilage of Outerbridge grade 2 produced a smooth cartilaginous surface via scanning electron microscopy. Although these results were promising, the use of lasers for treatment of chondromalacia has declined because of cost, inconvenience, and concerns for safety. The major drawback of lasers is the difficulty in controlling application temperatures during thermal chondroplasty. It is well known that chondrocytes begin to die at approximately 50° to 55°C.[4-7] Once chondrocytes are dead, the treated site has very limited ability to regenerate or maintain the local mileau.[8] Lane et al.[9] and Mainil-Varlet et al.[10] demonstrated that chondroplasty using with the Holmium:YAG laser caused significant proteoglycan loss and chondrocyte death.

Radiofrequency energy (RFE) has been used for medical applications for almost a century. Currently, two basic RFE systems are available for clinical application, monopolar RFE (mRFE) and bipolar RFE (bRFE) systems. In addition, temperature-controlled RFE probes/generators are available for clinical application with both monopolar and bipolar RFE systems. Both mRFE and bRFE were first investigated for thermal chondroplasty in 1996–1997.[11-13] The initial concept for treating chondromalacic cartilage with RFE was to use it to melt, seal, and smooth the fibrillated cartilaginous surface with only minimum chondrocyte death. However, the results of these studies were contradictory and controversial. Kaplan et al.[11] and Turner et al.[13] reported that bRFE appeared to be safe for use on chondromalacic articular cartilage with better histologic outcomes than traditional methods such as mechanical shaving. In contrast, Lu et al. and Edwards et al. reported that both mRFE and bRFE caused immediate chondrocyte death and should not be used for thermal chondroplasty until safe parameters were established.[12,14]

The principle of RFE heating with a monopolar probe utilizes an alternating current between the application probe and the grounding plate. This ionic current density produces molecular friction in tissue that results in tissue heating. Frictional or resistive heating of tissue around the probe tip is the primary source of heat, rather than the probe itself.[15,16] The specific amount of energy applied to the tissue and the current path resulting in energy application cannot be specifically determined even under these controlled conditions. When used arthroscopically, the mRFE path may pass from the probe through the cartilage surface and subchondral bone to the grounding plate on the skin, or from the probe through the irrigation solution to the joint capsule and then to the grounding plate. The path is most likely determined by the impedance encountered as the current passes along the cartilage surface and may be influenced by the cartilage thickness, water content, proteoglycan concentration, collagen content, subchondral bone thickness, position of the grounding plate, and the conductive characteristics of the irrigation solution. In contrast, energy produced by a bipolar probe follows the path of least resistance through a conductive irrigating solution around the probe tip. Consequently energy application by bRFE is different than mRFE.[15]

mRFE and bRFE are frequently used during arthroscopic techniques for thermal chondroplasty over the past several years.[17,18] RFE is an inexpensive surgical tool that may be delivered arthroscopically with a wide variety of probes that offer extended flexibility to surgeons.

INDICATIONS/CONTRAINDICATIONS

No single device or method is uniformly accepted for the treatment of diseased cartilage. RFE has the ability to smooth and contour the surface of articular cartilage, ablate cartilage fragments, stabilize loose cartilage edges, and stop bleeding of subchondral bone. However it must be emphasized that RFE achieves these effects via heat and that excessive and inappropriate application of the RFE will result in thermal injury to articular cartilage.[14,19] Currently, surgeons use both mRFE and bRFE mainly for ablation (i.e., subacromial decompression) and for the treatment of chondromalacic cartilage to smooth the rough surface and stabilize loose edges.

Chondromalacia is defined as softening of the cartilaginous surface. Chondromalacia lesions are divided into four grades based on the Outerbridge grading system[20]: grade 1, cartilage softening; grade 2, fibrillation or superficial fissures of the cartilage; grade 3, fibrillation and deep fissuring of the cartilage without exposed subchondral bone; and grade 4, cartilage erosion with exposed subchondral bone. Histologically, chondromalacic cartilage has a fibrillated surface with reduced proteoglycan staining and chondrocyte clones at the junction of normal and chondromalacic cartilage (Figure 5.1). Historically, when RFE was first used for chondromalacic lesions, some surgeons applied RFE for all Outerbridge grades. RFE was used to ablate large cartilage flaps, seal large clefts and fissures, and mold and seal delaminated cartilage on the edges of full-thickness cartilage defects. Although the gross appearance of the cartilaginous surface was smoothed in these applications, thermal damage to chondrocytes and the cartilage matrix likely occurred during these treatments (Figure 5.2). Currently, many authors recommend RFE treatment only for grades 2 or 3 and partial-thickness chondral defects with minor unstable borders.[17,21–25] Grade 1 lesions are not severe enough to warrant treatment with RFE, whereas grade 4 lesions are so severe that RFE treatment will likely be unsuccessful, and other treatment options such as cartilage restoration (e.g., microfracture, osteochondral grafting or autologous chondrocyte implantation), osteotomy, or arthroplasty should be considered.[18] In addition, acute cartilage

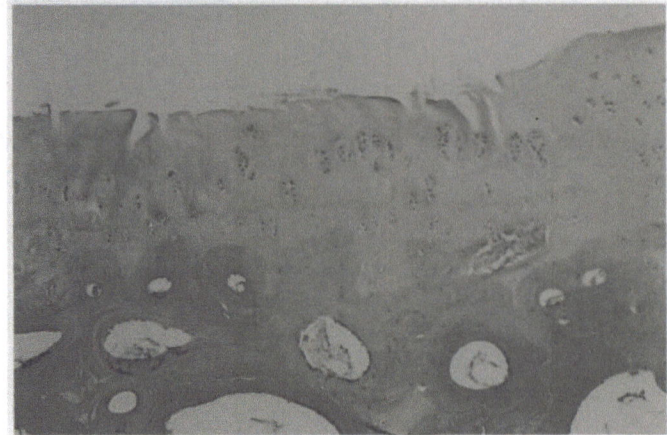

FIGURE 5.1 Chondromalacic articular cartilage of grade 2 with surface irregularities, fibrillation, and chondrocyte cloning. Hematoxylin and eosine. ×100.

injuries with wide fissures or thickened and large flaps are not recommended for treatment with mRFE or bRFE because prolonged times are necessary for RFE to smooth wide fissures or remove large flaps. With long treatment times, RFE inevitably results in full-thickness chondrocyte death, possibly affecting regions of the subchondral bone.

TECHNIQUE

Independent of the RFE device (either mRFE or bRFE) a surgeon uses, he or she should (1) understand the physical principles governing how the device works, including its safety parameters; (2) conduct sufficient diagnostic tests to understand that the patient's pathology would best be treated by RFE; and (3) apply the device in an appropriate manner. Currently, the three most commonly used RFE device systems available for arthroscopic application in thermal chondroplasty are the Vulcan EAS coupled with a TAC-C probe (Smith & Nephew Endoscopy, Menlo Park CA, USA), Mitek VAPR System coupled with a Flexible Side Effect Electrode (Mitek Surgical Products, Inc, Westwood, MA, USA), and ArthroCare 2000 System coupled with CoVac probe (ArthroCare Corporation, Sunnyvale, CA, USA) (Figure 5.3).

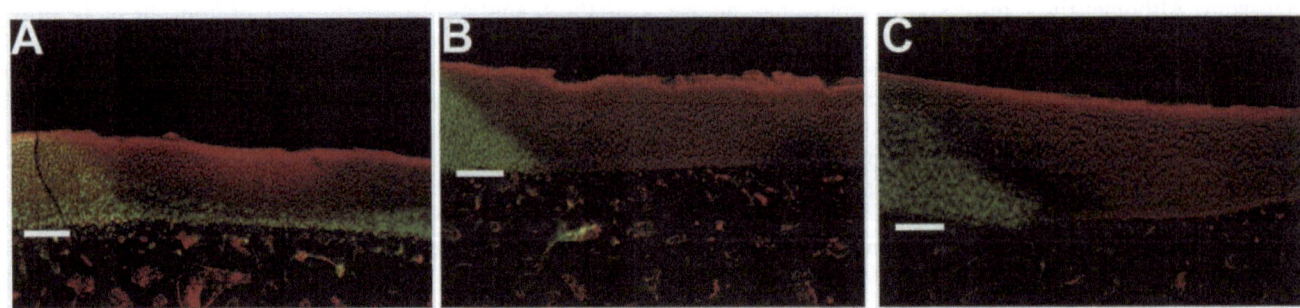

FIGURE 5.2 Confocal microscope images show cartilage surface treated with radiofrequency (*top* of each image) and subchondral bone (*bottom* of each image) following a paintbrush pattern application. *Green dots*, viable chondrocytes; *red dots*, dead chondrocytes ×20. **A.** Smith & Nephew mRFE treatment caused immediate chrondro-cyte death; penetration of cell death did not extend to subchondro-cyte bone. Both Mitek (**B**) and ArthroCare (**C**) bRFe treatment chondrocyte death and penetration of cell death to the subchondral bone. *White bar* demonstrates the boundary between the cartilage and subchondral bone.

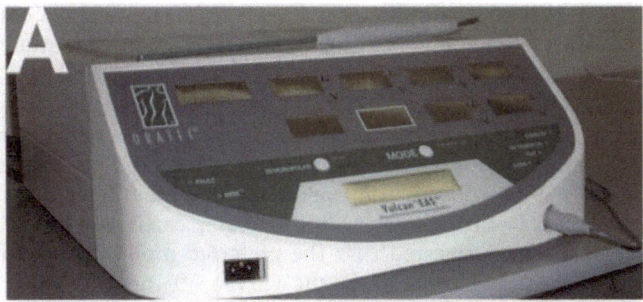

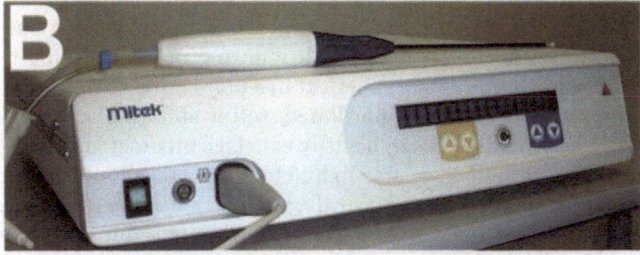

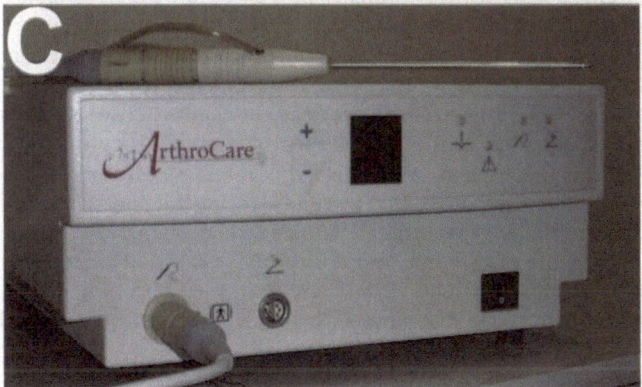

FIGURE 5.3 A. Smith & Nephew, Endoscopy, Vulcan EAS mRFE system. **B.** Mitek VAPR bRFE system. **C.** ArthroCare 2000 bRFE system.

The Smith & Nephew device is a mRFE system whereas the latter two are bRFE devices.

Electrosurgical RFE devices typically use frequencies between 300 kHz and 13 MHz. RFE oscillates the electrolytes in the intracellular and extracellular space, producing molecular friction.[16] RFE devices are selected to act above 300 kHz to avoid muscle fasciculation and nerve stimulation observed at lower frequencies.[15] The alternating current from the RFE generator is powered by a line source such as 110 volts at 60 Hz, and boosts the power as high as 600 volts at 460 kHz by oscillating a crystal tuned to 460,000 on/off cycles per second.[15] In mRFE heating, the alternating current passes from the RFE generator through the connecting cable, through the probe (positive electrode), and through the treated patient's body to the negative electrode (grounding plate). During bRFE heating, the alternating current passes from the RFE generator through the connecting cable, through the probe, and through the positive electrode to the negative electrode, where both positive and negative electrodes are on the probe tip. The conduction pass of the bRFE is within the irrigation fluid, resulting in vaporization of the physiologic saline in the joint. Therefore, the tissue effects with bRFE are secondary to thermal and ionic modification of the tissue.

The mRFE system currently used in clinical application (Smith & Nephew) is a temperature-controlled device. The mRFE system uses delivered power to control the tissue temperature reflected by a thermocouple within the mRFE probe tip. At the beginning of treatment, the RFE generator delivers full preset power to cause tissue heating. The thermocouple within the mRFE probe tip is subsequently heated, reaching the preset temperature relatively quickly. After reaching the preset temperature, the mRFE algorithm reduces the power to decrease tissue/probe-tip temperature and then uses minimum power output to maintain the tissue temperature near the preset temperature. This protocol may result in the mRFE generator delivering mean powers that are significantly less than preset powers (34% to 57% of preset power) to maintain the preset temperatures.[21]

Based on the unique design of mRFE, it should be applied in a contact mode for thermal chondroplasty. The treatment pattern is dependent on the surgeon's preference. It may be applied with paintbrush or pausing (dotted) pattern during treatment. The setting of the mRFE generator (Smith & Nephew) currently recommended by the manufacturer for thermal chondroplasty is 70°C/15W in a coagulation mode. When mRFE was first used for thermal chondroplasty, lavage flow was recommended during thermal chondroplasty. It was hypothesized that the lavage solution would cool the probe tip and the treated articular cartilage, reducing thermal injury to chondrocytes.[11,19] Edwards et al.[26] later determined that mRFE application combined with lavage flow would aggravate the thermal injury rather than alleviate it. The negative effect of lavage flow is secondary to how the device modulates power based on the probe tip's thermocouple. During lavage flow, the probe tip is actively cooled by the lavage solution, requiring increased power output by the mRFE generator to maintain the preset temperature. Delivered power output equals the electric current multiplied by electric voltage. Organ[16] reported that RFE current intensity had a strong influence on the size of the lesion generated; the lesion size increased as the square of current intensity. To minimize chondrocyte death during mRFE application, Lu et al.[21] evaluated the thermal penetration and surface smoothing of chondromalacic articular cartilage after mRFE treatment at one of two lavage temperatures, 22° and 37°C. The results of this study demonstrated that thermal chondroplasty performed with mRFE in the 37°C lavage solution caused significantly less chondrocyte death than that in 22°C lavage solution. The explanation for this decreased cell death is that less delivered power (energy) at the 37°C lavage temperature resulted in less chondrocyte injury compared to the 22°C lavage temperature.[21] A pilot study performed in the Comparative Orthopaedic Laboratory, University of Wisconsin-Madison, also compared the thermal injury for chondrocytes with mRFE used in two different treatment patterns, paintbrush versus pausing. This study revealed that there was no significant difference in depth of chondrocyte death between these two treatment patterns, although some viable cartilage regions were present among the treated portions in the pausing treatment pattern.

Most bRFE systems such as the Mitek VAPR System and ArthroCare 2000 System are power-controlled devices. These devices produce uniform and direct power output or a variable amplitude sinusoidal waveform while the bRFE probes are activated. With power-controlled devices, no thermocouples are embedded in the probe tip to monitor and adjust the temperature at the interface between the probe tip and treated tissue. According to the manufacturers' recommended power settings for thermal chondroplasty, the temperatures measured in the cartilage matrix treated by these two devices are in the range of 90° to 100°C.[26] Recently, Mitek introduced a new bRFE generator (VAPR II Electrosurgical System and VAPR TC Electrode) with a temperature-controlled mode for thermal chondroplasty. Shellock reported that this new bRFE maintained the temperature at the RFE electrode–tissue interface relatively close to the RFE preset temperature and may be useful for thermal-assisted chondroplasty.[27] ArthroCare uses a process the company terms "coblation" (cooler, controlled ablation), which is theoretically a nonheat driven process. Instead, bRFE is applied to a conductive medium (usually saline), causing a highly focused plasma field to form around the electrodes; this plasma field is comprised of highly ionized particles. These ionized particles have sufficient energy to break organic molecular bonds within the tissue. Some investigators described that this process replaces the thermally damaging vaporization and pyrolysis of standard electrosurgery with molecular disintegration via a cold ablative process most closely resembling that of excimer lasers, achieved by employing an electrically conductive fluid in the physical gap between the electrode and tissue. They have also stated that coblation enables volumetric removal of target tissue while producing minimal necrosis of collateral tissue. The results of the study by Lu et al.[6] contradicts this theory by demonstrating that at each subsequently higher power settings (2 versus 4 versus 6) in noncontact as recommended by ArthroCare corp., a greater depth of chondrocytes are killed in addition to a greater volume of tissue removal. This study concluded that higher power settings should be avoided due to the high likelihood of creating full-thickness chondrocyte death. Even at setting 2, the ArthroCare bRFE device killed more than a 1.5-mm thickness of chondrocytes and caused full-thickness chondrocyte death in 100% of specimens treated in a paintbrush pattern.

The settings and application methods recommended for bRFE thermal chondroplasty by the manufacturers (Mitek & ArthroCare) have changed over the past several years. Initially, the setting for the Mitek VAPR bRFE generator was V2-40 by the manufacturer whereas the setting for the ArthroCare 2000 bRFE was a setting of 2. It was suggested that both bRFE devices be applied in contact. The treatment patterns used were either paintbrush or pausing (dotted or interrupted in a very short time). Later, these manufacturers recommended that bRFE be applied in noncontact mode for thermal chondroplasty. The authors' research, however, does not support this recommendation. The bRFE probes should not be placed in direct contact with diseased cartilage, but instead should be held at a distance of approximately 1 mm from the cartilage surface. Lu et al.[14] compared the thermal effects of contact and non-contact modes on bovine cartilage with bRFE, showing that bRFE (ArthroCare) caused more chondrocyte death in noncontact mode than in contact mode. The possible reason for increased depth of thermal penetration for the noncontact mode is that a larger volume of tissue is heated, perhaps allowing the tissue to serve as a thermal mass, resulting in increased conductive heating similarly to using the laser in a defocused mode.

As stated previously, the temperature-controlled VAPR 2.3-mm TC electrode was introduced by Mitek in 2000, which utilized an algorithm along with a sensitive thermistor

to provide temperature control. There are few clinical reports about this product for chondroplasty except one in vitro study performed by Shellock on bovine articular cartilage.[27] Currently, the settings for this product for clinical chondroplasty have not been reported and the manufacturer is not uniformly recommending its use for thermal chondroplasty.

In 1999 to 2000, ArthroCare introduced the ArthroCare System 2000 with coblation for articular cartilage surgery. The company suggested that the preferred probe to use for articular cartilage surgery is the CoVac 50° or TriStar 50° probe in ablation mode. These probes were designed to provide good access to cartilage defects in joints, and their suction capability enhanced visibility during use. According to the company, the coblation effect in a non-contact mode readily removes the looser, fibrillated, softer abnormal cartilage while leaving the denser, healthy cartilage unaffected. During probe activation, an orange light (electrical arc) should appear at the tip of the probe. Recently, ArthroCare corp. and some researchers have recommended the setting of 3–4 for thermal chondroplasty as the company proposes that the setting of 2 is too low to produce ablative effects. Conversely, higher settings such as 3–4 may be less conductive and cause less chondrocyte death with more ablative effects. As stated earlier, the study by Lu et al. contradicts these concepts because higher power settings kill a greater depth of chondrocytes.[6] The ArthroCare company also stated that it was very important to avoid using any of the CAPS Wands (Wands for soft tissue) for chondroplasty, since these Wands are designed for tissue shrinkage, not ablation, and thus produce thermal effects that may damage cartilage. Similarly, the system should not be operated in coagulation mode, which is a thermally mediated process.

SURGICAL PEARLS AND PITFALLS

Radiofrequency energy thermal chondroplasty usually is performed via arthroscopy. Proper application of RFE is critical to safely accomplish the surgery and avoid collateral tissue damage. As with any surgical device, improper use can cause injury, especially with RFE. The purpose of thermal chondroplasty is smoothing the cartilaginous surface with minimum chondrocyte injury. To successfully accomplish this aim, several principles should be considered in advance before applying RFE for chondroplasty.

Device Selection

Choosing the proper RFE device (mRFE or bRFE) for thermal chondroplasty is dependent on the surgeon's preference and experience. The experience of the surgeon with the technique and the response of the tissue to the surgical application greatly affect the ultimate surgical outcome. The significant differences observed between mRFE and bRFE system are more dependent on whether the device is temperature controlled rather than if it is bRFE based or mRFE based. mREF is applied in contact and the RFE temperature can be preset whereas most bRFE devices are applied in noncontact without preset temperatures. Based on the manufacturers' recommended settings for thermal chondroplasty, the temperature of the probe tip for bRFE (90°–100°C) is significantly higher than that for mRFE (70°C).[26] Surgeons who prefer using bRFE

TABLE 5.1 The effects of lavage temperature.

Treatment time:	10s		15s	
Lavage temperature (°C)	22	37	22	37
Depth of chondrocyte death (μm)	620 ± 106	420* ± 219	930 ± 236	590* ± 214
Mean power (watts)	8.5 ± 0.6	5.9* ± 0.9	7.6 ± 0.8	5.1* ± 0.4
Time to set temp (s)	1.8 ± 0.5	0.7* ± 0.2	1.3 ± 0.5	1.0* ± 0.5
Mean probe temp (°C)	67.5 ± 1.1	70.1* ± 0.8	68.7 ± 0.6	70.3* ± 0.4

Data are means ± SD.
* Significant difference between lavage temperatures at each treatment time ($p < 0.05$).

rather than mRFE for chondroplasty must be more cautious because the higher operating temperatures of the bRFE can cause greater chondrocyte death and deeper thermal penetration.

Lavage Solution Selection

Based on the Lu et al. study,[21] mRFE for thermal chondroplasty using 37°C lavage solution can significantly decrease thermal penetration compared to using 22°C (room temperature) lavage solution (Table 5.1). The reason for this is based on the mRFE temperature control algorithm as described previously. The key point for this technique is keeping the lavage temperature in the joint at a relatively constant 37°C before mRFE application. The preparation of 37°C lavage solution and continuous flushing of the joint with this solution is somewhat inconvenient compared to a routine procedure using 22°C (room temperature) lavage solution. A temperature-controlled water bath and a water pump are necessary to successfully achieve precise lavage solution temperature. The lavage temperature should be monitored carefully, because at lavage solution temperatures higher than 45°C damage to all the cartilage within the joint may occur. Using a microwave to heat the lavage solution is not recommended because it is very hard to control temperatures. Alternatively, a controlled-temperature delivery system should be developed to maintain a constant temperature of 37°C. In addition, it is recommended that fluid flow rates during the period of mRFE probe activation be reduced or stopped to decrease the RFE power output required to maintain preset temperature. On the contrary, bRFE devices are directly power-controlled. Based on a pilot study performed by our research group, bRFE application for chondroplasty using hypothermic lavage solution (5°C) significantly decreased the thermal penetration of the device compared to using 22°C lavage solution. This result suggested that chondrocyte mortality might be limited through the use of hypothermic lavage when performing chondroplasty with bRFE. The results of this study need to be further validated.

Appropriate RFE Treatment Area

To locate an appropriate treatment area for RFE, it is very important for surgeons to use arthroscopy, as its magnification (2–4×) gives a much clearer and detailed image than the naked eye. The cartilage lesion that responds best to RFE treatment is fibrillated cartilage with protruding fine fronds and absence of wide and deep fissures (Outerbridge grades 2–3) (Figure 5.4). For areas with thickened fronds or large,

loose flaps, mechanical devices such as a motorized shaver and/or long grasping forceps should be used to debride these fronds or flaps before applying RFE. If RFE is used as the ablative tool rather than mechanical means, both mRFE and bRFE will easily denature the treated cartilage and cause full-thickness chondrocyte death, and perhaps even damage the subchondral bone because of the long treatment times required to remove these large lesions. In addition, cartilage thicknesses in different locations of the knee joint vary, ranging from 1.65 to 5.0 mm for normal cartilage.[28] Awareness of the cartilage's thickness in the RFE treatment area also is very important to evaluate the potential deleterious effect RFE treatment may have in the treated area. For example, in the patella where cartilage can range from 3 to 5 mm thick, RFE has a wider range of safety than in the femoral condyle or tibial plateau where cartilage thickness is much less. Before surgery, X-rays or magnetic resonance imaging (MRI) may be used to estimate cartilage thickness in the areas to be treated. Based on the experimental RFE studies, the mRFE device appears to be safer than the bRFE devices during chondroplasty. When considering thermal chondroplasty with any RFE device, surgeons should avoid treating the regions with cartilage thickness less than 1.5 mm.

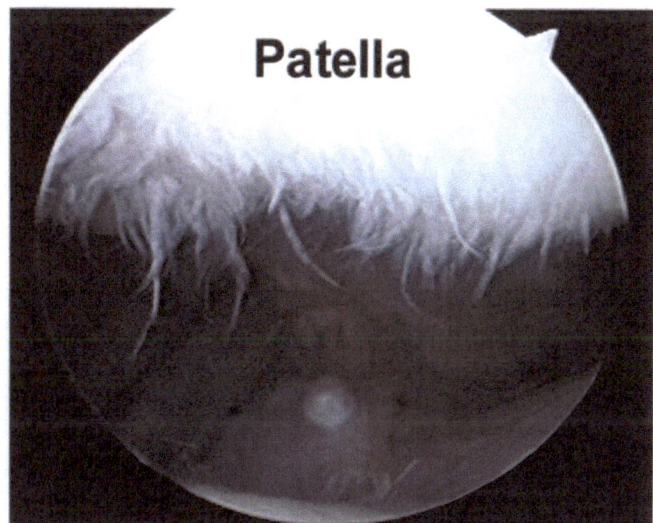

FIGURE 5.4 Arthroscopic image of chondromalacic grade 2 patella with fibrillated surface and protruding fronds.

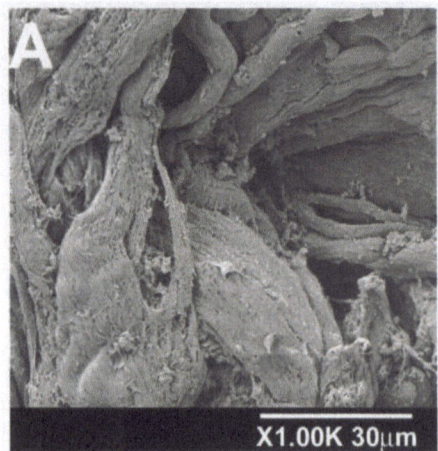
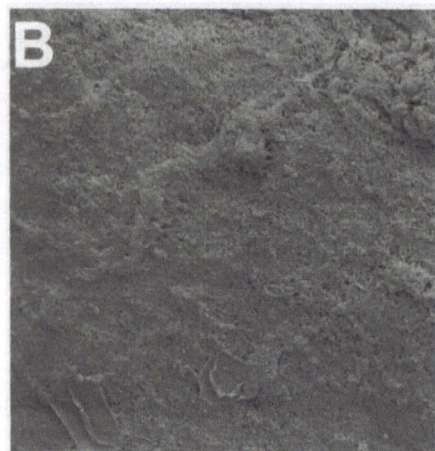
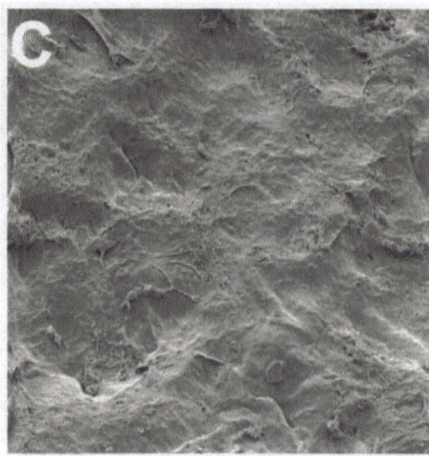

FIGURE 5.5 Scanning electron microscope images show control and RFE-treated cartilaginous surfaces. **A.** Control cartilage with fibrillated and irregular surface. **B.** Chondromalacic cartilage surface was smoothed after 15-s mRFE treatment. **C.** Chondromalacic cartilage surface was smoothed after 15-s bRFE treatment.

RFE Treatment Time

The effect that RFE produces in the tissue is also time dependent. Lu et al.[22] evaluated the effect of RFE treatment time on chondrocyte death and surface contouring. Lu et al. concluded that 10 to 15 seconds of RFE application for a 1-cm^2 area of chondromalacic cartilage with Outerbridge grade 2 resulted in a relatively smooth cartilaginous surface with depth of chondrocyte death ranging from 0.8 to 2.0 mm (Figure 5.5). If the treatment time for either mRFE or bRFE is longer than 15 s, the depths of chondrocyte death for mRFE and bRFE exceeded 1.0 mm and 2.2 mm, respectively (Figure 5.6). It is reasonable to prolong the treatment time for areas larger than 1.0 cm^2, but this should be done cautiously. Surgeons should keep this point in mind: prolonged treatment time for a fixed treatment area will cause more chondrocyte death and deeper thermal injury, especially for bRFE devices.

RFE Treatment Mode

Because the design, algorithm, and energy-delivery path for mRFE are different from for bRFE, the treatment modes for the two types of devices are different. mRFE should be applied in light but full contact. Chondromalacic cartilage is softer than normal cartilage and if high pressure is applied to the probe tip, the contact area of the probe tip with the cartilage increases, causing greater chondrocyte death and deeper thermal penetration. Lu et al. reported that a 50-g pressure applied to the mRFE probe and bRFE probe tip resulted in depths of chondrocyte death of 0.8 mm and 1.6 mm, respectively.[14] To achieve a smooth surface, the pressure applied to the mRFE probe tip should be as light as possible while maintaining full contact. However, it is extremely challenging for surgeons to control the pressure of the probe tip during the treatment of clinical cases because of the influences of several factors, such as the angle of probe insertion, the location and access of treatment area within the joint, and unevenness of the chondromalacic surface. The current recommendation for bRFE is application in noncontact with the probe tip 1 mm away from the cartilage surface.

RFE Treatment Pattern

Both mRFE and bRFE should be applied in a paintbrush pattern, which is a continuous application in a uniform manner using a brushing motion. The probes should not remain sta-

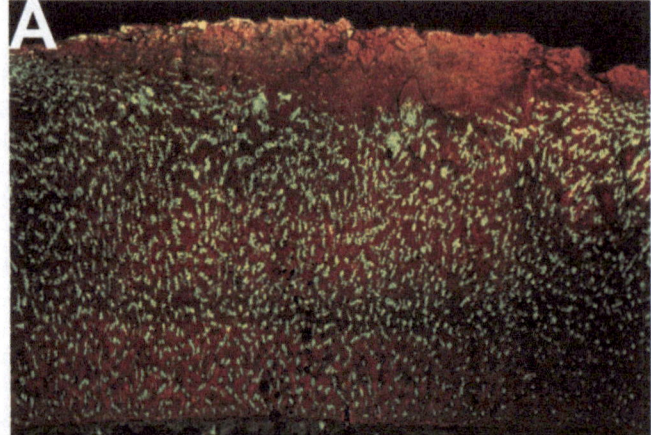
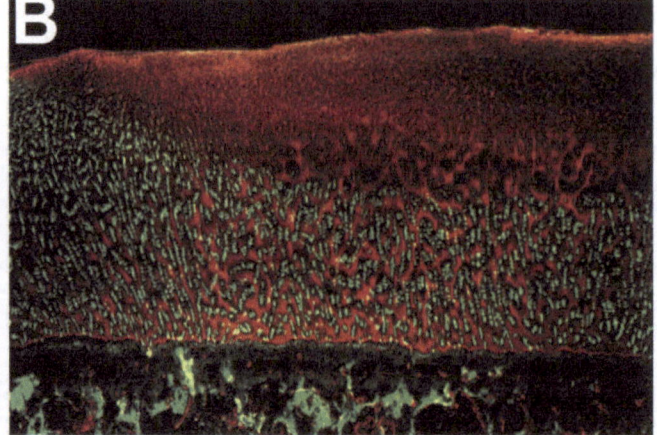

FIGURE 5.6 Confocal images demonstrate thermal penetration (chondrocyte death) after 15-s RFE treatment. *Top,* cartilage surface; *bottom,* subchondral bone. *Green dots,* live chondrocytes; *red dots,* dead chondrocytes. **A.** mRFE treatment. **B.** bRFE treatment. ×20.

tionary in one location for more than 1 to 2 s. Initially, the probe is placed near the surface, but not activated. The probe is then turned on and the chondromalacic cartilage is treated. Overlapping passes or repeated treatment of the same area should be avoided because repeated treatment equals prolonged treatment times and increased cell death. Recently, some surgeons have suggested that a "heat shock" treatment pattern (short bursts and dotted contact RFE application on one small spot) be used by bRFE to avoid deep thermal penetration. The results of this bRFE treatment pattern have not been reported.

REHABILITATION

The rehabilitation procedure following thermal chondroplasty is identical to that for mechanical debridement. Typically, thermal chondroplasty performed simultaneously with other nonthermal procedures requires rehabilitation. Some surgeons recommend that postoperative treatment consist of 10 to 14 days of toe-touch partial weight bearing on crutches, followed by a progressive physical therapy program. Theoretically, if only thermal chondroplasty is performed, a patient should be able to fully weight-bear immediately postoperatively. Continuous passive motion (CPM) may be used to reduce the pain and swelling of the knee joint for the first several days after surgery. It may take 3 to 6 months for patients to experience maximum medical improvement from the surgery. Adjuvant efforts to control postoperative effusion and swelling, such as NSAIDS (nonsteroidal antiinflammatory drugs), cryotherapy, and compressive sleeves, should be used. Additionally, patients should be strongly advised on the importance to their recovery of physical conditioning and exercise. Healthy and fit muscles of the lower extremity can effectively relieve stress on the operated joint. Regular aerobic exercise for the degenerative joint can also help maintain

the outcome of the arthroscopic surgery. If possible, patients may be reassessed rarely by a second arthroscopic look or more commonly, a clinic visit at 6, 12, and 24 months after surgery. This plan may help surgeons better direct a patient's rehabilitation protocol and understand long-term treatment outcomes.

COMPLICATIONS AND MANAGEMENT

There are no peer-reviewed publications describing complications of RFE chondroplasty. Hogan and Diduch presented one case report describing progressive articular cartilage loss following bRFE treatment of a partial-thickness lesion.[29] The case involved a 32-year-old female patient who had grade 2 chondromalacia of her medial femoral condyle, and was treated with bRFE (ArthroCare) set at the lowest power (setting 1). The bRFE probe was gently and briefly brushed over the affected area. Six months after surgery, the patient developed recurrent anterior knee pain and significant quadriceps atrophy compared to preoperation. An arthroscopic evaluation performed 1 year after surgery found that the treated area of the medial femoral condyle was markedly recessed and that significant cartilage loss had occurred (Figure 5.7). For mRFE, there have been no case reports describing complications of thermal chondroplasty.

Although few complications following thermal chondroplasty have been reported, experimental studies have demonstrated significant thermal injury to treated cartilage (chondrocyte death) following RFE application. If surgeons apply RFE improperly or excessively, RFE may not only cause greater chondrocyte death but also possibly kill the subchondral bone, resulting in subchondral bone necrosis. If this complication occurs, depending on the size and extent of thermal damage, cartilage transplantation or total knee replacement may be required.

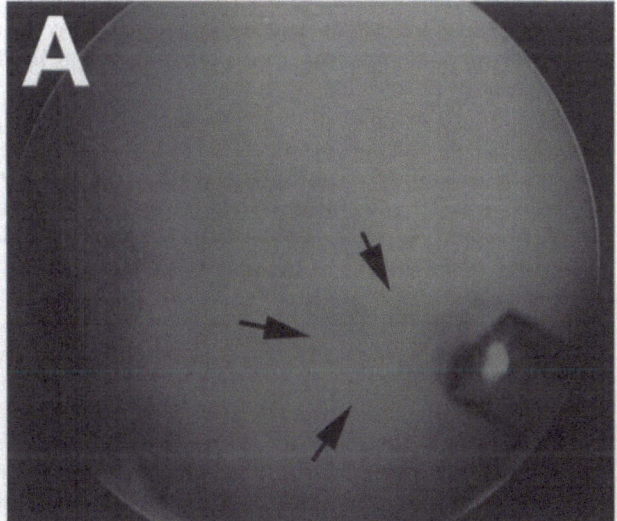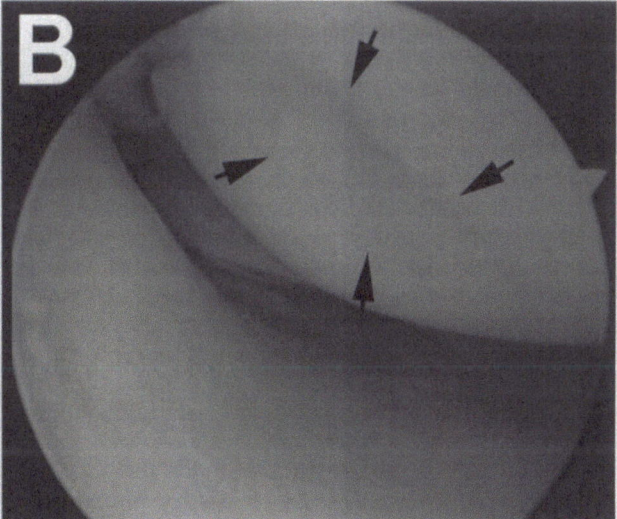

FIGURE 5.7 Arthroscopic images of articular cartilage after bRFE treatment. **A.** Lesion immediately after treatment. **B.** Treated area of medial femoral condyle showing progressive articular cartilage loss 12 months after initial RFE treatment. Arrows indicate RFE-treated area. (From Hogan and Diduch,[29] with permission.)

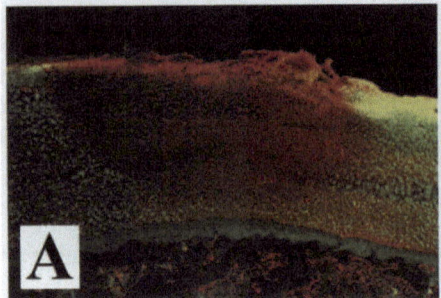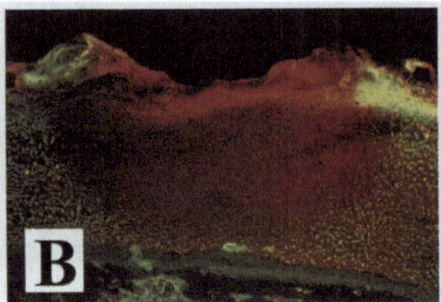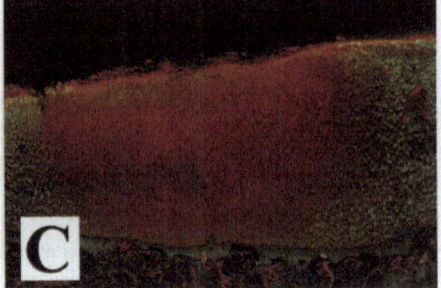

FIGURE 5.8 Confocal images indicate thermal damage with clear demarcation in ArthroCare bRFE treatment group. **A.** Setting 2. **B.** Setting 4. **C.** Setting 6. ×20 (From Lu et al.,[6] with permission.)

RESULTS

The experimental and clinical results of RFE for cartilage injury are controversial and confusing. In 1998, Turner et al.[13] described the first in vivo study regarding the effects of bRFE (Bipolar Arthroscopic Probe, Electroscope, Boulder, CO, USA) on ablated cartilage in an in vivo ovine model. The investigators concluded that bRFE allowed surface contouring without damaging adjacent normal cartilage and produced a better subjective histologic appearance than conventional mechanical shaving methods. No evidence of chondrocyte death or subchondral bone necrosis was reported, although chondrocyte viability was not evaluated and abraded, normal cartilage instead of naturally occurring chondromalacic cartilage was used as the experimental model in this study. In 2000, Kaplan et al. examined the acute effects of bRFE (ArthroCare) on human osteochondral explants with naturally occurring chondromalacia.[11] The authors concluded that bRFE smoothed the articular cartilage surface and was safe for use on articular cartilage even at the highest power settings. In the same year, Lu et al.[12] reported the first negative results of mRFE (ORA-50 Electrothermal System, Oratec Interventions, Menlo Park, CA, USA) chondroplasty on partial-thickness cartilage defects in an in vivo sheep model. Confocal laser microscopy (CLM) was used for the first time to evaluate chondrocyte viability after RFE chondroplasty. A clear zone of chondrocyte death was present in all RFE-treated areas. The researchers reported that mRFE caused immediate chondrocyte death and that the zone of chondrocyte death progressed to full-thickness death over time although the cartilage surface was contoured and smoothed. The interesting finding in this study was that the cartilage matrix was maintained over time although all chondrocytes were dead within the cartilage at 6 months after surgery. This study concluded that RFE did not appear to have the beneficial effects reported in previous studies and that RFE should be used cautiously.

In 2001, Lu et al. published work comparing the three commonly used RFE devices for clinical application.[14] Two bRFE (ArthroCare and Mitek) devices and one mRFE (Smith & Nephew) device were compared in an in vitro study using normal bovine cartilage. This study revealed that clinical application using a paintbrush pattern resulted in chondrocyte death reaching to the subchondral bone in all samples treated with the bRFE devices and none of the samples with the mRFE device. The limitations of this study included the

use of normal cartilage that was abraded to simulate chondromalacia similar to the Turner et al. study.[13] The authors of this study concluded that RFE should not be used clinically until further studies developed methods to limit the thermal injury associated with RFE chondroplasty. Lu et al.[6] repeated the study by Kaplan et al., but also evaluated cell viability of cartilage after bRFE treatment with vital staining and CLM. The results of this work contradicted the previous findings by Kaplan et al. A treatment time of 3 s smoothed the cartilage surface, but even this momentary application resulted in significant thermal injury. With increased bRFE settings, the thermal injury was more severe (Figure 5.8). Concerns regarding this study raised by Yetkinler and McCarthy[7] were that some chondrocytes may not actually have been dead after treatment, but had been temporarily impaired following bRFE application. Yetkinler et al. reported that the technique of CLM combined with LIVE/DEAD cell assays may overestimate chondrocyte death by as much as 50% at temperatures below 50°C since some dead staining chondrocytes may later demonstrate viability, secondary to recovery from heat shock.[7] There are many bodies of work that support the validity of CLM and the fact that thermal treatment results in irreversible chondrocyte death.[6,10,14,30] In the previous Lu et al. sheep study with partial-thickness cartilage defects, chondrocyte death was identifiable at time 0 and persisted until the termination of the project 6 months after surgery.[12] In no case did the investigators observe return of cell viability in areas where previous cell death had been demonstrated. In addition, treatment temperatures for both mRFE and bRFE for chondroplasty are above 65°C.

In 2002, to evaluate the effects of the RFE devices on chondromalacic human cartilage, Edwards et al. compared the three RFE devices currently used clinically (Smith & Nephew, Mitek, and ArthroCare) on naturally occurring human chondromalacic articular cartilage.[19] The results of this study were similar to the previous study using bovine cartilage performed by Lu et al. and confirmed greater chondrocyte death for bRFE devices than for mRFE devices.[14] To further investigate the temperature at the interface between the RFE probe tip and cartilage surface, Shellock and Shields (2000) performed a study that recorded interface temperatures using fluoroptic thermometry during bRFE (Mitek) treatment.[24] The authors stated that interface temperature between the probe tip and the cartilage was 58.1°C at the manufacturer-recommended setting of V2-40 and that this bRFE device was suitable and safe for thermal chondroplasty. In 2002, Edward et al. determined the temperatures reached within the cartilage matrix rather than at the interface, during simulated arthroscopic treatment of articular cartilage.[26] This study compared matrix temperatures during thermal chondroplasty between mRFE (Smith & Nephew) and bRFE (ArthroCare) devices at three depths (200 μm, 500 μm, and 2000 μm) below the cartilage surface. The results of this study demonstrated that bRFE resulted in temperatures of 95°C to 100°C at 200 μm and 500 μm under the surface, with temperatures of 75°C to 78°C at 2000 μm. The investigators of this work concluded that bRFE resulted in sufficiently high temperatures at the deepest depth measured (2000 μm) to potentially cause chondrocyte death up to and including this depth.

Clinical results regarding the use of RFE for chondroplasty are few and often do not concur with experimental results. In 2002, Owens et al. compared mechanical shaving and bRFE for the treatment of focal chondromalacia (grade 2 and 3) in female patients within a middle age range.[23] The results of this study demonstrated that the use of bRFE for chondromalacic grades 2 and 3 produced better clinical outcomes than a mechanical shaver during a 2-year follow-up period, utilizing a subjective scoring system. Although prospective in nature, this study utilized a nonvalidated subjective scoring system and bRFE treatment only focused on the patella where the cartilage is much thicker than, for example, the femoral condyle or tibial plateau. On the contrary, another clinical case report already described[29] demonstrated that bRFE had a deleterious effect on cartilage during thermal chondroplasty.

FUTURE DIRECTIONS

RFE devices may have some significant advantages for cartilage treatment over conventional mechanical debridement methods: (1) a smoother surface may be produced, (2) injury to adjacent and untreated cartilage may be more easily avoided, and (3) rapid and easy contouring is achieved, which may result in a shortened operation. Currently, however, these potential advantages are outweighed by the significant chondrocyte death caused by all RFE devices. The most important focus in the future for the manufacturers of both mRFE and bRFE is to develop newer and safer RFE systems that further reduce chondrocyte death compared to the RFE systems currently used clinically. In addition, experimental studies investigating the effect of heat on cartilages' biomechanical properties and clinical studies investigating both-short and long-term outcomes after RFE chondroplasty must be performed before the devices can be recommended clinically.

Acknowledgements

The authors acknowledge Ryland B. Edwards, DVM, John Bogdanske, Vicki Kalscheur, Shane Nho, John Heiner, MD, and Brian J. Cole, MD for assistance with completed research; and Smith & Nephew, Endoscopy, for research support.

References

1. Miller DV, O'Brien SJ, Arnoczky SS, Kelly A, Fealy SV, Warren RF. The use of the contact Nd:YAG laser in arthroscopic surgery: effects on articular cartilage and meniscal tissue. Arthroscopy 1989;5:245–253.
2. Raunest J, Lohnert J. Arthroscopic cartilage debridement by excimer laser in chondromalacia of the knee joint. A prospective randomized clinical study. Arch Orthop Trauma Surg 1990; 109:155–159.
3. Grifka J, Boenke S, Schreiner C, Lohnert J. Significance of laser treatment in arthroscopic therapy of degenerative gonarthritis. a prospective, randomised clinical study and experimental research. Knee Surg Sports Traumatol Arthrosc 1994;2:88–93.
4. Benton HP, Cheng T, MacDonald MH. Use of adverse conditions to stimulate a cellular stress response by equine articular chondrocytes. Am J Vet Res 1996;57:860–865.
5. Li S, Chien S, Branemark P. Heat shock-induced necrosis and apoptosis in osteoblasts. J Orthop Res 1999;17:891–899.
6. Lu Y, Edwards RB, Kalscheur VL, Effect of bipolar radiofrequency energy on human articular cartilage: comparison of confocal laser microscopy and light microscopy. Arthroscopy 2001;17:117–123.
7. Yetkinler DN, McCarthy EF. The use of live/dead cell viability stains with confocal microscopy in cartilage research. Sci Bull 2000;1:1–2.
8. Hunter W. Of the structure and disease of articulating cartilage. 1743. Clin Orthop 1995;317:3–6.
9. Lane JG, Amiel MD, Monosov AZ, Amiel D. Matrix assessment of the articular cartilage surface after chondroplasty with the holmium:YAG laser. Am J Sports Med 1997;25:560–569.
10. Mainil-Varlet P, Monin D, Weiler C, et al. Quantification of laser-induced cartilage injury by confocal microscopy in an ex vivo model. J Bone Joint Surg Am 2001;83A:566–571.
11. Kaplan L, Uribe JW, Sasken H, Markarian G. The acute effects of radiofrequency energy in articular cartilage: an in vitro study. Arthroscopy 2000;16:2–5.
12. Lu Y, Hayashi K, Hecht P, et al. The effect of monopolar radiofrequency energy on partial-thickness defects of articular cartilage. Arthroscopy 2000;16:527–536.
13. Turner AS, Tippett JW, Powers BE, Dewell RD, Hallinckrodt CH. Radiofrequency (Electrosurgical) ablation of articular cartilage. a study in sheep. Arthroscopy 1998;14:585–591.
14. Lu Y, Edwards RB, Cole BJ, Markel MD. Thermal chondroplasty with radiofrequency energy: an in vitro comparison of bipolar and monopolar radiofrequency devices. Am J Sports Med 2001; 29:42–49.
15. Fanton, GS. Arthroscopic electrothermal surgery of the shoulder. Op Tech Sports Med 1998;6:139–146.
16. Organ LW. Electrophysiologic principles of radiofrequency lesion making. Appl Neurophysiol 1976;39:69–76.
17. Barber FA, Uribe JW, Weber SC. Current applications for arthroscopic thermal surgery. Arthroscopy 2002;18:40–50.
18. Edwards RB, Markel MD. Radiofrequency energy treatment effects on articular cartilage. Op Tech Sports Med 2001;11:96–104.
19. Edwards RB, Lu Y, Kalscheur VL, Nho S, Cole BJ, Markel MD. Thermal chondroplasty of chondromalacic human cartilage: an ex vivo comparison of bipolar and monopolar radiofrequency devices. Am J Sports Med 2001;30:90–97.
20. Lonner BS, Harwin SF. Chondromalacia patellae: review paper. Part I. Contemp Orthop 1996;32:81–85.
21. Lu Y, Edwards RB, Nho S, Cole BJ, Markel MD. Lavage solution temperature influences depth of chondrocyte death and surface contouring during thermal chondroplasty with temperature controlled monopolar radiofrequency energy. Am J Sports Med 2002;30:667–673.
22. Lu Y, Edwards RB III, Nho S, Heiner JP, Cole BJ, Markel MD. Thermal chondroplasty with bipolar and monopolar radiofrequency energy: effect of treatment time on chondrocyte death and surface contouring. Arthroscopy 2002;18:779–788.

23. Owens BD, Stickles BJ, Balikian P, Busconi BD. Prospective analysis of radiofrequency versus mechanical debridement of isolated patellar chondral lesions. Arthroscopy 2002;18:151–155.

24. Shellock FG, Shields CL. Radiofrequency energy-induced heating of bovine articular cartilage using a bipolar radiofrequency electrode. Am J Sports Med 2000;28:720–724.

25. Stein DT, Ricciardi CA, Viehe T. The effectiveness of the use of electrocautery with chondroplasty in treating chondromalacic lesions: a randomized prospective study. Arthroscopy 2002;18:190–193.

26. Edwards RB, Lu Y, Rodriguez E, Markel MD. Thermometric determination of cartilage matrix temperatures during thermal chondroplasty: comparison of bipolar and monopolar radiofrequency devices. Arthroscopy 2002;18:339–346.

27. Shellock, FG. Radiofrequency energy-induced heating of bovine articular cartilage: evaluation of a new temperature-controlled, bipolar radiofrequency system used at different settings. J Knee Surg 2002;15:90–96.

28. Adam C, Eckstein F, Milz S, Schulte E, Becker C, Putz R. The distribution of cartilage thickness in the knee-joints of old-aged individuals—measurement by A-mode ultrasound. Clin Biomech (Bristol, Avon) 1998;13:1–10.

29. Hogan CJ, Diduch DR. Progressive articular cartilage loss following radiofrequency treatment of a partial-thickness lesion. Arthroscopy 2001;17:E24.

30. Zuger BJ, Ott B, Mainil-Varlet P, et al. Laser solder welding of articular cartilage: tensile strength and chondrocyte viability. Lasers Surg Med 2001;28:427–434.

PART II

Surgical Techniques

6

Arthroscopic Debridement of the Degenerative Knee

Gregory C. Fanelli and Daniel R. Orcutt

Debridement was one of the first methods for dealing with damaged articular cartilage.[1] The next advance was open drilling.[2,3] The thought was that lavage, debridement, drilling, and microfracturing might stimulate mesenchymal stem cell metaplasia forming fibrocartilage. Ficat et al. demonstrated a repair response in the articular cartilage after debridement.[4]

The advent of the arthroscope facilitated the development of multiple techniques in debridement, drilling, and microfracturing.[5-9] Rodrigo et al. described the ice pick microfracture technique in 1994.[9] Rodrigo et al. also demonstrated an improvement of cartilagenous repair with passive range of motion that supported Salter's work.[9,10] Abrasion arthroplasty was initially introduced by Johnson in 1986.[11]

These techniques for cartilage repair allow the articular hyaline cartilage defect to fill with fibrocartilage. This fibrocartilage is different in chemical structure and mechanical properties. The articular cartilage, which is composed of predominantly type II collagen is replaced principally by the type I collagen and fibrocartilage.[12] Because of the poor wear characteristics of fibrocartilage the clinical results of debridement and drilling deteriorate over time, and proper patient selection is critical for the success of this surgical procedure.[13]

INDICATIONS

The main indication for arthroscopic debridement, synovectomy, and chondroplasty is knee pain that has been refractory to nonsteroidal inflammatory drugs, activity modifications, physical therapy, and injections. The typical patient is middle aged to geriatric with no recent history of significant trauma; the patient has tightness and pain at the joint line with a slight antalgic gait. On physical examination the patient should have a stable knee with near normal range of motion. The patient may have an effusion, and the radiographs may show squaring of the tibial joint line and sharpening of the tibial spines, and preferably minimal joint space narrowing. If there is significant joint space narrowing or deformity in regards to varus/valgus, arthroscopic treatment may not be indicated unless it will be used in conjunction with an osteotomy to correct the malalignment. Additional diagnostic studies that complement the history, physical examination, and plain radiographs include magnetic resonance imaging and bone scan.

CONTRAINDICATIONS

Knee pain refractory to conservative treatment may benefit from arthroscopic surgery that includes exploration, debridement, synovectomy, loose body excision, lateral retinacular release, and chondroplasty. Premature arthroscopic surgery should not be a substitute for proper clinical workup for infection, inflammatory arthritidies, or tumor. Arthroscopic debridement may be used as a temporizing measure for a significantly deformed arthritic knee before total knee arthroplasty in the well-informed patient who prefers a minimally invasive procedure to total knee replacement at a specific point in time.

SURGICAL TECHNIQUE

The patient is placed supine on the operating table. General or regional anesthesia is utilized for adequate muscle relaxation. A tourniquet is placed on the proximal thigh and may be utilized during the surgical procedure. The appropriate lower extremity is prepped and draped in a sterile fashion.

A superior medial or superior lateral patellar portal is utilized for insertion of inflow cannula. Our preference is to use gravity for fluid inflow; however, other surgeons may prefer an arthroscopic pump. The inferior lateral patellar portal is used for initial arthroscope placement, and the inferior medial patellar portal is utilized for initial instrument placement. The portals are interchanged throughout the procedure as needed. Additionally, posterior lateral and posterior medial portals are utilized. The multiple arthroscopic portal approach enhances extensive arthroscopic debridement and synovectomy procedures.

The medial compartment is most easily visualized with the knee slightly flexed with valgus stress. Once this is inspected, the intercondylar notch is visualized. The lateral compartment is visualized using the same portals with the probe inserted in the medial portal crossing the knee until the

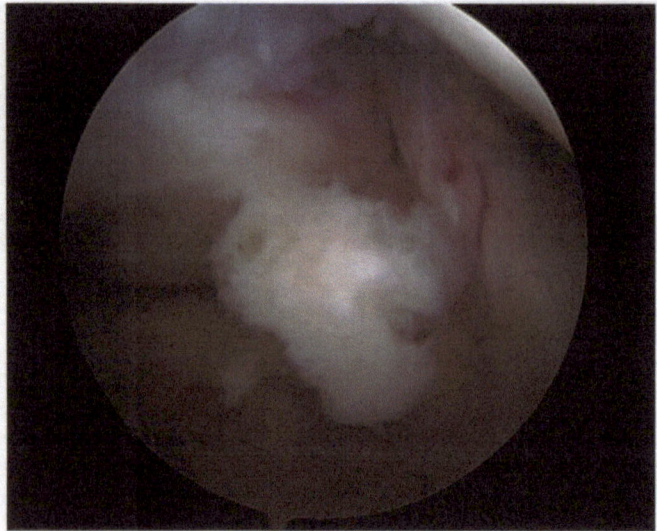

FIGURE 6.1 Arthroscopic excision of a loose body in a degenerative knee. Symptoms of mechanical locking and catching were eliminated after arthroscopic debridement and loose body excision.

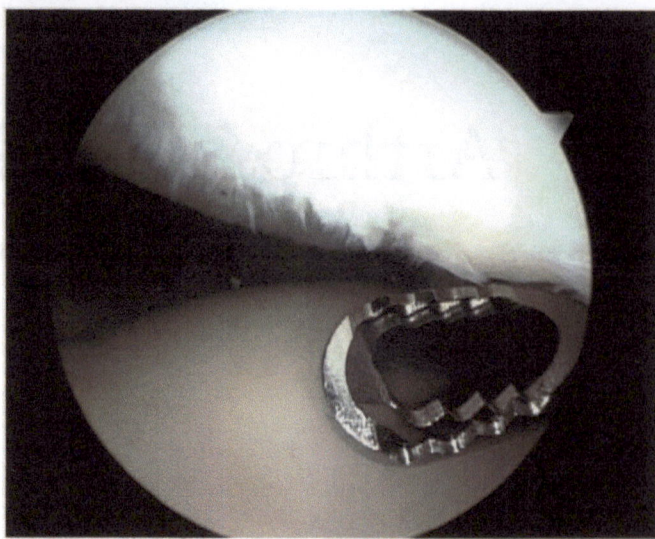

FIGURE 6.2 Arthroscopic patellar chondroplasty performed for chondromalacia of the patella.

tip is within the lateral compartment. The visualization of the lateral compartment is aided by positioning the knee in a "figure 4" position.

The knee is evaluated for synovitis, synovial impingement, meniscus pathology, loose bodies, osteophyte formation, and chondral injuries. The chondral lesions are graded, and the size documented and photographed. Chondroplasty is performed in the following fashion. A motorized shaver system is used to debride fibrillated articular cartilage, remove loose chondral flaps, and abrade exposed subchondral bone. The strategy is to decrease the volume of fragmentation of the degenerated articular cartilage in attempt to minimize reactive synovitis and to decrease the incidence of loose body formation. Care is taken not to remove more cartilage than necessary to debride and stabilize the articular cartilage lesion.

Exposed bare bone may be treated with arthroscopic abra-

sion arthroplasty using a motorized rotary burr or one of the newer bone-cutting synovial shavers. The goal of arthroscopic abrasion arthroplasty is to create a uniform bleeding surface for the ingrowth of fibrocartilage leading to a type of articular surface healing.

Synovectomy is performed through a multiple portal approach to debride the reactive synovitis that accompanies the articular surface breakdown in these degenerative knees, as well as to debride synovial impingement lesions. Degenerative meniscus tears are debrided either with partial, subtotal, or complete menisectomy as the pathology indicates. Loose bodies are excised, osteophytes are debrided, and in cases of patellofemoral arthrosis secondary to excessive lateral pressure syndrome, a lateral retinacular release is performed. Specific surgical procedures are demonstrated in Figures 6.1 through 6.5.

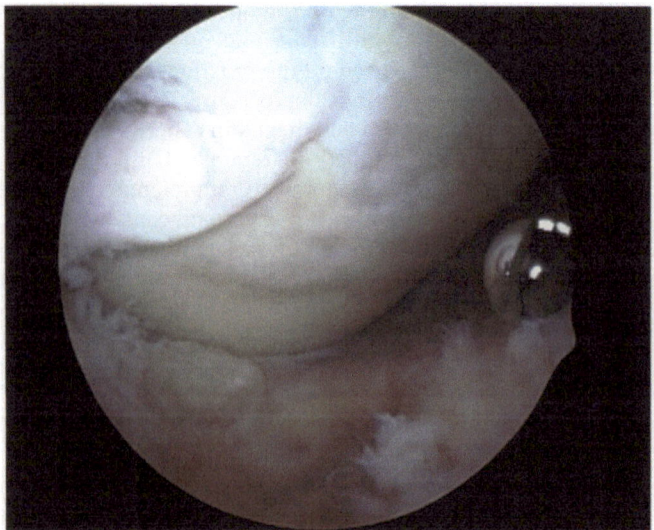

FIGURE 6.3 Arthroscopic synovectomy and debridement performed in a degenerative knee with chronic synovitis and synovial impingement.

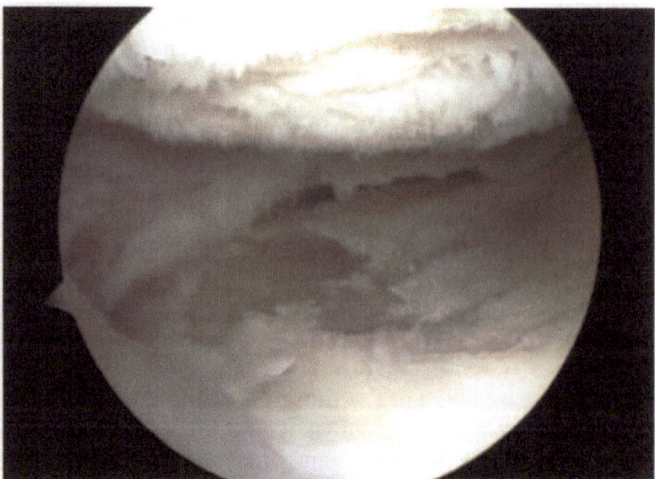

FIGURE 6.4 Severe medial compartment degenerative joint disease in a patient with relatively normal weight bearing radiographs. Arthroscopic chondroplasty was performed on the medial femoral condyle, and arthroscopic abrasion arthroplasty was performed on the medial tibial plateau.

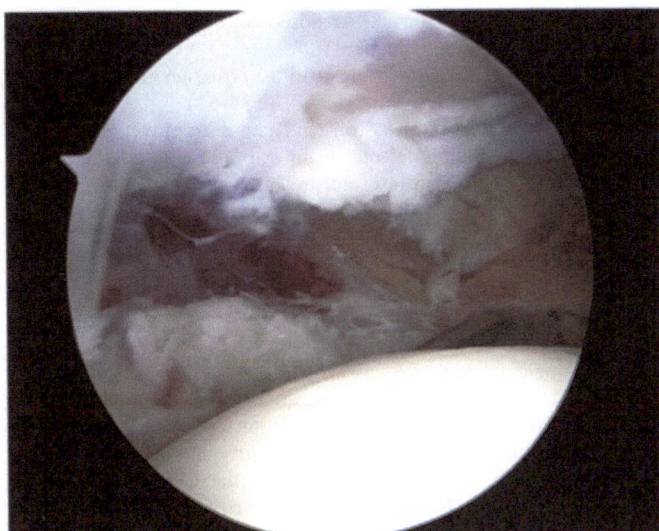

FIGURE 6.5 Lateral retinacular release performed in a patient with excessive lateral pressure syndrome, and patellofemoral degenerative joint disease. Lateral retinacular release will often decrease patellofemoral joint contact pressures to improve patients symptoms. Lateral retinacular release can be performed in conjunction with patellofemoral chondroplasty, and arthroscopic debridement procedures.

SURGICAL PEARLS AND PITFALLS

The use of the multiple portal technique is important to perform adequate debridement and synovectomy. Failure to gain access to all involved compartments may lead to a suboptimal result. The formation of a postoperative hematoma may occur and is successfully treated with aspiration and a compression dressing. Deep venous thrombosis may occur. Patients presenting in the postoperative period with excessive lower extremity swelling, calf pain, and a positive Homan's test should be evaluated with the appropriate vascular studies.

REHABILITATION

Postoperatively, a soft bandage and elastic wrap are applied. The patient is instructed in the use of crutches, and partial weight bearing on the affected side. The patient is advised to ice and elevate the knee, and protected range-of-motion exercises are initiated. The dressing may be changed the day after surgery.

Outpatient rehabilitation begins with range-of-motion exercises. The goal is full active extension and at least 120° of active flexion within the first 14 days. Techniques of limited arc and closed kinetic chain quadriceps strengthening and hamstring strengthening are shown to the patient, and these exercises are begun within 3 days of surgery. If abrasion arthroplasty was performed, the patient is modified weight bearing. If an effusion limits range of motion, the knee is aspirated. A significant number of patients lack the motivation or facility to rehabilitate. These patients need rehabilitation supervision by a physical therapist. Initially, isokinetic machines and full-arc exercises are not permitted.

COMPLICATIONS AND MANAGEMENT

The morbidity for arthroscopic knee surgery is low. Potential complications include anesthesia complications, infection, postoperative hematoma, overaggressive abrasion resulting in increased malalignment, arthrofibrosis, and continued pain. Additional iatrogenic complications include fractures, ligament rupture, and articular surface damage.

RESULTS

Several authors have presented their results with arthroscopic debridement in the degenerative knee. Bauer and Jackson[13] indicated that loose flaps and fibrillation with the articular cartilage still covering the subchondral bone provided better results with arthroscopic chondroplasty than when bare subchondral bone was present.

In a study of 202 knees in 166 patients with a minimum follow-up of 24 months, Jackson et al.[14] presented the following results. Of 65 patients undergoing arthroscopic lavage of their degenerative joint, 80% felt that significant improvement resulted from the procedure, and 45% felt the improvement was sustained at the minimum 2-year follow-up (3.5-year mean follow-up). In the same study group, 137 knees had arthroscopic surgical treatment (shaving and/or debridement) of articular cartilage and meniscal pathology. Of these cases, 12% had no improvement, 88% showed improvement initially, and 66% were still improved at a minimum 2-year (average 3.5 year) follow-up.

Johnson[15] has demonstrated improvement in 80% to 85% of patients following arthroscopic abrasion arthroplasty. This procedure appears to be most effective in small lesions with minimal malalignment and no instability. Thus, arthroscopic abrasion arthroplasty can play a reasonably effective role in resurfacing damaged areas of the joint that are relatively small.

Because of the poor wear characteristics of fibrocartilage, the clinical results of debridement and drilling deteriorate over time. Proper patient selection is critical for the best possible results with arthroscopic abrasion arthroplasty, chondroplasty, and debridement procedures.[14]

SUMMARY AND FUTURE DIRECTIONS

When proper patient selection is employed, arthroscopic debridement and lavage can be a valuable procedure in the treatment of degenerative arthritis of the knee and other joints. Of such patients, 80% to 85% show some improvement.[16] Chances of success with arthroscopic abrasion arthroplasty, chondroplasty, and debridement procedures are much less when bare bone is articulating with bare bone and the articular cartilage is worn away. When symptoms recur in patients who have had arthroscopic debridement, lavage, chondroplasty, and abrasion arthroplasty, these procedures can be repeated and may provide an additional limited period of symptom relief. It must be emphasized that arthroscopic lavage, debridement, chondroplasty, and abrasion arthroplasty are tools in the armamentarium of the arthroscopic surgeon in the treatment of degenerative joint disease and are utilized for the purpose of improving the patient's symptoms. The patient and surgeon must realize the procedure is designed to acquire a time of improved symptoms in patients not able or willing to undergo tibial or femoral osteotomies or total joint replacement and will not cure degenerative joint disease.

The future of arthroscopic surgery in the treatment of degenerative joint disease will most likely expand as surgical techniques and instrumentation advance. Currently available techniques in addition to arthroscopic lavage, debridement, chondroplasty, and abrasion arthroplasty include arthroscopic microfracture, and arthroscopic osteochondral transplantation. Arthroscopic autologous cartilage implantation and arthroscopically assisted arthroplasty may become routine surgeries in the future.

References

1. Magnusson PB. Technique of debridement of the knee joint for arthritis. Surg Clin North Am 1946;26:226–249.
2. Pridie KH. A method of resurfacing osteoarthritic knee joints [abstract]. J Bone Joint Surg 1959;41B:618–619.
3. Insall J. The Pridie debridement operation for osteoarthritis of the knee. Clin Orthop 1974;101:61–67.
4. Ficat RP, Ficat C, Gedeon P, et al. Spongialization: a new treatment for diseased patellae. Clin Orthop 1979;144:74–83.
5. Sprague NF III. Arthroscopic debridement for degenerative knee joint disease. Clin Orthop 1981;160:118–123.
6. Ogilvie-Harris DJ, Jackson RW. The arthroscopic treatment of chondromalacia patella. J Bone Joint Surg 1984;66B:660–665.
7. Schonholtz GJ, Ling B. Arthoscopic chondroplasty of the patella. Arthroscopy 1985;1:92–96.
8. Rae PJ, Noble J. Arthroscopic drilling of osteochondral lesions of the knee. J Bone Joint Surg 1989;71B:534–541.
9. Rodrigo JJ, Steadman RJ, Silliman JF, et al. Improvement of full-thickness chondral defects healing in the human knee after debridement and microfracture using continuous passive motion. Am J Knee Surg 1994;7:109–116.
10. Salter RB, Simmonds DF, Malcolm BW, et al. The biological effect of continuous passive motion on the healing of full thickness defects in articular cartilage. J Bone Joint Surg 1980;62A:1232–1251.
11. Johnson LL. Arthroscopic abrasion arthoplasty. Historical and pathologic perspective: present status. Arthroscopy 1986;2:54–69.
12. Buckwalter JA, Rosenberg LC, Hunziker EB. Articular cartilage: composition, structure, response to injury and methods of facilitating repair. In: Ewing JW (ed) Articular Cartilage and Knee Joint Function: Basic Science and Arthroscopy. New York: Raven Press, 1990.
13. Bauer M, Jackson RW. Chondral lesions of the femoral condyles: a system of arthroscopic classification. Arthroscopy 1988;4:97–102.
14. Jackson RW, Marans HJ, Silver RS. Arthroscopic treatment of degenerative arthritis of the knee. J Bone Joint Surg 1988;70B:332–336.
15. Johnson LL. Diagnostic and surgical arthroscopy. St. Louis: Mosby, 1981.
16. Jackson RW. Arthroscopic treatment of degenerative arthritis. In: McGinty JB, et al. (eds) Operative Arthroscopy. New York: Raven Press, 1991.

7

Bone Marrow Stimulation Techniques: Microfracture, Drilling, and Abrasion

Thomas J. Gill and J. Richard Steadman

BACKGROUND

Bone marrow stimulation techniques for the treatment of chondral defects include abrasion arthroplasty, debridement and drilling, and microfracture. The underlying premise of these techniques is that the body is capable of producing a repair tissue for a chondral defect if undifferentiated mesenchymal cells from the subchondral bone can be accessed. Proponents of these techniques advocate their technical simplicity, low patient morbidity, and cost-effectiveness. Critics argue that any clinical improvements obtained from these procedures are short lived and that the repair tissue generated is largely fibrous in nature with poor durability.

ABRASION ARTHROPLASTY

Arthroscopic abrasion arthroplasty is a modification of an open Magnusson debridement arthroplasty that was popularized by Lanny Johnson.[1] In this procedure, sclerotic exposed bone in the degenerative knee joint is abraded to access the abundant blood supply that is present less than 1 mm below its surface. The goal is to perform a superficial abrasion/debridement that will result in a fibrocartilaginous healing yet preserve the structural integrity of the subchondral bone. The resultant fibrocartilage has shown durability for many years, as confirmed during second-look arthroscopy.[2] In contrast, overly aggressive abrasion that violates the subchondral bone plate can destabilize the joint and result in distortion of the mechanical axis. The resultant varus or valgus deformity will inhibit repair tissue growth and maturation, and the procedure therefore results in early failure. Intraarticular debridement or abrasion alone in the malaligned knee is not recommended in view of the biomechanical forces, and the fact that the original hyaline cartilage deteriorated under these same forces.[3]

Abrasion arthroplasty is meant to relieve symptoms, not "cure" arthritis.[2] It can be used as an alternative to total knee replacement, delaying the surgery in a high percentage of patients for as long as 5 years.[2] Others have stated that long-term results are poor because of the inferior biomechanical structure of the repair cartilage[4] and that arthroscopic debridement alone is preferable to abrasion arthroplasty.[5] Johnson stated that it is not clear whether the abrasion or the general tissue debridement is responsible for the symptomatic relief.[1]

MICROFRACTURE

The technique of microfracture was developed by Dr. Richard Steadman.[6-9] The premise of the technique is to stimulate the underlying bone marrow, and rely on the stereotyped vascular response to injury to heal the full-thickness chondral defect.[10] The theory behind the mechanism of healing has been previously discussed.[10] Briefly, cartilage undergoes the same necrotic phase as any other body tissue. However, it cannot heal itself due to its lack of a blood supply and the resultant inability to mount the inflammatory phase necessary for healing.[11] The processes of transudation, exudation and hematoma formation are absent, and no fibrin clot exists to serve as a scaffold for repair. Microfracture and other bone marrow stimulation techniques allow the inflammatory phase to occur by accessing the underlying blood supply in the subchondral bone. This blood supply is rich undifferentiated mesenchymal cells capable of differentiation and modulation to the fibroblasts or chondroblasts required for repair.[3]

Initially, the full-thickness chondral defects caused by injury or drilling fill with blood and quickly organize into a fibrous clot. Undifferentiated bone marrow elements, blood, and platelets organize in the defect.[12] These cells differentiate into fibroblasts, which produce a reparative granulation tissue. The defect forms a scar at 10 days, which becomes less vascular and more firm. The fibrous tissue undergoes a progressive hyalinization and chondrification to produce a fibrocartilaginous mass that "heals" the defect.

Abrasion arthroplasty and drilling are less popular today than 10 years ago. Currently, the microfracture technique is the primary bone marrow stimulation technique utilized. The microfracture technique is unique when compared to cell-based or biologic therapies in that microfracture is indicated for both traumatic, focal chondral defects as well as more extensive, chronic degenerative lesions.[6-11,13] Both unipolar and bipolar lesions can be treated by microfracture. It can be performed in both primary treatment and revision settings.

Indications and Contraindications

The microfracture technique is indicated as a first line of therapy for the majority of chondral defects encountered at arthroscopy. There are no size or location constraints on its use, as evidenced in a study by Steadman and Gill.[14] Second-look arthroscopy may be helpful following microfracture for lesions greater than 3 cm in diameter. If healing is incomplete, a repeat microfracture to the exposed areas can be performed, or a different resurfacing technique can be considered. Microfracture is safe, technically straightforward, and has a very low rate of associated patient morbidity. In the event that the procedure fails, microfracture does not "burn any bridges" with regard to future surgical procedures such as mosaicplasty or autologous chondrocyte transplantation.

There are no absolute contraindications to the microfracture technique. However, relative contraindications do exist. It is often cited in discussions of other chondral resurfacing techniques that microfracture is not indicated for "large" lesions. To date, there has only been one study that has investigated this question. In a review of more than 100 patients operated on by the senior author, lesions less than $400 \, mm^2$ tended to have less pain than larger lesions, although this was not statistically significant.[10,14,15] In contrast, chronicity of a cartilage injury has a direct effect on its outcome from microfracture. Lesions treated by microfracture within 12 weeks of injury have significantly better outcomes than more chronic lesions,[14] although even degenerative lesions can have excellent outcomes.

Defect location in the knee serves as a relative contraindication for other chondral resurfacing techniques. Procedures such as mosaicplasty can not be performed for most tibial lesions, whereas the results of autologous chondrocyte implantation (ACI) for patellofemoral lesions has not been as good as for tibiofemoral lesions. Although there is no statistical difference in the outcome of microfracture based on defect location in the knee, femoral and trochlear lesions seem to have a more predictable "fill" than tibial or patellar lesions; this is especially true in microfractures performed in arthritic knees. The personal experiences of the authors with second-look arthroscopy following microfracture of the medial compartment done in conjunction with a high tibial osteotomy typically show a well-covered medial femoral chondyle but more patchy coverage of the tibial plateau (Figure 7.1), which may be due to the dense, sclerotic bone present in the plateau in the setting of varus gonarthrosis.

Perhaps the single most important contraindication for microfracture concerns its use in deep osteochondral lesions. Microfracture alone has limited indications for lesions deeper than 5 mm, and, generally, it should not be used for defects over 10 mm deep. The authors typically debride and bone graft these deeper defects, using either iliac crest graft or bone harvested from the intercondylar notch. At times, a fibrocartilaginous covering will form, especially in smaller lesions, much as is seen in the donor sites from mosaicplasty procedures. Depending on the size of the lesions, a mosaicplasty or autologous chondrocyte transplantation may be preferred. Microfracture can be used in the treatment of osteo-

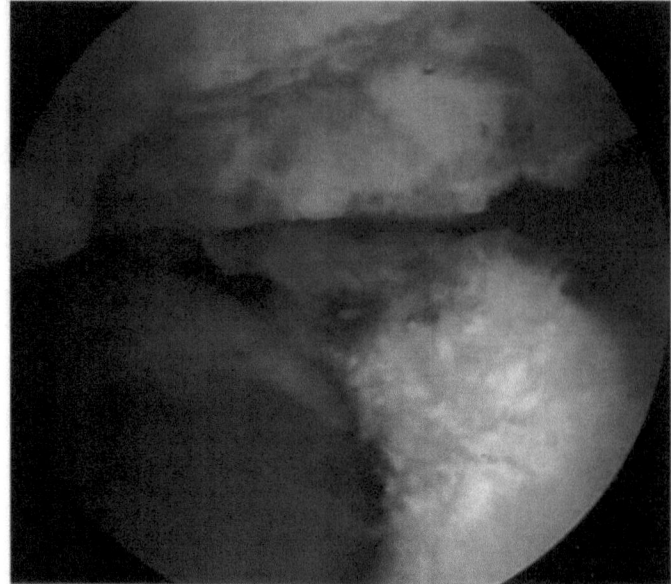

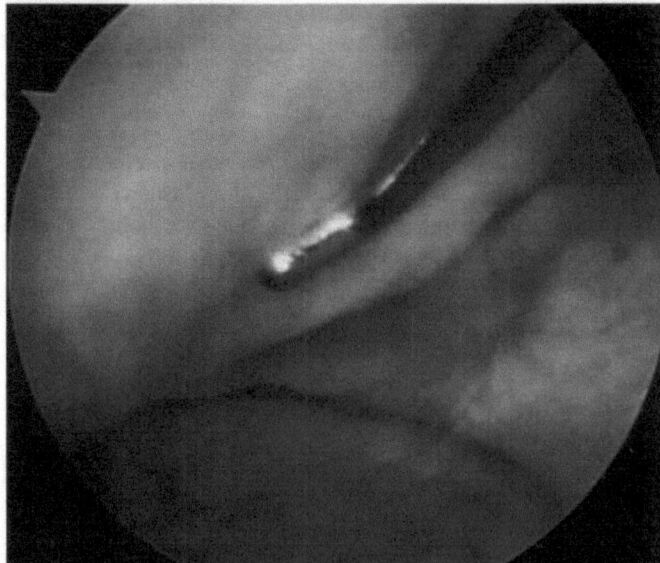

FIGURE 7.1 A 67-year-old man with medial gonarthrosis and a varus knee. He is an active tennis player and skier. **A.** Focal osteonecrosis of the medial femoral condyle and grade 4 defect of the tibial plateau **B.** Three months s/p high tibial osteotomy and microfracture of the medial compartment demonstrating excellent fill of the medial femoral condyle defect and more patchy coverage of the sclerotic tibial plateau.

chondritis dissecans. However, it is not indicated if marrow bleeding cannot be produced from the base of the defect after debridement or the depth of the lesion is greater than 10 mm.

The only absolute contraindication to the microfracture technique is a malaligned knee (Figure 7.2). Microfracture of the medial compartment in the setting of varus alignment almost always fails, as will almost any other resurfacing technique. In this situation, a microfracture should be performed in conjunction with a high tibial osteotomy to reestablish a neutral mechanical axis. Similarly, lateral patellofemoral lesions have a worse prognosis in the setting of patellar maltracking, and consideration should be given to a tibial tubercle osteotomy at the same time as treatment for the chondral injury.

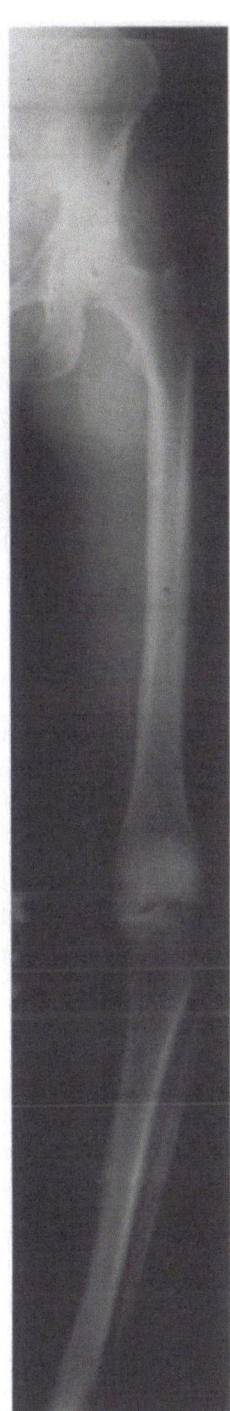

FIGURE 7.2 Three-foot standing radiograph demonstrating the mechanical axis of a varus knee.

TECHNIQUE

Debridement and Drilling

The technique for debridement and drilling is straightforward. In this procedure, an arthroscopic debridement is performed, removing any loose chondral fragments or flaps that may be present around a chondral defect. A Kirschner wire is then used on a motorized drill to penetrate the subchondral

bone and encourage bleeding into the defect. The difficulty with the technique lies in the fact that not all regions of the knee can be accessed using this technique. The wires are rigid, and because a perpendicular entry into bone is needed for the drill, the posterior aspects of the tibia and femur, as well as the patella and trochlea, cannot be reached arthroscopically. No attempt is made to remove the calcified cartilage zone of the defect, and patients are typically allowed to be weightbearing as tolerated in the immediate post-operative period.

Abrasion Arthroplasty

During an abrasion arthroplasty, a motorized shaver or burr is used to debride the sclerotic bone in the base of a chondral defect (Figure 7.3). This process is continued until punctate bleeding can be identified. Care is taken not to penetrate deeply into the subchondral plate, or the compartment can become destabilized, thereby leading to an angular deformity in the knee.

Microfracture Surgical Technique

The microfracture technique has been previously described by the authors. A standard diagnostic arthroscopy is performed, paying careful attention to examining the posterior aspects of the medial and lateral femoral condyles. If any surface changes are noted on the articular surfaces, a probe is used to assess the quality of the cartilage (Figure 7.4). Any unstable flaps are sharply debrided using an arthroscopic shaver or currette. Next, a currette is used to debride the calcified cartilage layer from the base of the full-thickness defect (Figure 7.5). A shaver is generally not used, as it is difficult to control the amount of bone removed and the subchondral bone is more likely to be violated.

The importance of removing this calcified cartilage layer has been studied in horses by Frisbie et al.[7] Removal of the calcified cartilage layer greatly enhances the percentage of the

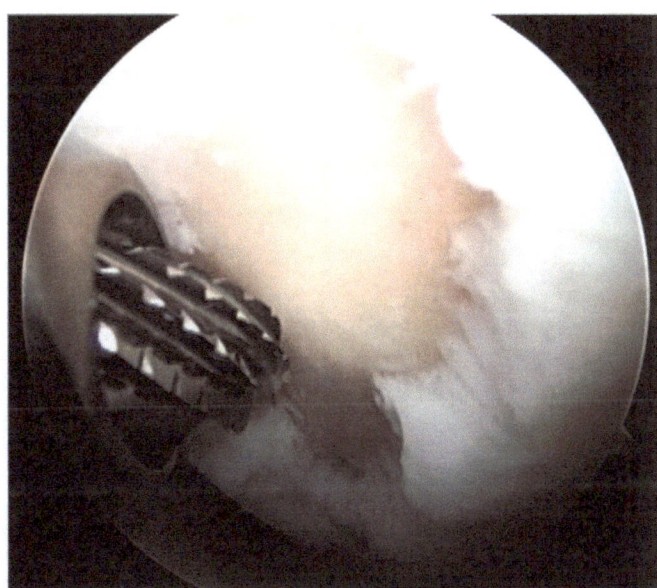

FIGURE 7.3 Arthroscopic burr used to perform an abrasion arthroplasty.

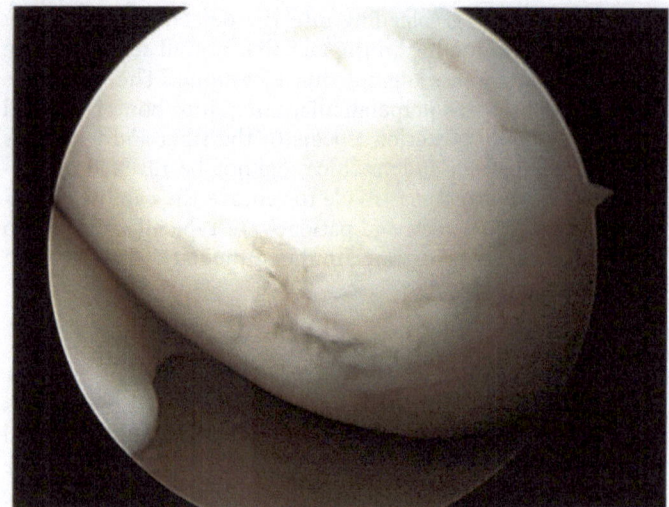

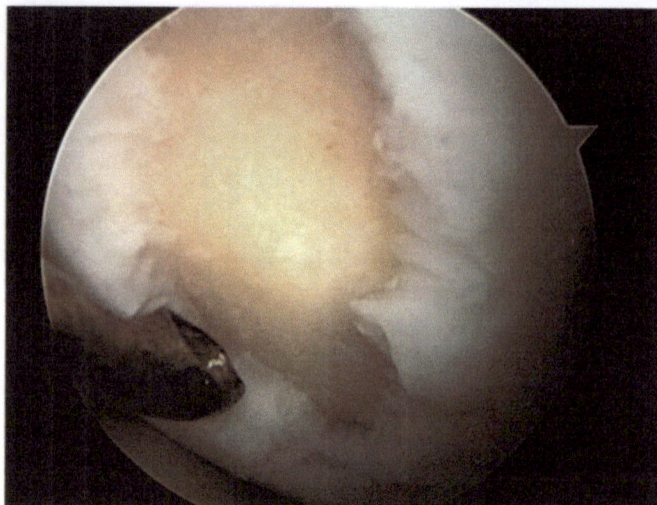

FIGURE 7.5 Curette us used to debride the base and periphery of the lesion.

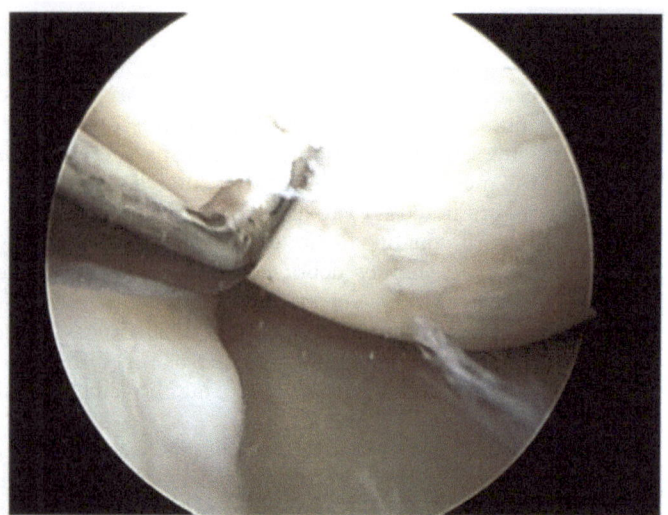

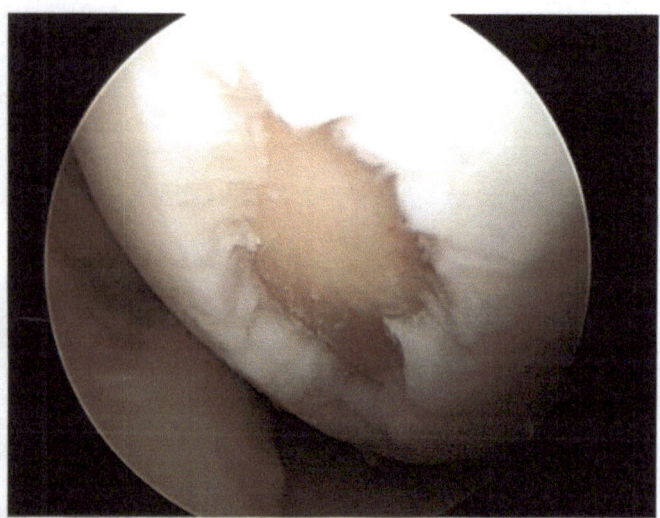

FIGURE 7.4 A. Initial arthroscopic view of a chondral defect of the medial femoral condyle in a 41 year old man. **B.** Probing of the lesion demonstrates unstable marginal flaps. **C.** View after debridement to a stable rim.

defect that is filled. This improvement presumably results from providing a better surface for the "superclot" to adhere to while allowing improved chondral nutrition through subchondral diffusion. The calcified zone is separated from the tangential, transitional, and radial zones by the tidemark. In the immature animal, the basal layers of cartilage are partially nourished by diffusion from the vasculature of the subchondral bone. In the adult, little if any nutrient is able to diffuse across the tidemark because of heavy deposition of apatites in the calcified zone.[12,17] The calcified zone also functions as an efficient barrier to cellular invasion, which has been used to explain the apparent immunity of cartilage transplants to the allograft rejection process (i.e., mechanical rather than immunologic).[18]

Once the chondral defect has been adequately debrided, any associated intraarticular pathology is addressed before performing the microfracture. A surgical awl (Linvatec, Largo, FL, USA) is then used to make multiple small holes ("microfractures") in the exposed bone of the chondral defect spaced 1 to 2 mm apart (Figure 7.6). Care is taken not to connect the holes. The microfracture method is preferred because it creates less thermal injury than drilling, can access difficult areas of the articular surface, and provides controlled depth penetration. On completion, a rough surface is generated for adherence of the ensuing blod clot containing the undifferentiated mesenchymal cells from the subchondral bone (Figure 7.7). The most peripheral aspects of the lesion must be penetrated by the awl to aid the healing of the repair tissue to the surrounding articular surface (Figure 7.8). Once the area has been microfractured, the arthroscopic pump is turned off. Marrow bleeding is observed flowing from the small holes and filling the defect (Figure 7.9).

SURGICAL PEARLS AND PITFALLS

Microfracture is not technically difficult to perform. However, several technical criteria must be followed if optimal results are to be obtained. First, the defects must be appropriately debrided. A curette is used to remove unstable

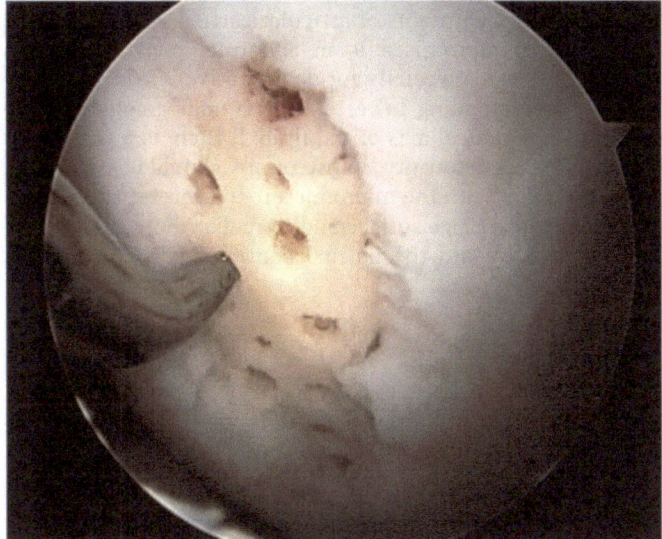

FIGURE 7.6 Spacing of microfracture holes approximately 1–2 mm apart. The goal is to make the holes as close as possible without connecting them.

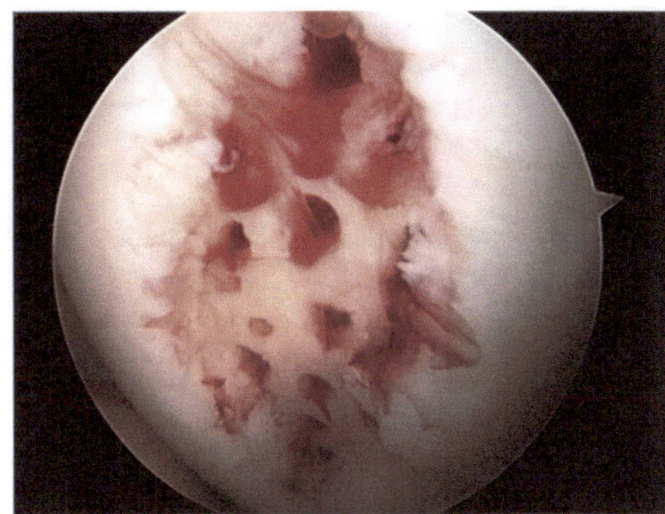

FIGURE 7.7 Rough surface for adherence of the ensuing clot.

flaps and leave a sharp edge in the ensuing defect. A stable, vertical edge leaves a better surface for adherence of the ensuing repair tissue.

Next, the calcified cartilage layer must be removed, paying attention not to significantly abrade the subchondral bone. In the equine study by Frisbie et al.,[7] full-thickness chondral defects were made arthroscopically; 50% were treated by microfracture and 50% were treated by debridement alone. Five horses were harvested at four months, and five were harvested at twelve months. It was clearly demonstrated that removal of the calcified cartilage layer greatly enhances the percentage of the defect that is filled.

Once the calcified cartilage layer is removed, the subchondral bone must be penetrated by the awl with a 1 to 2 mm spacing of the holes to allow connective tissue to fill the defect and adhere to the base of the defect. The periphery of the defect is microfractured first to ensure that the repair tissue contacts the host cartilage around the defect. Holes placed too closely will potentially destabilize the compartment by weakening the subchondral bone plate. A good rule of thumb is to place the holes as closely as possible without allowing them to connect with each other. Placing the holes too far apart limits the ability of the microfracture clot to fill the entire defect. After the defect is fully treated, the arthroscopic pump pressure should be lowered and suction applied over the holes. Bleeding should be visualized coming out of the microfracture sites. If no active bleeding is identified, the holes should be penetrated again with the awl to a slightly deeper level.

Perhaps of equal importance to the surgical technique is the postoperative protocol. Postoperative articular function must be maintained through early continuous passive motion. Strict protected weightbearing is enforced, as discussed in the next section (Table 7.1).

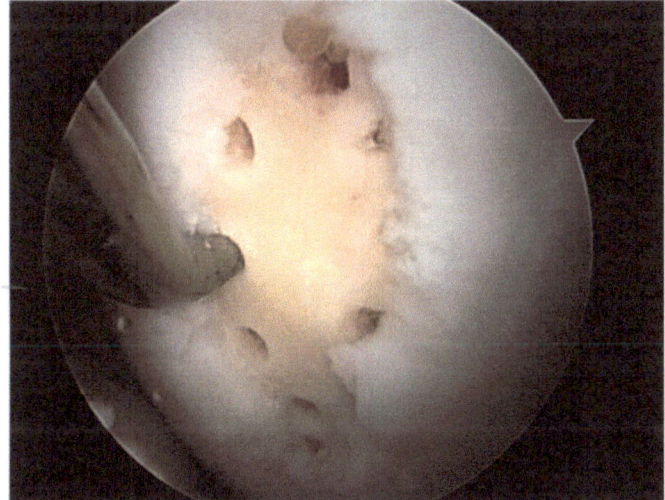

FIGURE 7.8 The microfracture is begun at the periphery of the defect to ensure that the repair tissue heals to the surrounding cartilage.

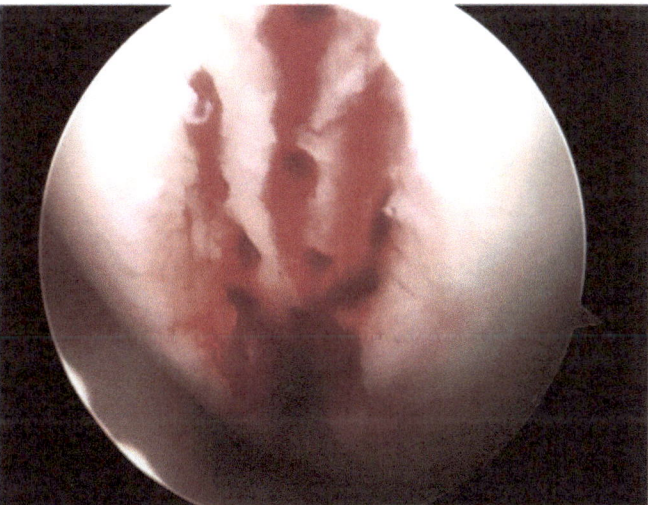

FIGURE 7.9 The pressure on the arthroscopic pump is lowered and blood is seen filling the defect. If no blood is seen in a given hole, the microfracture can be repeated in that area.

TABLE 7.1   Classification of traumatic chondral defects.

Classification	Prognosis	Treatment
I-A	Excellent	None; debridement
I-B	Excellent	None; debridement
II-A	Excellent/good	Microfracture; 6–8 weeks CPM/TDWB
II-B	Excellent/good	Microfracture; 8 weeks CPM/TDWB
III-A	Good	Microfracture; 6–8 weeks CPM/TDWB
III-B	Good/fair	Microfracture; 8 weeks CPM/TDWB

I, partial thickness; II, full thickness (<400 mm²); III, full thickness (>400 mm²);
A, acute (<12 weeks from injury); B, chronic (>12 weeks from injury).
CPM, continuous passive motion; TDWB, touch-down weight bearing.

Lastly, all treatments of articular cartilage defects can be potentially compromised if an abnormal mechanical axes is not corrected, especially for degenerative lesions. We routinely check standing lower extremity radiographs to measure the mechanical axis of the limb. If there is a significant varus or valgus deformity, an osteotomy should be performed in conjunction with the microfracture to decrease the load on the repaired cartilage surface and to re-distribute the weight-bearing axis toward the normal contralateral compartment (Figure 7.10).

REHABILITATION

The postoperative management following microfracture and other marrow stimulation techniques is as critical as the respective surgical procedure.[9,19] Postoperative weight-bearing

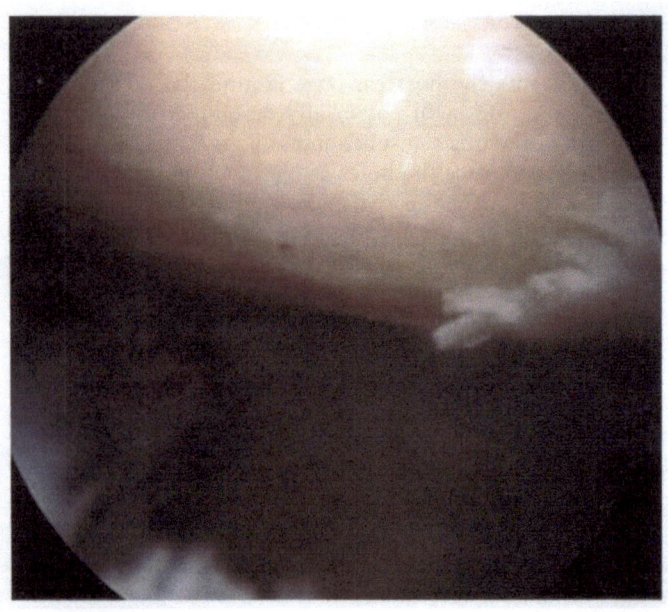

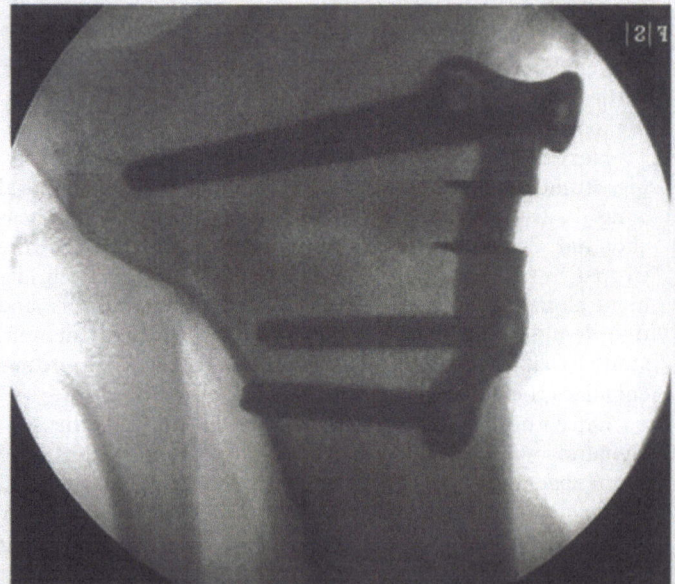

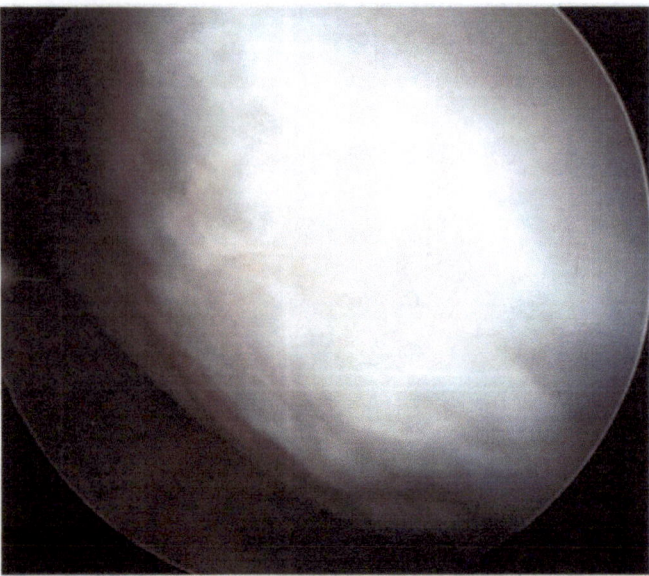

FIGURE 7.10 A. Degenerative medial compartment in a 55-year-old man seen after debridement. **B.** An opening wedge high tibial osteotomy is performed in conjunctions with an extensive fracture. **C.** View of the medial femoral condyle seen at 16 weeks.

status depends on the location of the lesion. Following microfracture of tibiofemoral lesions, patients are kept at touch-down weightbearing (15% weight bearing) for 6 to 8 weeks. If the lesions are in nonweight-bearing regions of the compartments, weightbearing may begin as early as 6 weeks postoperatively, depending on the size of the affected area. Additionally, they are provided with a continuous passive motion (CPM) machine for home use for 8 weeks set at one cycle per minute using the largest range of motion (ROM) tolerated.[19] If CPM is unavailable, patients are instructed to perform full knee passive range of motion 1500 times per day.

Patellar and trochlear groove lesions may be weightbearing as tolerated in a hinged brace with a 30° flexion stop; this protects the lesions, because the patella does not engage the trochlear groove until after 30° of flexion. Patients remove their brace when they are not weightbearing. A CPM machine is used from 10° to 90° for at least 8 hours per day (generally at night) similar to the protocol for the tibiofemoral compartment. If a CPM machine unavailable, patients are instructed to cycle their knee over the edge of a table 1500 times per day.

Following the 6- to 8-week period of protected weightbearing, patients are instructed to begin active ROM exercises and progress to fullweight bearing. No cutting, twisting, or jumping sports are allowed until at least 6 months post-operatively.

This protocol is supported by the recent work of Gill et al.[30] In their animal model using cynomolgous macaques, microfractured defects provided fibrocartilaginous repair tissue that dramatically improved from 6 to 12 weeks postoperatively. Similarly, Johnson reported on more than 6000 cases of arthroscopic debridement, concluding that weightbearing or joint loading delays healing of both partial- and full-thickness defects. Up to 2 months of non-weightbearing was required to promote early fibrous tissue maturation.[1]

The beneficial effect of motion on the healing of articular injuries is well documented.[19,21–24] The principles of CPM include enhanced nutrition and metabolic activity of articular cartilage, the stimulation of pluripotential mesenchymal cells to differentiate into articular cartilage rather than fibrous tissue or bone, and the acceleration of healing of both articular cartilage and periarticular tissues.[23] A slower rate of motion is superior to a faster rate.

Other studies demonstrate that in animals, CPM promotes early and more complete cartilage metaplasia and that pressure-dependent matrix flow from the surrounding articular surfaces may positively influence this metaplasia.[22,25] Additionally, defects exposed to CPM rather than immobilization or intermittent motion exhibit greater defect fill.

Synovial fluid is a source of nutrition for cartilage proliferation, and may contain chondrotrophic properties.[26,27] The pumping action of CPM improves articular cartilage nutrition and helps to clear hemarthroses.[3,23,28] Moreover, physiologic exercise increases the volume of synovial fluid and immobilization is associated with reduced synovial fluid.[29]

COMPLICATIONS AND MANAGEMENT

Complications related to the procedure are minimal. One patient in the series reported by Steadman et al.[14] who had an anterior cruciate ligament reconstruction at the time of the initial microfracture developed arthrofibrosis postoperatively which improved with an aggressive rehabilitation program. In essence, complications associated with microfracture are those associated with standard arthroscopy. To date, there is no data that clearly refutes the implementation of additional cartilage resurfacing techniques following a failed microfracture.

RESULTS

Results of Abrasion Arthroplasty

One of the earliest reports following abrasion arthroplasty was by Friedman et al. who reported on a retrospective survey of 73 procedures with an average follow-up period of 1 year.[30] Overall, 60% showed improvement; 34% reported that the knee was unchanged and 6% were worse. The results were best in patients younger than 40 years of age. In a comparable group of 37 patients treated with medial compartment debridement and medial meniscectomy without abrasion, only 32% showed improvement. Johnson reported lasting fibrocartilage repair tissue and clinical outcomes at up to 6 years postoperatively following abrasion arthroplasty.[1]

Akizuki et al. reported on the results of high tibial osteotomies performed with and without abrasion arthroplasty.[31] Although significantly more repair tissue was seen in the abrasion group, there was no difference in clinical outcome at 2- to 9-year follow-up. Rand et al.[32] studied the role of abrasion arthroplasty in the salvage of failed high tibial osteotomies. Only one of eight patients had any lasting relief at 34 months, and they concluded that abrasion arthroplasty is not a satisfactory salvage for a failed upper tibial osteotomy. Others have reported that the results of abrasion arthroplasty are inferior to the results of arthroscopic debridement alone.[5,33,34]

Menche et al. studied the differences in healing of full-thickness articular cartilage defects treated with abrasion arthroplasty versus subchondral drilling in a rabbit model.[35] Rabbits subjected to subchondral drilling had increased fibrocartilaginous healing with time, with a slight increase in degenerative changes. Abrasion arthroplasty resulted in cartilaginous coverage of the exposed surface as well as progressive increase in degenerative changes. Although both techniques were suboptimal, the authors concluded, based on histology of the repair sites, that subchondral drilling may result in a longer-lived repair than abrasion arthroplasty.

Results of Microfracture for Traumatic Chondral Defects

The first study on the long-term results of microfracture for traumatic chondral defects was presented at the first meeting of the International Cartilage Repair Society.[10,14] More than 100 patients treated by the senior author (J.R.S) with microfracture for full-thickness chondral defects were reviewed. The average follow-up was 6 years. Using a scoring system designed specifically for the treatment of chondral defects, patients were objectively assessed based on their pre- and postoperative examinations. Microfracture resulted in statistically significant improvements (p < 0.05) in pain,

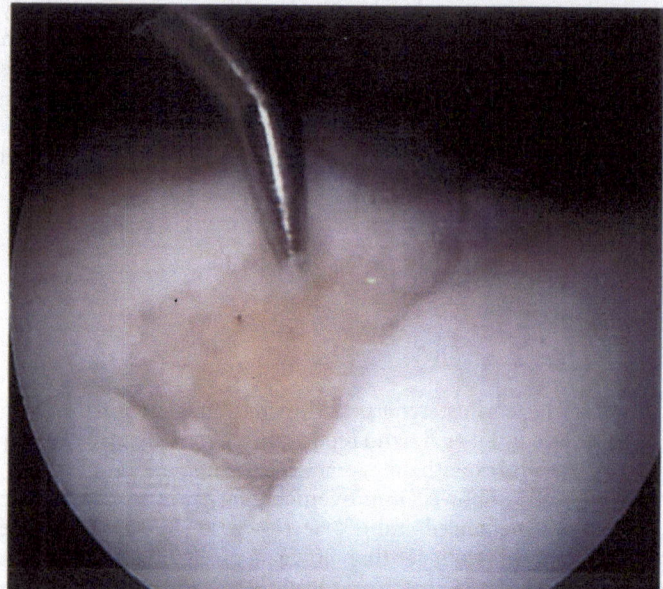

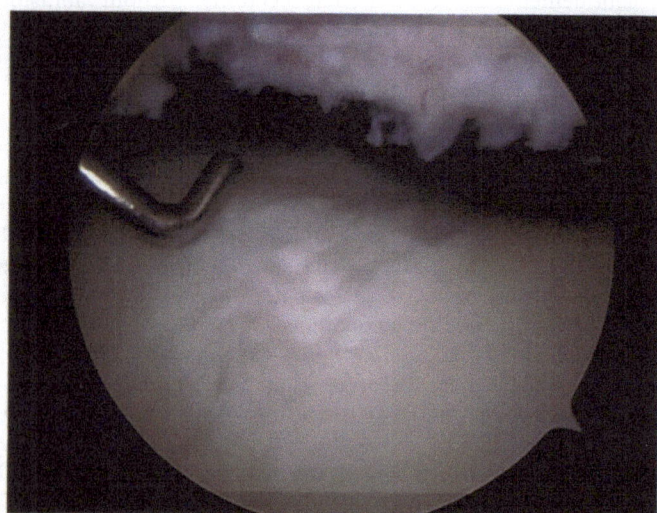

FIGURE 7.11 A. Trochlear lesion seen in a 27-year-old female soccer player. **B.** Second look at the defect at 2.5 year follow-up demonstrating complete fill and firm texture of the defect.

More recently, Gill and MacGillivray reviewed the results of microfracture for isolated chondral defects of the medial femoral condyle at The Hospital for Special Surgery.[15] Nineteen patients were studied at a mean follow-up of 3 years. The mean size of the chondral defects was 3.2 cm². The calcified cartilage layer was not routinely debrided, and patients did not routinely use CPM or limited weight bearing for 6 weeks. Subjectively, 74% had minimal or no pain, and 63% rated their overall condition as good or excellent using the modified Cincinnati questionnaire. Objectively, 1 patient had swelling and all patients had either mild or no crepitus on examination.

Follow-up magnetic resonance imaging (MRI) was performed on all patients employing a special cartilage sequence. Despite the good subjective results, only 42% of the patients had 67% to 100% defect fill, 21% had 31% to 66% fill, and the remaining 37% had 0% to 30% fill. There was no correlation between the size of the defect and the percent fill. Four patients had a smooth transition at the fibrocartilage–articular cartilage interface whereas the rest had a fissure.

At the time of second look arthroscopy, half the knees had firm, well-fixed, normal-appearing cartilaginous tissue which completely filled the site of the previous defect (Figure 7.12). A mildly fibrillated or discolored cartilaginous-appearing tissue was found in 16% of the previous defects. The defect was completely filled but uneven or slightly fragmented in 18%; 16% of the defects had at least one area of exposed bone in their base.

Steadman et al. have published their results on the outcome of microfracture for isolated chondral defects in the knee.[3] Seventy-five knees in 72 patients treated by microfracture were reviewed at 7- to 17-year follow-ups. Inclusion criteria included (1) traumatic full-thickness chondral defect, (2) no menisci or ligament injury, and (3) under 45 years of age (range, 13–45). These criteria were designed to ensure that there were no confounding variables associated with the outcomes measures for the procedure. There was a statistically significant improvement in Lysholm, Tegner, SSF-36, and Western Ontario and McMaster Universities Arthritis Index (WOMAC) scores. However, not everyone improved following the procedure. Although 80% rated themselves as improved, 15% were unchanged from their preoperative scores and 5% were worse. A multivariate analysis demonstrated that age was the only predictor of functional improvement. The study concluded that over the 7- to 17-year (average 11.3 years) follow-up, patients less than 45 years old treated with microfracture for a full-thickness chondral defect without associated ligament or cartilage pathology demonstrated statistically significant improvement in pain and function.

Results of Microfracture in Osteoarthritic Knees

The use of microfracture in 80 patients over the age of 50 with osteoarthrosis of the knee was reported by Steadman and Gill.[10,14] Outcome analysis was performed using the International Knee Documentation Committee (IKDC) scoring system as an objective assessment of the long-term clinical results. There was a significant improvement in outcome with regard to subjective complaints of pain and swelling. Microfracture resulted in a statistically significant improvement in the ability to walk 2 miles, run, climb stairs, perform

swelling, and all functional parameters studied. The ability to walk 2 miles, descend stairs, perform activities of daily living, and participate in strenuous work and sports also improved. Symptoms of pain and swelling improved up to 2 years postoperatively and maximum functional improvement was not achieved until 2 to 3 years postoperatively. Eighty-six percent of patients rated their knee as feeling normal to nearly normal following their microfracture. Only 14% of patients had their level of sports participation reduced following microfracture. There was no statistically significant difference in outcome between patellofemoral lesions, medial compartment lesions, and lateral compartment lesions (Figure 7.11). Larger lesions tended to have more pain at final follow-up than smaller lesions, although this was not statistically significant. Chondral defects treated within 3 months of injury had significantly less pain and better scores for activities of daily living regardless of lesion size.

FIGURE 7.12 A. Defect of the medial femoral condyle in a 29-year-old female skier. **B.** View of the defect after debridement. **C.** Second look at the defect at 2 year follow-up.

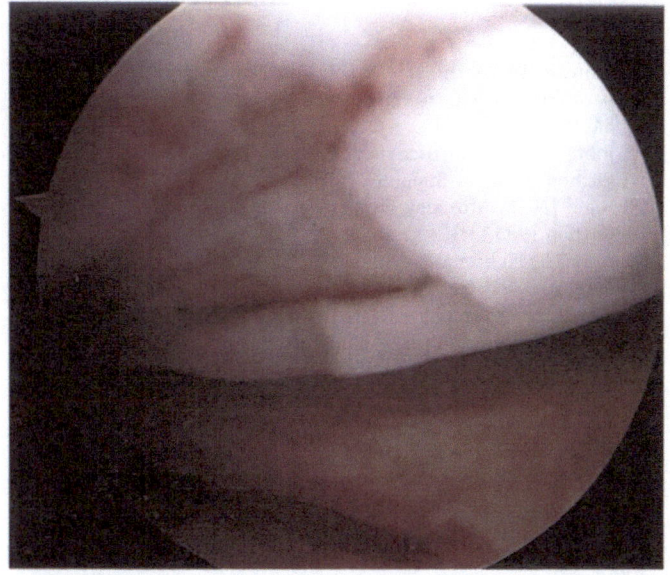

A

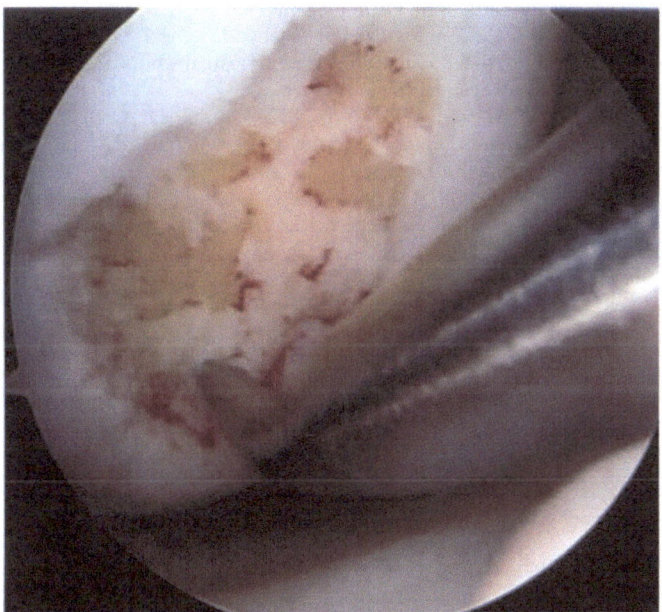

B

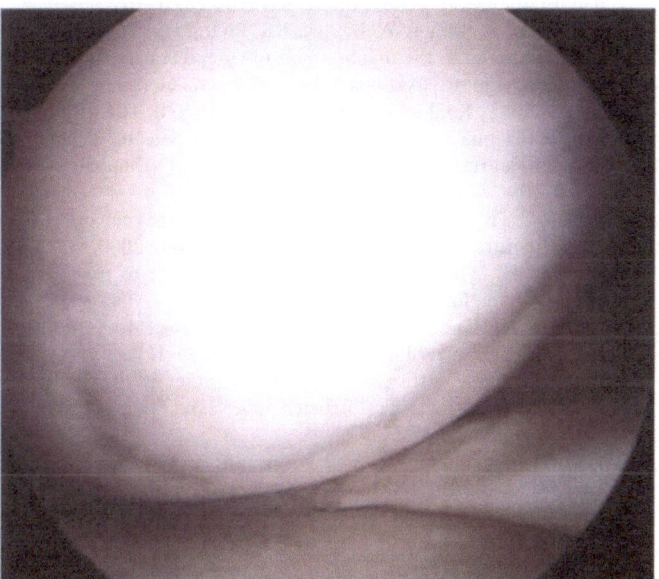

C

strenuous work, perform strenuous sports, and perform activities of daily living. Maximum functional improvement was not achieved until 2 to 3 years post-operatively.

Seven microfractures were classified as a failure because of the need for a subsequent procedure, including five total knee arthroplasties. Risk factors for a poor result included chronicity of the lesions and severity of preoperative joint space narrowing. Alignment also played a significant role in outcome following microfracture.

FUTURE DIRECTIONS

As in many areas of orthopedic surgery, it is clear that biochemical and genetic modulators play a significant role in the treatment of chondral defects. Studies demonstrating the ben-

eficial effect of growth factors such as bone morphogenetic protein (BMP) on the healing of chondral defects have recently been performed.[37] In a study being completed by Gill et al.,[14] the use of BMP-2 in a primate model is being investigated with regard to its effect on the quality of the repair tissue following the microfracture technique. The use of such growth factors may play a significant role in the future of treatment for chondral defects, particularly when combined with a technique such as microfracture. Altering the environment to which the early repair cells are exposed may further influence the differentiation of the mesenchymal cells.[5,28] Gene therapy may be able to contribute to the healing of these injuries as well. By influencing the maturation of the "superclot" along a chondroid line, it is hoped that a repair tissue more closely resembling normal articular cartilage may be able to be achieved.

References

1. Johnson LL. Arthroscopic abrasion arthroplasty historical and pathologic perspective: present status. Arthroscopy 1986;2:54–69.
2. Johnson LL. Arthroscopic abrasion arthroplasty: a review. Clin Orthop 2001;391 Suppl:S306–S317.
3. Rand JA. Arthroscopy and articular cartilage defects. Contemp Orthop 1985;11:13–30.
4. Minas T, Nehrer S. Current concepts in the treatment of articular cartilage defects. Orthopedics 1997;20:525–538.
5. Goldman RT, Scuderi GR, Kelly MA. Arthroscopic treatment of the degenerative knee in older athletes. Clin Sports Med 1997;16:51–68.
6. Steadman JR, Rodkey WG, Briggs KK, McIlwraith CW, Briggs KK. Microfracture procedure for treatment of full-thickness chondral defects: Technique, clinical results and basic science status. In: Harner CD, Vince KG, Fu FH (eds) Techniques in Knee Surgery. Media, PA: Williams and Wilkins, 2000.
7. Steadman JR, Rodkey WG, Briggs KK, Rodrigo JJ. The microfracture procedure: Rationale, technique and clinical observations for treatment of articular cartilage defects. Journal of Sports Traumatology and Related Research 1998;20:61–70.
8. Steadman JR, Rodkey WG, Briggs KK, Rodrigo JJ. [The microfracture technique in the management of complete cartilage defects in the knee joint.] Orthopade 1999;28:26–32. German.
9. Steadman JR, Rodkey WG, Briggs KK, Rodrigo JJ. The microfracture technique for full-thickness chondral defects: Technique and clinical results. Operative Techniques in Orthopedics 1997;7:300–304.
10. Gill TJ. The treatment of articular cartilage defects using microfracture and debridement. Am J Knee Surg 2000;13:33–40.
11. Mankin HJ. The response of articular cartilage to mechanical injury. J Bone Joint Surg 1982;64-A:460–465.
12. Mankin HJ. The reaction of articular cartilage to injury and osteoarthritis. New Eng J Med 1974;291:1285–1292.
13. Gill T. The role of the microfracture technique in the treatment of full-thickness chondral injuries. Oper Tech Sports Med 2000;8:2,138–140.
14. Gill TJ, Steadman JR, Rodrigo JJ, Briggs KK, Rodkey WG. Indications and long-term clinical results of microfracture. Presented at the 2nd Symposium of the International Cartilage Repair Society; November, 1998; Boston, Massachusetts.
15. Gill TJ, MacGillivray JD. The technique of microfracture for the treatment of articular cartilage defects in the knee. Operative Techniques in Orthopedics 2001;11:105–107.
16. Frisbie DD, Trotter GW, Powers BE, Rodkey WG, et al. Arthroscopic subchondral bone plate microfracture technique augments healing of large chondral defects in the radial carpal bone and medial femoral condyle of horses. Vet Surg 1999;28:242–255.
17. Mankin HJ. The articular cartilages: a review. AAOS Instructional Course Lectures. 1969;204–224.
18. Brown KLB, Cruess RL. Bone and cartilage transplantation in orthopaedic surgery. J Bone Joint Surg 1982;64-A:270–279.
19. Rodrigo J, Steadman JR. Improvement of full-thickness chondral defect healing in the human knee after debridement and microfracture using continuous passive motion. Am J Knee Surg 1994;7:109–116.
20. Glasson S, Powers J, Blanchet T, Peluso D, et al. Microfracture in non-human primates is the preferred model for repair of human cartilage defects. Presented at the 48th Annual Meeting of the Orthopedic Research Society; 2002; Dallas, TX.
21. Amiel D, Coutts RD, Abel M, Stewart W, Harwood F, Akeson WH. Rib perichondrial grafts for the repair of full-thickness articular cartilage defects. A morphological and biochemical study in rabbits. J Bone Joint Surg 1985;67-A:911–920.
22. O'Driscoll SW, Salter RB. The induction of neochondrogenesis in free intra-articular periosteal autografts under the influence of continuous passive motion. An experimental investigation in the rabbit. J Bone Joint Surg 1984;66-A:1248–1257.
23. Salter RB. The biologic concept of continuous passive motion of synovial joints. The first 18 years of basic research and its clinical application. Clin Orthop 1989;242:12–25.
24. Salter RB, Simmonds DF, Malcolm BW, Rumble EJ, MacMichael D, Clements ND. The biological effect of continuous passive motion on the healing of full-thickness defects in articular cartilage. J Bone Joint Surg 1980;62-A:1232–1250.
25. Kettunen KO. Effect of articular function on the repair of a full-thickness defect of the joint cartilage. An experimental study of mature rats. Ann Chir Gynaec Fenniae 1963;52:627–642.
26. Rubak JM. Reconstruction of articular cartilage defects with free periosteal grafts. Acta Orthop Scand 1982;53:175–180.
27. Rubak JM, Poussa M, Ritsila V. Chondrogenesis in repair of articular cartilage defects by free periosteal grafts in rabbits. Acta Orthop Scand 1982;53:181–186.
28. Frank C, Akeson WH, Woo SL-Y, Amiel D, Coutts RD. Physiology and therapeutic value of passive joint motion. Clin Orthop 1984;185:113–125.
29. Rubak JM, Poussa M, Ritsila V. Effects of joint motion on the repair of articular cartilage with free periosteal grafts. Acta Orthop Scand 1982;53:187–191.
30. Friedman MJ, Berasi CC, Fox JM, Del Pizzo W, Snyder SJ, Ferkel RD. Preliminary results with abrasion arthroplasty in the osteoarthritic knee. Clin Orthop 1984;182:200–205.
31. Akizuki S, Yasukawa Y, Takizawa T. Does arthroscopic abrasion arthroplasty promote cartilage regeneration in osteoarthritic knees with eburnation? A prospective study of high tibial osteotomy with abrasion arthroplasty versus high tibial osteotomy alone. Arthroscopy 1997;13:9–17.
32. Rand JA, Ritts GD. Abrasion arthroplasty as a salvage for failed upper tibial osteotomy. J Arthroplasty 1989;4 suppl:S45–S48.
33. Bert JM, Maschka K. The arthroscopic treatment of unicompartmental gonarthrosis: a five-year follow-up study of abrasion arthroplasty plus arthroscopic debridement and arthroscopic debridement alone. Arthroscopy 1989;5:25–32.
34. Rand JA. Role of arthroscopy in osteoarthritis of the knee. Arthroscopy 1991;7:358–363.
35. Menche DS, Frenkel SR, Blair B, Watnik NF, et al. A comparison of abrasion burr arthroplasty and subchondral drilling in the treatment of full-thickness cartilage lesions in the rabbit. Arthroscopy 1996;12:280–286.
36. Steadman JR, Briggs K, Rodrigo J, Kocher M, Gill TJ, Rodkey WG. Outcomes of microfracture for traumatic chondral defects of the knee: Average 11-year follow-up. Accepted for publication Arthroscopy.
37. Sellers RS, Peluso D, Morris EA. The effect of recombinant human bone morphogenic protein-2 (rhBMP-2) on the healing of full-thickness defects of articular cartilage. J Bone Joint Surg 1997;79-A:1452–1463.

8

Osteochondral Autograft Replacement

Andrew S. Levy and Steven W. Meier

BACKGROUND

Analytical studies have shown that both blunt and shear stress are manifest at the tidemark that separates the calcified and uncalcified cartilage in the articular surface.[1] This "essential lesion" of articular cartilage damage has subsequently been substantiated by cadaver and animal studies.[2,3] The development of focal lesions of the articular surface is attributed to the progression of this essential deep lesion. Thus, the rationale behind osteochondral transfer is to replace the damaged cartilage bone unit with a healthy one.

In 1908, Judet[4] first reported the use of autogenous osteochondral grafting. He reported on the transplantation of osteochondral fragments after trauma and noted clinical relief of pain. In 1961, Pap and Krompecher published canine data that showed that cartilage transplanted on bone less than 5 mm survived more than 2 years without deterioration.[5] Similar data were published by Campbell et al. in 1963 that showed that 1- to 2-cm osteochondral plugs with less than 5 mm bone survived more than 1 year.[6] Other authors further showed that bone, not cartilage, is replaced in whole joint grafts.[7,8] In 1985, McDermott et al.[9] confirmed the efficacy of wafer grafts (2–3 mm bone) in osteocartilage replacement and noted "the fate of the bone portion of graft directly effects the fate of cartilage."

The recent enthusiasm for osteochondral grafting of cartilage lesions can be traced to the development of instrumentation that allows for careful harvest and placement of graft to fill focal lesions. The term mosaicplasty has evolved to describe the use of multiple small-diameter osteochondral plugs to fill chondral holes. At present, at least three orthopaedic companies market instruments to assist the surgeon in performing osteochondral grafting.

INDICATIONS AND CONTRAINDICATIONS

Osteochondral grafting is recommended for the treatment of symptomatic focal chondral and osteochondral lesions. As in most other chondral lesion treatment options, it is con-traindicated in cases of fulminate arthritis. Lesion size and location limit the application of osteochondral autografts.

Grafts must be placed perpendicularly into the recipient site, which makes application virtually impossible for posterior condylar and tibia lesions unless indirect techniques are utilized. Although some investigators have reported use on the patella, this is not recommended because of cartilage thickness mismatch (5–10 mm for patella and 2–3 mm for graft). Consequently, the preferred lesion is on the femoral condyle in the anterior or middle third. Trochlea lesions are potentially treatable with this technique, but extra care must be taken to match the curvature of the groove.

Because the grafts are harvested from within the patient's own knee, there is a limited supply of donor tissue. Furthermore, the larger lesions present a loss of containment over 2 cm² and radius mismatch of plugs increases. Although some authors have reported using this technique for large lesions, these results are unpredictable. Consequently the ideal lesion for osteochondral grafting is a lesion less than 2.5 cm² located on the femoral condyle.

TECHNIQUE

The available systems differ on their technique of harvest, depth of harvest, and mechanism for ease of graft delivery. No system has shown superior clinical outcomes when compared and no randomized trials have been completed to assess for differences in outcome. All differences in equipment or technique should be considered as theoretical advantages or disadvantages, and surgeons should choose accordingly.

Consistent Osteochondral Repair (COR) System (Mitek Inc, Norwood, MA)

ADVANTAGES

Harvest depth, 8 mm (5 mm bone), consistent with basic science.

Tooth on harvester allows cutting of base of graft with a twisting motion, thus preventing toggling damage during extraction. During implantation, resulting bevel *or groove* on graft may also allow water to pass out from recipient hole during arthroscopic impaction, thus decreasing force needed to impact. Clear delivery tubes allow full, unobstructed inspection of graft so that obliquity can be controlled during graft impaction.

DISADVANTAGES

Preparation of recipient site is through use of a drill. Some surgeons are concerned with potential thermal effect. Maintaining an awareness of this and drilling at relatively lower rpm may be helpful. Impaction occurs with mallet. Overzealous impaction may damage graft. Plastic impactors help reduce impaction forces.

Osteochondral Autologous Transplantation System (OATS; Arthrex Inc, Naples FL)

ADVANTAGES

Slotted delivery tubes allow inspection of graft, and obliquity can be controlled for during graft impaction. Impaction (graft placement) can be performed with a screw mechanism, preventing graft damage by reducing impaction forces. "Coring"-type harvesting device lessens potential thermal concerns. Perpendicular placement of recipient site is aided with a coring-type recipient site device. Relying on the tactile as well as visual feedback provided by placing the rim of the device concentrically on the recipient surface can facilitate perpendicular placement.

A "Corkscrew device" is available for removal of unacceptable grafts.

DISADVANTAGES

Harvest depth, 10 to 15 mm (8–12 mm bone), inconsistent with basic science, but can be controlled to obtain lesser depths. Harvest cutters employ toggling to remove graft; this exposes graft to potential shearing and fracture during harvest.

Mosaicplasty (Acufex Microsurgical, Inc., Mansfield, MA)

Recommended graft sizes are 2.7, 3.5, and 4.5 mm in diameter and 15 mm in length. Instrumentation for graft diameters of 6.5 and 8.5 mm are also offered.

ADVANTAGES

Reported ability to fill larger defects (up to 9 cm²) because of the use of more numerous, smaller-diameter grafts from both medial and lateral femoral condyle of the patellofemoral joint.

Better ability to recreate contour of femoral condyle using numerous, smaller grafts.

DISADVANTAGES

Smaller grafts are weaker and more susceptible to fracture and chondral delamination from shear stresses. Harvest depth (15 mm) is inconsistent with basic science. Higher ultimate ratio of fibrocartilage (20%–40%) to hyaline cartilage (60%–80%) results from the placement of small and numerous grafts, creating more interstices that then fill with fibrocartilage "grout".

Harvest cutters employ toggling to remove graft, which exposes graft to potential shearing during harvest. Preparation of recipient site is through use of drill. Some surgeons are concerned with potential thermal effect. Impaction occurs with mallet. Overzealous impaction may damage graft.

Consistent Osteochondral Repair Technique

The Consistent Osteochondral Repair (COR) System introduced in 1997 is the technique presented here.

STEP I: PREPARATION OF CHONDRAL LESION

Once a chondral lesion is identified, it must be debrided to a stable border for all cartilage repair techniques. It has been noted that the initial appearance of the chondral lesion is usually one third of the final size once debrided.[10] Debridement is best performed by using a bent curette or osteotome (Arthrex, Naples, FL, USA). It is important to achieve vertical walls at the edge of the chondral lesion (Figure 8.1) to provide stability and prevent synovial exposure of deep chondral layers. Because osteochondral grafting relies on fibrocartilage stimulation to provide "the mortar" around the plugs, punctate bleeding is achieved at the base of the lesions using microfracture or limited abrasion. Drilling should be avoided during this step because it can interfere with socket creation.

Recipient site sizing is initially performed with calibrated probes. The metal graft impactors are then used to delineate plug size and array. This step can also be used to determine perpendicular alignment of portal and lesion. It is often advisable to resect the ligamentum mucosum and debride the fat pad to maximize exposure and prevent entrapment when delivering the graft.

STEP II: SELECTION OF DONOR SITE

Although there is no true completely nonweight-bearing articular cartilage of the knee, contact studies have revealed sites with significantly less contact pressure including the femur at the outer edges of the patellofemoral joint and the intercondylar notch. The donor site at the periphery of the lateral femoral condyle donor site, for instance, can be easily accessed from a standard lateral portal with the leg at or near extension. The intercondylar notch site is best accessed from a standard medial or transpatellar tendon portal (Figure 8.2). Factors that influence donor site choice include concomitant anterior cruciate ligament (ACL) reconstruction (harvest as part of notchplasty), previous ACL reconstruction (previous notchplasty), size of lesion, donor cartilage thickness, and apparent radius of curvature of recipient site.

STEP III: GRAFT HARVEST

The appropriate size cutter (with tooth) is placed on the harvester and introduced into the knee (Figure 8.3). Graft diameter options with the COR system are 4, 6, and 8 mm, depending on the harvester used. The authors' preference for graft diameter is 6 mm.

Insertion of the harvesting device is best performed with the plunger fully inserted to prevent synovial tissue from

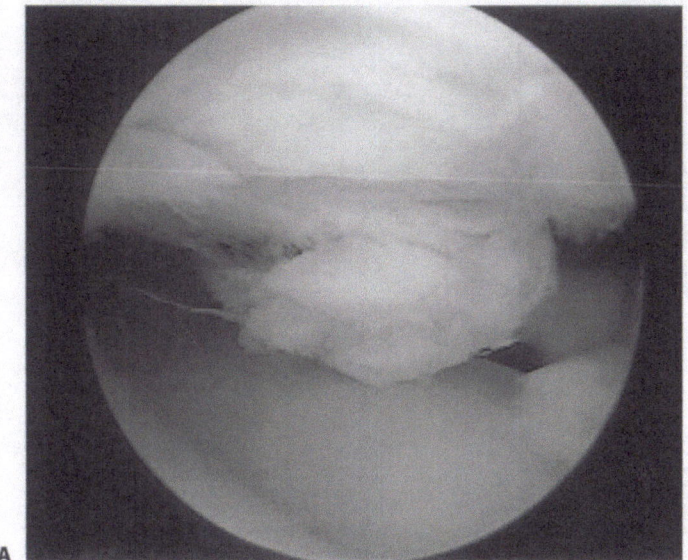

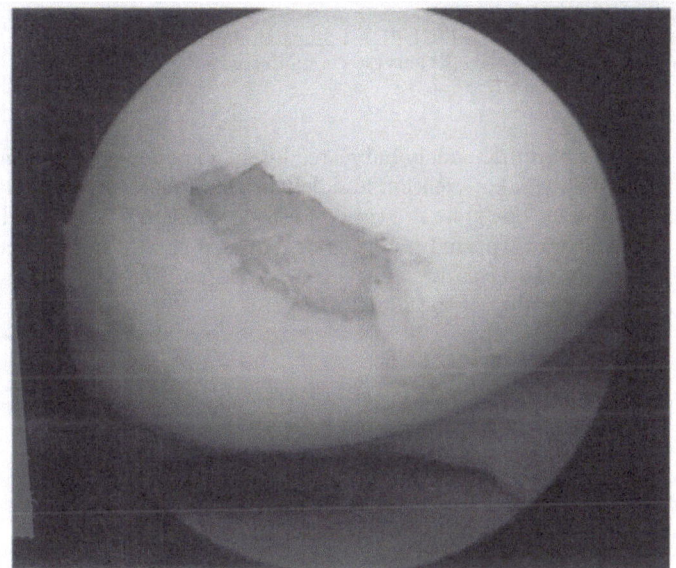

FIGURE 8.1 Curettes (**A**) or bent osteotomes (**B**) are used to debride lesion to stable borders and verticle walls.

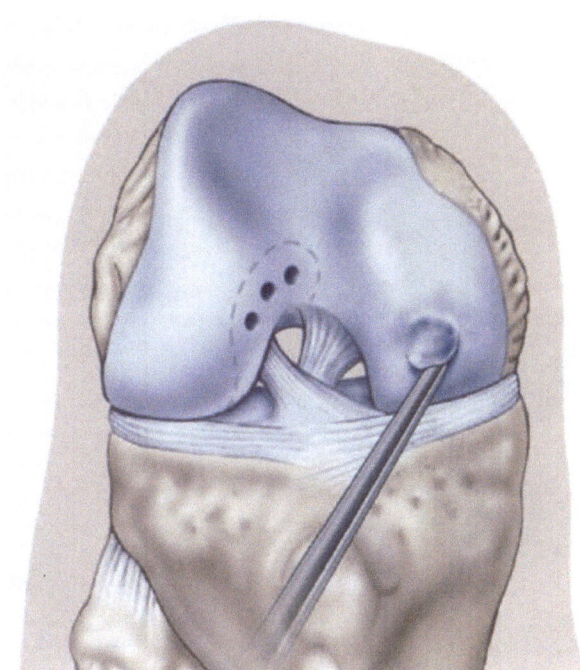

FIGURE 8.2 Notch site for graft harvest.

STEP IV: BACK TABLE HARVEST ASSESSMENT

Once harvest is complete, the graft/harvest assembly is taken to the back table where the cutter is removed. The graft can then be plunged with a metal plunger into a clear delivery tube (Figure 8.5), which should be done with the open end of the clear delivery tube stabilized on the table to prevent inadvertent graft loss. The graft is then measured for final determination of obliquity and depth to better prepare the recipient site.

STEP V: CREATION OF RECIPIENT SOCKET

The arthroscope is placed in the portal contralateral to the side of the lesion. The drill is brought in through the appropriate portal. It is advisable to first deliver the drill into the notch region to prevent iatrogenic chondral damage. The drill is positioned as perpendicularly as possible to the lesion. Occasionally, a midpatellar portal may be necessary to achieve perpendicular alignment. In cases of multiple plugs, the most posterior graft is placed first. Once the location is chosen, the drill nipple is pressed into the subchondral plate to prevent skiving (Figure 8.6). The recipient site is then drilled so that the flange is equal to the cartilage surface. The drill is removed, and the socket is cleaned with a shaver to remove bony debris.

being caught in the cutter during entry into the knee. The plunger is removed and replaced by the anvil for impacting the assembly. The cutter assembly is placed over the desired hyaline cartilage donor site. Care is required to assure that alignment is as perpendicular as possible; this should be checked by visualization around the entire harvesting device. It is important to remember that the use of a 30° arthroscope will result in some distortion of perpendicular appearance. The cutter/harvester is impacted to the 8-mm depth using a mallet (Figure 8.4A). The harvester is then rotated 360° so that the cutting tooth scores and cuts the graft 8 mm below the surface (Figure 8.4B). The device is then withdrawn and taken to the back table with the graft held in the cutter.

Donor sites may be left open or may be filled with either cancellous bone or a graft substitute. If left open, they are rapidly filled with cancellous bone and are covered with a layer of fibrocartilage.

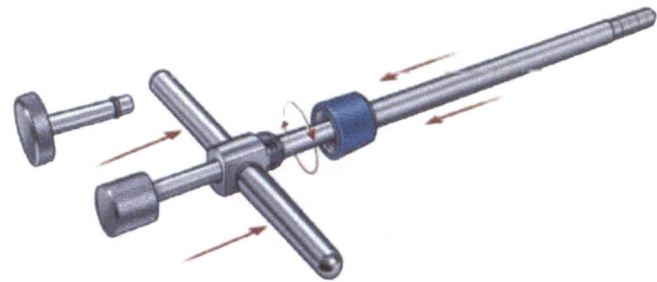

FIGURE 8.3 Assembly of graft cutter/harvester.

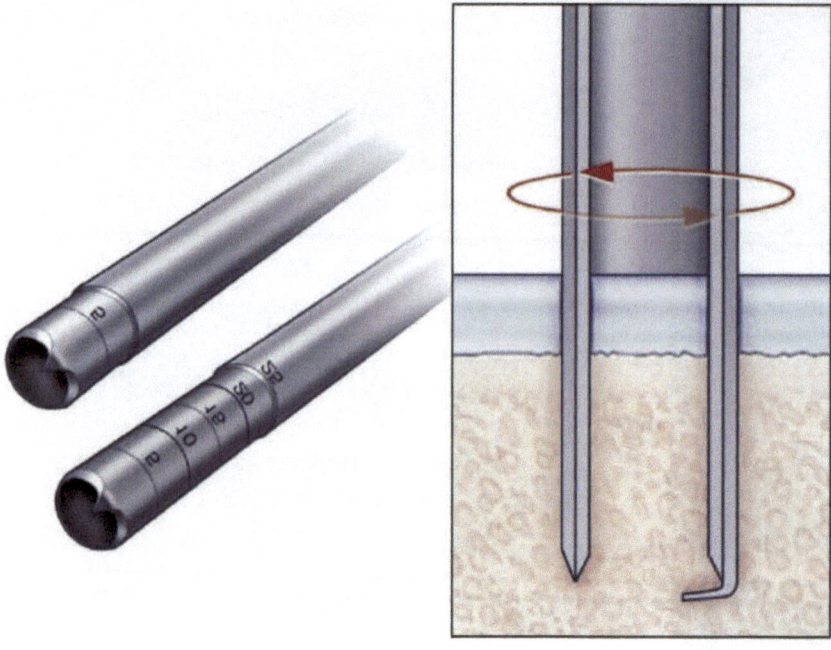

A

B

FIGURE 8.4 Impaction of **(A)** graft cutter and **(B)** harvest via tooth rotation.

STEP VI: DELIVERY OF GRAFT

The clear delivery sleeve holding the graft is placed into the knee. The sleeve is rotated to align any obliquity with the curvature of the stable surrounding cartilage. The graft is then gently impacted into position by using a plastic plunger (Figure 8.7). The graft is delivered so that all bone is below the surrounding cartilage. The sleeve is removed (Figure 8.8) and final impaction is performed to bring the graft cartilage parallel and flush with the surrounding cartilage (Figure 8.9). This alignment should be assessed with a probe.

STEP VII: MULTIPLE PLUGS

Multiple small plugs allow better radius curvature matching, but each graft will be weaker in torsional strength and more susceptible to delamination during impaction. Grafts greater than 8 mm in diameter raise concerns with harvest morbidity and radius mismatch.[11] Consequently, multiple plugs are more commonly used to fill defects. Although multiple grafts

can be simultaneously harvested by the experienced surgeon, recipient socket creation and delivery should be successfully completed one graft at a time. It is acceptable to partially drill the edge of a placed secure graft, but this should not exceed 10% of the circumference of the graft as this could cause destabilization of the remaining graft.

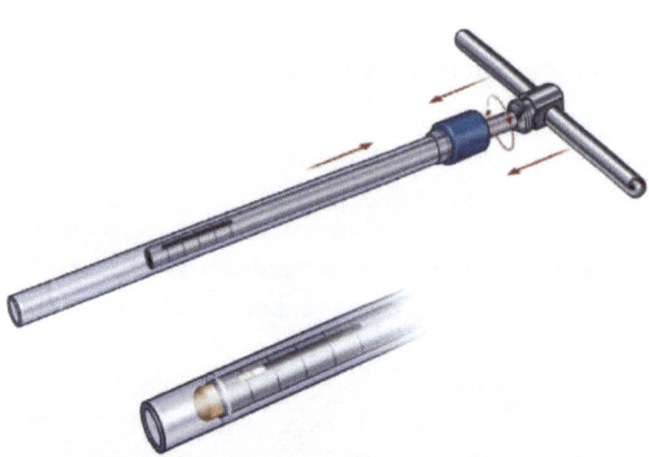

FIGURE 8.5 Deposition of graft into clear delivery tube.

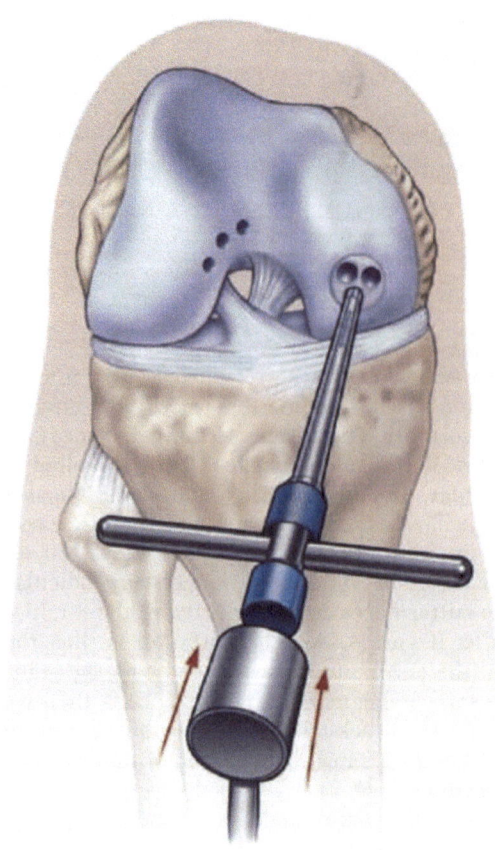

FIGURE 8.6 Schematic of drill alignment.

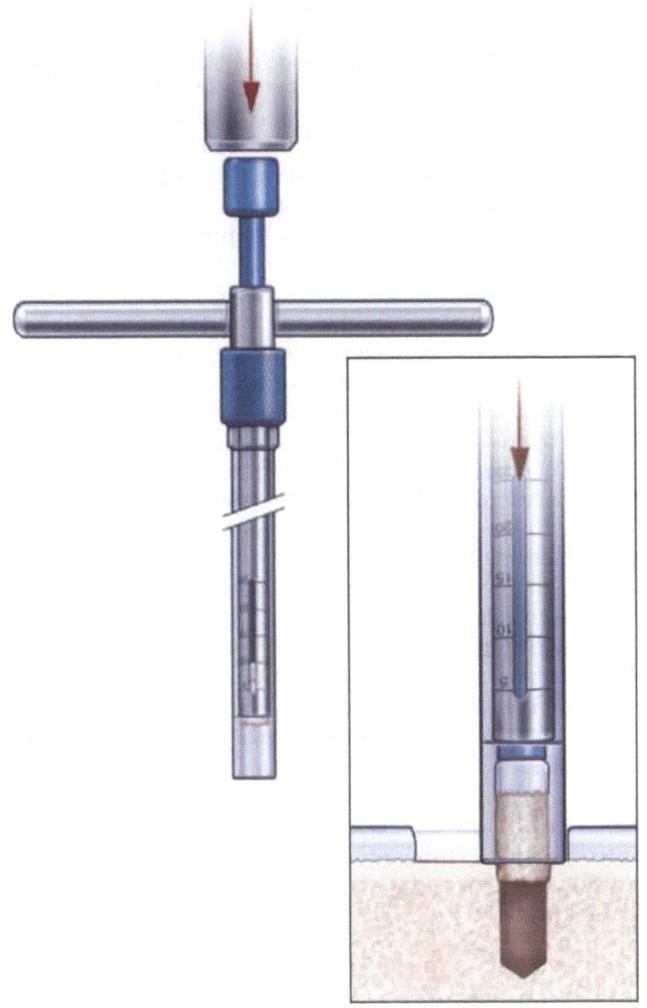

FIGURE 8.7 Schematic of graft insertion.

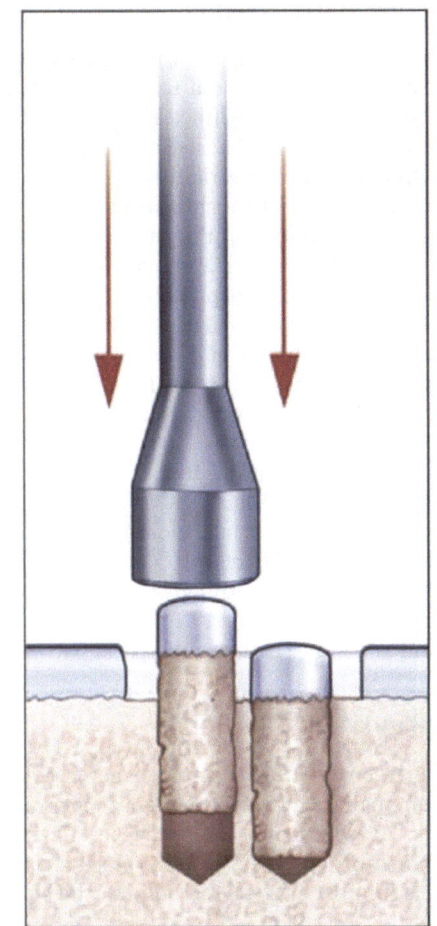

FIGURE 8.8 Schematic of final impaction of graft.

TECHNICAL PEARLS

1. Perpendicular is the rule for both harvest and implantation. Graft obliquity results in incongruent transplant that may be proud on one side and depressed on the other.

2. Miniarthrotomy does not increase surgical morbidity and can be extremely useful for achieving proper graft orientation and placement for lesions requiring multiple plugs and difficult locations.

3. Generously excise anterior synovitis and hypertrophic fat pads at the beginning of the case to facilitate visualization and prevent entrapment during graft delivery.

4. "Microtap" grafts in place to avoid heavy pressure on graft that could cause chondral delamination.

5. Visualize plug before insertion; this allows conformation of actual graft depth before drilling. Clear delivery tubes also allow for assessment of any graft obliquity. In many cases, obliquity of less than 20° can be used to match the radius of curvature of the femoral condyle if matched at insertion.

6. Remove unacceptable plugs. Do not accept poorly placed plugs. A sharp osteotome should be used to trim any proud component. In many cases, the resultant 2-mm fibrocartilage rim is acceptable, or additional smaller plugs can be used around a plug whose surface has been cut.

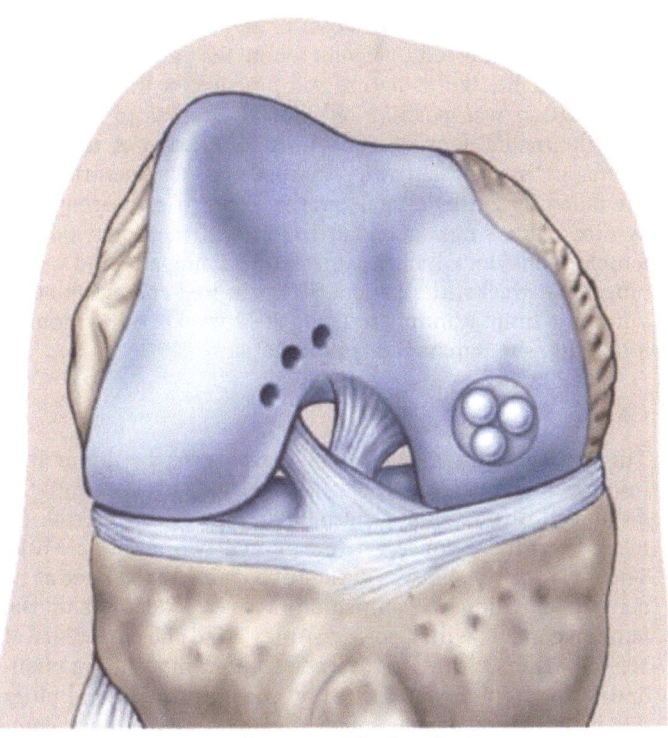

FIGURE 8.9 Schematic of final graft placement.

POSTOPERATIVE REHABILITATION

Early range of motion is important for cartilage viability and prevention of stiffness. Several factors may determine the optimal progression of weightbearing status, and treatment should be individualized. The use of a single graft plug with precise depth match and a rigid back–wall interface may allow immediate partial weightbearing, which should continue for 4 to 6 weeks. On the other hand, placement of multiple adjacent plugs or absence of a rigid back–wall interface may warrant more protection and nonweightbearing for the full 4 to 6 weeks. The following is a general protocol recommended by the authors:

0–3 weeks: nonweightbearing; full active/active assisted range of motion; passive extension; isometric strengthening

3–6 weeks: 50%, weightbearing; full range of motion, cycling, short-arc quad strengthening

6–9 weeks: full weightbearing; closed-chain and eccentric strengthening; stepper; treadmill

9–12 weeks: open-chain strengthening; activity-specific conditioning

12 weeks and beyond: return to full sports participation.

Complications

Potential early complications include hemarthrosis, persistent effusion, pain, graft fracture, graft delamination, and loose bodies. Avascular necrosis must be considered a risk, particularly if multiple deep (1–2 cm) plugs are harvested or deposited. As in most surgical techniques, the best treatment is prevention.

CASE 1

This patient is a 34-year-old woman who was a recreational runner with no acute injury. She began developing pain with running accompanied by occasional swelling. Eventually, symptoms progressed to a point where the pain was constant and toothache-like in nature and produced a limp. Clinical examination was positive only for tenderness to palpation over the medial femoral condyle at 90° flexion. A magnetic resonance image (MRI) was obtained that was negative and she failed 2 months of conservative care. At arthroscopy, an 11-mm × by 8-mm chondral lesion was identified on the femoral condyle, which was treated by using a 6- and 4-mm plug. By 6 weeks, the patient was pain free and ambulating without a limp. Running resumed at 12 weeks. At 36 months follow-up, she remained asymptomatic.

CASE 2

This patient is a 26-year-old man who was the driver in a motor vehicle accident. He reported banging his knee into the dashboard during this accident. Before surgical referral, he had 4 months of conservative care and two negative MRIs. The major complaint was of painful popping in the knee as he bent down. Clinical examination revealed tenderness on the femoral condyle with a positive Apley grind and crepetence at 45° of flexion. Arthroscopy revealed a 15-mm × 15-mm chondral lesion, which was treated by three osteochondral plugs (Figure 8.10). At 2 year follow-up, the patient's only complaint is of mild pain with weather change.

Clinical Results of Osteochondral Grafting

In 1997, Hangody et al. reported 102 cases of "mosaicplasty" using 4.5-mm-wide and 15-mm-deep cylinders obtained from the medial and lateral trochlea. At 32 months follow-up, 102 of 107 results were rated good to excellent on Hospital for Special Surgery scoring.[12,13] Using a similar technique, other investigators have reported 86% good to excellent results by using 15-mm-deep grafts.[14,15] In a multicenter study, several investigators used plugs 8 mm deep and reported marked improvement in pain and activity level in 85% of patients studied.[16,17]

In an effort to provide continuing clinical data and outcome analysis using this technique, we initiated a prospective multicenter study to follow-up 200 patients for 5 years. Lesions treated averaged 143 mm^2 (range, 80–250 mm^2). A total of 81% of repairs were performed by arthroscopy, with 19% requiring miniopen technique. All patients reported improvement with the technique and no deterioration of results has been noted at 2-year follow-up.

The long-term goal of treating chondral lesions is the prevention or delay of osteoarthricic progression. To date, no treatment option for this complex problem has shown an ability to prevent arthritic progression. The short-term goal, however, is to diminish symptoms of pain and swelling and improve function. Although additional long-term follow-up is needed, the early results presented so far have shown an overall 85% efficacy of osteochondral autografts to diminish symptomatology associated with focal chondral lesions. Osteochondral grafting offers a cost-effective, clinically successful treatment option for small (<2.5 cm^2) chondral lesions of the knee.

Recent Research

In the original descriptions of osteochondral grafting by Hangody et al., harvest sites included the femur at the medial, lateral, and superior aspects of the patellofemoral joint.[18,19] The rationale was that these areas were presumed to be "nonarticulating" and would be protected from harvest site morbidity such as accelerated cartilage degeneration. The intercondylar notch was also described as a potential harvest site in a case report by Matsusue et al. who harvested from the "lateral wall of the patellar groove, located outside the patellofemoral joint and the anterolateral side of the intercondylar area."[20]

In 1998 Simonian and coworkers[21] conducted a study with pressure-sensitive film to detect possible articular contact pressures at commonly recommended harvest sites. Their purpose was to test the theory that "nonarticulating" articular cartilage actually exists. The authors only tested the intercondylar notch and outer aspect of the lateral femoral condyle. Indeed, they did find significant contact stresses at these presumed nonarticulating areas through a functional range of knee motion. These pressures were not distributed evenly, however, and pressures in the medial intercondylar notch and superior portion of the outer aspect of the lateral femoral condyle were significantly lower than those in the inferior portion of the outer aspect of the lateral femoral condyle.

Several recent studies have called into question the conventional practice of harvesting grafts from the the lateral

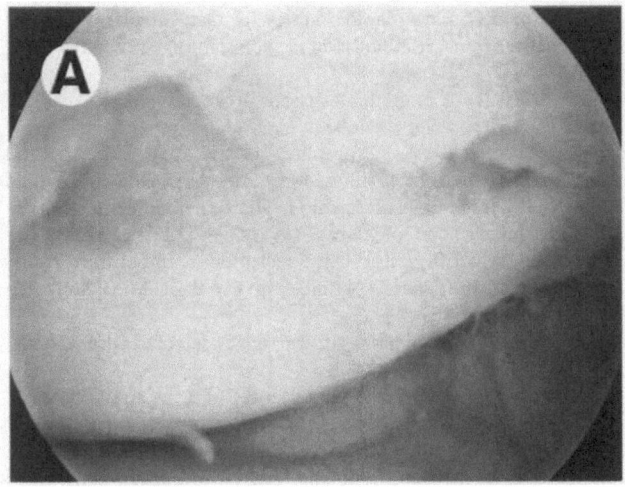
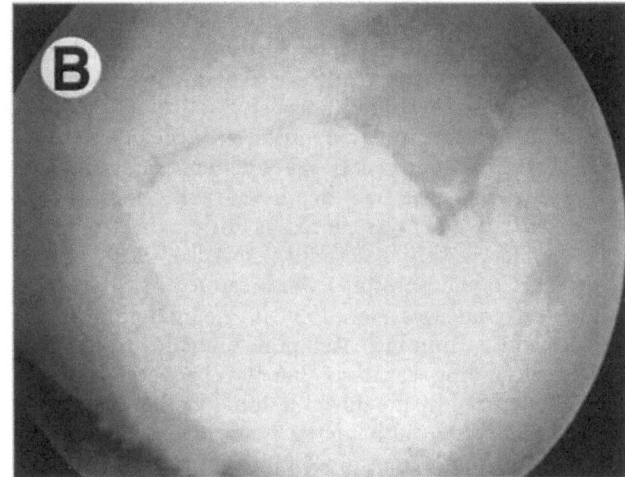
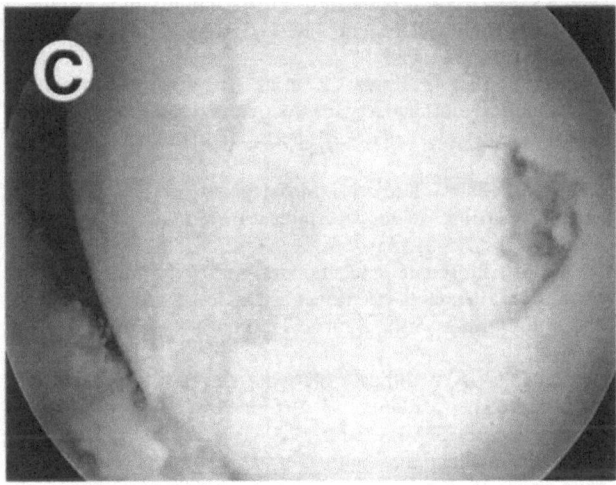

FIGURE 8.10 A. Chondral lesion after debridement to stable borders. **B.** Harvest site. **C.** Site of lesion after insertion of grafts.

femoral condyle. A cadaver study by Garretson et al.[22] on contact pressures in the patellofemoral joint revealed that although pressures are lower on the periphery of the patellofemoral articulation versus in the central trochlea, they are comparatively higher on the periphery of the lateral femoral condyle than the medial femoral condyle. Additionally, in contrast to the findings of Simonian et al., the pressures on the lateral side were found to be highest superiorly and decreased inferiorly toward the sulcus terminalis. These data suggest that perhaps grafts should be preferentially harvested from the outer aspect of the medial femoral condyle to minimize potential donor site morbidity. Furthermore, when grafts must be harvested from the lateral condyle, such as when an additional graft source is needed for large lesions, harvesting should be done inferiorly, near the sulcus terminalis.

The recommendation to harvest from the medial femoral condyle is supported by a study by Ahmad et al.[23] These investigators found that the distal medial condyle was virtually free of contact through a functional range of motion. They also found the intercondylar notch to be an acceptable graft source. Although their results lacked statistical significance, the pressures in the intercondylar notch were intermediate, being higher than the inferior medial condyle but less than the lateral femoral condyle or superior medial condyle. Further support for harvesting from the intercondylar notch lies in studies on notchplasty for ACL reconstruction that have revealed that up to 8 mm of lateral intercondylar notch can be removed without significant alteration in patellofemoral contact forces.[24]

Ahmad et al.[23] also presented the importance of matching the radius of curvature between graft and recipient site to potentially ensure better longevity of the graft. They found that central trochlear lesions were best matched by the concave grafts taken from the intercondylar notch whereas lesions on the weight-bearing surfaces of the medial and lateral femoral condyles were matched best with the convex grafts taken from the outer aspects of the medial and lateral condyles. These findings have been substantiated by Bartz et al.[25]

The importance of accuracy in placing the osteochondral grafts perpendicularly and to the correct depth cannot be overemphasized. When impacting the donor graft into the recipient site, the goal is to advance the donor graft so its chondral surface matches up with the surrounding recipient cartilage as closely as possible. Grafts that are placed proud may lead to high contact stresses on the graft, and counter-sunk grafts may not adequately provide the desired load-sharing role to the surrounding cartilage. Oblique insertion can lead to both mismatches simultaneously.

Improper graft placement may contribute to accelerated cartilage degeneration. Koh and colleagues demonstrated the effects of varying the insertion depth on joint contact pressures.[26] When the graft was placed as little as 0.5 mm proud, peak contact pressures actually exceeded those of the initial defect. Contact pressures were restored nearly to normal when the graft was placed flush. Countersinking the graft by 0.5 and 1.0 mm increased peak pressures to the immediately surrounding cartilage, but levels were still less than those produced by the initial lesion. One may conclude from this study that although it is optimal to place grafts as flush as possible, if the surgeon must err, such as in the case of a slightly oblique graft, it is preferable to counter-sink the low portion of the graft rather than leave the high side proud.

Pearce et al.[27] supported the importance of placing grafts flush with the surrounding cartilage. They performed osteo-chondral autografting in sheep and compared the bony incor-poration of plugs placed flush versus those placed proud. It has been the practice of some surgeons to place grafts slightly proud in an overreamed recipient site to allow the graft to naturally subside to an optimum level. The investi-gators found that the proud grafts produced inferior overall results. Although these grafts did settle to an acceptable level with weightbearing, they were associated with poor bony incorporation and peri-graft fissuring and fibroplasia, whereas the flush-placed grafts remained at the correct level and exhi-bited good incorporation.

Another consideration that may be important when plac-ing grafts is proper rotational orientation in regard to collagen fiber direction. Using a split-line technique, Below et al. have demonstrated that there exists a distinct longitudinal orien-tation pattern of collagen fibers in the superficial layer of hyaline cartilage.[28] Although it has yet to be proven experi-mentally, proper rotational alignment of osteochondral plugs with respect to collagen fiber direction may be important to optimize resistance to tensile forces and ensure better longevity of the graft.

FUTURE DIRECTIONS

The short-term goal of osteochondral autogenous graft trans-fer is to provide symptomatic relief from isolated chondral lesions and subsequent improvement in function. Short-term follow-up has been encouraging, and it is hoped that long-term follow-up will demonstrate continued favorable outcomes.

References

1. Ateshian GA, Lai WM, Zhu WB. An asymptotic solution for the contact of two biphasic cartilage layers. J Biomech 1994;27:1347–1360.
2. Radin EL, Ehrlich MG, Chernack R, et al. Effect of repetitive impulsive loading on the knee joints of rabbits. Clin Orthop 1978;131:288–293.
3. Thompson RC, Oegema TR, Lewis JL. Osteoarthritic changes after acute transarticular load. J Bone Joint Surg Am 1991;4:73:990–1001.
4. Judet H. Essai sur la greffe des tissus articulaires. C R Acad Sci III 1908;146:193–196, 600–603.
5. Pap K, Krompecher S. Arthroplasty of the knee. Experimental and clinical experiences. J Bone Joint Surg Am 1961;43:523–537.
6. Campbell CJ, Ishida H, Takashi H. The transplantation of artic-ular cartilage. J Bone Joint Surg Am 1963;45(1):579–1590.
7. Entin MA, Alger JR, Baird RM. Experimental and clinical trans-plantation of autogenous whole joints. J Bone Joint Surg Am 1962;44:1518–1536.
8. Campbell CJ. The healing of cartilage defects. Clin Orthop 1969;64:65.
9. McDermott AG, Langer F, Pritzker KP. Fresh small-fragment osteochondral allografts: long term follow-up study on first 100 cases. Clin Orthop 1985;197:96–102.
10. Levy AS, Lohnes J, Sculley S. Chondral delamination of the knee in soccer players. Am J Sports Med 1996;24:634–639.
11. Levy AS, Meier SW. Approach to cartilage injury in the anterior cruciate ligament-deficient knee. Orthop Clin North Am 2003;34:1–19.
12. Hangody L, Kish G, Karpati Z, et al. Arthroscopic autogenous osteochondral mosaicplasty for the treatment of femoral condy-lar articular defects. Knee Surg Sports Traumatol Arthrosc 1997;5:262–267.
13. Hangody L, Kish G, Karpati Z. Mosaicplasty for the treatment of articular cartilage defects: Application in clinical practice. Orthopedics 1998;21:751–756.
14. Bobic V. Arthroscopic ostcocliondral autograft transplantation in anterior cruciate ligament reconstruction: a preliminary clin-ical study. Knee Surg Sports Traumatol Arthrosc 1996;3:262–264.
15. Morgan CD: GAYS clinical experience and results. Presented at the American Academy of Orthopedic Surgeons Annual Conference, AOSSM Specialty. 1999; Traverse City, MI.
16. Bradley J: Osteochondral autograft transplantation clinical out-come study. In: Proceedings of the Metcalf Memorial Meeting; 1999; Sun Valley, ID.
17. Gambardella RA. Autogenous osteochondral grafting: a multi-center review of clinical results. Arthroscopy Association of North America (AANA); 1999; Vancouver, BC, Canada.
18. Hangody L, Karpati Z. [New possibilities in the management of severe circumscribed cartilage damage in the knee.] Magy Traumatol Ortop Kezseb Plasztikai Seb 1994;37:237–243. Hungarian.
19. Hangody L, Sukosd L, Szigeti I, et al. [Arthroscopic autogenous osteochondral mosaicplasty.] Magy Traumatol Ortop Kezseb Plasztikai Seb 1996;39:49–54. Hungarian.
20. Matsusue Y, Yamamuro T, Hama H. Arthroscopic multiple osteochondral transplantation to the chondral defect in the knee associated with anterior cruciate ligament disruption [case report]. Arthroscopy 1993;9:318–321.
21. Simonian PT, Sussman PS, Wickiewicz TL, Paletta GA, Warren RF. Contact pressures at osteochondral donor sites in the knee. Am J Sports Med 1998;26(4):419–494.
22. Garretson R, Katolik L, Verma N, Bach B, Cole B: Contact pres-sure at osteochondral donor sites in the patellofemoral joint. Presented at the American Academy of Orthopedic Surgeons Annual Conference, AOSSM Specialty; February, 2002; Dallas, TX.
23. Ahmad CS, Cohen ZA, Levine WN, Ateshian GA, Mow VC. Biomechanical and topographic considerations for autologous osteochondral grafting in the knee. Am J Sports Med 2001;29(2):201–206.
24. Morgan EA, McElroy JJ, DesJardins JD, et al. The effect of inter-condylar notchplasty on the patellofemoral articulation. Am J Sports Med 1996;24:843–846.

25. Bartz RL, KAmaric E, Noble PC, Lintner D, Bocell J. Topographic matching of selected donor and recipient sites for osteochondral autografting of the articular surface of the femoral condyles. Am J Sports Med 2001;29(2):207–212.

26. Koh J, Wirsing K, Lautenschlager E. The effect of graft height mismatch on contact pressure following osteochondral grafting: a biomechanical study. Presented at the American Academy of Orthopedic Surgeons Annual Conference, AOSSM Specialty Day; February, 2002; Dallas, TX.

27. Pearce SG, Hurtig MB, Clarnett R, Kalra M, Cowan B, Miniaci A. An investigation of 2 techniques for optimizing joint surface congruency using multiple cylindrical osteochondral autografts. Arthroscopy 2001;17:50–55.

28. Below S, Arnoczshy SP, Dodds J, Kooima C, Walter N. The split-line pattern of the distal femur: a consideration in the orientation of autologous cartilage grafts. Arthroscopy 2002;18: 613–617.

9

Osteochondral Allograft Transplantation

William D. Bugbee

BACKGROUND

Initial experimentation with fresh joint transplantation started with Erich Lexer in the early 1900s[1]; however, in the modern era, fresh small-fragment osteochondral allografting for the treatment of articular cartilage injury and disease began nearly three decades ago, in the 1970s. This clinical experience, along with basic scientific investigation, has provided an understanding of the rationale and support for the use of fresh osteochondral allografts. Currently, fresh osteochondral allografts are utilized to treat a broad spectrum of articular cartilage pathology, from focal chondral defects[2,3] to joints with established osteoarthrosis.[4] Most commonly, allografts have successfully treated osteochondritis dissecans (OCD),[5] osteonecrosis,[6] and posttraumatic reconstruction of the knee.[7,8] Allografts also have been utilized in the treatment of disease of the ankle joint,[9,10] as well as the hip joint.[11]

The fundamental concept governing fresh osteochondral allografting is the transplantation of architecturally mature hyaline cartilage, with living chondrocytes that survive transplantation and are thus capable of supporting the cartilage matrix. Hyaline cartilage possesses characteristics that make it attractive for transplantation. It is an avascular tissue, and therefore does not require a blood supply, meeting its metabolic needs through diffusion from synovial fluid. It is an aneural structure, as well, and does not require innervation for function. Third, articular cartilage is relatively immuno-privileged,[12] as the chondrocytes are embedded within a matrix and are relatively protected from host immune surveillance.

The second component of the osteochondral allograft is the osseous portion, which functions generally as a support for the articular cartilage as well as a vehicle to allow attachment and fixation of the graft to the host. The osseous portion of the graft is quite different from the hyaline portion, as it is a vascularized tissue, and cells are not thought to survive transplantation; rather, the osseous structure functions as a scaffold for healing to the host by creeping substitution (similar to other types of bone graft). Generally, the osseous portion of the graft is limited to a few millimeters; however,

depending on the clinical situation, the allograft may contain more extensive amounts of bone, required to restore injured or absent subchondral tissue, such as is seen in OCD, osteonecrosis, or posttraumatic reconstruction.

As a result of the foregoing concepts, it is helpful to consider a fresh osteochondral allograft as a composite graft of both bone and cartilage, with a living mature hyaline cartilage portion and a nonliving subchondral bone portion. It is also helpful to understand the allografting procedure in the context of a tissue or organ transplantation, as the graft essentially is transplanted as an intact structural and functional unit replacing a diseased or absent component in the recipient joint. The transplantation of mature hyaline cartilage obviates the need to rely on techniques that induce cells to form cartilage tissue, which are central to other restorative procedures; however, the allograft has its own set of clinical issues, including the following: complexities of acquisition, processing, and storage of the donor tissue, safety concerns with respect to disease transmission from donor tissue, immunologic behavior of the allograft, and the allograft-host bone interaction.

The cornerstone of an allografting procedure is the availability of fresh osteochondral tissue. It is important to note that currently, in fresh osteochondral allografting, the small-fragment allografts are not HLA or blood-type matched, and are utilized fresh, rather than frozen or processed. This is in contrast to grafts used in other bulk allografting or tumor-reconstructive procedures. The rationale for fresh tissue is predicated on the concept of maximizing the quality of the articular cartilage in the graft. This concept is in distinction to cases of large osseous reconstructions, where restoration of the osseous defect is the primary goal, and therefore, frozen tissue may be more appropriate. Despite numerous efforts at cryopreservation that maintains some chondrocyte viability, it has been demonstrated that the freezing process effectively eliminates more than 95% of viable chondrocytes.[13] Furthermore, clinical experience has shown that the articular matrix in frozen allografts deteriorates over time, presumably because there are no cells within the matrix to maintain tissue homeostasis.[14]

Conversely, with fresh osteochondral allografts, it has been demonstrated through retrieval studies that viable chondrocytes and relatively preserved cartilage matrix are present many years after transplantation.[15,16] These experiences have generally supported the use of fresh versus frozen tissue for small osteochondral allografts in the setting of reconstruction of chondral and osteochondral defects.

Understanding the process of tissue procurement, testing, and storage is critically important in the allografting procedure. Historically, the obstacles presented by these fundamental components have led to the development of fresh allograft programs only at specialized centers that have not only a close association with an experienced tissue bank but have put significant investment of resources into setting up protocols specific for safe and effective transplantation of fresh osteochondral tissue.

Recently, fresh osteochondral grafts have become commercially available and thus more accessible to the orthopaedic surgical community. Procurement, processing, and testing of donor tissue follows guidelines established by the American Association of Tissue Banks.[17] These guidelines include extensive donor histories as well as serologic and bacteriologic testing. The age criterion for the donor pool for fresh grafts is generally between 15 and 40 years of age. The joint surface must also pass a visual inspection for cartilage quality. These criteria ensure, but do not guarantee, acceptable tissue for transplantation. Experienced allograft surgeons often discuss particular donor characteristics with tissue bank personnel. It is extremely important to acknowledge that fresh human tissue is unique and that no two donors have the same characteristics. Therefore, strict adherence to tissue banking standards and adherence to protocols and processes in quality control are paramount. Furthermore, an essential part of the informed consent process is a discussion of the risk of bacterial or viral disease transmission.

As with any transplantation of allogeneic organs or tissue, there exists risk of transmission of infectious disease, despite donor screening and testing. Advances in serologic testing for human immunodeficiency virus (HIV) and hepatitis have improved safety, but a measurable risk does remain and both the surgeon and the patient should be well aware of the possibility for the transmission of serious disease.

In 1999, 650,000 musculoskeletal allografts, primarily processed grafts, were distributed. The number of graft-associated infections is not known with certainty, but likely represents less than 0.1%.[18] In a 20-year experience at our institution, utilizing more than 350 fresh allografts, there have been no documented cases of transmission of disease from donor to recipient. Historically, concerns about transmission of viral disease, such as HIV or hepatitis, have been most important; however, the risk of bacterial contamination and subsequent infection exists as well. The need for viable tissue precludes the ability to sterilize fresh osteochondral grafts; therefore, graft safety requires adherence to procurement protocols and results of bacterial cultures that can take up to 14 days.

The storage of osteochondral allografts, after harvesting and before implantation, is an emerging issue. Historically, centers with experience in allografting have transplanted tissue within 7 days of procurement in an effort to maximize articular cartilage health and cellular viability. Although this time frame allows for completion of most testing, it does not allow for completion of all bacteriologic tests. Recently, many tissue banking and distribution entities have developed protocols for refrigerated storage of fresh grafts for up to 42 days in an effort to improve graft availability and ease the logistic obstacles encountered in successfully completing a fresh allograft procedure. Recent studies on allograft storage have shown significant deterioration in cell viability, cell density, and metabolic activity of grafts in culture medium up to 28 days.[19,20] Conversely, the hyaline matrix appears to be relatively unperturbed. The clinical consequences of these storage-induced graft changes are yet to be determined.

The immunology of fresh osteochondral allografts is another important consideration. While it appears that hyaline cartilage is relatively immunoprivileged,[12] it is also evident that fresh unmatched osteochondral allografts do elicit a variable immune response. In a canine study comparing the immune response to fresh and frozen leukocyte antigen matched and mismatched allografts, Stevenson demonstrated that fresh mismatched osteochondral allografts generated the largest immune response.[21] Conversely, in humans, allograft retrieval studies[14,22] have consistently shown little or no histologic evidence of immunomediated pathology. In another study of fresh osteochondral allografts, 50% of individuals generated serum anti-HLA antibodies.[23] The presence of the anti-HLA antibodies correlated with inferior appearance of the graft–host interface on magnetic resonance imaging studies, suggesting that humoral immunity may play a role in the outcome of fresh allografting. Current clinical practice does not include either HLA or blood type matching of donor and recipient; however, the issue of immune behavior may ultimately become clinically relevant, and it is clearly an area where more knowledge is necessary to improve outcomes from fresh osteochondral allografting.

INDICATIONS AND CONTRAINDICATIONS

Fresh osteochondral allografts possess the ability to restore a wide spectrum of articular and osteoarticular pathology. As a result, the clinical indications cover a broad range of pathology. As is true for other restorative procedures, the careful assessment of the patient and the entire joint in addition to the defect is critical. Many proposed treatment algorithms suggest the use of allografts for large lesions (>2 or 3 cm) or for salvage in difficult reconstructive situations. In our experience, allografts can be considered as a primary treatment option for osteochondral lesions >2 cm (approximately) in diameter, as is typically seen in OCD and osteonecrosis. Additionally, allografts often are used primarily for salvage reconstruction of posttraumatic defects of the tibial plateau or the femoral condyle.[7,8] Allografts also have been utilized in the treatment of epiphyseal tumors where a significant amount of joint surface requires reconstruction. Other indications for allografting in the knee include treatment of patellofemoral chondrosis or arthrosis[24] and select cases of unicompartmental tibiofemoral arthrosis.[6] Additionally, allografts are useful as a salvage procedure when other cartilage-restorative procedures, such as microfracture, osteochondral autograft transplantation or autologous chondrocyte implantation have previously been performed.

In the ankle joint, fresh allografts are indicated in posttraumatic reconstruction, including resurfacing of the tibiotalar joint with posttraumatic arthrosis, osteonecrosis of the

TABLE 9.1 Indications for fresh osteochondral allografting.

Knee
1. Chondral lesions
   Traumatic
   Degenerative
2. Osteochondritis dissecans
3. Posttraumatic reconstruction
   Tibial plateau fracture
   Femoral condyle fracture
4. Osteonecrosis
5. Salvage of previous cartilage procedure
6. Patellofemoral chondrosis or arthrosis
7. Unicompartmental arthrosis (selected cases)

Ankle
1. Osteochondritis dissecans
2. Osteonecrosis
3. Posttraumatic arthrosis

Hip
1. Osteonecrosis
2. Osteochondral fracture

talus, and OCD lesions not amenable to other restorative procedures.[9,10] Unlike our experience in the knee, the use of fresh allografts for bipolar resurfacing of the tibiotalar joint is uniquely successful for the younger individual with end-stage arthrosis of the tibiotalar joint.

In the hip, osteochondral allografts have been utilized in the treatment of osteonecrosis of the femoral head, with mixed results.[11] Current indications are evolving and include symptomatic Ficat stage II or III lesions with limited head involvement (Steinberg classification B) that have not responded to other treatments. Fresh osteochondral allografts also may be useful in posttraumatic reconstruction of femoral head fractures or treatment of large chondral lesions, although clinical experience is limited and no published data are available.

Relative contraindications to allografting include uncorrected joint instability or uncorrected malalignment of the limb. An allograft may be considered in combination or as part of a staged procedure in these settings. In the knee, allografting should not be considered an alternative to prosthetic arthroplasty in an individual with symptoms and acceptable age and activity level for prosthetic replacement. In the younger individual, bipolar and multicompartmental allografting have been modestly successful. Advanced multicompartment arthrosis, remains a relative contraindication. to the allografting procedure. The presence of inflammatory disease, crystal-induced arthropathy, and unexplained synovitis are also considered relative contraindications. The use of fresh osteochondral allografts in individuals with altered bone metabolism, such as is seen in chronic steroid use, smoking, or even nonsteroidal antiinflammatory agents, has not been studied extensively. Results in the knee and in the hip have demonstrated mixed results in the treatment of steroid-induced Avascular Necrosis (AVN), but this may represent the extent of disease rather than the effect of steroid usage (Tables 9.1, 9.2).

TABLE 9.2 Contraindications to fresh osteochondral allografting.

1. Malalignment
2. Instability
3. Advanced osteoarthrosis of the knee
4. Inflammatory synovitis

PERIOPERATIVE CONSIDERATIONS

The surgical technique for fresh osteochondral allografting depends on the joint and surface to be grafted. Common to all fresh allografting procedures is matching the donor with recipient which is done on the basis of size. In the knee, an anteroposterior (AP) radiograph with a magnification marker is used, and a measurement of the medial-lateral dimension of the tibia, just below the joint surface, is made. This corrected measurement is utilized, and the tissue bank makes a direct measurement on the donor tibial plateau.

Alternatively, a measurement of the affected condyle can be performed. A match is considered acceptable at ±2 mm; however, it should be noted that there is a significant variability in anatomy, which is not reflected in size measurements. In particular, in treating OCD, the pathologic condyle typically is larger, wider, and flatter; therefore, a larger donor generally should be used (Figure 9.1). In the ankle, a similar measurement is made of the mediolateral dimension of the talus from an AP or mortise view, and a direct measurement is made on the talus at the time of tissue processing. Similarly, the diameter of the femoral head is measured from the radiograph and is correlated to a direct measurement on the donor.

Most femoral condyle lesions can be treated utilizing dowel-type grafts. Commercially available instruments (Arthrex, Inc, Naples, FL) to simplify the preparation, harvesting, and insertion of these grafts which may be up to 35 mm in size (Figure 9.2).

Surgical Technique

FEMORAL CONDYLE

For most femoral condyle lesions, allografting can be performed through a miniarthrotomy. If questions regarding the meniscal status, or the status of the other compartments exist, a diagnostic arthroscopy can be performed before the allografting procedure (Figure 9.3).

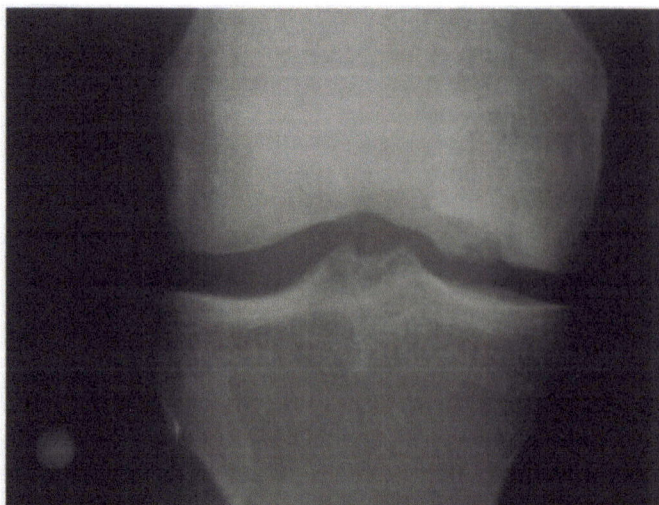

FIGURE 9.1 Osteochondritis dissecans of the medial femoral condyle. Note the relatively wide, flat contour of the condyle.

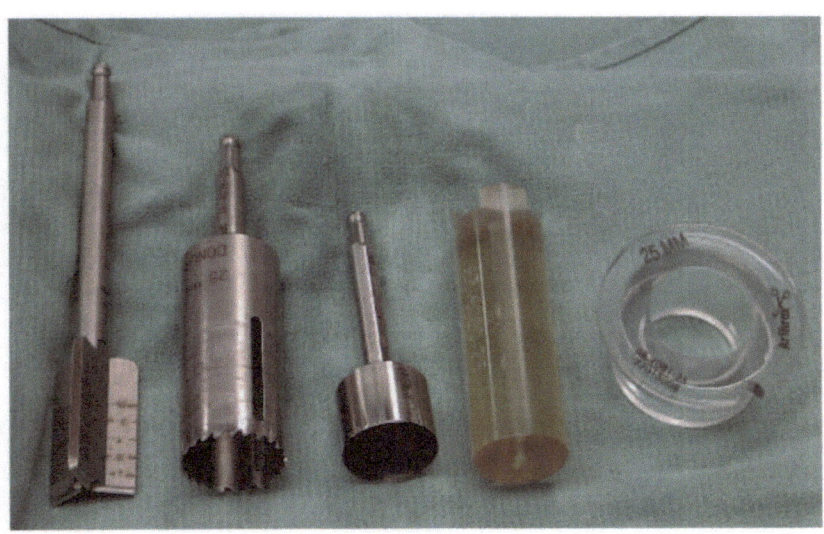

FIGURE 9.2 Surgical instruments for preparing dowel-type allografts.

The patient is positioned supine, with a tourniquet on the thigh. A leg holder is valuable in this procedure, to position the leg in between 70° and 100° of flexion to access the lesion. Before incision, the fresh graft is placed in chilled saline and inspected to confirm the adequacy of the size match and tissue quality.

A standard midline incision is made from the center of the patella to the tip of the tibial tubercle. Depending on the location of the lesion (either medial or lateral), a retinacular incision is then made from the superior aspect of the patella inferiorly. Great care is taken to enter the joint and incise the fat pad without disrupting the anterior horn of the meniscus. In some cases where the lesion is posterior or very large, the meniscus must be taken down; and generally, this can be done safely, leaving a small cuff of tissue adjacent to the anterior attachment of the meniscus for later repair.

Once the joint capsule and synovium have been incised and the joint has been entered, retractors are placed medially and laterally to expose the condyle (Figure 9.4). Care is taken for positioning the retractor within the notch to protect the cruciate ligaments and articular cartilage. The knee is then flexed or extended until the proper degree of flexion is noted that presents the lesion into the arthrotomy site. Excessive degrees of flexion limit the ability to mobilize the patella. The lesion is inspected and palpated with a probe to determine the extent, margins, and maximum size. A guidewire is driven into the center of the lesion, perpendicular to the curvature of the articular surface. The size of the proposed graft then is determine utilizing sizing dowels and a special reamer is used to remove the remaining articular cartilage and 3 to 4 mm of subchondral bone (Figure 9.5). In deeper lesions, the pathologic bone is removed until there is healthy, bleeding bone. Generally, the preparation does not exceed 6 to 10 mm, and usually bone grafting is performed to fill any deeper or more extensive osseous defects. After removal of the guide pin, depth measurements are made in the four quadrants of the prepared recipient site.

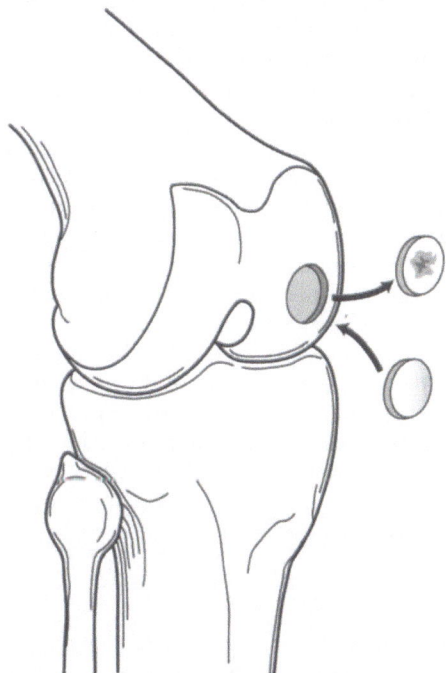

FIGURE 9.3 Femoral condyle allografting.

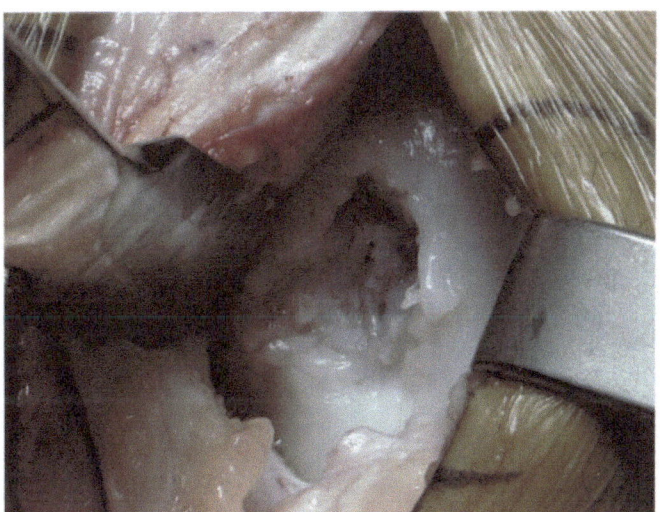

FIGURE 9.4 Exposure of lesion in medial femoral condyle.

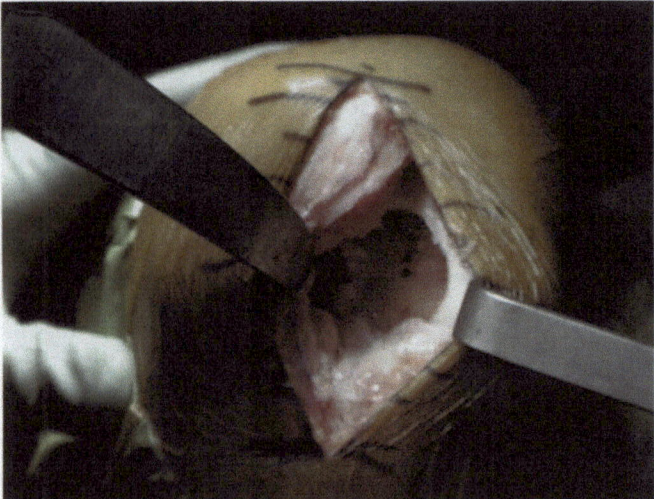

FIGURE 9.5 Recipient size after preparation and removal of diseased cartilage and bone.

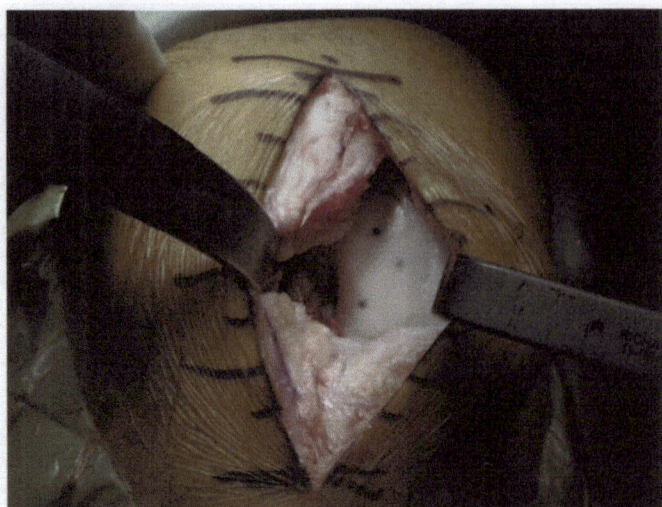

FIGURE 9.7 Graft is inserted and, in this case, fixed with three absorbable pins.

The corresponding anatomic location of the recipient site then is identified on the graft. The graft is placed into a graft holder (or alternately, held with bone-holding forceps). A saw guide then is placed perpendicular to the articular surface and the appropriate-sized tube saw is used to core the graft. Once the graft is removed, depth measurements are transferred to the graft. The graft is cut with an oscillating saw and then trimmed with a rasp to the appropriate thickness in all four quadrants (Figure 9.6). The graft should be irrigated copiously with high-pressure lavage to remove all marrow elements.

The graft is then inserted by hand in the appropriate rotation and gently tamped in place until flush. If the graft does not fit, the recipient site can be dilated or the graft modified as needed. Once the graft is seated, a determination is made whether additional fixation is required. Typically, absorbable pins are utilized, particularly for larger or uncontained grafts (Figure 9.7). Often, the graft needs to be trimmed in the notch region to prevent impingement. The knee is then brought through a complete range of motion to confirm graft stability and to assess for catching or soft-tissue obstruction.

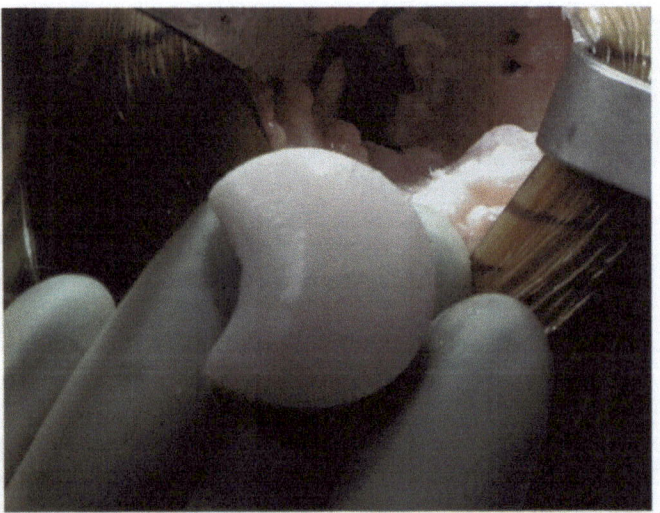

FIGURE 9.6 Prepared graft. Note the shape corresponds to the curvature of the medial femoral notch.

TROCHLEAR ALLOGRAFTS

The anatomy of the trochlea is more complex leading to technical issues in creating symmetric matching of the recipient and donor. In this setting, care is taken to match the anatomic location and the angle of approach as most larger grafts are elliptical in shape because of the anatomy of the trochlear groove. Cases of patellofemoral arthrosis where the entire trochlea is removed are performed similar to arthroplasty with resection of the anterior femur. The graft is osteotomized similarly and is fixed in place with interfragmentary screws both medially and laterally. Great care must be taken not to thin the graft in the central portion of the trochlea to prevent graft fracture.

PATELLAR ALLOGRAFTS

The patella is often resurfaced in its entirety when using an osteochondral allograft. In this setting, a technique similar to that used in arthroplasty resurfacing is utilized. Patellar thickness is first measured, and resection of the articular surfaces is performed, maintaining at least 12 to 15 mm of residual patellar bone. The graft is then osteotomized freehand in a similar fashion ensuring minimal thickness of the medial and lateral facets which generally results in a maximal thickness of 10 to 12 mm. The graft is seated in appropriate position and rotation, and tracking is noted. The patellar graft can be moved a few millimeters on the recipient surface to optimize patellar tracking. Fixation typically is performed with interfragmentary screw fixation from the anterior surface of the patella into the median ridge of the graft which has adequate bone for small-screw purchase. An extensive lateral release is routinely performed and proximal or distal patellar realignment is optional. Smaller patellar lesions can be treated with dowel-type grafts with a technique similar to that for the femoral condyle.

TIBIAL PLATEAU ALLOGRAFTS

Surgical technique of tibial plateau allografting utilizes principles similar to those in unicompartmental arthroplasty (Figures 9.8–9.10). The tibial plateau graft typically can be

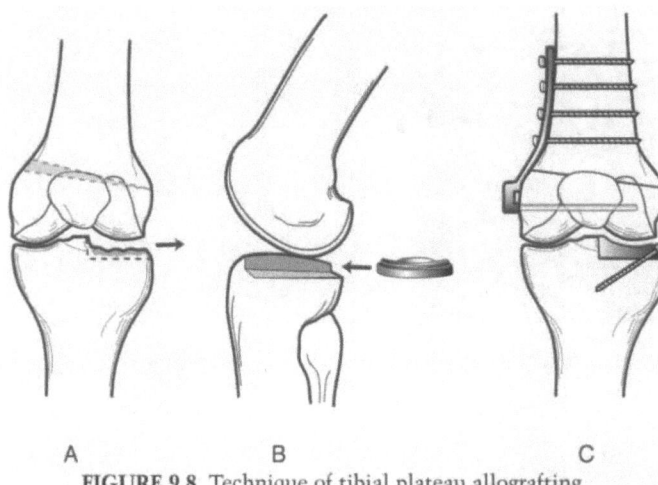

A   B   C

FIGURE 9.8 Technique of tibial plateau allografting.

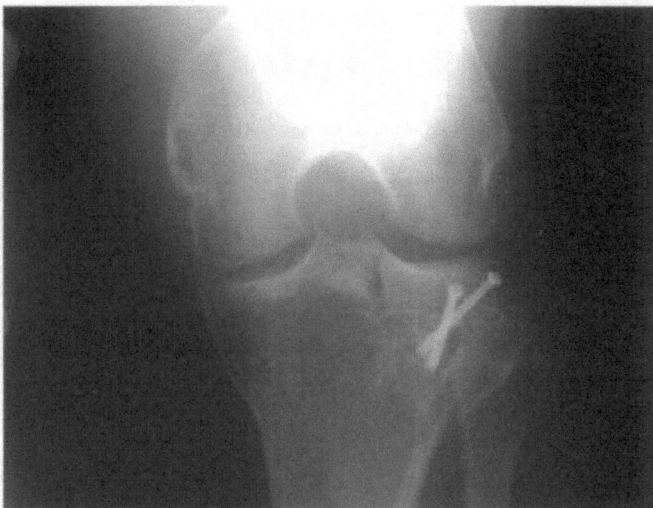

FIGURE 9.10 Post-operative radiograph after lateral tibial plateau allograft. Note restoration of height of plateau. No osteotomy was performed in this case.

performed through an arthrotomy that does not require patellar eversion. The cruciate ligament and meniscal attachments are preserved. Fluoroscopy is utilized extensively in this procedure. Two guidewires are placed in the tibial metaphyseal bone paralleling the desired slope and depth of resection of the diseased tibial surface. The more central pin also acts as a guide for the level of vertical resection of the tibia and the anteroposterior direction of the cut. After placement of the pins is confirmed, a freehand cut is made, resecting a minimal amount of subchondral bone. After removal of all diseased or damaged tissue, particularly in the back of the joint, the knee is brought into appropriate alignment and the width of the resected surface is measured as is the joint space gap from the femoral condyle to the resected surface. This provides an estimate of the required allograft thickness. The tibial allograft then is placed in the graft holder, and the desired thickness is measured and marked on the graft. Typically, grafts are at least 12 mm thick, with a minimum of 10 mm. A reciprocating saw cut is then made, and when meniscal transplantation is performed, this includes the meniscal attachments. An oscillating saw cut then is made, utilizing the guidemarks placed on the graft margins.

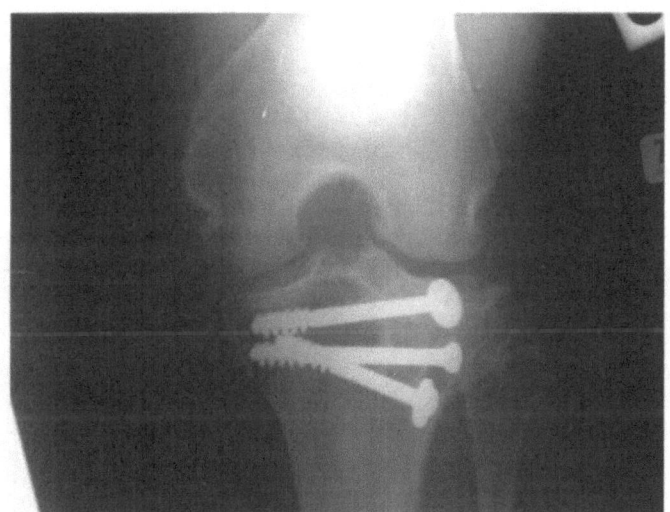

FIGURE 9.9 Radiograph of 42-year-old woman with malunion of lateral tibial plateau fracture.

At this point, the graft is measured for appropriate width and length and often needs to be thinned in the mediolateral direction. Trimming is performed as necessary and the graft is lavaged. The knee is brought into flexion and an unloading stress of the compartment is applied. The graft is gently placed under the femoral condyle taking care not to entrap the native meniscus or to ensure that the associated allograft meniscus is seated under the condyle. The knee is then brought through a range of motion, and the graft is visualized both clinically and under fluoroscopy for appropriate position and restoration of the joint line and slope. Revisions are made as necessary. Grafts are fixed with interfragmentary screw fixation from the submeniscal articular margin at the midcoronal and anterior positions. The meniscus is sutured in a standard fashion. It is vitally important to ensure graft stability and to prevent mechanical overload either by overstuffing or underfilling the compartment which may create an angular deformity with excessive graft stress.

ANKLE ALLOGRAFTS

The surgical procedure for ankle allografting depends on the surfaces to be grafted (Figures 9.11–9.14). Focal lesions of the talus are amenable to either anterior arthrotomy or in some cases may require a medial malleolar or fibular osteotomy to access more posterior medial or lateral talar lesions, respectively. These lesions generally can be treated with small dowel-type allografts as described in treating the femoral condyle lesions. In cases of extensive talar involvement such as large necrotic segments from osteonecrosis or large OCD lesions, half or the entire talar articular surface is replaced. An anterior arthrotomy is performed and the talar dome is resected under fluoroscopic guidance from the articular margin anteriorly to posteriorly. The talar graft then is resected freehand in a similar manner using the anterior articular margin to the posterior articular margin as landmarks. This generally creates a maximum graft thickness at the center of the talar dome of between 10 and 13 mm. The graft is inserted under the tibial plafond by bringing the foot into maximum

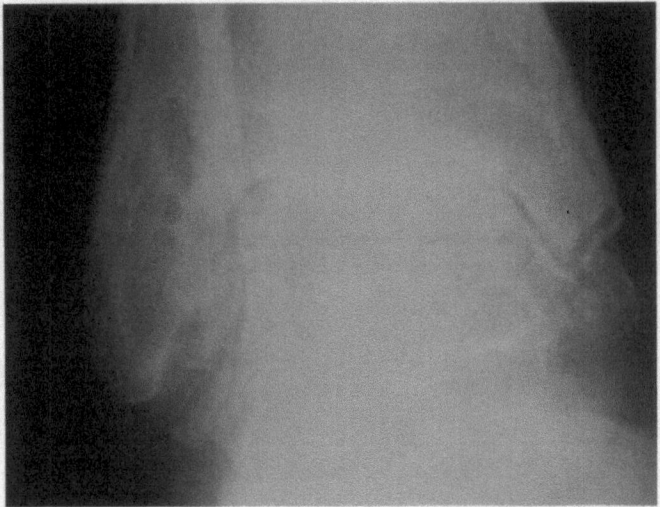

FIGURE 9.11 AP/lateral radiograph of posttraumatic tibiotalar arthrosis.

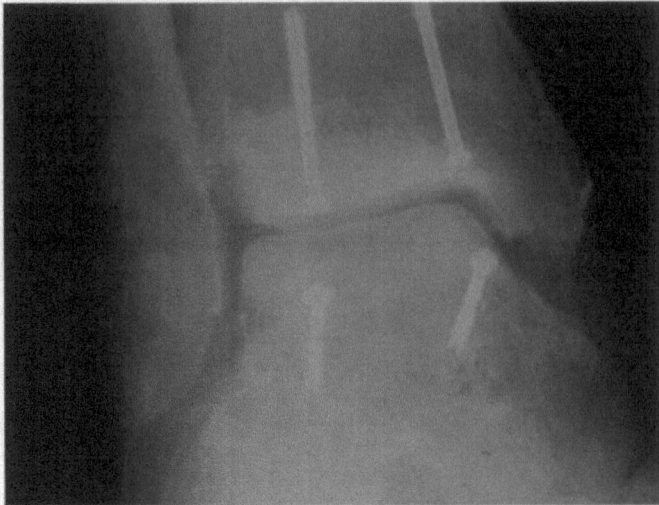

FIGURE 9.13 Postoperative radiograph after bipolar ankle allografting.

plantar flexion. In many cases, the use of an external fixator for distraction facilitates graft insertion.

Bipolar allografting of the tibiotalar joint is the most complex of the fresh allografting procedures. The procedure essentially parallels that utilized for prosthetic replacement of the ankle.[10] Initially, an external fixator is placed on the medial side of the ankle and the ankle is distracted. An extensile anterior arthrotomy is performed, and the joint is entered. Under fluoroscopic guidance, the Agility Ankle Jig with the appropriate-sized cutting block is placed on the ankle (DePuy, Warsaw, IN, USA). Matched resections of the tibial and talar surface are performed with the joint in neutral and the ankle distracted 6 mm to 10 mm. Great care is taken to avoid over-resection of the medial malleolus or injury to neurovascular structures.

The resected diseased surfaces are removed and the graft is measured. The tibia and talar grafts are prepared sepa-rately. The next larger size cutting jig (i.e., recipient cut with size 2, donor with size 3) is placed onto the tibial graft in appropriate position and rotation under fluoroscopic guidance. Great care is taken to match rotation, slope, and position as precise fitting of this graft is critical. The talus is resected freehand utilizing the anterior and posterior articular margins as a reference with a goal of resecting a maximum of 10 to 12 mm. Once these grafts are prepared, the composite thickness is measured and compared to the resection gap of the recipient. The grafts are irrigated and trial fittings are performed. Commonly, the medial malleolus requires trimming. The external fixation and distraction is removed and the ankle is brought through range of motion to help center the grafts. Fluoroscopy is used to ensure that the tibial and talar grafts are centered appropriately and a check for anteroposterior impingement is performed. The grafts are fixed with small-fragment screws or pins.

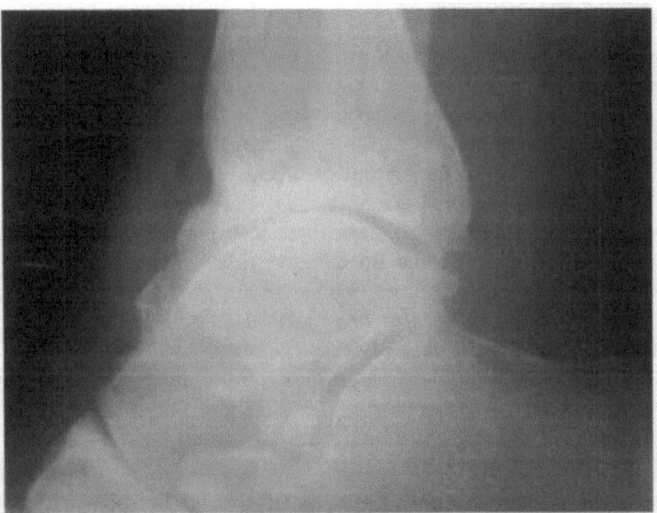

FIGURE 9.12 Posttraumatic AP/lateral radiograph of another tibiotalar arthrosis.

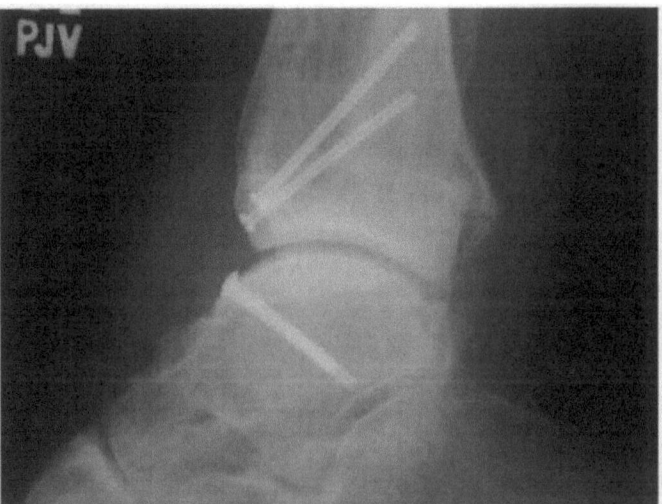

FIGURE 9.14 Another bipolar allografted ankle shown in postoperative radiograph.

TABLE 9.3 General surgical principles of allografting.
1. Careful consideration of patient and surgeon goals.
2. Assessment of biologic and mechanical environment of joint.
3. Adequate confirmation of appropriateness of lesion for fresh osteochondral allografting.
4. Careful informed consent process, including risks of infection and disease transmission.
5. Confirm graft recipient match, in both size and side.
6. Review other graft characteristics, including donor age, history, and length of graft storage time since harvest.
7. Inspect graft material before making incision.
8. Be prepared to prepare graft and recipient with a freehand technique, if necessary.
9. Utilize fluoroscopy to confirm the clinical perspective, particularly with tibia, patella, and ankle allografts.
10. Minimize the osseous portion of the allograft at 3–6 mm, except in the tibial plateau and tibiotalar joint, where minimal graft thickness should be 10 mm.
11. Always remove all soft tissue and perform pressurized lavage of graft before insertion.
12. Avoid excessive impacting of the graft during insertion.
13. Use adjunctive fixation, including absorbable pins or screws. Adequate fixation is essential.

TABLE 9.4 Femoral condyle allograft: postoperative regimen.
1. Nonweight bearing 6–12 weeks
2. Range-of-motion exercises
3. Quad sets
4. Stationary bicycle at 4 weeks
5. Progressive weight bearing beginning 8–12 weeks
6. Sports/recreation at 6 months

HIP ALLOGRAFTS

Allografting of the hip is generally performed through an anterior or anterolateral approach with gentle anterior dislocation of the femoral head. Typically most lesions are anterosuperior and this step facilitates visualization and exposure. Debridement of the lesion is performed and the graft is fashioned either utilizing instruments to create a dowel-type graft or performed freehand utilizing small power burrs and cutting instruments. Fixation of these grafts is typically with pins or screws through the articular surface (Table 9.3).

POSTOPERATIVE MANAGEMENT AND REHABILITATION

In the knee, early postoperative management includes reduction of pain and swelling and restoration of limb control and range of motion. Patients are made touch-down weight bearing for a minimum of 6 weeks and typically closer to 8 to 12 weeks depending on the size and stability of the graft. Patients with patellofemoral grafts are permitted to weight bear as tolerated in extension and generally are limited to 45° of flexion for the first four weeks utilizing an immobilizer or range-of-motion brace. Tibial or bipolar grafts and those with an associated osteotomy are fitted with a range-of-motion brace to control varus/valgus stress. Tibial grafts with associated meniscal allograft are often limited to 90° of flexion for the initial 6 weeks. Weight bearing is progressed slowly between the second and fourth month, with full weight bearing utilizing a cane or crutch. Full weight bearing and normal gait pattern are generally tolerated between the third and fourth month. Recreation and sports are not reintroduced until joint rehabilitation is complete and radiographic healing has been demonstrated which generally occurs no earlier than 6 months postoperatively (Table 9.4).

Continuous passive motion use is considered optional and often is used only in the hospital setting. Restoration of range of motion and quadriceps/hamstring function with isometrics and avoidance of open-chain exercises are empha-

sized early in the rehabilitation protocol. Stationary cycling and pool therapy are begun at 4 to 6 weeks.

Clinical follow-up includes radiographs at 4 to 6 weeks, 3 months, 6 months, and yearly thereafter. Careful radiographic assessment of the graft–host interface is important. Any concern of delayed healing should lead to a more cautious approach to weight bearing and other high-stress activities.

The protocol following ankle allografting includes the use of a bulky splint to control swelling and allow wound healing for the first 1 to 2 weeks. A fracture brace or removable cast is then employed and nonweight-bearing is maintained for as long as 3 months for large and bipolar allografts. Gentle range-of-motion exercises are performed three to four times a day with avoidance of excessive force at the extremes of motion which may stress the graft-host interface. At 6 weeks attention is given to increasing range of motion, particularly in dorsiflexion and to Achilles tendon stretching. Progressive weight bearing begins first in the fracture brace at 3 months and then out of the brace at 4 months. A cane is often utilized at this time. Unprotected weight bearing begins between 4 and 6 months if radiographic confirmation of interface healing is demonstrated.

Typically, patients will demonstrate continued incremental clinical improvement over the first postoperative year. A plateau in recovery typically can be expected at 1 year although patients often demonstrate continued functional improvement between years one and two. Often, this depends on patient motivation, desired activities, and persistence with the rehabilitation program.

COMPLICATIONS OF FRESH OSTEOCHONDRAL ALLOGRAFTING

Early Complications

Early complications unique to the allografting procedure are few. There does not appear to be any increased risk of surgical site infection with the use of allografts as compared with other procedures. The use of a miniarthrotomy in the knee decreases the risk of postoperative stiffness. Occasionally, one sees a persistent effusion which is typically a sign of overuse but may indicate an immune-mediated synovitis. Delayed union or nonunion of the fresh allograft is the most common early finding and is evidenced by persistent discomfort and/or visible graft–host interface on serial radiographic evaluation. Delayed union or nonunion is more common in larger grafts, such as those used in the tibial plateau or in the setting of compromised bone such as in the treatment of osteonecrosis. In this setting, patience is essential and complete healing or recovery may require an extended period. Decreasing activities, the institution of weight-bearing precautions, bracing, and possible use of external bone stimulators may be helpful in the early management of a delayed healing. In this setting, careful evaluation of serial radiographs can provide insight into the healing process; MRI scans are rarely helpful, particularly before 6 months postoperatively as they typically show extensive signal abnormality that is difficult to interpret.

It should be noted that with adequate attention to postoperative weight-bearing restrictions and adequate graft fixation, delayed union or nonunion requiring repeat surgical intervention within the first year is extremely uncommon. The natural history of the graft that fails to osseointegrate is unpredictable. Clinical symptoms may be minimal, or there may be progressive clinical deterioration and radiographic evidence of fragmentation, fracture, or collapse This is most commonly seen in grafts of the tibial plateau or ankle joint. Typical symptoms of this type of graft failure include a sudden onset of increased pain often associated with minor trauma. Effusion, crepitus, or focal, localized pain are commonly seen. Careful evaluation of serial radiographs typically will demonstrate collapse, subsidence, fracture, or fragmentation. CT scans or MRI also can be utilized to confirm graft failure. Treatment of this type of graft failure generally requires either allograft revision or, in cases of more extensive disease, conversion to arthroplasty or arthrodesis in severe cases in which the graft was used as a salvage.

Late Complications

Requisite of a successful fresh allograft procedure is healing of the host–graft bony interface and integration of the host bone into the osseous portion of the allograft (Figures 9.15–9.17). This process of so-called creeping substitution is well described in the paradigm of bone-graft healing. Revascularization of the allograft bone by the host may take many years and may occur incompletely.[22] The amount of bone within the allograft may be important in this process, and it is likely that thinner grafts will have more complete revascularization than thicker grafts. Retrieval studies of failed fresh osteochondral allografts have provided tremendous insight into the allograft healing process and have led to the understanding that fresh osteochondral allografts rarely fail because of the cartilage portion of the graft.[14–16,22] These studies suggest that most failures originate within the osseous portion of the graft or from progression of osteoarthrosis. It is likely that late allograft failure, which has been seen between 2 and 17 years, is the result of graft subsidence, collapse or fragmentation. Fragmentation may be due to fatigue failure very much like that seen with bulk allografts placed under repetitive loading situations.

The prospects of late failure underscores the need to pay close attention to joint alignment and stability in the initial treatment of the patient. Clinically, with late failure, the patient presents with new pain or mechanical symptoms of either insidious or acute onset. Radiographs may show cysts, sclerosis, or subchondral collapse. Collapse typically occurs in the center of the graft which may be most distant from the revascularization process or in an area that has been under excessive loads. Again, careful review of serial radiographs is important. MRI also may be useful and generally is obtained to confirm the allograft pathology and to rule out other sources of pain or sites of pathology in the knee joint. It is

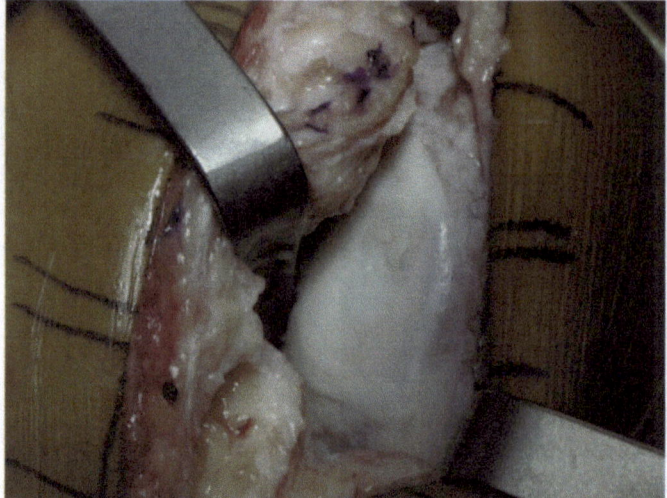

FIGURE 9.15 Failed medial femoral condyle allograft. Note relatively preserved cartilage and depressed central portion of graft.

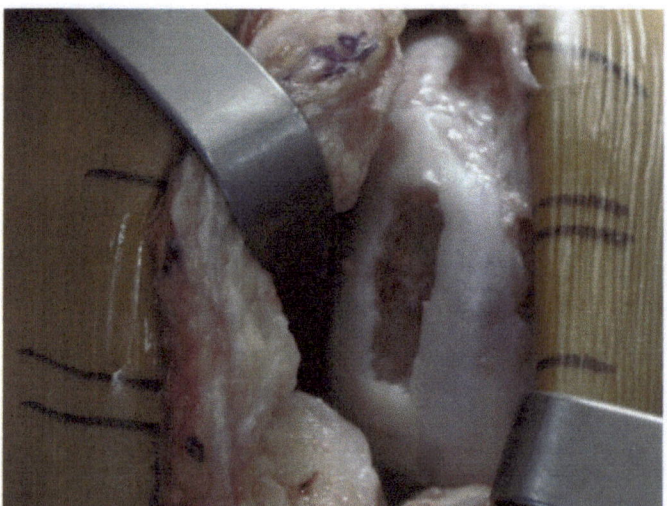

FIGURE 9.16 Failed graft after debridement to healthy, bleeding bone. The periphery of graft remains intact.

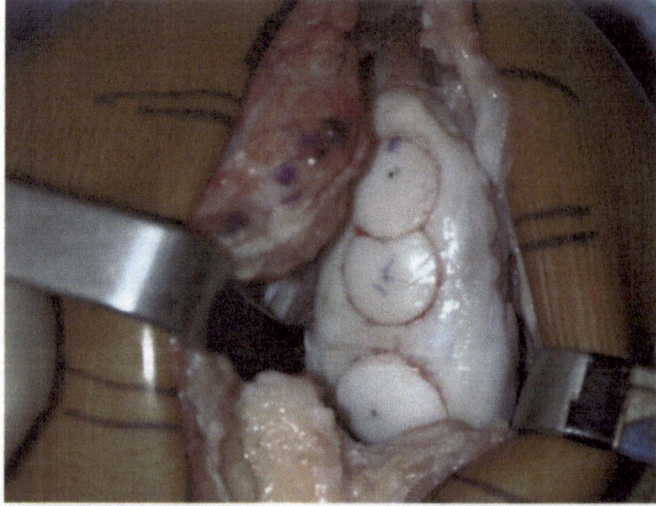

FIGURE 9.17 After revision allografting and primary grafting of satellite posterior lesion.

TABLE 9.5   Results of fresh osteochondral allografting.

Author	Site	Diagnosis	Number	Mean follow-up (years)	Successful outcome
Ghazavi[7]	Knee	Trauma	126	7.5	85% survivorship
Meyers[2]	Knee	Multiple	31	3.5	77%
Chu[3]	Knee	Multiple	55	6.2	84% G/E
Aubin[8]	Femur	Trauma	60	10.0	85% survivorship
Garrett[5]	f. c.	OCD	17	2–9	16/17
Bugbee[25]	f. c.	OCD	69	5.2	80% G/E
Bugbee[6]	Knee	Arthrosis	41	4.5	54% G/E
Jamali[24]	p-f	Multiple	29	4.5	52%
Gross[9]	Talus	OCD	9	12.0	6/9
Kim[10]	Ankle	Arthrosis	7	10.0	4/7

f. c., femoral condyle; (p-f, patellofemoral; OCD, osteochondritis dissecans; G/E, good/excellent.

important to note that the allografted joint may suffer from the same pathology that is present in any other joint, such as meniscus or ligamentous injury. It should also be noted that radiographic and magnetic resonance abnormalities are commonly noted even in well-functioning allografts[23] and therefore, decision making is guided by strict correlation of imaging studies with clinical findings.

Treatment options for failed allografts include observation if the patient is minimally symptomatic and the joint is thought to be at low risk for further progression of disease. Arthroscopic evaluation and debridement also may be utilized.[6,7] Fresh allografting does not preclude a revision allograft as a salvage procedure for failure of the initial allograft. In many cases, revision allografting is performed and generally has led to a success rate equivalent to primary allografting. In cases of more extensive joint disease, particularly in older individuals, conversion to prosthetic arthroplasty is appropriate (Table 9.5).

RESULTS

Fresh osteochondral allografts are most commonly utilized in the treatment of OCD of the femoral condyle (Figures 9.18–9.20). These lesions typically are large and involve the subchondral bone, characteristics that make allografting attractive because the graft can address both the osseous and the chondral components of the lesion.

Garrett[5] first reported on 17 patients treated with fresh osteochondral allografts for OCD of the lateral femoral condyle. All patients had failed previous surgery, and in a 2- to 9-year follow up period, 16 of 17 patients were reported as asymptomatic. Most recently, we reviewed our experience in the treatment of OCD of the medial and lateral femoral condyle.[25] Sixty-nine knees in 66 patients were evaluated at a mean of 5.2 years postoperatively. All allografts were implanted within 5 days of procurement. Patients were prospectively evaluated using an 18-point modified D'Aubigne and Postel scale, and subjective assessment was performed with a patient questionnaire. In this group, there were 49 males and 17 females, with a mean age of 28 years (range, 15–54). Forty lesions involved the medial femoral condyle and 29 the lateral femoral condyle. An average of 1.6 surgeries had been performed on the knee before the allograft procedure. Allograft size was highly variable, with a range

from 1 to 13 cm^2. The average allograft size was 7.4 cm^2. Two knees were lost to follow-up. Overall, 53/67 (79%) knees were rated good or excellent, scoring 15 or above on the 18-point scale; 10/67 (15%) were rated fair; and 6/67 (6%) were rated poor. The average clinical score improved from 13.0 preoperatively to 15.8 postoperatively (p < 0.01). Six patients had reoperations on the allograft: 1 was converted to total knee arthroplasty; and 5 underwent revision allografting at 1, 2, 5, 7, and 8 years after the initial allograft. Forty-nine of 66 patients completed questionnaires: 96% reported satisfaction with their treatment; 86% reported less pain. Subjective knee function improved from a mean of 3.5 to 7.9 on a 10-point scale.

Chu et al.[3] reported on 55 consecutive knees undergoing osteochondral allografting. This group included patients with diagnoses such as traumatic chondral injury, avascular necrosis, OCD, and patellofemoral disease. The mean age of this group was 35.6 years, with follow-up averaging 75 months (range, 11–147 months). Of the 55 knees, 43 were unipolar replacements and 12 were bipolar resurfacing replacements. On an 18-point scale, 42 of 55 (76%) of these knees were rated good to excellent, and 3 of 55 were rated fair, for an overall success rate of 82%. It is important to note that 84% of the

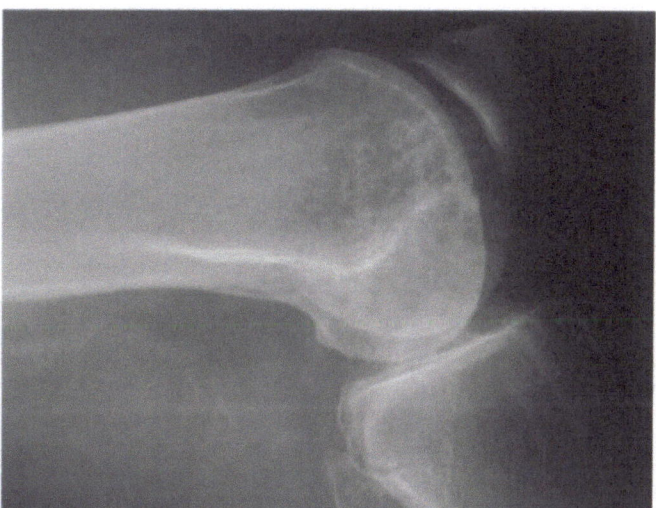

FIGURE 9.18 Femoral condyle allograft eight years post-operative. Note osseous incorporation of graft.

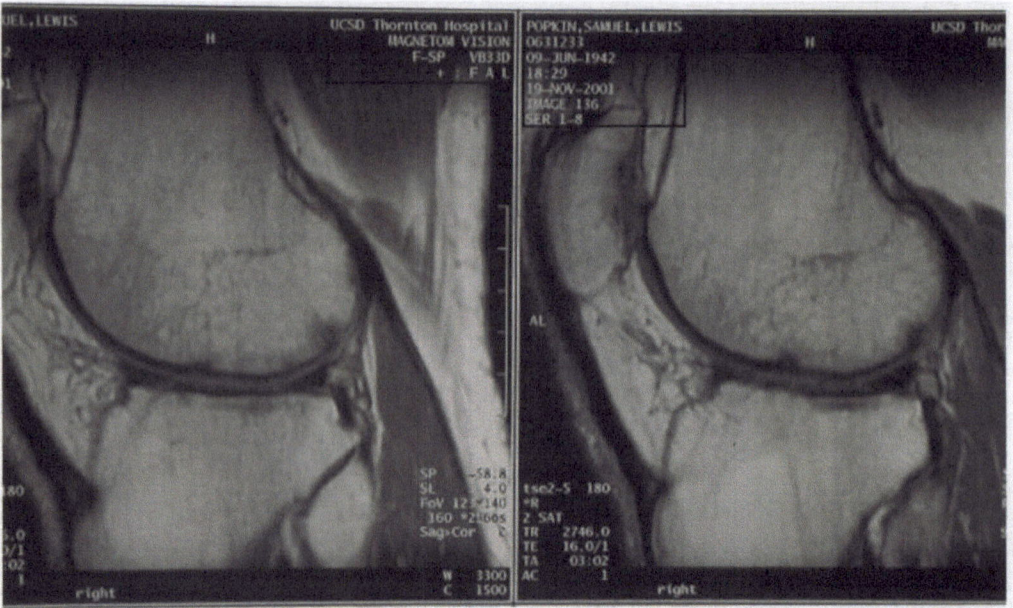

FIGURE 9.19 MRI of same graft shown in Fig. 18. Note the signal homogeneity and preservation of articular surface.

knees that underwent unipolar femoral grafts were rated good to excellent, and only 50% of the knees with bipolar grafts achieved good or excellent status.

Aubin et al.[6] reported on the Toronto experience with fresh osteochondral allografts of the femoral condyle. Sixty knees were reviewed with a mean follow-up of 10 years (range, 58–259 months). The etiology of the osteochondral lesion was trauma in 36, OCD in 17, osteonecrosis in 6, and arthrosis in 1. Realignment osteotomy was performed in 41 patients and meniscal transplantation in 17. Twelve knees required graft removal or conversion to total knee arthroplasty. The remaining 48 patients averaged a Hospital for Special Surgery Score of 83 points. The authors reported 85% graft survivorship at 10 years.

Fresh allografts are also effective primary treatment for smaller chondral femoral condyle lesions, but in our experience are often used as a salvage if other grafting procedures such as microfracture, osteochondral autografting, or autolo-gous chondrocyte implantation have failed. Fresh allografts also have been utilized in the treatment of osteonecrosis.[2,26]

Posttraumatic Reconstruction

Fresh osteochondral allografts have a particularly valuable role in the treatment of posttraumatic knee reconstruction after periarticular fractures of the tibial plateau or femoral condyle in individuals considered too young for prosthetic arthroplasty. The Toronto group has a large experience with allografts for posttraumatic reconstruction. Ghazavi et al.[7] reviewed 126 knees in 123 patients with osteochondral defects primarily secondary to trauma. The average age of these individuals was 35 years (range 15–64). There were 81 males and 42 females. In this group, 63 lesions involved in the tibial plateau, 50 involved the femoral condyle, and 7 were bipolar lesions. In 47 cases, the meniscus was included with the transplant, and 68 knees underwent osteotomy to correct alignment. Patients were evaluated both clinically and radiographically. Survivorship analysis demonstrated 95% survivorship at 5 years, 71% survivorship at 10 years, and 66% survivorship at 20 years. Among 18 failures, 1 underwent arthrodesis, 8 underwent total knee replacement, 1 graft was removed, and 8 failed because of low clinical score but still retained their grafts.

Tibiofemoral Resurfacing

Fresh osteochondral allografts also have been utilized for salvage of advanced tibiofemoral arthrosis in carefully selected cases.[4,27] Forty-one knees were reviewed at a mean of 4.5-years of follow-up. Twelve of these knees underwent unipolar or single-surface grafting, 26 underwent bipolar femoral and tibial grafting, and 3 underwent multisurface grafting. Fifteen of the tibial grafts had associated meniscal transplantation. In this group, 54% were considered successful and 47% were considered unsuccessful. Seven patients were revised to total-knee arthroplasty, 5 underwent revision allografting, and 5 failed due to low clinical scores. It is important to note that

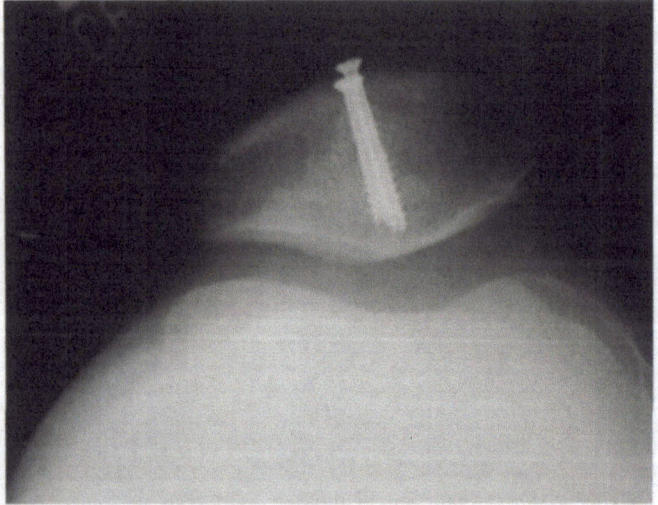

FIGURE 9.20 Patellar allograft.

in this group, unipolar grafts performed far better than bipolar grafts (70% versus 48% successful).

Patellofemoral Disease

In the patellofemoral joint, allografts have been used for treating patellar or trochlear chondral lesions, avascular necrosis, and patellofemoral arthrosis due to chronic malalignment (see Figure 9.20).[24] In this group, 29 knees have been evaluated at a mean of 4.5-years of follow-up. Twenty-two underwent complete patellar resurfacing, 1 underwent trochlear resurfacing, and 7 underwent combined patellar and trochlear grafting. In this difficult group, 57% were considered as having good or excellent results, and 40% were considered fair, poor, or underwent reoperation. The reoperations included 4 revision allografts, 3 total-knee arthroplasties, and 1 arthrodesis for sepsis. Four required no further surgery but failed due to a low clinical score.

Ankle Allografts

There are limited published data on ankle allografts. Gross et al.[9] reported on nine patients treated for osteochondral lesions of the talus caused by OCD or fracture. Six of nine grafts remained in situ at mean follow-up of 12 years (range, 4–20 years). Three ankles required arthrodesis.

Kim et al.[10] reported on bipolar tibiotalar allografting for posttraumatic arthrosis in seven patients. At mean 10-year followup, four of seven patients were rated good/excellent, one did not improve, and two underwent arthrodesis (see Table 9.5).

FUTURE DIRECTIONS

Clinical experience with fresh, small-fragment osteochondral allograft transplantation extends nearly three decades. The value of this procedure in reconstructing large or difficult chondral and osteochondral lesions is reflected in the increasing utilization of allografts in cartilage and joint reconstructive procedures. Despite the extensive clinical experience and basic scientific investigation, there are large gaps in our understanding of fresh osteochondral allografts. As with other cartilage-restorative procedures, the indications for the use of fresh osteochondral allografts are still evolving with respect to the use of allografts in the treatment of focal femoral condyle lesions, as well as the use of allografts in more extensive disease states that typify the arthritic joint. One can envision applying allografting techniques to other anatomic locations in special circumstances. The technical aspects of the procedure are evolving rapidly and it is anticipated that improved surgical instrumentation, techniques, and innovations will allow more reproducible results and decrease the number of technically related early failures. With respect to the fresh grafts, we can anticipate further improvements in tissue banking techniques—not only to improve safety, but also to enhance the graft quality. Innovations in allograft storage will prolong the useful life of fresh allografts allowing more widespread access to this procedure.

Further understanding of the immunologic behavior of fresh allografts is clearly needed. Modulating the immunologic response, either by donor–recipient matching or other therapies, may lead to breakthroughs in short- and long-term success of allograft procedures. The rapidly emerging field of growth factors and other bioactive substances could provide new methods that would serve to enhance bone healing and may improve the integration of the allograft bone to the recipient, which is currently the most important event for clinically successful allografting. Processing or manipulation of the osseous portion of the allograft with addition of growth factors may allow the allograft bone to act more like an autograft and enhance or facilitate osseous integration considered vital to the success of the allograft. We may also envision the application of growth factors or other substances to the hyaline cartilage portion of the graft to improve matrix properties or cellular function, effect integrative cartilage repair of allograft to host, and limit the detrimental effect of storage on the allografts. When one compares the knowledge and understanding of fresh osteochondral allograft transplantation in comparison with the body of knowledge available for the transplantation of other organs and tissues, one recognizes that we are in the very early beginnings of understanding the osteochondral transplant procedure. There can be no doubt that many questions have yet to be answered.

References

1. Lexer E. Joint transplantations and arthroplasty. Surg Gynecol Obstet 1925;40:782–809.
2. Meyers MH, Akeson WA, Convery FR. Resurfacing of the knee with fresh osteochondral allograft. J Bone Joint Surg Am 1989; 71A:704–713.
3. Chu CR, Convery FR, Akeson WA, et al. Articular cartilage transplantation: Clinical results in the knee. Clin Orthop 1999; 36:159–168.
4. Bugbee WD, Jamali A, Rabbani R. Fresh osteochondral allografting in the treatment of tibiofemoral arthrosis. Proceedings of the 69th meeting, AAOS, February 2002, Dallas, TX.
5. Garret JC: Fresh osteochondral allografts for treatment of articular defects in osteochondritis dissecans of the lateral femoral condyle in adults. Clin Orthop 1994;303:33–37.
6. Bugbee WD: Fresh osteochondral allografts. Semin Arthroplasty 2000;11(4):1–7.
7. Ghazavi MT, Pritzker RP, Davis AM, et al. Fresh osteochondral allografts for post-traumatic osteochondral defects of the knee. J Bone Joint Surg Br 1997;79B:1008–1013.
8. Aubin PP, Cheah HK, Davis AM, Gross AE. Long term follow-up of fresh femoral osteochondral allografts for post-traumatic knee defects. Clin Orthop 2001;391S:318–327.
9. Gross AE, Agnidis A, Hutchison CR. Osteochondral defects of the talus treated with fresh osteochondral allograft transplantation. Foot Ankle Int 2001;22:385–391.
10. Kim CW, Tontz WL, Jamali A, et al. Treatment of post-traumatic ankle arthrosis with bipolar tibiotalar osteochondral shell allografts. Foot Ankle Int 2002;23:1091–1102.
11. Meyers MH. Resurfacing of the femoral head with fresh osteochondral allografts: long-term results. Clin Orthop 1985;197: 111–114.
12. Langer F, Gross AE. Immunogenicity of allograft articular cartilage. J Bone Joint Surg Am 1974;56A:297–304.
13. Ohlendorf C, Tomford WM, Mankin HJ. Chondrocyte survival in cryopreserved osteochondral articular cartilage. J Orthop Res 1996;14:413–416.
14. Enneking WF, Campanacci DA. Retrieved human allografts: a clinicopathological study. J Bone Joint Surg Am 2001;83: 971–986.

15. Czitrom AA, Keating S, Gross AE. The viability of articular cartilage in fresh osteochondral allografts after clinical transplantation. J Bone Joint Surg Am 1990;72:574–581.

16. Convery FR, Akeson WH, Meyers MH. The operative technique of fresh osteochondral allografting of the knee. Oper Tech Orthop 1997;47:340–344.

17. American Association of Tissue Banks. Standards for tissue banking. Arlington, VA: American Association of Tissue Banks, 1987.

18. Centers for Disease Control. Morbidity and Mortality Weekly Report 2002:51(10);207–210.

19. Ball S, Chen AC, Tontz WL Jr, et al. Preservation of fresh human osteochondral allografts: effects of storage conditions on biological, biochemical, and biomechanical properties. Trans Orthop Res Soc 2002;27:441.

20. Williams SK, Amiel D, Ball ST, et al. Fresh osteochondral allografts: time-dependent storage effects. Session 57: Podium Presentation #6, International Cartilage Repair Society Annual Meeting, June 2002, Toronto, Canada.

21. Stevenson S. The immune response to osteochondral allografts in dogs. J Bone Joint Surg Am 1987;69:573–582.

22. Oakeshott RD, Farine I, Pritzker KP, et al. A clinical and histologic analysis of failed fresh osteochondral allografts. Clin Orthop 1988;233:283–294.

23. Sirlin CB, Brossman J, Boutin RD, et al. Shell osteochondral allografts of the knee: comparison of MR imaging findings and immunologic responses. Radiology 2001;219(1):35–43.

24. Jamali A, Bugbee WD, Chu C, et al. Fresh osteochondral allografting of the patellofemoral joint. Paper #177, Presented at the AAOS 68th Annual Meeting, February 2001.

25. Bugbee WD, Emmerson BC, Jamali A. Fresh osteochondral allografting in the treatment of osteochondritis dissecans of the femoral condyle. Paper #054, presented at the AAOS 70th Annual Meeting, February 2003.

26. Gross AE, McKee NH, Pritzker KP: Reconstruction of skeletal deficits of the knee: a comprehensive osteochondral transplant program. Clin Orthop 1983;174:96–106.

27. Gross AE, Silverstein EA, Falk J. The allotransplantation of partial joints in the treatment of osteoarthritis of the knee. Clin Orthop 1975;108:7–14.

10

Autologous Chondrocyte Implantation for Focal Chondral Lesions

Scott D. Gillogly and Mats Brittberg

BACKGROUND

Articular cartilage trauma is extremely common, and, until recently, methods for treatment of the cartilaginous lesions have not produced good long-term results. A better understanding of how articular cartilage responds to injury has produced various techniques that hold promise for long-term success. Among such techniques is autologous chondrocyte implantation (ACI), in which a patient's own cartilage cells are harvested, expanded in vitro, and reimplanted in a full-thickness articular surface defect.[1] Results are available with up to 11 years follow-up, and more than 80% of the patients have shown improvement with relatively few complications.[2] Since the presentation of the first series of chondrocyte-treated patients in 1994,[3] much discussion and debate around this technique has fueled the current interest and excitement around cartilage repair. This chapter reviews the indications, technical considerations, and clinical findings, and addresses many of the questions raised about autologous chondrocyte implantation.

INDICATIONS AND CONTRAINDICATIONS

Autologous chondrocyte implantation is the only treatment option approved in the United States by the Federal Food and Drug Administration (FDA) for symptomatic, full-thickness chondral lesions and osteochondritis dissecans (OCD) lesions of the femoral condyles and trochlear groove. The presence of coexisting pathology that might adversely affect cartilage repair, such as ongoing ligamentous instability, tibiofemoral malalignment, bone deficiency, patellofemoral malalignment, or complete meniscal deficiency should be carefully evaluated. Deficiencies in any of these areas must be addressed before or concomitant with ACI.

The gold standard for determining if a patient is a suitable candidate for ACI must be at the time of the arthroscopic evaluation, as magnetic resonance imaging (MRI) still does not have enough sensitivity or specificity for secure cartilage injury evaluation. Location, depth, and size of the lesion, quality of the surrounding cartilage, degree of undermining cartilage, and status of opposing chondral surface can all be evaluated at the time of arthroscopy. The ideal chondral lesion to treat with ACI is one from a symptomatic patient with a full-thickness defect surrounded by healthy, normal cartilage in an otherwise healthy knee. However, the ideal defect is more the exception than the rule, as many defects occur in knees with concomitant pathology and some degree of uncontainment. In general, the defects treated with ACI are greater than $2\,cm^2$,[3–5] and are for physically high-demand patients who want to return to an active lifestyle.

Autologous chondrocyte implantation is not approved as a treatment option for advanced osteoarthritis, such as in the presence of bipolar bone-on-bone lesions. Therefore, in addition to a comprehensive physical examination, standing anteroposterior (AP), 45° bent-knee, and patellar alignment radiographs should be obtained[6] to rule out advanced degenerative joint disease. The knee radiographs should also be fully evaluated for bony deficiency and malalignment, in addition to evidence of arthritic changes. Other contraindications include active rheumatoid arthritis, autoimmune connective tissue disease and patients with concomitant malignancies.

ACI SURGICAL TECHNIQUE

The surgical technique for autologous chondrocyte implantation has been well defined in numerous publications.[3,7–10] The steps include an initial cartilage biopsy which is sent for chondrocyte culture, followed by a procedure for cell implantation. Implantation consists of arthrotomy, defect preparation, periosteal procurement, fixation of periosteal tissue to defect, securing a watertight seal with fibrin glue, implanting the chondrocytes, and wound closure.

Chondral Biopsy for Chondrocyte Culture

If a chondral lesion is considered appropriate for ACI, a biopsy site for cartilage harvesting is chosen. The most common sites for a cartilage biopsy are the superomedial edge of the femoral condyle and the lateral intercondylar notch in the same location in which a notchplasty is performed during anterior cruciate ligament (ACL) reconstruction. The other recommended area is the superolateral edge of the femoral condyle that is nonarticulating with the tibia or patella. An arthroscopic gouge or ring curette is used to obtain two or three small slivers of full-thickness cartilage, the size of a fingernail clipping (5 by 10 mm). It is often helpful to try to leave an end of the biopsy attached to the subchondral bone so it can be grasped with an arthroscopic grasper and torn off. After the biopsy is arthroscopically removed from the knee, it is placed in the biopsy medium/shipping vial in sterile fashion. Two or three slices of cartilage will yield between 300,000 to 500,000 chondrocytes that can be cultured. The cartilage is shipped under sterile conditions to Genzyme Biosurgery, (Cambridge, MA), for cell culturing in USA, or shipped to the chosen cell laboratory facility in Europe. Currently five European companies offer this cell culturing service. The goal in culturing cells is to expand the number of chondrocytes by 20 to 50 times the initial cell amount. Routinely, the cultured cells are cryopreserved and a surgical date is scheduled.

Surgical Approach

A standard medial or lateral parapatellar incision and arthrotomy is used for exposure of the defect. As with any surgical procedure, good exposure is essential. If the lesion is located on the central portion of the condyle, a miniarthrotomy can be used. For larger and hard-to-reach chondral injuries, typically a medial or lateral incision with a medial or lateral parapatellar arthrotomy and eversion of the patella are required, especially when the lesion is on the posterior portion of the lateral condyle.

Debridement of the Defect

After adequate exposure is obtained, the defect must be thoroughly debrided of all unhealthy cartilage surrounding the lesion, including all fissures and undermined cartilage in addition to any fibrocartilage present in the base of the defect. Attempting to secure the periosteal patch to soft, damaged cartilage, can compromise the host–graft interface, potentially allowing the sutures to pull loose during the early motion phase of rehabilitation. This zone of damaged cartilage surrounding the chondral defect needs to be fully excised using a fresh scalpel blade, cutting vertically through the cartilage down to the level of, but not into the subchondral bone. A ring curette can be used to remove the damaged cartilage or any fibrocartilage in the base of the defect.

During debridement, care is taken to avoid penetrating the subchondral bone plate which might cause unwanted bleeding which can compromise the quality of the repair tissue. There are three steps to control hemostasis. The first is to place neuropatties diluted with a combination of epinephrine and thrombin into the base of the defect. A second method is to apply fibrin glue to the point of penetration, followed by the surgeon holding pressure over the defect for a minute or two. A third method is electrocautery with a needle tip Bovie at a low setting, 5 to 8 W, using it only at the point of perforation.

Internal osteophytes in the subchondral bone can be the result of penetration of the subchondral bone from either injury or prior surgical procedures such as drilling, abrasion, or microfracture. These bony prominences, if small, can be addressed by gently tapping them back into the subchondral bone plate with a smooth, noncorrugated bone tamp.[11] Fibrous

plugs in the subchondral bone plate may also be encountered during debridement, usually as a result of prior surgical procedures (drilling or microfracture). These fibrous plugs should be debrided from the defect; however, the fibrous tissue should not be removed from the drill holes in the subchondral bone, as this can also result in loss of hemostasis.

Once the defect is prepared, the dimensions are measured and recorded. To help assist obtaining the right size periosteal patch, a template made from either sterile paper or aluminum can be placed over the defect and outlined with a sterile marking pen, oversizing by 1 to 2 mm. The template is then cut out and used during the periosteal patch harvest to help ensure an accurate size and shape. Adding 1 to 2 mm in size when cutting the periosteal graft allows for the tendency of the periosteum to shrink after harvest.

Periosteal Harvesting

The periosteal patch is obtained through a separate incision from the proximal medial tibia, two fingers distal to the pes anserinus and medial collateral ligament insertion on the subcutaneous border.[12] All fat and fascia layers must be removed from the periosteum. Leaving the thin fascia layer on the periosteum is one of the most common mistakes made with harvesting the periosteal graft.[13] A sharp dissection with scissors is recommended to remove this thin fascial layer. A wet sponge also assists in removing any redundant tissue over the periosteum. The periosteum is a white glistening tissue; if there is an off-white or shaded appearance to the periosteum, the fascia may still remain over the periosteum. If the fascia layer is not removed, the is increased risk of periosteal hypertrophy.[2]

The outer surface should then be marked with a marking pen to help distinguish it from the inner cambium layer. The template is placed over the periosteum and carefully outlined with a sharp 15 blade down to the bone, and a sharp periosteal elevator is used to slowly dissect the periosteum from the bone. Smooth forceps can be used on the leading edge of the periosteum to avoid penetration.[12] If the proximal medial tibia periosteum is too thin and fragile, an alternate site for periosteal procurement must be used. The distal femoral periosteum, just proximal to medial and lateral femoral condyle articular surfaces, can serve as a second source of periosteum. Although this periosteum is thicker, making it easier to handle, it should be used as a last resort. The rule of thumb is to have the thinnest periosteum possible; this will reduce the number of adverse events.

If the tissue is harvested from the femur, a synovial incision and subsynovial dissection are used to obtain the distal femoral periosteum. A T-incision is recommended, pulling back the synovial lining, thus exposing the periosteum. The periosteum is frequently covered with small blood vessels, which can be carefully cauterized with a needle-point Bovie on a low setting before harvesting. After periosteum procurement, the synovium should be repaired in its original location to discourage hemarthrosis.[11] The proximal tibia should serve as the primary source of periosteal tissue.

Securing the Periosteal Patch

The periosteum should always be kept moist, preserving the viability of the cambium layer, and should not be handled with surgical gloves. The cambium layer has chondrogenic cells, which in combination with the implanted chondrocytes may assist with the development of the repair tissue.[13] The periosteum should be attached to the defect using 5-0 or 6-0 Vicryl sutures (Ethicon Vicryl polyglactin 910 P-1 cutting needle, Johnson & Johnson, New Brunswick, NJ) using interrupted sutures with the cambium layer facing into the defect. The suture needle should be passed through the periosteum from outside to inside, approximately 2 mm from the edge of the periosteum. The needle should then be passed through the cartilage from inside to outside with the needle entering the cartilage approximately 2 mm in the defect and perpendicular to the defect wall. It is recommended to have approximately 2- to 3-mm bites from the edge of the defect. To allow the sutures to easily pass through the periosteum, they should first be immersed in sterile glycerin. The periosteum should be flush and taut across the defect, having a manhole-cover appearance with the graft up to, but not extending over, the cartilage rim. Any redundant tissue should be trimmed with sharp scissors to keep appropriate tension on the graft.

The sutures are then placed alternately around the defect, spaced approximately 3 to 4 mm from each other. The knots should be tied on the side of the periosteum, not on the surface of the cartilage, thus avoiding any frictional force that could cause loosening of the knots. A short 2- to 3-mm tail should be left when cutting the suture because cutting the sutures at the base of the knot also can result in knot loosening. A variety of needle choices is recommended to handle the many situations that may arise. A smaller needle with a shorter radius works best around thick normal cartilage, and a thin needle with a greater radius allows a longer pass through thinner cartilage or when required to suture into soft tissue.

After fully securing the graft, except for a small 5- to 6-mm opening to accommodate an angiocatheter, the watertight integrity of the graft should be tested. An 18-gauge catheter attached to a saline-filled tuberculin syringe is placed under the periosteum and slowly filled with saline. Any leakage is reinforced with additional sutures. The suture line is then sealed with fibrin glue to assure watertightness.

Implantation of Autologous Chondrocytes

The cultured cells are returned in a non-sterile vial with the cells being sterile within it. Therefore, strict sterile procedures must be followed when resuspending the cells. The vial is held in a vertical position, the top of the vial is wiped with alcohol, and a sterile 18-gauge catheter with needle is used to penetrate the rubber stopper. The syringe is then attached to the angiocatheter for cell aspiration after the metal needle is withdrawn, leaving the plastic catheter tip within the vial. Aspirating and injecting back into the vial several times will resuspend the pellet at the bottom of the vial. The total volume of cells is typically between .25 and .35 cc. When all the cells are aspirated in the syringe, the hub of the catheter and syringe are grasped by the surgeon's sterile hand and withdrawn from the vial. The catheter is then placed through the small opening of the defect and advanced to the distal end of the defect. The cells are slowly injected under the periosteal patch as the catheter is slowly withdrawn to the opening of the defect. The small opening is then closed with one or two additional sutures, and then sealed with fibrin glue (Figure 10.1).

Any concomitant procedures should be completed before implanting the chondrocytes, and the knee should not be placed through a range of motion after the cell implantation. The arthrotomy is then closed in a layered fashion, and a soft sterile dressing is applied to the knee. If a drain is applied, it should not be placed inside the joint.

COEXISTING KNEE PATHOLOGY

With any cartilage repair method, good results cannot be expected if coexisting knee pathology is not thoroughly addressed. Biomechanical malalignment and ligamentous insufficiency can lead to excessive forces and abnormal compressive loads that can destroy neorepair tissue.[14,15] Therefore, it is critical that any associated knee pathology responsible for or contributing to the chondral defect be identified and corrected before or in conjunction with the cells being implanted. Coexistent knee pathology can be addressed in a staged surgical procedure before ACI, or concomitantly with ACI. Concomitant procedures facilitate the healing process of the hyaline-like repair tissue by unloading overloaded compartments, ensuring proper tracking, and balancing soft tissues.

Biomechanical Alignment

If physical examination or initial radiographs (weight-bearing AP, 45°, and axial views) indicate any malalignment, full-length films from hip to ankle should be obtained. If the mechanical axis passes through the compartment in which the chondral injury is located, an unloading osteotomy is recommended to shift abnormal forces away from that compartment. If the osteotomy is done concomitantly with ACI, it is recommended that stable fixation of the osteotomy be obtained before securing the periosteal graft to the chondral defect. Unloading osteotomies should also be considered when the lesions on the condyles are large, even without a malalignment; an alternate method is protected weight bearing with the use of a custom-made unloader brace.

Patellofemoral Malalignment

Any abnormal patellar tracking not only is the likely source of the patellar or trochlear injuries but also would create a hostile environment for the implanted chondrocytes, as was thought to be the case with the initial seven patellae reported by Brittberg et al.[3] In addition to the concerns of maltracking of the patella, decreasing the patellofemoral contact forces also is desirable.[16] Depending on the degree of lateral maltracking, the amount of medialization can be adjusted accordingly. The anteromedialization of the tibial tubercle as described by Fulkerson[17] offers the option of adjusting the degree of medialization while still elevating the tubercle anteriorly. In some cases, without lateral maltracking, anterior transfer of the tibial tubercle alone may be sufficient to reduce the contact pressure of the patellofemoral compartment. Both authors routinely decompress the patellofemoral joint when treating larger lesions to help provide the chondrocytes with an optimal environment for maturation.

Patellar chondral defects can occur in a variety of different patterns, which require different techniques for repair to reconstruct the normal contour of the patella. Patellar cartilage lesions can be isolated to one of the facets, or they can be diffuse large central defects involving both facets, crossing the median ridge. Clinical experience has shown that lesions isolated to one facet have better outcomes than central defects

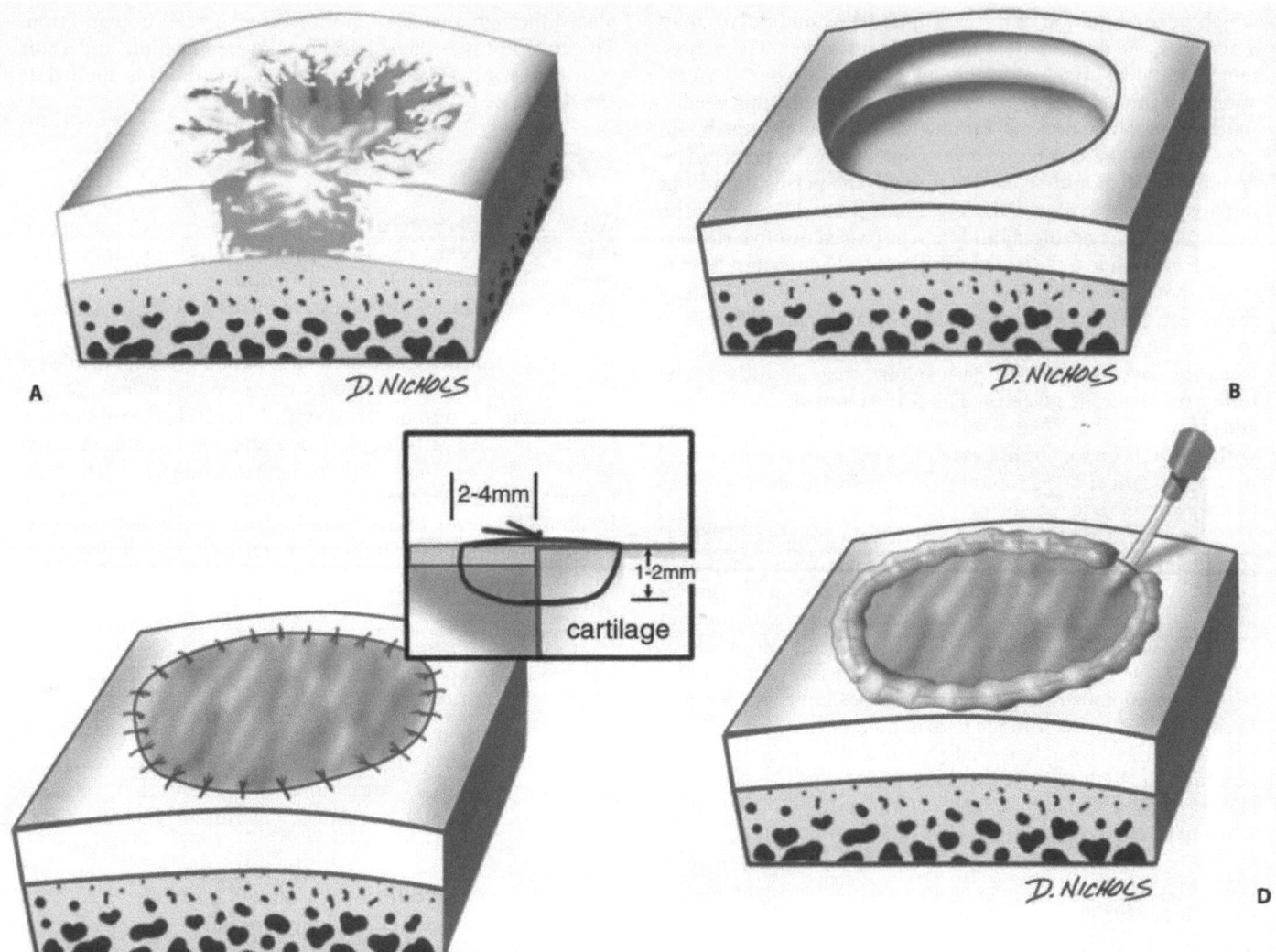

Figure 10.1 A. The defect is debrided to the edge of normal articular cartilage down to the subchondral bone, removing any fibrous debris from the bone. **B.** Debridement should result in a slightly oval, well-delineated defect, with good vertical borders down to a clean subchondral bone. **C.** The periosteal patch is sutured over the defect with the cambium layer facing the defect and sutured to the remaining cartilage with the interrupted sutures creating a manhole appearance. The needle should be placed a 1 mm bite into the periosteum. The needle should be placed 1 to 2 mm deep into the defect with a bite of 2 to 4 mm through the cartilage, finishing by tying the knot on the side of the periosteum. A water test is performed to ensure the patch is watertight. Fibrin glue is then applied along the suture line. **D.** The autologous chondrocyte suspension is injected under the patch through a small portal at the superior part of thee graft. A final suture is then passed and additional fibrin glue is applied.

that cross the median ridge, and lesions that have a good cartilage border around the periphery do better than uncontained lesions.[2] Therefore, when debriding a patellar lesion, a peripheral rim of cartilage should be preserved whenever possible. For defects that are isolated to one facet, the same technique used for the condyle is recommended, leaving the periosteum flush to the host cartilage surface. However, for patellar defects crossing the median ridge, it is more challenging to recreate the normal contour of the patella when suturing the periosteum over a centralized defect (Figure 10.2). The periosteum should be oversized in both the medial and lateral directions by 3 to 4 mm, as opposed to the standard 1 to 2 millimeters. The apex of the medium ridge (at the highest point of the patella) should be sutured first. Then, sutures should be placed in an alternating fashion medially and laterally and then extending peripherally to creat a tentlike appearance. This technique helps to recreate the complex normal articular facets and median ridge architecture of the patella.[10] Since the initial series was reported,[3] the long-term Swedish experience has improved. At the 2002 ICRS meeting, it was reported that 83 patients with a follow-up between 3 to 13 years, showed an 83% good to excellent result when all the background factors are addressed.[18]

Trochlear lesions can also be challenging because of the concave geometry of the trochlear groove. The key to avoiding excessive tension and shear stresses across the repair tissue is to recreate the normal contour of the sulcus. The periosteum should be oversized by about 3 to 4 mm in the proximal to distal dimension, and suturing should begin at the central sulcus and then progress medially and laterally in an alternating fashion. This method helps to recreate the concave topography of the sulcus, avoiding central wear and minimizing the risk of delaminating the periosteal graft (see Figure 10.2C).

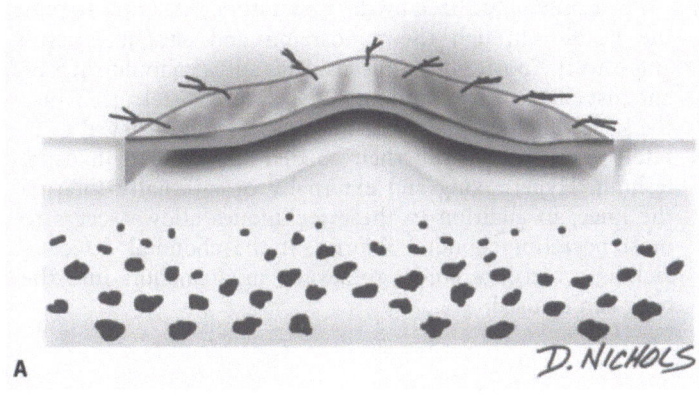

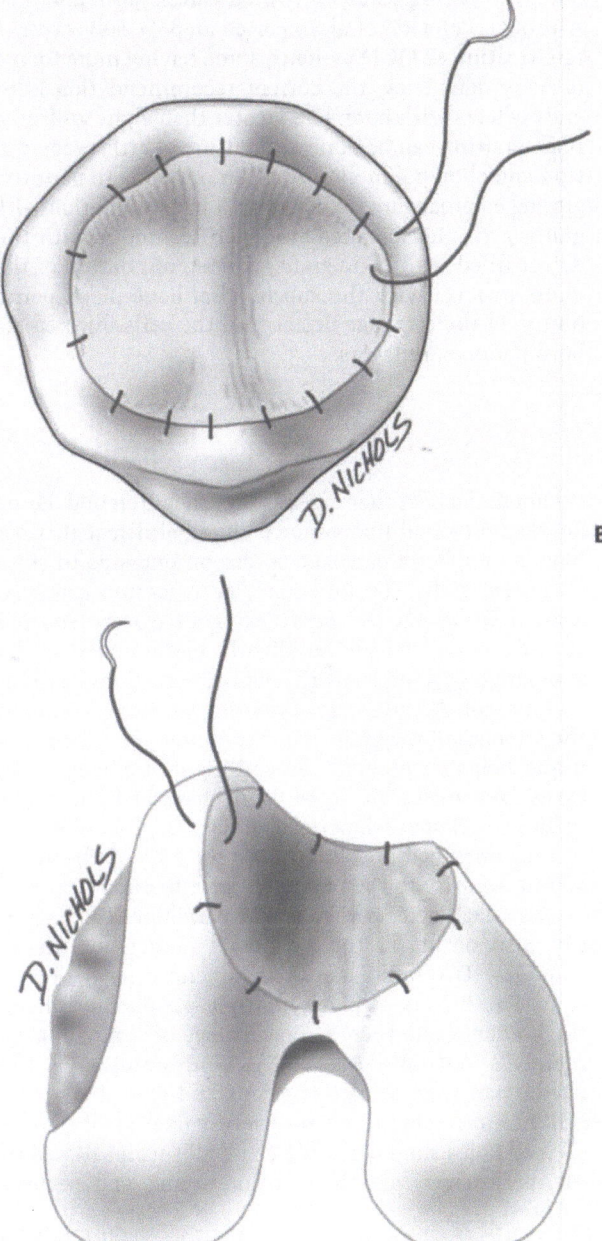

Figure 10.2 A. When dealing with a large central patella, the periosteum is sutured over the defect to recreate a normal triangular shape. The central ridge is reconstituted by starting the sutures at the highest point and then alternating side to side, allowing the periosteum to flow into the facets establishing the normal convex shape. **B.** Frontal view shows the periosteum following the contour of the facets. **C.** When suturing the periosteum over a trochlear defect that crosses the midline, involving both facets, the normal concave surface should be reconstituted to avoid overloading the central trochlear surface.

Ligamentous Insufficiency

Ligamentous insufficiency produces excessive shear forces in the knee which would irreversibly jeopardize the maturing repair tissue. If performed concomitantly, ACL reconstruction should precede autologous chondrocyte implantation and should be performed using the surgeon's standard technique. Regardless of the technique used, it is beneficial to wait for final fixation until the ACI procedure is completed. The obvious advantages of performing both procedures at the same time are that there is only one surgery, one rehabilitation, and a lower cost. Postoperatively, the ACI rehabilitation program is more limiting and is the overriding guidance postoperatively.

Meniscal Deficiency

The importance of a functional meniscus with ACI cannot be overstated. Whenever possible, it should be preserved or repaired.[19] In the presence of a total meniscectomy, or when the meniscal function is equivalent to a total meniscectomy, a meniscus transplantation should be considered. The meniscal allograft will help to reduce the concentrated forces in the involved compartment and help protect the newly formed repair tissue. When performing a meniscal allograft concomitantly with ACI, the meniscal allograft should be placed and secured, followed by completion of the ACI. The experience and indications of ACI and meniscal allografts is discussed in Chapter 13.

Bony Deficiency

Shallow bony lesions to 8 millimeters have been shown clinically to do well with only implanting the autologous chondrocytes.[9,12] The sclerotic bottom of these shallow defects should be debrided gently, but one must be careful not to elicit a bleeding response, which can be difficult to control. Although Peterson et al.[2] reported an 83% subjective success rate treating 42 OCD patients, some having more than 10 mm of bony deficiency, the current recommendation is to bone graft defects with bony loss greater than eight millimeters.[4,15] Bone grafting can be done at the time of arthroscopic evaluation and chondral biopsy. Another option is to perform a single staged procedure involving ACI in combination with bone grafting via the so-called sandwich technique with the bony defect filled with bone grafts, periosteum on top of the bone grafts in level with the subchondral bone plate, periosteum on top of the cartilage defect, and the cells injected between both periosteum layers.

UNCONTAINED CHONDRAL LESIONS

A chondral defect that extends into the intercondylar notch is an example of an uncontained chondral defect that does not have a peripheral cartilage border on one side to suture the periosteal graft. The intercondylar synovium can serve as a margin to which the periosteal graft can be sutured. The sutures should be placed slightly closer together than the standard 3 to 4 mm when using the synovium as the peripheral margin. Additionally, a running suture helps to reinforce the strength of the graft–synovium interface. Using this technique helps to prevent the spilling of implanted chondrocytes, minimizes any type of mechanical friction and thus redues the chances of periosteal hypertrophy. A longer needle is recommended to obtain a larger bite of the soft tissue adding security to the periosteal graft fixation.

Cartilage defects that lack a peripheral cartilage margin can also occur on the peripheral borders of the femoral condyles. Two options are recommended for periosteal fixation. The first is to place multiple peripheral drill holes at the border where there is no cartilage or synovium, approximately 3 to 4 mm apart, with a Keith needle. A P-1 cutting needle can then be flattened out and passed through these drill holes. To obtain the most secure fixation of graft to bone, all drill holes should be drilled and all sutures passed through the periosteum and bone before tying and securing the sutures.

The second option is to utilize the mini-Mitek (Mitek, Inc, Norwood, MA) suture anchors. The nonabsorbable suture should be removed and replaced with a 6-0 Vicryl suture before placing the anchors. Each anchor should be placed approximately 3 to 5 mm apart. Again, all suture anchors should be passed through the periosteum before tying to allow adjustment of the periosteal tension.

One of the authors (M.B.) suggests using two or three cylindrical autologous osteochondral plugs to build up the wall to which the periosteum could be sutured when the cartilage is quite thick in one direction and uncontained on the opposite side.[7]

Defects that extend far posteriorly, especially in the lateral compartment, can be difficult to fully expose and secure the periosteal graft to the posterior chondral margin with the standard anterior approach to the knee. These hard-to-reach compartments can be maximally opened by hyperflexing the knee and externally or internally rotating the leg. Also, smaller needles with a shorter radius of curvature allow for a quicker bite of cartilage, which may be necessary in these difficult lesions.

A technique utilized by the first author (S.D.G.) is to pass the needle through the periosteum and chondral tissue and into the posterior meniscus. The suture should then be cut just above the needle and the suture is retrieved into the knee. The needle can then be grasped and retrieved separately. The sutures can then be tied and secured in usual fashion. Hyperflexing and externally or internally rotating the knee, in addition to these techniques allows access to most posterior chondral injuries. If the chondral defect is lacking a cartilage border to suture, microanchors into the bone can be used.

REHABILITATION

The concept of a slow gradual time course of healing is critical to understand for rehabilitation following ACI. If the intraarticular environment is protective, the remodeling and maturation of this tissue will continue. However, if the graft is overloaded, failure can occur. As there is a degree of individual variation with the rehabilitation process, the program should be designed according to the patient's status and needs, as well as such factors as the size and location of the lesion and any possible concomitant procedures performed. It is critical that there is regular dialogue between the physician, patient, and therapist, especially during the first 3 to 12 months following ACI.

The foundation principles of a successful ACI rehabilitation program are centered around graft protection, mobility and motion exercises, muscle strengthening, progressive weight bearing, and patient education. Protection of the repair tissue from excessive intraarticular force is critical during the early postoperative period with avoidance of twisting and rotational shear forces. Continuous passive motion and a gradually increased weight-bearing status should be the initial steps of the rehabilitation process. Isometric quadriceps training, straight leg raises, and hamstring strengthening should be introduced early and progressively advanced to resisted exercises and return to greater degrees of functional activities. After 3 weeks, progressive closed-chain exercises with light resistance is begun. Open-chain exercises are initiated around the 8th week. Running is not advised until the 8th or 9th month post-ACI with high level activities being initiated at the 12th month.

Rehabilitation for patellar or trochlear lesions requires special considerations to obtain early motion while protecting the forces across the repair tissue. Contact pressure of the patellofemoral articulation is maximized between 40° and 70° of knee flexion, and thus should be avoided during active knee flexion until the graft is mature enough to withstand these shear stresses. Exercises to promote patella mobility should be initiated early to help prevent adhesions. Additionally, patients should not be allowed to perform active knee extension during the first 10 to 12 weeks following repair of a patellar or trochlear lesion. Passive motion with continuous passive motion (CPM) or by using the contralateral leg to extend the involved leg is allowed and encouraged. The gradual progression of active extension exercises depends on the size and location of the defect as observed in the operating room; therefore, it is essential that the surgeon provide guidance and reassurance to the patient and the therapist. If the defects are large, one may consider using an unloader brace for the first 3 to 5 months.

Management of Complications

The complications that occur with ACI can be classified as being associated with the periosteum, the arthrotomy, or concomitant procedures being performed. Periosteal overgrowth or hypertrophy is the most common adverse event that occurs with the graft.[4,15] Symptoms include catching, popping, or swelling, which may or may not be painful, and tend to occur between 5 to 9 months post-ACI.[11] When a patient presents with any of these symptoms, associated activities need to be altered accordingly. If symptoms still persist despite a modification in the patient's activities and rehabilitation, arthroscopic evaluation should be considered. If the periosteum appears to protrude above the level of the surrounding host cartilage, it can be managed by using an arthroscopic shaver blade to remove any loose fibrillating periosteal repair tissue that is protruding from the cartilage margin. Radiofrequency energy ablation should not be used to manage periosteal hypertrophy, as its variable depth of penetration can cause irreversible damage to the maturing repair tissue (Figure 10.3).[20]

Graft failure can occur as a result of graft delamination. Total delamination of the graft is uncommon and is most often an early event within the first year posttransplantation. The two most common causes of graft failure are mechanical overload and the genetic disposition of the patient.[2] Loosening can occur as a marginal, partial, or complete delamination. In case of a marginal or partial loosening, the loose part of the graft is debrided with a sharp knife and the defect area is abraded or microfractured to create interpositional ingrowth of fibrocartilage tissue to stabilize the graft against the adjacent cartilage to avoid further delamination (Figure 10.4).

Overload of the maturing graft involves unexpected or sudden trauma to the knee or noncompliance of the patient with the rehabilitation protocol during the early postoperative period. Both these scenarios underscore the importance of a protected gradual rehabilitation course and educating the patient and family to follow this protocol stringently. It must be reiterated to patients that the purpose of the rehabilitation protocol is to optimize their results, and as they start to feel more comfortable with their knee, they must still follow it. These issues are less concerning at 6 months postoperatively. Although the repair tissue has not fully matured at this point, it is usually firm enough and sufficiently integrated to host bone and cartilage to withstand higher levels of force.

Intraarticular adhesions or arthrofibrosis is a risk of any type of knee arthrotomy; this occurs in about 2% of autologous chondrocyte implantations and has a higher risk of occurring in those patients who are undergoing concomitant procedures.[10,11] The best way to avoid stiffness is early motion. CPM should be started in the immediate postoperative period.[19]

When arthrofibrosis does occur, the first line of treatment should be an aggressive range of motion therapy program. If the patient has not shown signs of recovering motion, then arthroscopic lysis of adhesions is indicated. Adhesions are best released with arthroscopic electrocautery or gentle shaving with a large resector shaver blade, taking extreme caution to not contact the repair tissue. Following resection of adhesions and visualization of the graft, the knee should be placed through a gentle manipulation. Postoperatively, the patient resumes an aggressive motion and weight-bearing protocol. Normal or near-normal range of motion of the knee can almost always be regained.

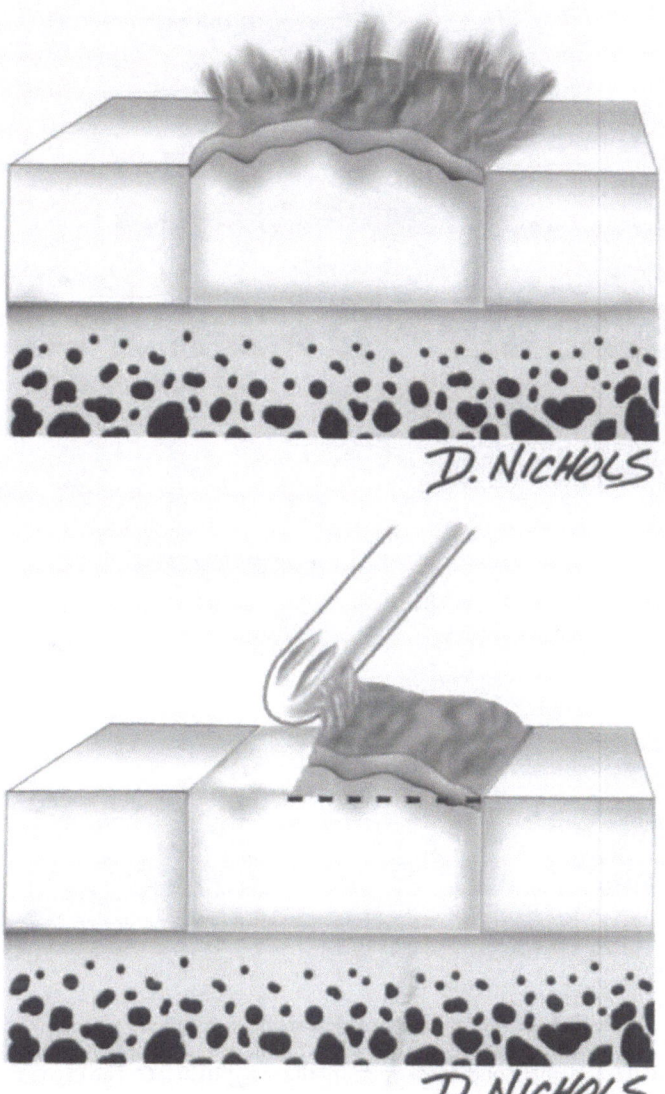

Figure 10.3 A. Hypertrophy of the periosteal patch can cause a pseudo-locking or pain. The mechanism of this of this overgrowth is thought to be from mechanical friction; it usually occurs 6 to 9 months postimplantation. **B.** Using a turbowhisker, the overgrowth tissue is trimmed down to the level of the adjacent cartilage, resolving the mechanical symptoms.

Clinical Results

Since the report from the first 23 patients in 1994,[3] ACI has been performed in more than 8000 patients throughout the world by more than 1000 orthopaedic surgeons, with more than 12 years of followup.[21] The clinical results have been reported from numerous centers worldwide. Bahuaud et al.,[22] Cole and D'Amoto,[8] Gillogly and Hamby,[9] Minas,[23] Brittberg et al.,[3] and Gersoff[24] all reported outcomes more than 85% successful. From European centers, Lohnert,[25] Richardson et al.,[26] and Knutsen et al.[27] have all reported outcomes comparable to the Swedish experience. Peterson et al.[12] recently reported a retrospective analysis on the first 100 patients treated with ACI. At follow-up ranging from 2 to 9 years, 23 of 25 (92%) patients with isolated femoral condyle chondral lesions had successful outcomes, and 16 of 18 (89%) patients with osteochondral defects had good to excellent results. They reported a

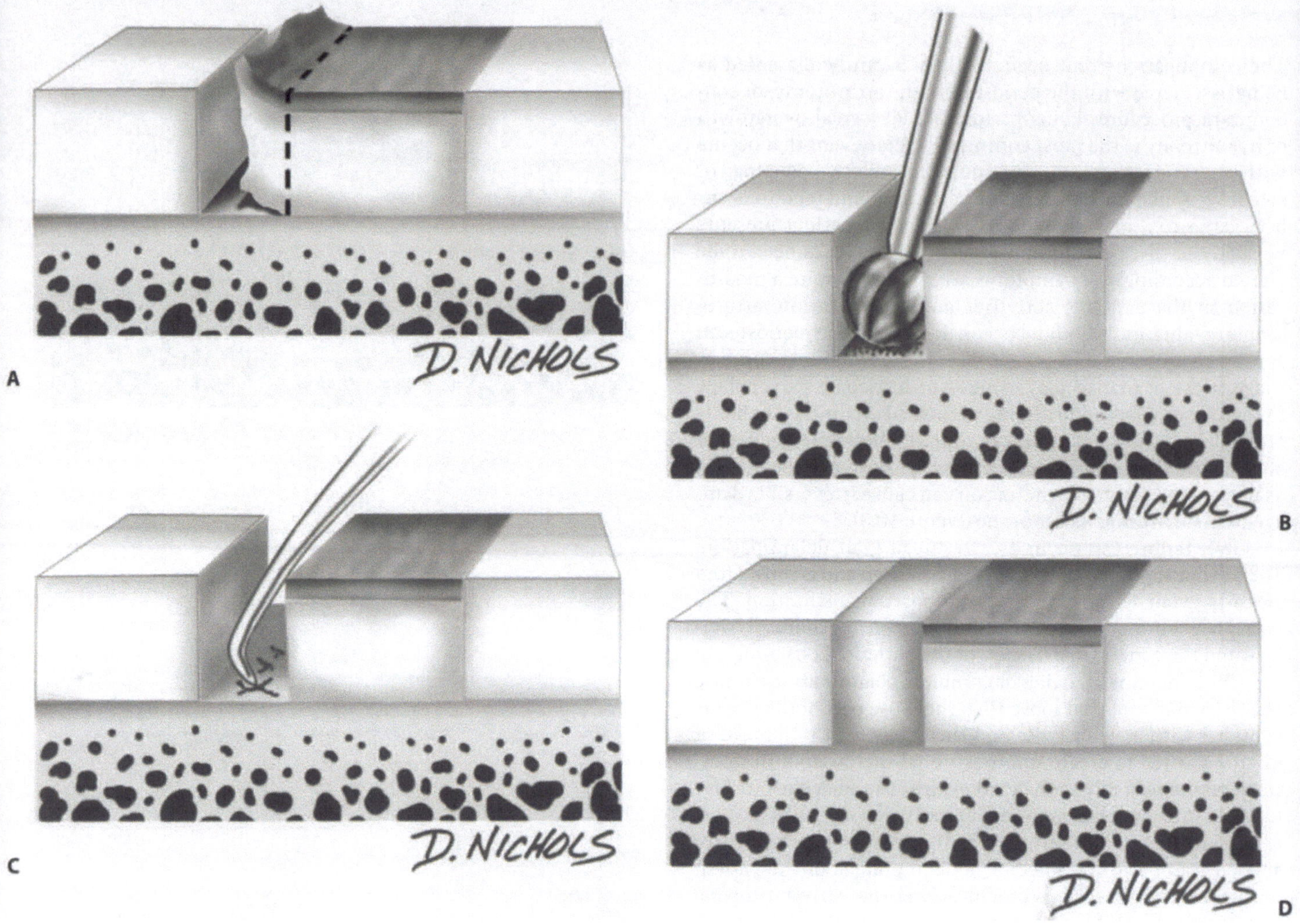

D. NICHOLS

A

D. NICHOLS

B

D. NICHOLS

C

D. NICHOLS

D

Figure 10.4 A. Partial detached periosteal patch (line of resection is *hatched*) can occur with early trauma to the repair tissue. **B.** Debridement of the loose piece of the repair tissue. **C.** The exposed bone can be microfractured or abraded to induce a marrow response. **D.** Ingrowth of fibrocartilaginous tissue provides a interpositional stabilization for the graft.

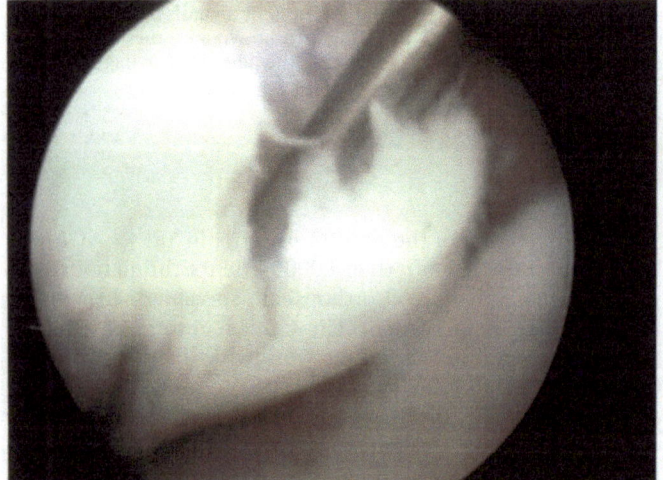

A

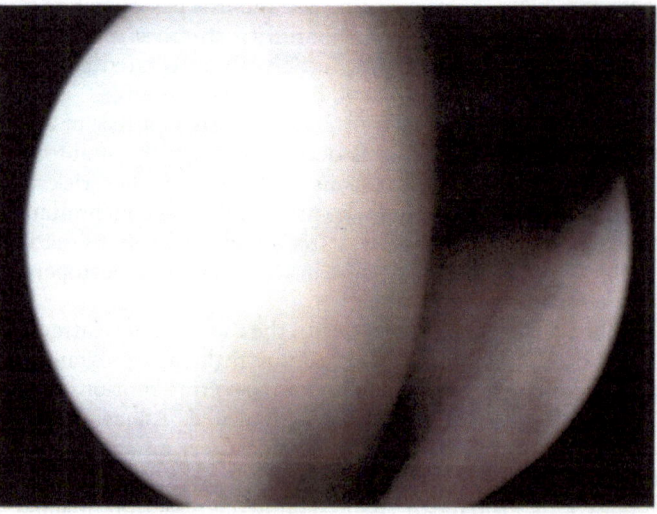

B

Figure 10.5 A. A 22-year-old man sustained traumatic injury in the fall of 1994. In October, he underwent an arthrocopic assessment for autologous chondrocyte implantation (ACI) showing 4.5–5 cm² defect on the medial femoral condyle. He was implanted in November 1994. **B.** Second-look arthroscopy at 36 months postimplant shows complete filling of the defect and integration of the repair tissue.

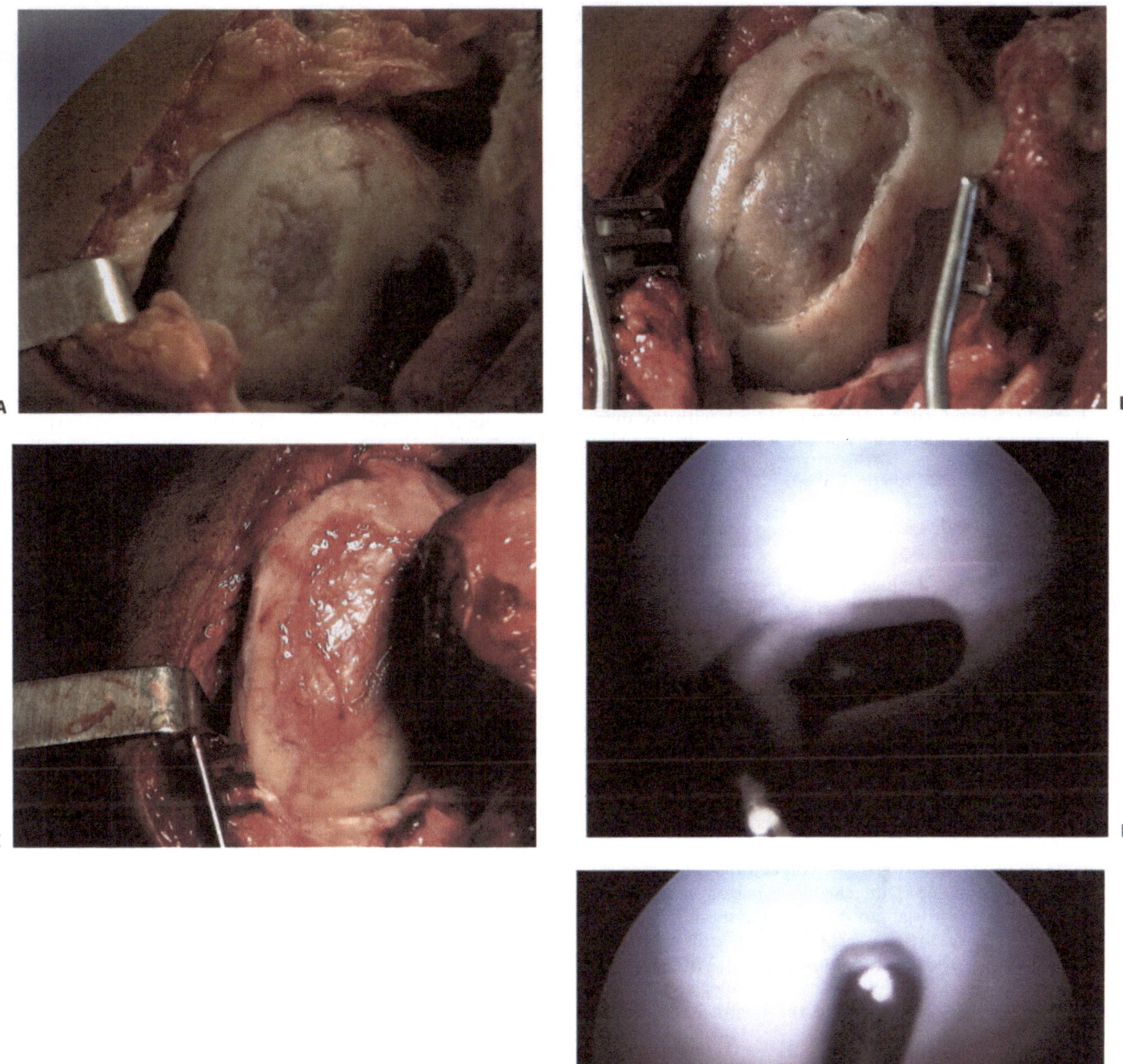

Figure 10.6 A. A 36-year-old laborer who used heavy equipment experienced significant pain and swelling upon exertion and obtained leave with worker's compensation. He had a large medial femoral condyle lesion, 6.5 cm. **B.** Defect was prepared with vertical borders back to a stable rim. **C.** Periosteal patch sutured over the defect. **D.** Second-look arthroscopy at 14 months postimplant showed defect was filled and well integrated. Patient returned to work with full activity. **E.** In the body of the lesion, firmness is comparable to adjacent cartilage; in the posterior edge of the lesion, tissue is softer than in the body of the lesion.

67% success rate in patients with multiple chondral lesions or for salvage scenarios (one-third of the patients had lesions involving bipolar lesions) (see Figures 10.5).

Peterson et al.[2] also published their long-term durability biomechanical data, showing a 96% durability factor with the first 62 consecutive patients treated at 2 years and then again at 7.5 years. The clinical outcomes remained constant (80% good-to-excellent results at 2 years, and 78% at 7.5 years) and second-look arthroscopies did not show signs of tissue breakdown.[2]

Minas et al.[15] has reported results on 235 patients treated with ACI, with an 87% success rate over a 6-year period. The

Atlanta Sports Medicine and Orthopaedic Center reported the clinical results of 112 patients treated with ACI, showing a 91% good-to-excellent success rate.[9] There was a statistical difference for better results with lesions treated within 1 year from injury or onset of symptoms than in chronic defects present for more than 1 year.

The Cartilage Registry Report,[21] an international multi-center observational assessment of patients treated with ACI indicated that by patient assessment, 78% of all defects treated with ACI improvement, whereas 81% of isolated femoral condyle defects had improved. Clinician evaluations have shown a 79% improvement for all lesions and an 85% improvement in femoral condyle lesions; 80% of the trochlea lesions also showed good improvement. The most common adverse event reported with ACI is intraarticular adhesions (2%). The other most common adverse events include detachment/delamination of graft (1.4%), hypertrophic tissue (1.3%–17 %) and catching/popping (1.0%), with the overall adverse event rate and safety profile less than 7% (see Figure 10.6).[28]

SUMMARY

ACI allows for resurfacing of large defect areas and a high percentage of the tissue produced has a similarity to the histology and mechanical properties of hyaline cartilage. Good to excellent results are reproducible, as a number of independent centers have reported high degrees of satisfaction achieved across a broad spectrum of knee pathology. The consensus among the leaders in this technology is that ACI may be considered as a primary treatment for lesions greater than 2 cm^2 in active individuals and as a secondary option for all other lesions, regardless of size.

We have come into a new era of tissue-engineered repair for musculoskeletal injuries, and future cartilage repair methodology is likely to be based on cultured cells supported in engineered tissue. Different biodegradable matrices that could support cartilage growth for some months while the cartilage cells or the mesenchymal stem cells and matrix become established are being investigated. With additional growth factors and with emerging technologies using cell-based repair, the indications for the treatment of cartilage injuries should expand.

References

1. Grande DA, Pitman MI, Peterson L, Mench D, Klein M. The repair of experimentally produced defects in rabbit articular cartilage by autologous chondrocyte transplantation. J Orthop Res 1989;7:208–218.
2. Peterson L, Lindahl A, Brittberg M, Kiviranta I, Nilsson A. Autologous chondrocyte transplantation: biomechanics and long-term durability. Am J Sports Med 2002;30:2–12.
3. Brittberg M, Lindahl A, Nilsson A, Ohlsson C, Isaksson O, Peterson L. Treatment of deep cartilage defects in the knee with autologous chondrocyte transplantation. N Engl J Med 1994;33 1:889–895.
4. Minas T, Chiu R. Autologous chondrocyte implantation. Am J Knee Surg 2000;13:41–50.
5. Mandelbaum BR, Browne JE, Fu F, et al. Articular cartilage lesions of the knee. Am J Sports Med 1998;26:853–861.
6. Rosenberg TD, Paulos LE, Parker RD, Coward DB, Scott SM. The forty-five-degree posteroanterior flexion weight-bearing radiograph of the knee. J Bone Joint Surg 1998;70A:1479–1483.
7. Brittberg M. Die transplantation autogener knorpelzellen in gelenkflachendefekte. Oper Orthop Traumatol 2001;3:198–207.
8. Cole BJ, D'Amato M. Autologous chondrocyte implantation. Oper Tech Orthop 2001;11:115–131.
9. Gillogly SD, Hamby TH. Clinical results of autologous chondrocyte implantation for large full-thickness chondral defects of the knee: five-year experience with 112 consecutive patients. Presented at the American Orthopaedic Society for Sports Medicine, June 28, 2001, Keystone, CO.
10. Minas T, Peterson L. Advanced techniques in autologous chondrocyte transplantation. Clin Sports Med 1999;18:13–44.
11. Peterson L. Cartilage cell transplantation. In: Malek MM (ed) Knee Surgery: Complications, Pitfalls, and Salvage. New York: Springer-Verlag 2001.
12. Peterson L, Minas T, Brittberg M, Nilsson A, Sjorgren-Jansson E, Lindahl A. Two- to 9-year outcome after autologous chondrocyte transplantation of the knee. Clin Orthop 2000;374:212–234.
13. Brittberg M. Autologous chondrocyte transplantation. Clin Orthop 1999;367(suppl):S147–S155.
14. Minas T. Nonarthoplasty management of knee arthritis in the young individual. Curr Opin Orthop 1998;9:46–52.
15. Minas T. Autologous chondrocyte implantation for focal chondral defects of the knee. Clin Orthop. 2001;391(suppl):349–361.
16. Fulkerson JP. Patellofemoral pain disorders: evaluation and management. J Am Acad Orthop Surg 1994;2:124–132.
17. Fulkerson JP. Anteromedialization of the tibial tuberosity for patellofemoral malalignment. Clin Orthop 1983;177:176–181.
18. Bjornun S, Peterson L, Brittberg M, Lindahl A. Patellar defects treated with autologous chondrocyte implantation. Presented at the International Cartilage Repair Society (ICRS) Meeting, 2002, Toronto, Canada.
19. Salter RB, Simmonds DF, Malcolm BW, Rumble EJ, MacMichael D, Clements ND. The biological effect of continuous passive motion on the healing of full-thickness defects in articular cartilage. An experimental investigation in the rabbit. J Bone Joint Surg 1980;62A:1232–1251.
20. Lu Y, Edwards RB, Cole BJ, Markel MD. Thermal chondroplasty with radiofrequency energy: an in vitro comparison of bipolar and monopolar radiofrequency devices. Am J Sports Med 2001; 29:42–49.
21. Anderson AF, Browne JE, Ergglet C, et al. Cartilage repair registry. Vol 7. Cambridge, MA: Genzyme Biosurgery; 2001;7:1–7.
22. Bahuaud J, Maitrot RC, Bouvet R, et al. Autologous chondrocyte implantation for cartilage repair. Presentation of 24 cases. Chirurgie 1998;123:568–571.
23. Minas T. Autologous cultured chondrocyte implantation in the repair of focal chondral lesions of the knee: clinical indications and operative technique. J Sports Traumatol 1998;20:90–102.
24. Gersoff W. Clinical experience with autologous chondrocyte implantation: a preliminary report. Presented at the Western Orthopaedic Society Meeting; July 21, 2001; Steamboat Springs, CO.
25. Lohnert J. Regeneration of hyalin cartilage in the knee joint by treatment with autologous chondrocyte transplantation. Langenbecks Arch Chir Suppl Kongressbel 1998;115:1201–1207.
26. Richardson JB, Caterson B, Evans EH, Ashton BA, Roberts S. Outcomes of autologous chondrocyte implantation in 40 patients. Presented at the ICRS Meeting; 2000; Toronto, Canada.
27. Knutsen G, et al. Autologous chondrocyte implantation versus microfracture: a prospective randomized norwegian multicenter trial. Presented at the ICRS Meeting; 2002; Toronto, Canada.
28. Micheli L, et al. Autologous chondrocyte implantation of the knee: multicenter experience and minimum 3-year follow-up. Clin J Sports Med 2001;11:223–228.

11

Autologous Chondrocyte Implantation in the Osteoarthritic Knee

Tom Minas

BACKGROUND

This chapter discusses the role of autologous chondrocyte implantation (ACI) for the treatment of full-thickness cartilage injuries of the knee. The use of ACI for more damaged knees with early osteoarthritis has been relatively contraindicated. However, before U.S. Food and Drug Administration (FDA) approval,[1] the only cases approved for treatment by this technique in the author's practice were on the basis of failed prior cartilage repair procedures or for compassionate reasons in severely injured knees of young patients. Hence, the author has a large experience in the management of the young patient with advanced chondrosis. Interestingly, patient satisfaction and self-perception of improvement after treatment has been the highest in this category of treatment (see Results).

The salvage category of treatment has been defined as the osteoarthritic knee.[2,3] Osteoarthritis has been defined as radiographic evidence of joint space narrowing on standing X-rays, peripheral osteophyte formation, or intraarticular osteophyte formation. Arthroscopically, it is defined as generalized chondromalacia, Outerbridge classification[4] stage II or greater with focal chondral defects, or focal chondral defects that are "kissing" in nature; that is, patella and trochlea, or tibia and femur.

The prevalence of chondral defects is frequent with sporting injuries and advancing age. Full-thickness chondral injuries secondary to work-related and sporting activities have an incidence between 5%–10% of acute hemarthrosis.[5] A retrospective review of 31,516 knee arthroscopies demonstrated the presence of Outerbridge grade III (41%) and grade IV (19.2%) lesions. In patients less than 40 years of age, only 5% had unipolar grade IV injuries to the medial femoral condyles.[6] The article pointed out that only 5% of cases were suitable for treatment with ACI based on FDA guidelines. This study found lesions were more common in patients over 40 years of age, leaving a large patient population with symptomatic chondral defects who are considered too young for total knee replacement and who do not obtain adequate pain relief and functional improvement after arthroscopic debridement alone.

Patients over the age of 40 are especially difficult to manage by marrow stimulation techniques, as the defects are often large, chronic in nature, and there is evidence to suggest that intrinsic marrow stem cell population is low[7] and repair capacity poorer in this age group.[8–10] ACI would therefore be an alternative over total knee arthroplasty, theoretically maintaining a higher quality of life in the young patient.

Osteoarthritis is a spectrum of diseases. Multiple focal defects with a well-maintained joint space are likely an early manifestation of this process. The arthritic process may be caused by inherent biologic failure (Figure 11.1) or secondary to trauma (Figures 11.2 and 11.3). Posttraumatic examples of cartilage injury include ligamentous instability, postmeniscectomy chondrosis, long-standing axial malalignment, recurrent patellar instability, or a combination of these or acute trauma. Osteoarthritis secondary to anterior cruciate ligament (ACL) disruption, in the author's opinion, is considered the knee at highest risk. Acute chondral injuries with ACL disruption and medial meniscus injury are frequent. ACL disruption with magnetic resonance imaging (MRI) evidence of bone bruising occurs in 80% of tears. Articular cartilage injury to the area of bone bruising is frequent[11]; the incidence of full-thickness chondral defects occurring chronically in ACL-injured knees approaches 20%. Hence, at least 20% of cases are predisposed to osteoarthritis.[2]

Traditional marrow stimulation techniques—drilling, abrasion, and microfracture—have had limited success for small defects and especially with large defects with the production of a fibrocartilage repair.[12–16] However, the repair tissue tends to be mechanically soft and degenerates over time.[17] Similarly, autologous periosteal grafts have had good results in the short term but results were poor in the long term.[18] Perichondrial grafts have a tendency to undergo enchondral ossification and fail between 2 and 5 years postoperatively.[2,19] Autologous osteochondral grafts are also used for small lesions but suffer from the problem of donor site morbidity when lesions become large.[20–25] ACI has had durable results in the midterm follow-up of 2 to 9 years postoperatively in Sweden.[26,27] ACI has the advantage of not disrupting the osteochondral unit and of utilizing end-differentiated chondrocytes to resurface large areas.

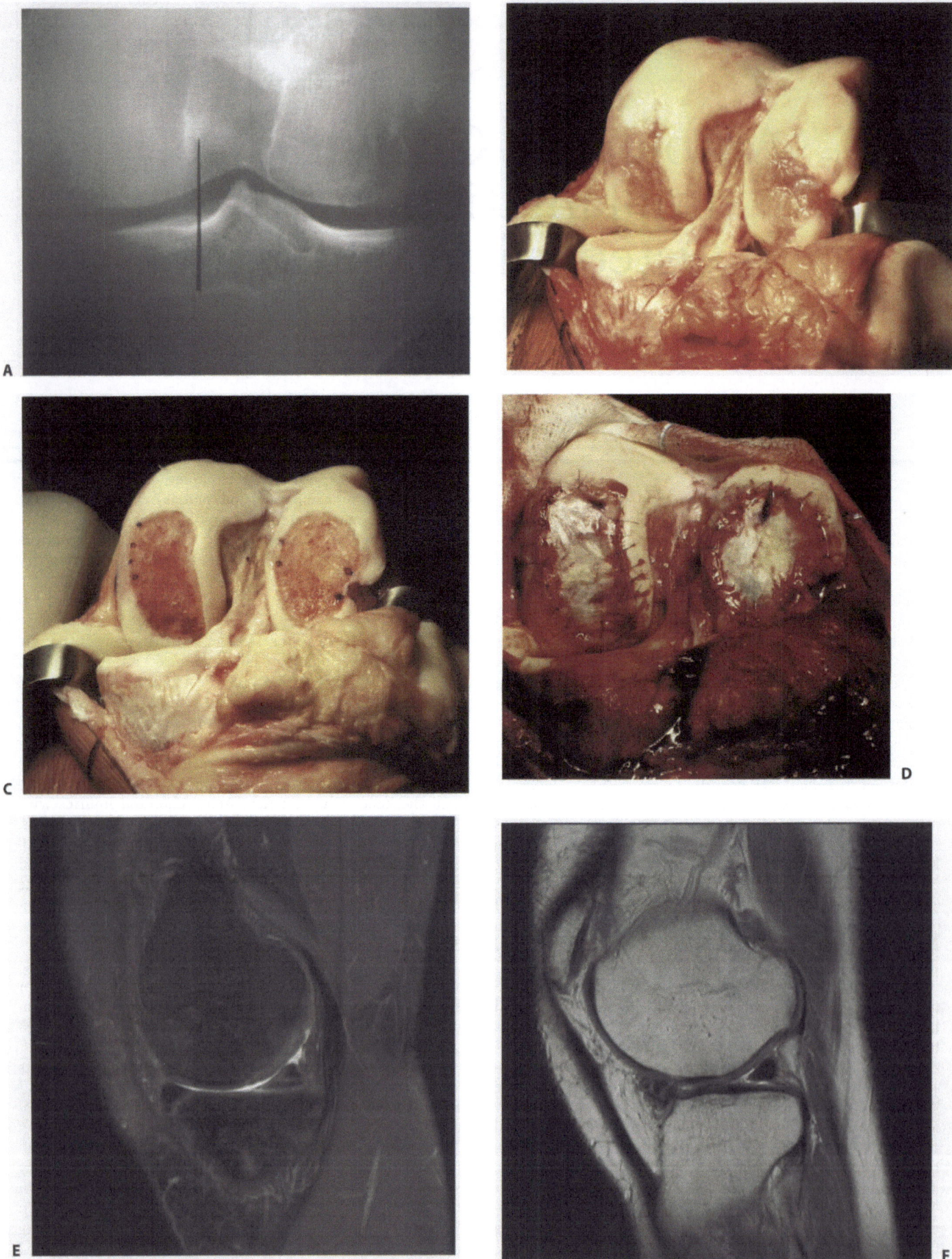

FIGURE 11.1 37-year-old manual laborer with a 10-year history of gradual left knee pain without perceiving injury. Persistent effusion at the end of an 8- to 12-h workday, accompanying limp, unable to participate in recreational activities. Rheumatologic workup negative for inflammatory arthritis. **A.** Standing X-ray demonstrates well-maintained joint space, mechanical axis, falls into medial joint compartment. **B.** Open arthrotomy with medial meniscus taken down to expose posterior aspect of chondral defects demonstrates uncontained large erosive femoral condylar lesions. Tibial plateau articular surfaces are healthy. Osteotomy surgery is not indicated due to mild varus alignment and lateral condylar disease. **C.** Radical debridement of articular damage reveals focal chondral defects with stable margins. Punctate peripheral markings indicate entrance and exit sites of drill holes made for suture passage to secure periosteum to uncontained margins. Sclerotic subchondral bone has been removed back to normal subchondral bone with curettes and a high-powered burr. **D.** Autologous chondrocyte implantation (ACI) grafts sutured and peripherally sealed with allogeneic fibrin glue. Note the *pen markings* on the leading edge of both periosteal patches to orient the superficial periosteal fibrous layer and the leading edge of the defect that was templated. **E.** One-year postoperative MRI scan of the medial condylar graft with fat suppression indicates no bone marrow edema, completely filled cartilage graft. **F.** One-year postoperative MRI scan of the lateral condylar graft without fat suppression demonstrates complete fill, integration, and equal cartilage appearance to adjacent native cartilage.

INDICATIONS AND CONTRAINDICATIONS

There are many considerations in the management of a young arthritic with biologic repair. As prosthetic arthroplasty obtains better long-term results, the age at which arthroplasty is being performed is decreasing. However, it is still desirable for the orthopedist "not to burn bridges" by proceeding to total knee replacement unless advanced tricompartmental disease is present. Absolute contraindications to repair with ACI include ongoing inflammatory arthropathy, unresolved septic arthritis, tricompartmental arthritis, or tricompartmental avascular necrosis. However, if there is less than 50% joint space narrowing on a standing X-ray or skyline patellofemoral view, the patient may still be a candidate for treatment by ACI even if bipolar kissing lesions are noted arthroscopically. The patient must thoroughly understand the rehabilitation process and consider carefully the time commitment involved to achieve a successful outcome.

The preoperative assessment must include patient factors and joint factors. The factors to consider for the patient include the desired level of activity to be obtained, the emotional well-being of the patient including his level of social functioning, and sense of vitality as determined by the Short Form 36 Health Survey[28] which is prognostic for clinical outcome. Patients must be free of dependency on narcotics, be nonsmokers, and have realistic expectations. A family history of osteoarthritis may be a bad prognostic indicator for cartilage failure secondary to intrinsic biologic mechanisms not yet understood. Other joint involvement may be important in determining a biologic versus prosthetic option. Preoperative assessment of the joint includes a complete radiographic examination and physical examination to correlate symptoms to objective pathology. A standard radiographic evaluation should include a 54-in standing axial alignment AP X-ray of both knees, to include hips, knees, and ankles, a standing AP and lateral, skyline patellofemoral, and standing 45° bent-knee (Rosenberg) views.[29] MRI scanning, when performed with gadolinium enhancement, and an advanced cartilage sequencing[30,31] will improve the sensitivity and specificity of diagnosing cartilage injuries to greater than 95%. However, arthroscopic evaluation remains the gold standard for assessing the degree of articular cartilage damage.

The clinical examination should document ligamentous stability, crepitation, joint line tenderness, and subtle patellofemoral maltracking that may become pronounced after open knee surgery if not recognized and corrected at the time of reconstruction. Before entering the operative theater for arthroscopic evaluation and possible cartilage biopsy for cell culturing, the surgeon should have a clear idea of the localization of damage as well as the other factors previously mentioned.

In order of importance, the factors to consider for successful reconstruction are axial alignment/patellofemoral alignment, ligamentous stability, defect size, and the presence or absence of a meniscus. Algorithms have been published regarding treatment options for defect size and patient activity levels.[32–35] Axial alignment with a mechanical axis devia-

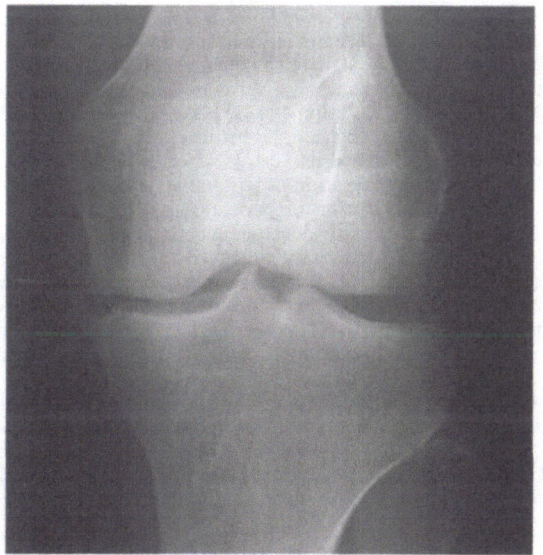
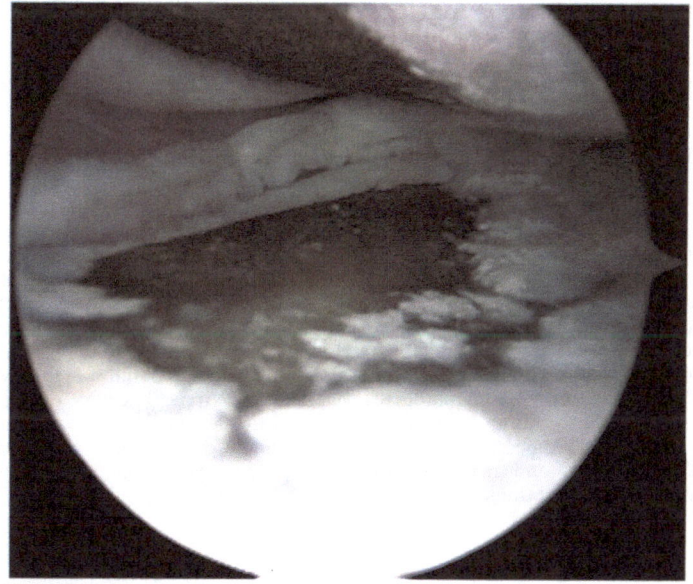

A   B

FIGURE 11.2 Continued

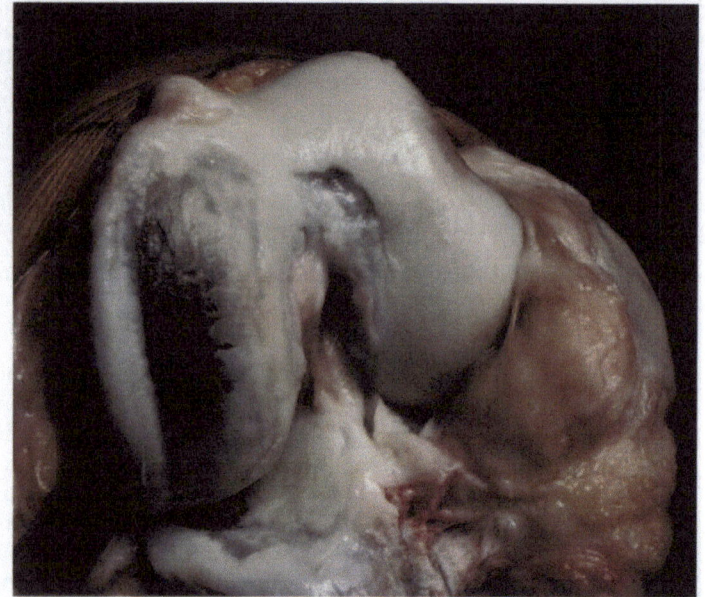

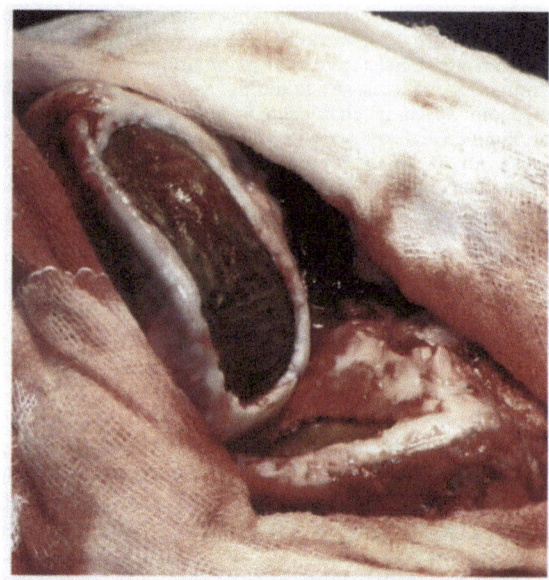

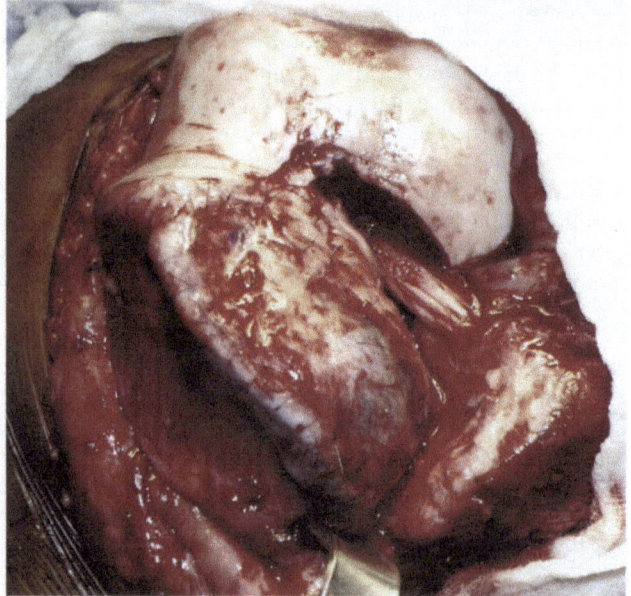

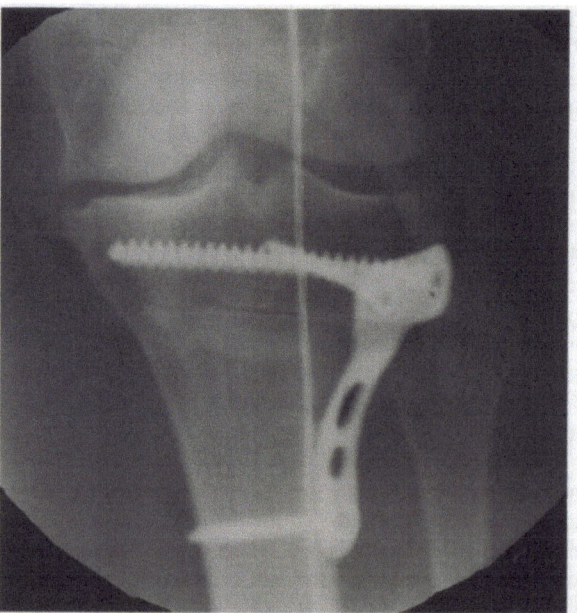

FIGURE 11.2 This eighteen year old female had persistent medial left knee joint pain, inability to walk comfortably on campus, frequent swelling, and sensation of instability when descending hills. She was unable to participate in any sports. Problems started 3 years earlier when she sustained an ACL tear while playing soccer. Surgical reconstruction was performed with patellar tendon bone tendon bone. She returned to sports and sustained a medial meniscus tear, repaired surgically with failure and meniscal excision. Medial joint pain progressed rapidly after this. **A.** AP X-ray demonstrates greater than 50% joint space narrowing, peripheral osteophyte formation, and subchondral tibial sclerosis. **B.** Arthroscopic appearance of medial joint compartment with grade IV chondromalacia of medial tibial plateau, medial femoral condyle, and absent medial meniscus. Examination under anesthesia demonstrated ACL laxity grade 3, with posteriorly placed tibial tunnel. Lateral joint compartment and patellofemoral compartment appeared normal. Intercondylar notch biopsy for culture articular chondrocytes was taken. **C.** Appearance at time of open arthrotomy Note severe loss of articular cartilage, lack of ACL. **D.** Appearance of debrided chondral defects on medial tibial plateau and medial femoral condyle. The subchondral bone was sclerotic and thickened requiring removal with high-speed burr. Note minimal bleeding from bone bed with tourniquet let down. **E.** Appearance of ACI grafts sutured into place with cell suspensions injected. ACL reconstructed by open technique using cadaver patellar tendon bone tendon bone. Varus malalignment corrected with HTO. Order of reconstruction was (1) HTO with midshaft fibular osteotomy and internal fixation; (2) arthrotomy, debridement of chondral defects, and periosteal harvest; (3) open ACL tunnel placement, graft placement, and fixation of femoral bone plug; (4) tourniquet was let down for suturing of periosteal patches, fibrin glue sealant, culture chondrocyte suspension injection, and closure; (5) relocation of patella and arthrotomy closure; and (6) tensioning and fixation of tibial ACL bone plug. **F.** Intraoperative mechanical axis correction to lateral intercondylar spine. **G.** Standing AP of both knees 6 months postoperative. Note restoration of medial joint compartment joint space on AP standing X-ray. **H, I.** One year postoperative MRI sagittal and coronal views demonstrate complete fill of chondral defects to medial femoral condyles and medial tibial plateau, respectively. **J, K.** One-year second-look arthroscopy performed at the time of hardware removal demonstrates complete fill of medial femoral condyles ACI graft posteriorly, and anteriorly, respectively, with equal firmness to adjacent articular cartilage.

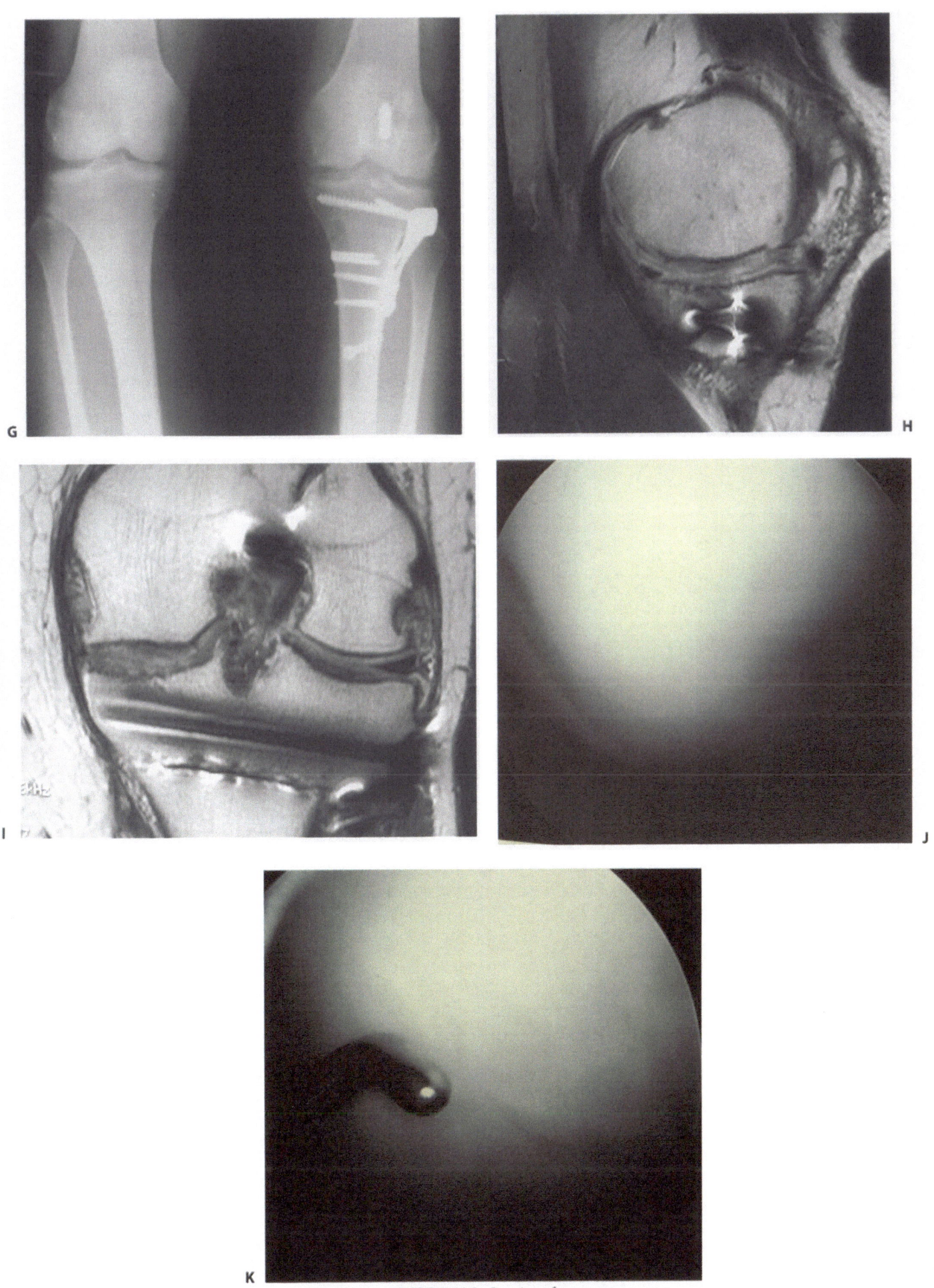

FIGURE 11.2 *Continued*

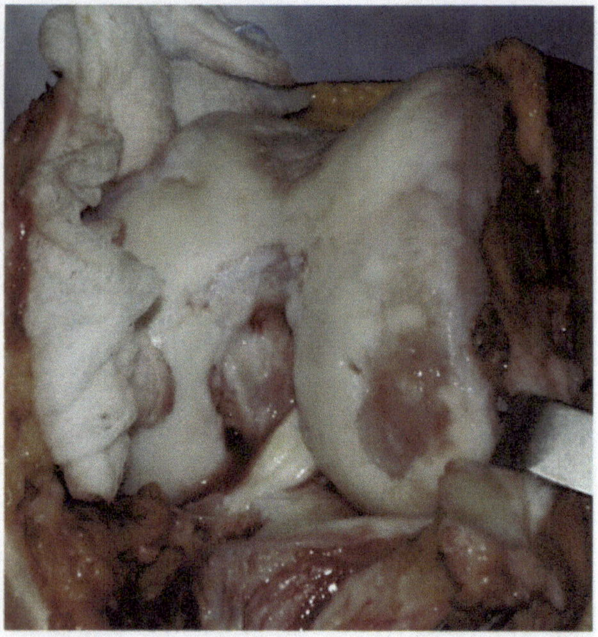

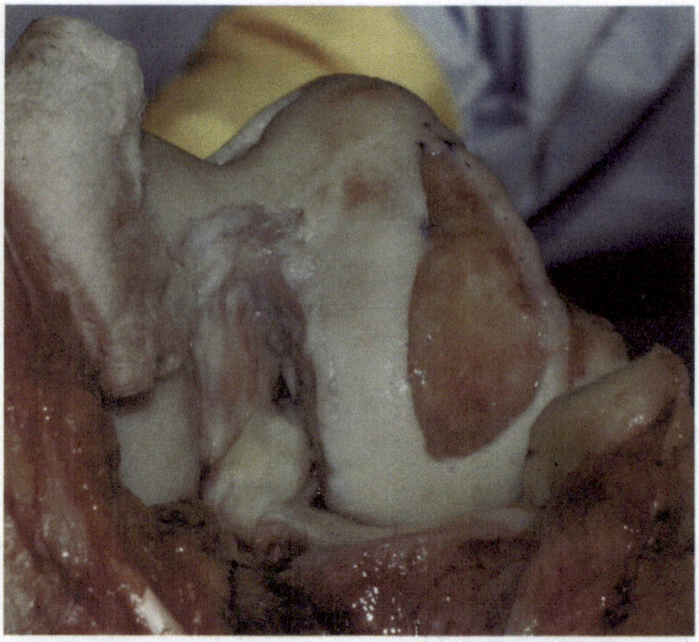

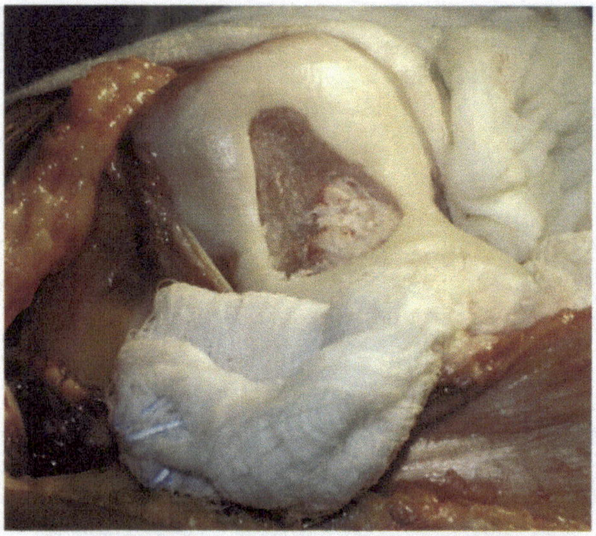

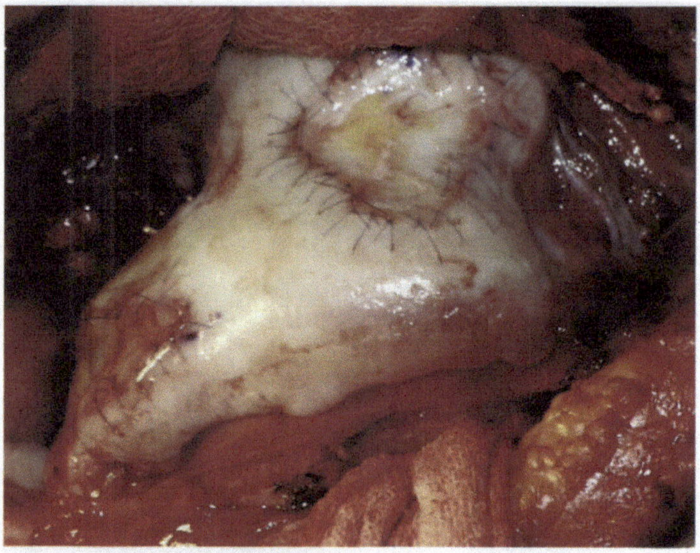

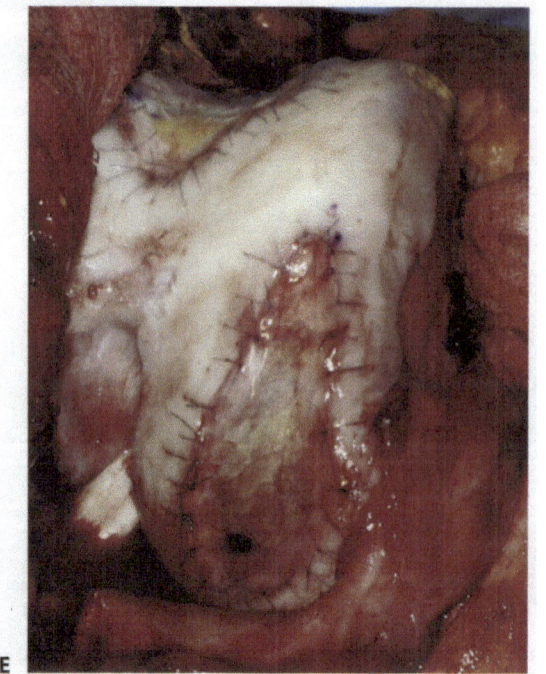

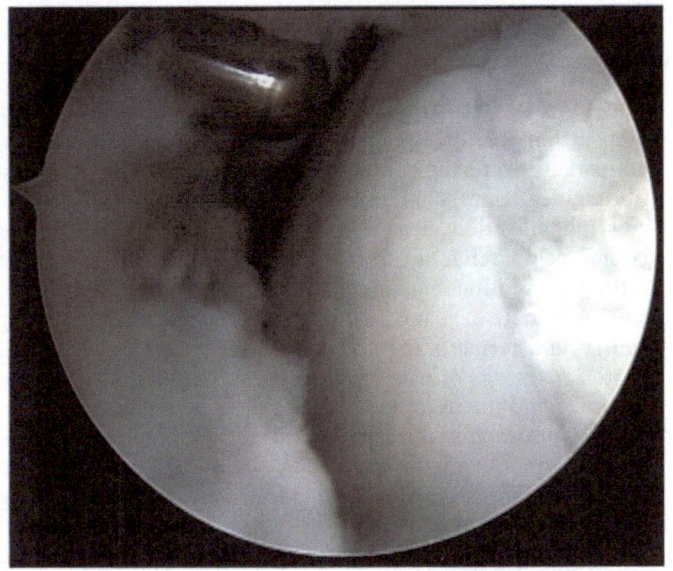

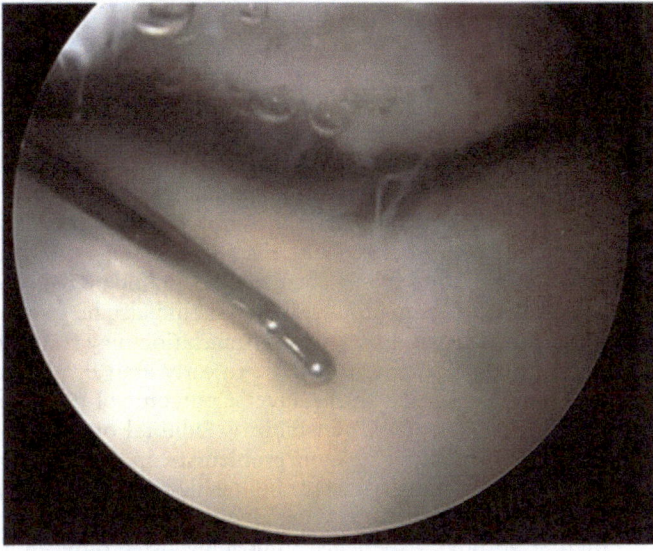

F

G

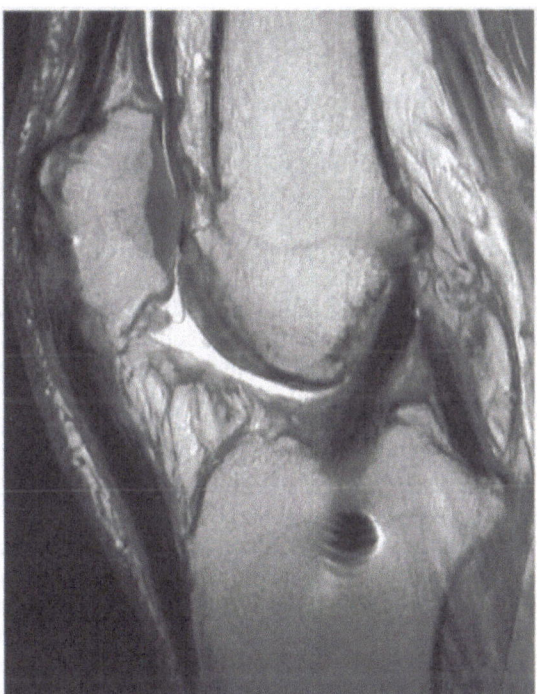

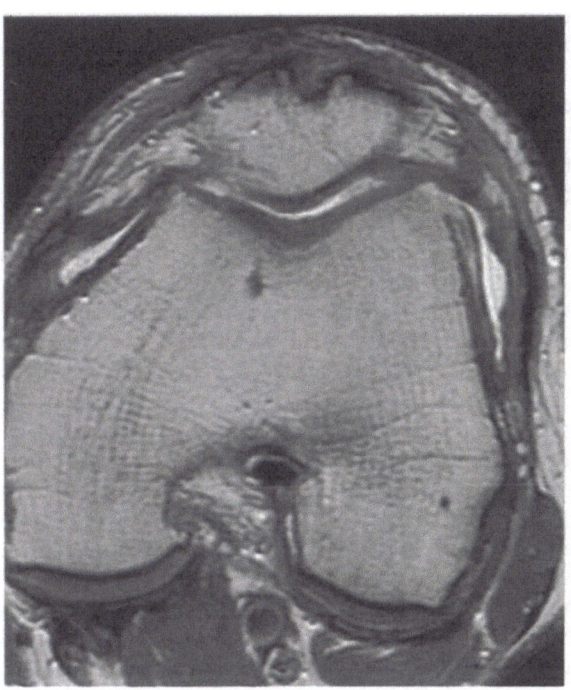

H

I

FIGURE 11.3 Thirty-two-year-old male, with prior ACL disruption from playing football 5 years earlier underwent patellar tendon bone tendon bone ACL reconstruction 1 year after injury and subsequently had a partial medial meniscectomy. Since then, he has had persistent crepitations in the patellofemoral joint accompanied by marked effusions after activity with generalized aching. Finds the need to be missed trustworthy and is having pain on a daily basis, rated at 6 of 10. **A.** Appearance at the time of open arthrotomy for ACL reconstruction. Note the very large, poorly contained lateral femoral condyle injury, and the large intralesional osteophytes in the trochlea, more apparent after debridement. **B.** Debrided lateral femoral condyle, leaving peripheral osteophyte intact to contain the defect; multiple drill holes are marked with a sterile marking pen, and defect is deepened with a high-speed burr to contain the chondrocytes in a cavity. **C.** Demonstration of large intralesional osteophytes in the debrided trochlea; these must be removed before chondrocyte implantation, to prevent the periosteum from eroding through the osteophytes. **D.** Appearance of ACI graft to the trochlea. **E.** ACI graft to the lateral femoral condyle. **F.** Second-look arthroscopy 18 months following ACI for removal of adhesions in the infrapatellar fat pad region. Appearance of lateral femoral condyle ACI graft, is firm, smooth repair site. **G.** Eighteen months after ACI to the trochlea, graft is smooth, firm, and well integrated to adjacent cartilage and underlying bone. **H, I.** MRI appearance of trochlea on sagittal and oblique axial films, respectively, demonstrating complete fill and cartilage appearance to native cartilage.

tion greater that 25% from the midline requires correction when associated with a chondral defect. The degree of correction depends radiographic evidence of joint space narrowing, sclerosis and defect size. If the chondral defect is associated with 50% joint space narrowing and subchondral sclerosis of the bone in that compartment, a mechanical axis overcorrection to the opposite intercondylar spine is the appropriate correction, that is, 2° to 3° of overcorrection. If the chondral defect is associated with malalignment and the joint space is normal, then the mechanical axis should be restored back to neutral. Ligamentous stability should also be present before cartilage repair. Excessive AP translation may result in shearing forces that may predispose to early graft delamination and failure, similar to the adverse outcome of meniscal repair with persistent ACL instability. Subtotal or extruded nonfunctioning menisci are more problematic in the decision-making process. The absence of the medial meniscus with a chondral defect is usually associated with a varus knee.

In the author's experience, unloading osteotomy alone with ACI has had excellent long-term results even in the absence of a medial meniscus. However, if the medial condyle injury is large (e.g., 6 to 10 cm^2), the alignment is neutral, and the meniscus is absent, the author would recommend cartilage repair with meniscal allograft transplantation. Absence of the lateral meniscus has usually been associated with a neutrally aligned knee or a varus knee. In this situation, ACI to the lateral femoral condyle has usually been performed combined with a lateral meniscus allograft. It has been unusual, in the author's case series, to have a combination of an absent lateral meniscus and a valgus knee with an articular cartilage defect without severe end-stage bone-on-bone disease considered not suitable for ACI.

The other factor to consider before reconstruction is the risk of arthrofibrosis. Patient-related factors predisposing to arthrofibrosis include race (i.e, fair-skinned Caucasian redheads are more prone to arthrofibrosis) or the very muscular mesomorph phenotype. Multiple ACI grafts, combined with multiple intraarticular procedures, may also predispose to arthrofibrosis. When the reconstruction requires multiple procedures, it may be advantageous to stage the reconstruction if the patient is considered at high risk for arthrofibrosis. Osteotomy and ligament reconstruction should be performed first before ACI and meniscal transplantation. In this way, the risk of arthrofibrosis is minimized.

TECHNIQUE OF AUTOLOGOUS CHONDROCYTE IMPLANTATION

Surgical Correction of Factors Predisposing to Chondral Injury

Several predisposing factors to chondral injury must be assessed so that these may be either corrected in a staged or concomitant fashion with ACI. Tibial femoral malalignment, patellofemoral malalignment, and ligamentous, meniscal, or bone insufficiency must be assessed before definitive cartilage cell re-implantation. These techniques are discussed after the technique of open surgical transplantation of autologous chondrocytes is reviewed. The technique has been illustrated in more complete detail in previous publications.[36–38]

Surgical Transplantation of Autologous Chondrocytes: Pearls and Pitfalls

The steps in open implantation include arthrotomy, defect preparation, periosteum procurement, periosteum fixation, periosteum watertight integrity testing, autologous/allogenic fibrin glue sealant, chondrocyte implantation, wound closure, and rehabilitation. For a unicondylar injury, a medial or lateral parapatellar arthrotomy is used, usually performed through a midline incision or a longitudinal parapatellar incision. Adequate exposure is crucial to good periosteal suturing and several retractors are often required to obtain this goal. Posterior lesions on the femur often require hyperflexion of the knee and meniscal takedown; this is performed by incising the intermeniscal ligament anteriorly, releasing the coronary ligament below the meniscus, and then taking down the entire sub-periosteal envelope posteriorly. A repair during closure involves reduction of the meniscus anatomically and repair of the anterior horn with a nonabsorbable suture via a bone suture. For multiple lesions, a traditional medial parapatellar arthrotomy is often required with subluxation or dislocation of the patella and hyperflexion of the knee for patch suturing.

Defect preparation is critical. Radical debridement of all fissured and undermined articular cartilage surrounding the full-thickness chondral injury to healthy contained cartilage is desirable. Oval or curvilinear excisions with a 15 blade are done by incising the articular cartilage vertically down to the subchondral bone plate without penetrating the bone. Small ring or closed curettes and periosteal elevators are used to debride the degenerating articular cartilage back to healthy host cartilage. Maintaining an intact subchondral bone plate without subchondral bone bleeding is important. However, removing intralesional osteophytes in all sclerotic bone is equally important,(see Figure 11.3). An intralesional osteophyte will tent the periosteum, leading to possible erosion of the periosteum and loss of cells, or a bony prominence without cartilage cover during the repair process, leading to persistent pain and failure. The subchondral bone may be polished and sclerotic. In this situation, a high-speed burr is required to remove the bone until healthy-appearing subchondral cancellous bone is visualized (see Figure 11.2). Usually 1 to 2 mm of bone is removed to achieve this; not only does this allow for better cell integration to the subchondral bone, it also prepares a cavity in which cells can proliferate. This step is usually performed with the tourniquet applied; surprisingly, there is little bleeding when the tourniquet is let down in this situation. Any bleeding is usually easily controlled with thrombin and epinephrine-soaked neural patties. If bleeding persists, a pinpoint electrocautery or a dab of fibrin glue usually stops bleeding in the small vessels.

A contained lesion is desired, and it is better to leave a minimally chondromalacic cartilage border than to remove it and provide an uncontained lesion that would require suturing to synovium or small drill holes in bone (see Figures 11.1, 11.3). Once a healthy defect bed is prepared, it is templated with sterile tracing paper (sterile glove packaging paper works well). A sterile marker can be used to template the defect and can then be cut out to fit the defect perfectly. This pattern can then be oversized by approximately 2 mm in both length and width as a template on the periosteal site when it is prepared because some shrinkage of the periosteum occurs as it is procured.

Tibiofemoral and Patellofemoral Malalignment

When varus or valgus malalignment is concomitant with a medial or lateral condyle injury, respectively, a corrective osteotomy is paramount to the success of the chondral transplantation. This step can be done either in a staged or concomitant fashion. However, if it is done concomitantly, a stable fixation must be obtained at the time of osteotomy surgery so that continuous passive motion (CPM) and early active range of motion may be pursued immediately postoperatively. Otherwise, a staged reconstruction should be performed.

Patellofemoral maltracking combined with a trochlear or patellar chondral injury requires careful pre-operative assessment with physical examination and CT or MRI imaging techniques. Tibial tubercle osteotomy combined with soft tissue realignment to ensure proper tracking is paramount to successful graft healing.

Congenital trochlea dysplasia, an uncommon factor contributing to patellofemoral maltracking or recurrent instability is best assessed by a preoperative CT scan demonstrating a flattened or convex proximal trochlea. Treatment is by surgical trochleoplasty combined with patellar realignment as necessary.[38] Results of trochleoplasty for trochlear dysplasia have been excellent.[39] Twenty-one patients (25 knees) with recurrent dislocation of the patella due to patellofemoral dysplasia were treated with a combination of proximal and distal realignment in conjuction with a trochleoplasty (deepening of the intercondylar sulcus on the proximal joint surface of the femur). At follow-up, on average 6 years later, there were 21 good and excellent results, and 3 fair or poor.

Ligament Insufficiency

Anterior cruciate insufficiency may jeopardize a newly regenerating cartilage graft. Staged or concomitant surgery should be performed with the goal of preventing shear forces and instability episodes from damaging a regenerating graft. When a medial femoral condyle injury is present with ACL insufficiency, the author performs an open ACL reconstruction with an ACI to the medial femoral condyle. Medial arthrotomy allows direct visualization for ACL tunnel placement and ACI repair is straightforward. For lateral sided injuries, ACL tunnel placement is poorly visualized through a limited lateral arthrotomy. Thus, when a lateral femoral condyle injury is present with ACL insufficiency, the author performs an arthroscopic ACL reconstruction to ensure exact tunnel placement, which is then followed by an open ACI reconstruction through a limited lateral arthrotomy.

The rehabilitation follows that for ACI, which is the rate limiting process in recovery. Anterior cruciate rehabilitation is modified to exclude closed-chain resisted strengthening exercises until 3 months after combined surgery to prevent excessive compressive load to the chondral repair site. Six to 9 months are required before these exercises may be instituted.

Bone Deficiency

In the case of bony deficiency, such as after an osteochondral fracture or with osteochondritis dissecans (OCD) or avascular necrosis, the depth of the bony lesion should be assessed preoperatively by radiography or tomography. Osteochondritis dissecans defects, on average, are 6 to 8 mm deep including cartilage and bone. These defects often will do well without bone grafting using ACI alone. However, defects that are greater than 1 to 2 cm deep clearly need preliminary bone grafting and healing before cartilage resurfacing, which may be performed either arthroscopically or by open techniques. Following bone grafting, weight bearing is protected for the initial 8 weeks and CPM is utilized. An interval of 6 to 9 months is required before second-stage articular resurfacing to allow the cancellous bone graft to form a new subchondral bone plate which is generally associated with minimal if any bleeding at the time of ACI.

Special Considerations for the Trochlea, Patella, and Tibia

The results of ACI when treating the patella are 62% good and excellent overall, and when malalignment is corrected, the results improve to 85%.[17] The trochlea does best when only one facet is treated, and as with the patella, results approach 85%. Results when treating the tibia are not known at this time because few cases have been performed, with a short follow-up. However, the techniques for all three lesions require some special considerations.

When harvesting periosteum for trochlea repair, templating is especially useful as defects are irregularly shaped. The concave medial to lateral curvature is best reconstituted by oversizing the periosteum in the same direction by several millimeters. Suturing is then performed to recreate this topography, starting at the central sulcus and moving peripherally, restoring the concave topography of the trochlea. ACI of the patella requires unique technical considerations in addition to correction of maltracking. Early failures were thought to be partly due to inadequate debridement of softened and undermined tissue. In addition, the technique of debridement should leave behind a defect whose leading and trailing margins are angled so as to not produce an abrupt interface between sutured periosteum and host cartilage. The angle may be more gradual when the articular cartilage is thick, but must be more vertical when cartilage is thin, so that suture fixation is secure. Similarly, the contour of the patella must be reproduced by the suture technique. This is most easily performed by oversizing the periosteal patch in the medial to lateral direction and then starting the suturing at the apex of the median ridge alternating from side to side, much like "pitching a tent."

The tibial plateau is largely covered by meniscus. Exposure therefore involves takedown of the meniscus for debridement and suturing. The lateral tibial plateau is easier, involving a lateral arthrotomy, incision of the intermeniscal ligament and the coronary ligament while retracting the meniscus laterally as the knee is hyperflexed and internally rotated. Further subperiosteal dissection of the coronary ligament–lateral meniscus attachment gives excellent exposure. Rarely does the posterolateral complex origin from the lateral epicondyle require takedown with a bone block to gain posterolateral exposure.

The medial tibial plateau, however, is not so easily accessed. Except for smaller anterior lesions, the medial epicondyle–medial collateral ligament complex routinely must be taken down in addition to the medial meniscus. A bone block with stable fixation is required to start early CPM. A prefitted unloader brace is used postoperatively for 6 months to protect the graft, which experiences point loading with femoral rollback.

REHABILITATION

The concept of a time course of healing of ACI (Table 11.1) resulted from the clinical observations of improving patient symptomatology and arthroscopic second looks to assess graft appearance and for mechanical indentation. Animal models that assess the histologic appearance of healing transplants also support this time course.[40–43] Stages of healing include proliferation (0–6 weeks), transition (7–26 weeks), and remodeling (27 weeks onward). Proliferation denotes a rapid response of defect fill with a primitive repair tissue by 6 weeks, which is soft. The transitional phase demonstrates macromolecular matrix production histologically; clinically the graft starts to firm up, taking on the texture of a gelatin (3–6 months). The remodeling stage demonstates further cellular activity with matrix production, accompanied by further mechanical hardening as time goes on, usually achieving a putty-like consistency by 6 to 7 months clinically.

The grafts are vulnerable to injury during these stages of healing, when mechanically the grafts are not as firm as the adjacent articular surfaces. Excessive activity at these early time points may result in graft delamination or overload and degeneration. Protected and graduated functional rehabilitation results in graft maturation over the ensuing months preventing graft injury. This process also depends upon defect size, depth and site (i.e, taking up to 24 to 36 months for the patella). Joint catching, pain, or increased swelling indicate that the activity is excessive and should be lessened until a pain free smooth joint function returns.

The following principles are emphasized as guidelines to successful functional rehabilitation:

1. Range of motion exercises (passive/active-assisted) to enhance chondrocyte regeneration and decrease the likelihood of intraarticular adhesions
2. Protected graft loading for 6 to 12 weeks after surgery to prevent the likelihood of delamination or periosteal overload and central degeneration of the graft
3. Restoration of muscle tone with isometric muscle exercises to prevent atrophy, followed by light functional resisted activities

Continuous passive motion is instituted after 6 hours when cell attachment has occurred or starts the next day. With weight-bearing femoral condyles, CPM is increased to regain a full range of motion as the patient tolerates, with a very slow cycle setting of approximately 2 per minute. CPM is utilized approximately 6 to 8 hours daily for up to 6 weeks postoperatively. This period is based on experimental work [44,45] that has demonstrated an enhancement of the quality of repair tissue via this modality as well as clinical work[15] which has demonstrated increased repair tissue fill with CPM 6 to 8 h/day for 6 to 8 weeks postoperatively. At this time, the exact quantity and duration of CPM for ACI have not been determined. Patients are comfortable while on CPM and it does decrease the likelihood of intraarticular adhesions. Deep friction and patellar mobilizations start immediately after surgery to prevent infrapatellar adhesions and patellar maltracking and to improve range of motion. CPM for defects of the trochlea is less aggressive. Initially, CPM is used for a range of 0° to 40° maximum. The remainder of the motion is obtained by allowing the patient to dangle the leg hourly over the edge of the bed to regain further motion. CPM from 40° to 70° degrees is not recommended because maximal patellofemoral contact forces occur in this range.

Femoral condyle ACI is protected with touch down weight-bearing for 6 weeks postoperatively on crutches. Weight bearing is then increased to full body weight by 12 weeks postoperatively. Thereafter, the patient is instructed to

TABLE 11.1   Time course of healing for ACI.

Stage	Proliferation (0–6 weeks)	Transition (7–12 weeks)	Remodeling and maturation >13 weeks–3 years
Histology	Rapid proliferation of spindle-shaped cells with defect fill; mostly type I collagen with early formation of colonies of chondrocytes forming type II collagen	Matrix formation, mostly chondrocytes producing type II collagen and proteoglycans; poor integration to underlying bone and cartilage	Ongoing remodeling of matrix with reorganization and quantity of collagen type II, with integration to bone (arcades of Benninghoff), and adjacent host cartilage; large-chain aggregates of proteoglycans, with increased water content of cartilage
Viscoelastic arthroscopic appearance	Filled, soft, white tissue	Jelly-like firmness, with "wavelike" motion when probed, not yet firm, and integrated to underlying bone	Firm "indentable," but not "wavelike," when probed by 4–6 months after ACI; graft whiter than host cartilage, may demonstrate periosteal hypertrophy (20%); equal firmness to host cartilage 9–18 months after ACI
Activity level	CPM starts 6 h after surgery for 6–8 h/day × 6 weeks Touch WB Isometric muscle exercises and ROM	Discontinue CPM Active ROM Partial graduated WB to full WB by 12 weeks Functional muscle usage, stationary bicycle, treadmill, elliptical trainer, and isometrics	Discontinue assistive devices 4–5 months postoperative if free of pan, catching, swelling Distance walking, hiking, cross-country skiing, inline skating Nonpivoting running 14–18 months Pivoting allowed 18–24 months

ACI, autologous chondrocyte implantation; CPM, continuous passive motion; ROM, range of motion; WB, weight bearing.

use one crutch in the opposite arm and switch to a cane when comfortable. Each patient's progress is individualized and is guided by symptoms. If weight-bearing discomfort, catching, locking, or swelling of the knee occurs, weight-bearing status and activity level are decreased as tolerated by the patient. These symptoms may indicate that the graft is undergoing overload, with stimulation of the subchondral bone, resulting in pain for the patient. On average, it is 4 to 4.5 months before patients have discarded their canes and are walking relatively comfortably with a small effusion. Larger lesions require longer recovery time. If a patient has a lesion 6 to 10 cm^2 or larger, kissing transplants, or a deep OCD lesion, then an unloader brace is used early after surgery when swelling subsides and is discontinued at 6 to 9 months postoperatively when pain has resolved. With the use of a brace, the rehabilitation is the same as for a weight-bearing femoral condyle. At this time, nonimpact activities such as long-distance walking, cycling, swimming, and cross-country skiing are encouraged. Running is not permitted until graft hardness is similar to adjacent cartilage which takes approximately 18 to 24 months.

Lesions of the trochlea are slower in the rehabilitation process and healing. Full weight-bearing is allowed early with a knee immobilizer. Isometric straight-leg lifts are instituted immediately. Rehabilitation to decrease patellofemoral contact pressure is encouraged. At 6 to 8 weeks following surgery, treadmill walking backward, straight-leg lifts, active flexion, and passive extension are encouraged. Effusion is more common with trochlea repairs for up to 6 months after surgery. Stationary bicycling with low resistance is allowed at 4 to 6 weeks. Kneeling, squatting, and so forth are not permitted until 12 to 18 months following surgery, at which time graft hardness is similar to that of adjacent cartilage.

COMPLICATIONS, MANAGEMENT, ADVERSE EVENTS, AND FAILURES

The overall need for second-look arthroscopy was 25% of cases for symptoms from arthrofibrosis and periosteal hypertrophy, 20% for periosteal problems, and 5% for adhesions. If a patient's recovery lacks range of motion or develops painful catching during the course of rehabilitation, an MRI scan with gadolinium intravenous enhancement is performed for an indirect arthrogram effect. The MRI scan has become a valuable tool. Using a computer workstation, the status of adhesions and grafts can be assessed before arthroscopy, allowing a guided arthroscopic lysis of adhesions or chondroplasty of periosteal hypertrophy of the ACI graft. Graft delamination, when recognized by this method preoperatively, allows for a planned cartilage repair depending on the size of the defect remaining.

Early complications are generally related to adhesions and knee stiffness. If there is a painful limitation of motion that does not progress with physical therapy, then early arthroscopic lysis of adhesions in the first 3 months after surgery results in an excellent outcome. Blind manipulation is not recommended because of the frequent incidence of adhesions attached to the grafts.

Periosteal problems, when they occur, are generally at more than 3 months after surgery. Hypertrophy manifests itself as a new onset of painful catching that does not

improve. If the crepitation on examination is minimal, then observation often results in spontaneous relief of symptoms. However, if the clinical examination reveals a very palpable or audible crepitation or snapping, early arthroscopic intervention and chondroplasty are recommended to prevent graft detachment or delamination. Typically, rehabilitation resumes with limited discomfort.

Failure was defined as failure to clinically improve, and/or complete delamination or removal of the graft, or surgical retreatment of the same defect that violated the subchondral bone. Failures generally occurred early (<12 months postimplantation). Of 169 patients treated, 22 patients (13%) were considered failures. The failures by category of treatment were simple 2 of 12 (16.7%); complex 8 of 86 (9.3%); and salvage 12 of 71 (16.9%). Of the patients considered to have failed, 8 underwent successful re-ACI, 1 required patellectomy, 1 underwent cadaveric allograft replacement, 2 went on to total knee replacement (TKR), and 9 underwent arthroscopic debridement alone and wished no further treatment at the last clinical review. No patients considered themselves worse than before initial ACI treatment.

RESULTS

Overall, 87% of cases were considered successful with clinical improvement as of December 1999. These results have been maintained at the most recent update in August 2002. After approval by the human ethics committee, a prospective evaluation of ACI-treated patients was undertaken in March 1995. At publication,[2] 169 patients had been treated, and 260 patients as of August 2002.

Demographic data, prior surgical history, defect characteristics, and baseline evaluation including completion of four validated rating scales were collected (Tables 11.2–11.4): SF-36 (Short Form 36, Quality of Life questionnaire), WOMAC (Western Ontario and MacMaster Universities Osteoarthritis Index), KSS (Knee Society Score), and the modified Cincinnati Knee Rating System. Patient outcome questionnaires were chosen to be complementary to capture both high- and low-demand goals of patients with differing stages of severity of disease. A patient satisfaction survey included these questions: "Rate the results," "Compared to preoperative," "Overall satisfaction," and "Choose surgery again" with four categorical responses for each. In this way, it was hoped that both highly functional and severely involved patients would be captured by the instruments utilized as they were complementary to both high- and low-demand goals.

Follow-up evaluation was completed using these same four scales at 12, 18, and 24 months and at yearly intervals

TABLE 11.2 Clinician Cincinnati Knee Rating System score comparison by osteotomy type: salvage category patients with minimum 12-month follow-up.

Group	n	Baseline score	Follow-up score	p value
No osteotomy	26	3.1	5.2	<0.001
High tibial osteotomy	15	3.9	5.5	0.02
Tibial tubercle osteotomy	10	3.1	3.8	0.09

Note: Higher score indicates improved condition.

TABLE 11.3   Knee Society Score comparison by osteotomy type: salvage category patients with minimum 12-month follow-up.

Group	n	Knee Score Baseline	Knee Score Follow-up	p value	Function Score Baseline	Function Score Follow-up	p value
None	26	54.0	73.6	<0.001	65.0	71.3	0.05
High tibial osteotomy	15	54.1	65.8	0.07	70.1	70.7	1.0
Tibial tubercle osteotomy	10	52.1	60.1	0.11	66.7	69.5	0.32

Note: Higher score indicates improved condition.

thereafter. Data were collected independent of the implanting surgeon by trained research staff using standardized case report forms, and statistical analysis were conducted by an unbiased third party (AACT-Abt Associates Clinical Trials, Cambridge, MA, USA). Data on adverse events were also collected.

As of December 1999, 169 patients were treated for 295 full-thickness Outerbridge grade IV chondral defects. Patients were categorized into three groups for outcome evaluation. The salvage group ($n = 71$) with focal defects and early radiographic osteoarthritis (OA) had unexpectedly good results. The results to follow have been updated as of August 2002 and they continue to be maintained and improved. The results are being prepared for peer-review publication.

Statistically significant clinical improvement with a minimum follow-up of 24 months (average, 42 months) has been noted. Patients were 69% male and averaged 39 years of age (range, 13–58 years) for the salvage cases. More than half of the patients with complex and salvage lesions had failed previous attempts at surgical repair with alternative treatments; these included marrow stimulation techniques, perichondrial grafting, periosteal grafting, and osteochondral autografting. The areas treated were large, $11.66\,cm^2$ ($5.3\,cm^2$/defect × 2.2 defects/case; range, $5\,cm^2$–$31\,cm^2$). Salvage category patients frequently had adjuvant treatments including valgus tibial or tibial tubercle osteotomies or ligament reconstruction (see Tables 11.2–11.4). Salvage category patients had dramatic improvements in SF-36 quality of life scores (physical summary at 24 months, $p < 0.01$). Sporting activities increased, as noted by improvement in the Cincinnati rating scale, when the patellofemoral joint was not involved. Patient satisfaction at 24 months for salvage cases was 90%.

Outcome Measure Results

Patients experienced dramatic improvement in pain and functionality as well as general well-being. In general, there was a time-dependent improvement with a maximal improvement by 24 months with femorotibial resurfacing and 36 months with patellofemoral resurfacing.

TABLE 11.4   Western Ontario and MacMaster Universities Osteoarthritis Index (WOMAC) score comparison by osteotomy type: salvage category patients with minimum 12-month follow-up.

Group	n	Baseline score	Follow-up score	p value
No osteotomy	26	34.1	19.6	<0.001
High tibial osteotomy	15	33.2	24.1	0.12
Tibial tubercle osteotomy	10	36.2	28.6	0.15

Note: Lower score indicates improved condition.

Patellofemoral improvements were not as dramatic as for the tibiofemoral joint. Time-dependent improvements were evident on all scales used.

When chondral defects were treated by ACI alone, the results appeared superior to those accompanied by osteotomy (see Tables 11.2–11.4), which may in part be explained by indications for the need for osteotomy correlating with lessened results. High tibial osteotomy (HTO) in the salvage category group was used for large defects on the weight-bearing femoral condyle (>8–$10\,cm^2$/$>8\,mm$ deep) or mechanical axis deviation ($>25\%$ of the width of the tibial plateau), in addition to treatment of kissing femoral and tibial ACI grafts. Tibial tubercle osteotomies (TTO), usually Fulkerson type anteromedializations, were employed when symptomatic maltracking was present, or in association with a chondral defect to the trochlea or patella in addition to kissing patella and trochlea defects.

When results are evaluated by osteotomy type (see Tables 11.2–11.4), it is apparent on all outcome scales that patients with ACI-treated chondral defects that are treated alone do better than those who also require HTO, which in turn do better than those for whom treating the patellofemoral joint is treated with TTO. TTO was not performed routinely for trochlea or patella defects undergoing ACI unless maltracking coexisted.

SUMMARY

To date, clinical improvement in patients treated by ACI has been 87% in the first 169 consecutive patients treated by the author. The lesions have been substantial, with $11.66\,cm^2$ per salvage treatment case. These are challenging cases for which no easy answer exists. No patients were made worse by treatment with ACI.

At present, ACI involves an open technique with the inherent disadvantages of adhesions and a more prolonged recovery. However, these disadvantages must be weighed against the procedure's ability to produce a tissue with greater durability than repairs produced by traditional marrow stimulation techniques. Rationale for the treatment of cartilage damage in younger patients depends on an understanding of the predisposing factors for the chondrosis, patient expectations, and procedure matching.

Implantation with autologous cultured chondrocytes allows for resurfacing of larger defect areas or revision chondral surgery with reproducible improvement on the femur. Patellar lesions may also be successfully treated, but strict attention must be given to correction of maltracking. Two failures in 43 resurfaced patellas to date remains encouraging.

When tibiofemoral disease was treated in salvage categories using ACI alone, results demonstrated marked functional improvement including return to sporting activities. Large lesions (>8–$10\,cm^2$) when unloaded with HTO also improved with patients frequently returning to sporting activities. These patients, however, did not have as large a clinical improvement compared to those patients treated with ACI alone. Finally, when TTO was used in conjunction with patellofemoral lesions in isolation or with kissing lesions (salvage category), pain relief was reproducible but high levels of functionality were not (i.e., sports with high-level pivoting).

To date, assessment of repair tissue histologically has been difficult in the United States due to a lack of patient willingness to undergo a 2-mm core biopsy for histologic and mechanical evaluations. However, the few biopsies that have been performed have demonstrated the same four-layer pattern noted in Sweden: a fibrous periosteal remnant cover, a transitional repair tissue, and a deep hyaline-like repair tissue well integrated to subchondral bone through a calcified layer.[3,26,27,46] The usual markers for cartilage are present by histochemical and immunochemical staining. The deep layers are positive for type II collagen and proteoglycans and lack a fibrous-appearing component to the matrix. The grafts frequently demonstrate a thickened hypertrophic fibrous periosteal remnant that may be several millimeters thick.

Refinements in patient selection, surgical technique, rehabilitation, and methods to enhance graft maturation through physical modalities and nutritional supplements are presently being investigated. However, ultimately a tissue-engineered repair tissue that is delivered by a minimally invasive technique with good graft–host integration is ideal. Until then, ACI offers a good treatment for the young individual with large chondral injuries.

Acknowledgments

I thank Tim Bryant R.N., for his collection of patient data and patient education; Brenda Surowiec, for obtaining patient approvals for treatment and for her devotion to my patients' well-being; Thomas Thornhill, M.D., and James Herndon, M.D., for recognizing the importance of this newly developing field of cartilage repair in orthopedics and supporting the development the Cartilage Repair Center.

References

1. U.S. Food and Drug Administration, Biologics Application #1233, August 22, 1997.
2. Minas T, Nehrer S. Current concepts in the treatment of cartilage defects. Orthopedics 1997;20:525–538.
3. Minas T. Autologous chondrocyte implantation for focal defects of the knee. Clin Orthop 2001;391(suppl):S349–S361.
4. Outerbridge RE. The etiology of chondromalacia patellae. J Bone Joint Surg 1961;43B:752–767.
5. Noyes FR., Bassett RW, et al. Arthroscopy in acute traumatic hemarthrosis of the knee: Incidence of anterior cruciate tears and other injuries. J Bone Joint Surg Am 1980;62A:687–695.
6. Curl W, Krome J, et al. Cartilage injuries: a review of 31,516 knee arthroscopies. Arthroscopy 1997;13(4):456–460.
7. Caplan AI. Mesenchymal stem cells. J Orthop Res 1991;9:641–650.
8. Dzioba RB. The classification and treatment of acute articular cartilage lesions. Arthroscopy 1988;4:72–80.
9. Friedman MJ, Berasi CC, Fox JM, et al. Preliminary results with abrasion arthroplasty in the osteoarthritic knee. Clin Orthop 1984;182:200–205.
10. Bert J, Maschka K. The arthroscopic treatment of unicompartmental gonarthrosis: a five-year follow-up study of abrasion arthroplasty plus arthroscopic debridement and arthroscopic debridement alone. Arthroscopy 1989;5:25–32.
11. Johnson DL, Urban WP, Caborn NNP, et al. Articular cartilage pathology associated with MRI detected "bone bruises" after ACL rupture. Presented at the American Academy of Orthopedic Surgeons Society for Sports Medicine Specialty Day, February 25, 1996, Atlanta, GA.
12. Pridie KH. A method of resurfacing osteoarthritic knee joints. J Bone Joint Surg 1959;41B:618–619.
13. Ficat RP, Ficat C, Gedeon P, Toussaint JB. Spongialisation: a new treatment for diseased patella. Clin Orthop 1979;144:74–83.
14. Aizukiki S, Yasukawa Y, Takizawa T. Does arthroscopic abrasion arthroplasty promote cartilage regeneration in osteoarthritic knees with eburnation? A prospective study of high tibial osteotomy with abrasion arthroplasty versus high tibial osteotomy alone. Arthroscopy 1997;13:1, 9–17.
15. Rodrigo J, Steadman JR, et al. Improvement of full-thickness chondral defect healing in the human knee after debridement and microfracture using continuous passive motion. Am J Knee Surg 1994;7(3):109–116.
16. Steadman JR, Rodkey WG, et al. Microfracture technique for full-thickness chondral defects: technique and clinical results. Oper Tech Orthop 1997;7(4):300–304.
17. Nehrer S, Spector M, Minas T. Histological analysis of failed cartilage repair procedures. Clin Orthop 1999;365:149–162.
18. Angermann P, Riegels-Nielsen P, et al. Osteochondritis dissecans of the femoral condyle treated with periosteal transplantation. A preliminary study of 14 patients. Orthopedics 1999;1194(2):425–428.
19. Homminga G, Bulstra S, Bouwmeester P, van der Linden AJ. Perichondral grafting for cartilage lesions of the knee. J Bone Joint Surg Br 1990;72B:1003–1007.
20. Yamahita F, Sakakida K, Suzu F, et al. The transplantation of an autogeneic osteochondral fragment for osteochondritis dissecans of the knee. Clin Orthop 1985;201:43–50.
21. Matsusue Y, Yamamuro T, Hama H. Arthroscopic multiple osteochondral transplantation to the chondral defect in the knee associated with anterior cruciate ligament disruption. Arthroscopy 1993;9(3):318–321.
22. Outerbridge HK, Outerbridge AR, Outerbridge RE, et al. The use of lateral patellar autologous graft for the repair of a large osteochondral defect in the knee. J Bone Joint Surg Am 1995;77A(1):65–72.
23. Bobic V. Arthroscopic osteochondral autograft transplantation in anterior cruciate ligament reconstruction: a preliminary clinical study. Arthroscopy 1996;3:262–264.
24. Hangody L, Kish G, Karpati Z, et al. Autologous osteochondral graft technique for replacing knee cartilage defects in dogs. Orthopaedics 1997;5(3):175–181.
25. Hangody L, Kish G, et al. Osteochondral plugs: autogenous osteochondral mosaicplasty for the treatment of focal chondral and osteochondral articular defects. Oper Tech Orthop 1997;7(4):312–322.
26. Brittberg M, Lindahl A, Nilsson A, et al. Treatment of full-thickness cartilage defects in the human knee with cultured autologous chondrocytes. N Engl J Med 1994;331:889–895.
27. Peterson L, Minas T, Brittberg M, et al. Two- to 9-year outcome after autologous chondrocyte transplantation of the knee. Clin Orthop 2000;374:212–234.
28. Minas T, Marchie A, Bryant T. SF-36 score and outcome for autologous chondrocyte implantation of the knee. Presented at the International Cartilage Repair Society Meeting; June 15–18, 2002; Toronto, Canada.

29. Rosenberg T, Paulos L, Parker R. The forty-five-degree posteroanterior flexion weight bearing radiograph of the knee. J Bone Joint Surg 1988;70A(10):1479–1483.
30. Winalski CS, Minas T. Evaluation of chondral injuries by MRI: repair assesments. Oper Tech Sports Med 2000;8(2):108–119.
31. Alparslan L, Winalski CS, Boutin RD, Minas T. Postoperative MRI of articular cartilage repair. Semin Musculoskelet Radiol 2001;5(4):345–363.
32. Minas T. Treatment of chondral defects in the knee. Orthopedics (special issue) 1997:69–74.
33. Minas T. The role of cartilage repair techniques, including chondrocyte transplantation, in focal chondral knee damage. In: Zuckerman JD (ed) Instructional Course Lectures. vol 48 Rosemont, IL: American Academy of Orthopaedic Surgeons; 1999:629–643.
34. Mandelbaum BR, Seipel PR, Teurlings L. Articular cartilage lesions: current concepts and results. In: Arendt EA (ed) Orthopaedic Knowledge Update. Rosemont, IL: American Academy of Orthopaedic Surgeons: 1999.
35. Minas T. A practical algorithm for cartilage repair. Oper Tech Sports Med 2000;8(2):141–143.
36. Minas T, Peterson L. Chondrocyte transplantation. Oper Tech Orthop 1997;7(4):323–333.
37. Minas T, Peterson L. Advanced techniques in autologous chondrocyte transplantation. Clin Sports Med 1999;18:13–44.
38. Minas T, Peterson L. Autologous chondrocyte transplantation. Oper Tech Sports Med 2000;8(2):144–157.
39. Peterson L, Karlsson J, et al. Patellar instability with recurrent dislocation due to Patellofemoral dysplasia results after surgical treatment. Bull Hosp Joint Dis 1988;48(2):130–139.
40. Grande DA, Pitman ML, et al. The repair of experimentally produced defects in the rabbit articular cartilage by autologous chondrocyte transplantation. J Orthop Res 1989;7;208–218.
41. Brittberg M, Nilsson A, Lindahl A. Rabbit articular cartilage defects treated with autologous cultured chondroctye. Clin Orthop 1995;326:270–283.
42. Breinan H, Minas T, Hsu HP, et al. Effect of cultured articular chondrocytes on repair of chondral defects in a canine model. J Bone Joint Surg 1997;79A:1439–1451.
43. Breinan H, Minas T, Barone L, et al. Histological evaluation of the course of healing of canine articular cartilage defects treated with cultured chondrocytes. Tissue Eng 1998;4(1):101–114.
44. O'Driscoll SW, Salter R. The induction of neochondrogenesis in free intra-articular periosteal autografts under the influence of continuous passive motion. J Bone Joint Surg Am 1984;66A(8):1248–1257.
45. O'Driscoll SW, Keeley FW, Salter RB, et al. Durability of regenerated articular cartilage produced by free autogneous periosteal grafts in major full-thickness defects in joint surfaces under the influence of continuous passive motion. J Bone Joint Surg 1988;70A:595–606.
46. Richardson JB, Caterson B, Evans EH. Repair of human articular cartilage after implantation of autologous chondrocytes. J Bone Joint Surg Br 1999;81:1064–1068.

12

Osteochondritis Dissecans: Current Treatment Options

Lyle J. Micheli and L. Pearce McCarty, III

BACKGROUND

Osteochondritis dissecans (OCD) is a pathologic process that results in destruction of subchondral bone with secondary damage to overlying articular cartilage. It has a typical clinical presentation involving pain and clicking in the affected joint, and demonstrates characteristic radiographic findings (Figures 12.1–12.3). OCD likely represents a common endpoint for multiple possible pathologic pathways, including trauma, ischemia, and genetic predisposition. Although the literature most commonly reports on cases involving the distal femoral articular surface, talus, and capitellum, there are case reports involving the patella, distal tibia, scaphoid, humeral head, and metatarsal heads as well, and bilaterality in some locations is not uncommon.[1,2]

Certain authors have delineated juvenile and adult forms of OCD as distinct entities with different prognoses,[2-9] but the essential lesion remains injury to the subchondral plate, resulting in destabilization of overlying articular cartilage, increased susceptibility to stress and shear, and eventual fragmentation and loss of articular integrity leading to early degenerative changes and loss of function. The deterioration of subchondral bone is central to the pathologic process, as the biomechanics of the underlying subchondral plate has been shown to influence the status of overlying articular cartilage.[10] Green and Banks[5] perhaps said it best in their classic study: "...the basic process in osteochondritis dissecans is an aseptic necrosis involving the subchondral bone and ... all other changes are secondary." This sequence of subchondral deterioration followed by articular injury differentiates OCD from processes that involve direct, primary insults to articular cartilage, a difference that proves conceptually important when entertaining treatment options.

Injury to cartilage in OCD may range in severity from early softening of the articular surface to separation of a fragment or fragments of articular cartilage from the subchondral plate, as suggested by Konig's[11] use of the term *dissecans*, from the Latin *dissec*, "to separate." Furthermore, damage to articular cartilage, whether juvenile (JOCD) or adult in nature, has the potential to produce arthrosis at an early age leading to progressive pain and disability and making early intervention imperative.[2,8,12-18]

Recognition of the limited capacity for articular cartilage to self-repair is not recent.[19] In his 1743, treatise, "Of the structure and disease of articulating cartilages,"[20] William Hunter makes an often-cited statement that more than 250 years later remains frustratingly accurate: "...from Hippocrates down to the present age, we shall find that an ulcerated cartilage is universally allowed to be a very troublesome disease; that it admits of a cure with more difficulty than a carious bone; and that, when destroyed, it is never recovered." However, the development of new biologic resurfacing strategies, together with evolution of arthroscopic technique, has led to the development of aggressive new surgical therapies.[21] As mentioned, alteration in subchondral biomechanics remains central conceptually to one's approach to OCD, and one must answer the question of fragment stability as accurately as possible before being able to select the appropriate treatment. Modalities tend to fall into one of two camps. On one hand, strategies such as nonoperative treatment, activity modification, marrow stimulation, and fragment reduction and fixation attempt to restore native subchondral bone to a healthy state thereby preserving native articular cartilage. On the other hand, strategies such as autologous chondrocyte implantation (ACI) that attempt to regenerate articular cartilage, and autologous osteochondral transfer and allogenic osteochondral grafting each attempt to resurface an osteochondral defect with hyaline or hyaline-like articular cartilage, thereby reproducing joint congruity. As detailed by Ambroise Paré in *Oeuvres Complets*,[22] operative treatment of OCD appears in the literature as early as 1558, comprising removal of loose bodies from affected joints (Figure 12.4).

With respect to current treatment alternatives, less aggressive operative options include simple arthroscopic lavage, removal of loose bodies, and debridement to a stable rim in hopes of preventing further delamination and lesion expansion. Marrow stimulation techniques include drilling, microfracture, and abrasion arthroplasty, although the last of these may not have as clear an indication in the treatment of OCD lesions. Common to all marrow stimulation techniques is the recruitment of pluripotential stem cells from bone mar-

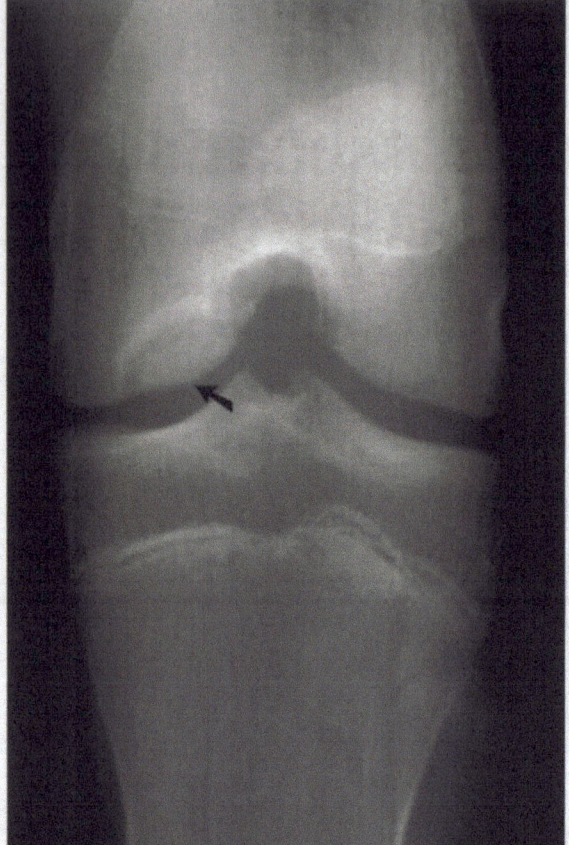

FIGURE 12.1 AP radiograph shows large OCD lesion in "classic" site, along lateral aspect of the medial femoral condyle. Note the lucent radiographic line surrounding the defect (*arrow*).

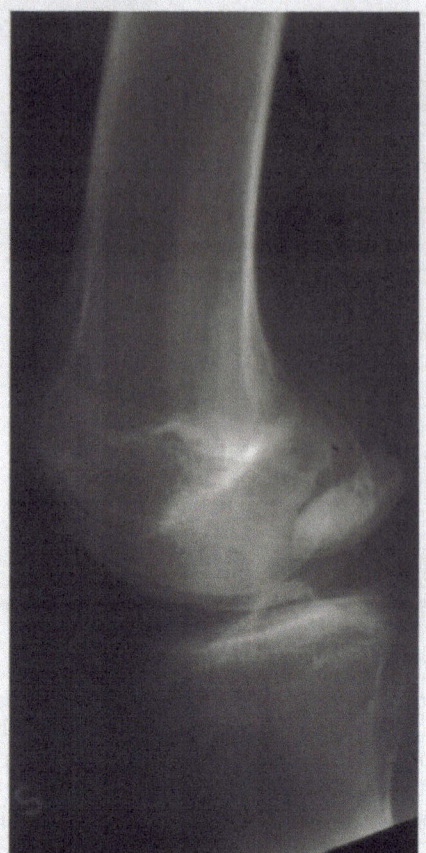

FIGURE 12.2 Lateral radiograph of a large, unstable OCD fragment along the posterior aspect of the femoral condyle.

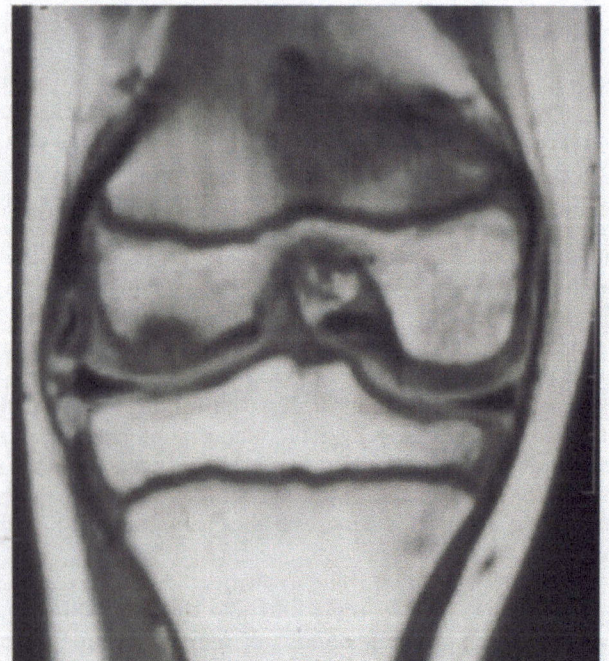

FIGURE 12.3 Coronal, T1-weighted MRI of a femoral condylar OCD lesion shows subchondral edema.

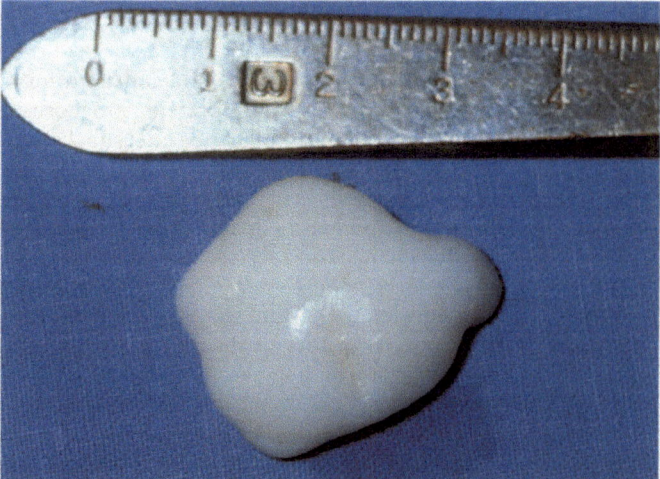

FIGURE 12.4 Example of the type of loose body that can be produced by detachment of an osteochondral fragment. This large specimen was removed from a patient's knee.

row underlying the subchondral plate into the affected area to enhance the native capacity for cartilaginous self-repair.[19,21] Antegrade or retrograde drilling may offer distinct advantages in the treatment of OCD lesions when a layer of devitalized bone exists over viable bone in the base of the defect and where deeper penetration may be necessary to reach the viable bone. The communication between viable bone (and associated marrow) and devitalized bone permits revitalization of the latter by "creeping substitution," in addition to setting the stage for fibrocartilage to fill the articular defect.

In the setting of OCD, the goal of marrow stimulation techniques such as drilling is not so much the production of fibrocartilage within an articular defect as it is the restoration of viable subchondral bone and stabilization of the osteochondral fragment in question. An additional restorative technique is that of rigid fixation of an osteochondral fragment. The use of bioabsorbable rods, Herbert screws, cannulated screws, Kirschner wires, and bone pegs have all been described for the this purpose,[2,23–30] all with the common goal of producing "fracture" healing, restoring normal subchondral plate dynamics and creating an optimal environment for survival of articular cartilage.

On the more aggressive end of the spectrum, incorporation of biologic strategies into orthopaedic techniques has given rise to autologous chondrocyte implantation (ACI), autologous osteochondral autografting, and other developments holding promise with respect to the restoration of congruous, near physiologic joint surfaces. ACI was first introduced in Sweden in 1987 after animal studies had demonstrated the formation of hyaline-like repair cartilage when chondrocytes were implanted beneath periosteal patches in vivo.[21,31,32] Initial reports of its use in humans with full-thickness cartilage defects, including but not limited to those caused by OCD, are encouraging.[31,33,34] Autologous osteochondral grafting in the form of cylindrical grafts harvested from minimally weight-bearing regions of the knee and transferred to a full-thickness cartilage defect in a single plug fashion or in a mosaic-like pattern was popularized by Hangody et al. in Hungary in the late 1990s. As with ACI, initial reports of the use of autologous osteochondral grafting in the treatment of full-thickness articular lesions show promise.[1,35–41] One advantage of the latter technique is that it does not require the presence of viable bone at the base of the lesion, and the depth of the harvested bone plug can to some extent be adjusted to compensate for the depth of the defect. Lexer first reported the use of fresh osteochondral allografts for biologic resurfacing of damaged articular surfaces in the early 1900s. Techniques in the harvesting, preservation and implantation processes have improved since that time.[23,42–45]

The ultimate goal of all surgical strategies that address the lesions of OCD is to restore a healthy, durable, and congruous articular surface, avoiding progression to osteoarthritis and permitting early range of motion with return to premorbid level of activity. Perhaps more important than the technique employed, however, is "timely operative intervention," as emphasized by Smillie in his 1957 review of the state of the art in surgical treatment of OCD.[30] Early treatment remains the key factor in preservation of the subchondral plate and therefore of native hyaline cartilage.

INDICATIONS AND CONTRAINDICATIONS

Indications for operative versus non-operative treatment of OCD, as well as for specific operative techniques vary according to patient age, functional demands, motivation, location and severity of lesion (i.e., fragment stability, diameter, depth, etc.). Issues such as patient motivation and functional demand cannot be overemphasized, as the more complex reparative and regenerative techniques entail extended periods of limited weight bearing and relative disability requiring a firm commitment to rehabilitation by both patient and surgeon.

First, contrary to traditional belief and particularly as one approaches epiphyseal closure, certain juvenile cases may be better treated early with operative means. One often-cited study reports a 50% failure rate of "conservative management" of juvenile OCD.[3,4] In part, such results may derive from an inability of radiographs to discriminate accurately between early cases of OCD that could respond well to nonoperative treatment and more advanced cases that demand operative intervention. Takahara et al.[46] reported 24 patients with clinical and radiographic findings consistent with OCD of the capitellum and divided their cohort into two groups based upon plain radiographic findings. The first group comprised "early" OCD lesions and the second "advanced" lesions. Both groups were treated with observation and activity modification, with a mean follow-up of 5.2 years. No statistically significant difference could be found between the number of poor outcomes within each subgroup. Poor results in greater than 50% were seen in both the "early" and "advanced" groups. There is evidence, however, that magnetic resonance imaging techniques may significantly improve the accuracy with which clinicians can delineate between early and advanced OCD lesions, permitting more appropriate decisions regarding those lesions meriting observation and those requiring intervention.[47]

Furthermore, several long-term studies have demonstrated that onset of OCD before epiphyseal closure does not obviate the eventual onset of arthrosis and depends upon factors such as size and location of the defect and method of treatment.[3,12,17,48] Nevertheless, Yoshida et al.[9] demonstrated with a mean follow-up time of 11.5 years, 100% healing rates for inferocentral medial condylar lesions of the femur, 89% healing for inferocentral lateral condylar lesions, and 55% healing rates for intercondylar lesions in juvenile OCD (JOCD) treated nonoperatively. Green and Banks[5] reported on 18 knees with a mean follow-up of 4.5 years treated with restricted weight bearing and/or cast immobilization, 17 of which had "excellent" results. Three of these 18 knees were opened for other reasons around the time of diagnosis which were remarkable only for softening of the overlying articular cartilage. Again, careful attention must be given to the presenting symptomotology, size, location, and stage (stability) of a JOCD lesion when weighing nonoperative versus operative treatment options.

Nonoperative treatment consisting of close observation, activity modification, and restricted weight bearing should serve as an appropriate first line of treatment in many cases of JOCD, but orthopaedists should take care not to extend a period of nonoperative treatment to a deleterious extent with the mistaken belief that all, or even most, JOCD lesions heal spontaneously. Additionally, when weighing nonoperative versus operative treatment, more advanced imaging studies such as magnetic resonance imaging may provide useful information regarding staging of the lesion. This being stated, operative treatment of JOCD can be problematic from the standpoint that many surgical strategies require, or at least involve the possibility of violating the growth plate. For JOCD cases in which the native osteochondral fragment cannot be re-implanted, a strategy such as ACI may present the best alternative, as violation of the growth plate is not required.

TABLE 12.1 Indications for nonoperative and operative treatment.	
Nonoperative	*Operative*
Stable lesion as determined by MRI	Instability of lesion as determined by MRI or arthroscopy
Absence of mechanical symptoms, such as locking or catching of the joint	Presence of mechanical symptoms, such as locking or catching of the joint
Open physes	Persistence of symptoms in patient approaching epiphyseal closure
	Persistence of symptoms following an appropriate trial of nonoperative treatment
	Epiphyseal closure

TABLE 12.2 Relative and absolute contradictions to operative treatment.	
Relative	*Absolute*
Advanced physiologic age	Osteoarthritis
Presence of significant medical comorbidities	Uncorrected instability of joint
No previous surgery (i.e., no trial of nonoperative therapy)	Uncorrected malalignment of joint
Early degenerative changes	Uncorrected patellar maltracking when treating trochlear or patellar lesions
	Patient inability to comply with rehabilitation protocol

Results have been poor with nonoperative treatment of adult, or postepiphyseal closure OCD and one should therefore follow a more aggressive operative strategy when approaching lesions in this population. General indications for operative versus nonoperative treatment in both the pre- and postepiphyseal closure populations are listed in Table 12.1. Relative and absolute contraindications to operative treatment are as listed in Table 12.2.

Chronologic age should not serve as an absolute contraindication for operative treatment. Aside from coexisting instability and mechanical malalignment which can be corrected with a staged or combined procedure before addressing a cartilage defect, diffuse osteoarthritis represents the only absolute contraindication against resurfacing procedures such as ACI and autologous osteochondral transfer. The ideal candidate for such procedures is the young (<30 years of age), motivated, otherwise fit individual with a focal, solitary osteochondral defect 20 mm or less in diameter that is surrounded by healthy articular cartilage. Appropriateness of a

given operative technique for a given patient must be determined on an individual basis according to the anatomic location of the lesion, the operating surgeon's personal experience and technical capacity, and the availability of appropriate resources and rehabilitation personnel in the treating facility. The general guidelines are illustrated in the decision tree in Figure 12.5.[49,50]

Lesion stability is most commonly assessed via arthroscopic visualization or by magnetic resonance imaging (MRI), with or without gadolinum-diethylenetriamine pentaacetic acid arthrography. Depending upon the criteria used during image interpretation, a high degree of accuracy using conventional MRI to predict lesion stability can be routinely achieved.[47,51–53] Likewise, "lesion instability" is determined via the presence of mechanical symptoms including locking and catching (the presence of additional mechanical pathology such meniscal tears must be ruled out), radiographic (MRI), or direct arthroscopic examination that reveals a break in the cartilage surface or a displaced fragment.

Simple arthroscopic lavage and debridement, although potentially indicated when dealing with unstable lesions of the talus or capitellum, probably does not have a place in the treatment of unstable lesions of the femoral condyles. A frag-

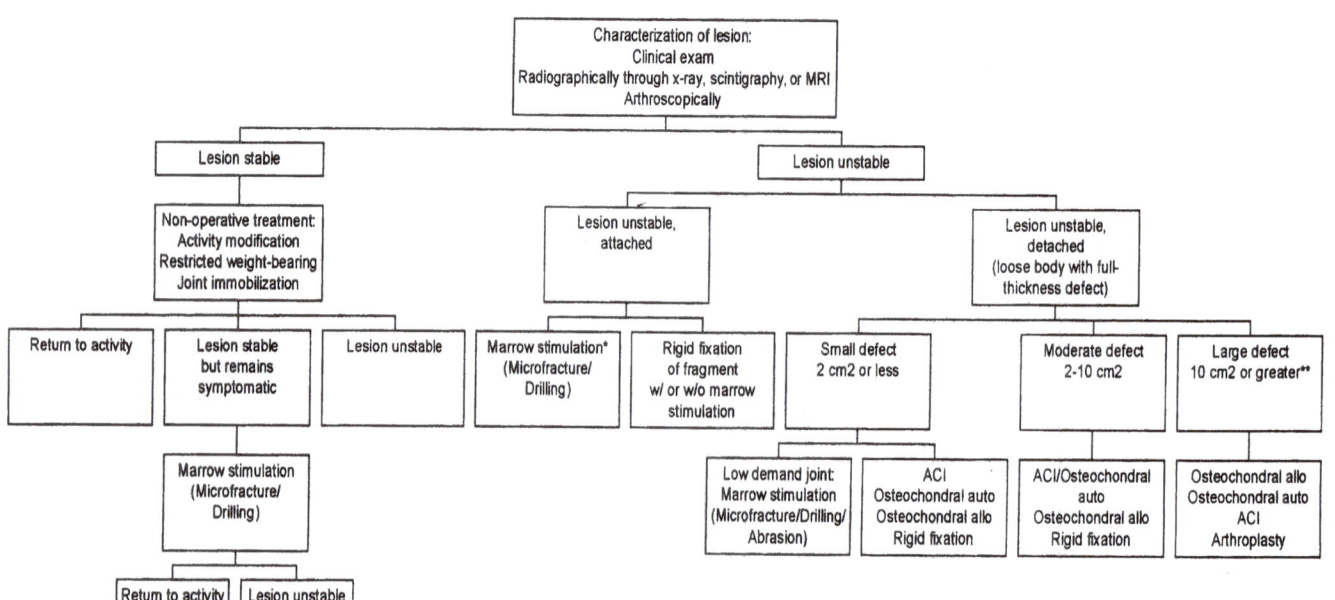

FIGURE 12.5 Decision tree for treatment of OCD lesions. Particularly if they measure <1 cm, such lesions are rarely encountered. When seen, however, every effort should be made to fix the native fragment in place.

ment judged to be unstable via MRI or arthroscopic evaluation, but that remains attached in its crater, represents the ideal candidate for in situ fixation. Marrow stimulation techniques provide a useful adjunct in this setting. In particular, the technique of antegrade drilling is probably most appropriate under these circumstances, as it affords adequate depth of penetration and avoids the risk of fragment displacement, theoretically introduced by the use of retrograde drilling techniques. Defects involving substantial bone loss may be best treated with osteochondral transfer, either autologous or allogeneic, to restore bone stock. Allogeneic grafting may offer the best option for large, noncontained defects.[54] Alternatively, if ACI has been deemed a more appropriate treatment option, one may address bone loss with a staged procedure[55] in which the defect is first filled with autologous, cancellous bone graft (e.g., from iliac crest) and allowed to heal and restore the subchondral plate. Cartilage resurfacing can then be performed by the usual the ACI protocol. If a staged approach is not feasible, one may attempt a "sandwich" type procedure in which a combined periosteal and autologous bone graft is used to reconstitute the subchondral plate at the time chondrocyte implantation is performed. Finally, mechanical malalignment of the knee, including patellar maltracking, as well as ligamentous instability, must be addressed before (or concomitantly with) undertaking cartilage restoration procedures.

REVIEW OF TECHNIQUES

Nonoperative

Nonoperative treatment ranges from activity modification to strict limitation of weight bearing and temporary immobilization of the affected joint. At a minimum, activity should be reduced to a point at which the patient is no longer symptomatic. Range-of-motion and strengthening exercises can then be introduced as the individual's symptoms resolve. The duration of nonoperative treatment is more difficult to determine, although it should probably not be continued for more than 6 months without clear evidence of significant clinical and/or radiographic improvement. Extended periods of restricted weight bearing and/or joint immobilization should be avoided as these can produce muscular atrophy, joint stiffness, and lead to further degeneration of the articular surface.[48] However, when treating OCD of the capitellum, some authors report success with periods of immobilization up to 3 weeks in duration.[15]

Early acute lesion of the talus can also be treated with a 3 to 6 week period of cast or brace immobilization followed by aggressive physical therapy as tolerated for ankle rehabilitation.[40] Throughout the period of nonoperative treatment, the patient should be followed closely, both clinically and radiographically. A reasonable periodicity is 6 to 12 weeks with reevaluation for mechanical or worsening symptoms suggestive of lesion destabilization. With respect to imaging, the use of plain radiography may suffice, although there is evidence that scintigraphy and MRI provide earlier and more accurate characterization of OCD lesions and should be used at least during initial evaluation.[52] Return to unrestricted activity should be predicated upon a gradual increase in activity level through monitored physical therapy involving range of

motion and strengthening. In certain cases, such as OCD of the capitellum in a gymnast or high-level baseball pitcher, it is doubtful that the patient will ever be able to return to their previous level of competition.[15,17] Such eventualities should be addressed with parents and/or the patient at the initiation of treatment to avoid unrealistic expectations.

Operative

An increasing number of treatment options for OCD continue to appear in the literature. In addition to simple arthroscopic lavage and loose body removal, this section provides an overview of two methods for restoring the damaged subchondral plate to health, thereby preserving native, overlying articular cartilage: marrow stimulation, via either drilling or microfracture, and in situ fixation. The three techniques reviewed for resurfacing late-stage OCD defects are autologous cultured chondrocyte implantation, autologous osteochondral grafting, and allogeneic osteochondral grafting. It must be recognized that the applicability of each technique varies with individual patient considerations and surgeon experience. Conditions such as mechanical malalignment and ligamentous instability of the knee must without exception be addressed before embarking upon cartilage restoration. Similarly, a staged procedure may be required to correct pathologic ligamentous laxity in the ankle prior to addressing the osteochondral defect.[1]

ARTHROSCOPIC LAVAGE AND DEBRIDEMENT

Routine arthroscopy of the involved joint is performed, including careful examination for additional pathology such as meniscal tears or articular cartilage problems. The lesion is evaluated by inspection and probing. Unstable articular cartilage is sharply debrided back to a stable shoulder using an arthroscopic shaver or curette. The underlying crater is cleared of calcified cartilage and granulation tissue back to healthy, bleeding bone using an arthroscopic shaver or curette. Loose bodies are removed from the joint (Figure 12.6).

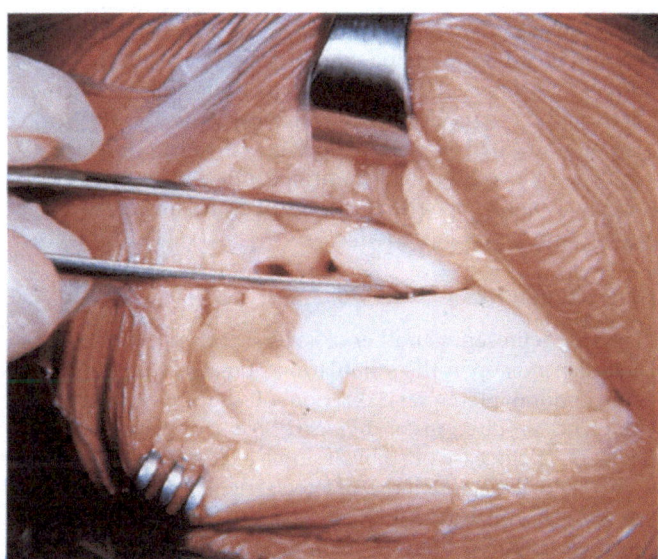

FIGURE 12.6 Removal of a large, detached osteochondral fragment from the knee.

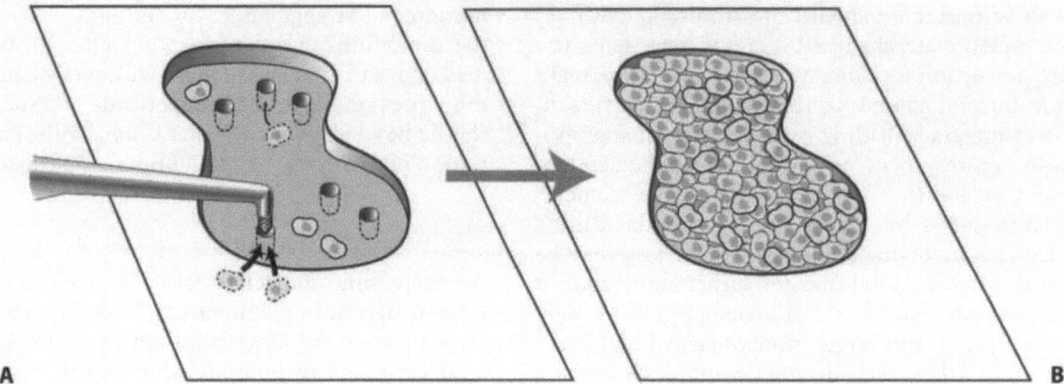

FIGURE 12.7 Conceptual illustration of microfracture technique. **A.** Penetration of subchondral plate with microfracture awl, permitting influx of pluripotent marrow cells. **B.** "Superclot" within defect, leading to formation of fibrocartilage.

MICROFRACTURE

Microfracture represents one of several techniques whose success depends upon access to marrow underlying the subchondral plate and the influx of pluripotent stem cells into the osteochondral defect resulting in the production of fibrocartilage to replace the articular deficiency (Figure 12.7). One of the reputed advantages of microfracture over marrow stimulation techniques such as drilling is the lack of thermal necrosis of subchondral bone during penetration of the subchondral plate with the microfracture awl.

Routine arthroscopy of the involved joint is performed, including careful examination for accompanying pathology such as meniscal tears. The lesion is characterized by inspection and probing, and an arthroscopic shaver or curette is used to sharply debride unstable cartilage flaps back to subchondral bone, so that the base of the defect is surrounded by a vertical shoulder of healthy articular cartilage. This shoulder will serve to contain the "superclot" generated by the microfracture technique, which in theory leads to establishment of a more stable, and therefore durable, repair cartilage. Calcified cartilage is further debrided from the base of the lesion, taking care not to violate subchondral bone. A surgical awl is then used to generate holes, or "microfractures," in the exposed bone of the defect. Holes are typically carried down to a depth of 2 to 4 mm and are spaced 3 mm apart. Care should be taken to include the periphery of the lesion immediately adjacent to the healthy cartilage shoulder when generating the microfractures to promote seamless integration of repair fibrocartilage into surrounding hyaline cartilage. The arthroscopic pump is then turned off and an efflux of fat droplets or blood from the microfracture sites ensures adequate depth of penetration.

TRANSARTICULAR DRILLING

Drilling represents another of several techniques whose success depends upon the stimulation of marrow underlying the subchondral plate, revitalization of the subchondral plate, and the production of fibrocartilage to fill any articular defects. In the case of stable lesions, a nonthreaded Kirschner wire is drilled through the affected articular surface to a depth of several millimeters (Figure 12.8). Drilling is performed through exposed bone of the debrided defect in the case of unstable lesion. A 1.6-mm Kirschner wire has been used successfully in the knee, whereas small diameters are more

appropriate for the ankle and elbow (e.g., 1 or 1.2 mm for the talus). Appropriate depth of penetration is confirmed by efflux of blood or fat from the drilled holes. Care should be taken to include the periphery of the lesion in the drilling as mentioned previously.

FIXATION OF NATIVE OSTEOCHONDRAL FRAGMENTS

Union of the fragment in question can restore normal subchondral plate biomechanics and preserve native hyaline cartilage with the potential of a return to premorbid joint function. Multiple means of fixation have been described, including cannulated screws, Kirschner wires (Figure 12.9), Herbert screws, and biodegradable rods.

The use of biodegradable implants or buried fixation, such as the Herbert screw, are preferred to obviate the need for a second operation and implant removal (Figure 12.10). Regardless of the technique employed, reduction and fixation is attempted arthroscopically to minimize morbidity associ-

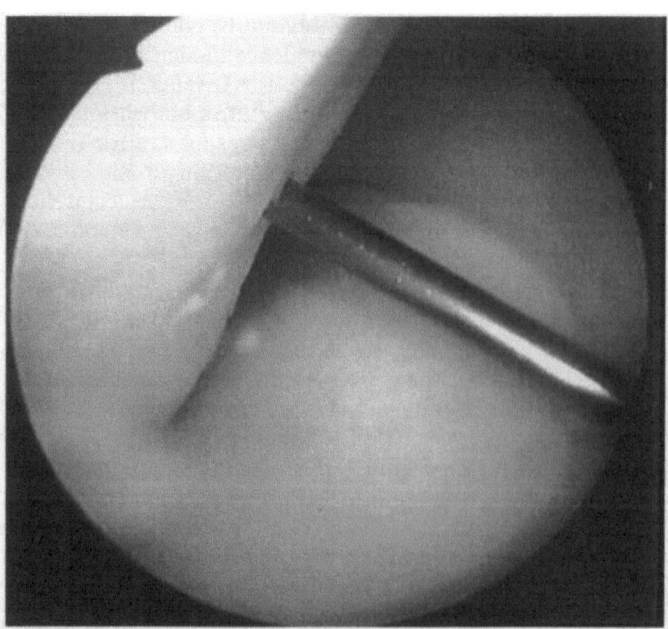

FIGURE 12.8 Intraoperative view of arthroscopic, transarticular, antegrade drilling of OCD defect.

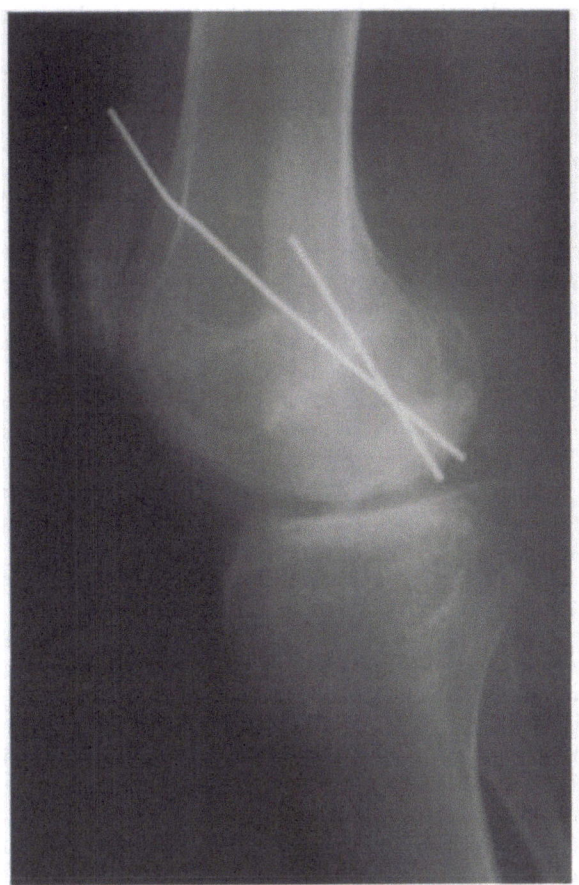

FIGURE 12.9 In situ fixation using Kirschner wires.

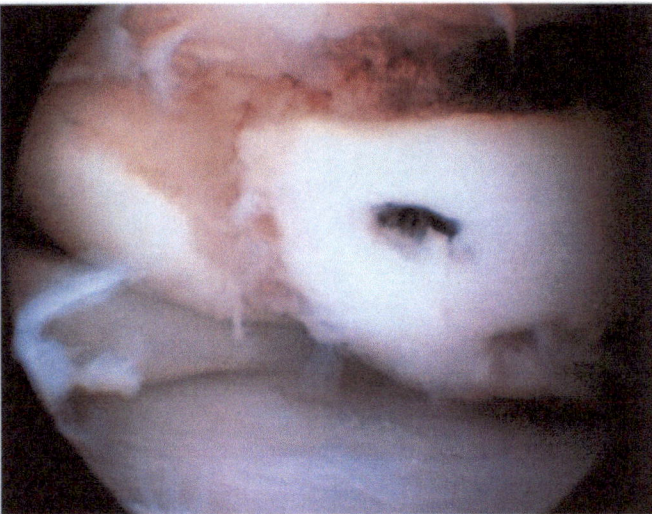

FIGURE 12.10 In situ fixation using cannulated Herbert screw placed arthroscopically.

ated with arthrotomy. Stable flaps are not extensively debrided but are drilled and fixed in situ (Figure 12.11).

Unstable or displaced fragments may necessitate open arthrotomy for reduction and fixation (Figure 12.12). In these cases the fragment and crater are debrided of granulation tissue and sclerotic bone. Bony defects are replaced with iliac crest cancellous autograft to prevent fragment subsidence. In the case of unstable or free fragments, a significant amount of sculpting may be necessary to establish a congruent joint surface after implantation. Marrow stimulation is then achieved through antegrade drilling of the reduced and pinned fragment using a small-gauge (1.6mm or smaller) non-threaded Kirschner wire. Healing of the fixed fragment is monitored with standard radiography postoperatively (Figure 12.13).

The number of implants needed varies with the type of implant and size of the defect, with as few implants used as possible without sacrificing stability of fixation. The exact technique of fixation varies with the type of implant selected.

AUTOLOGOUS CULTURED CHONDROCYTE IMPLANTATION

Implantation of autologous cultured chondrocytes attempts to resurface the defect with hyaline or hyaline-like articular cartilage. This technique necessitates two operations (Figure 12.14) as elaborated upon in chapters 10 and 11.[55] At the time of biopsy, marrow stimulation of the defect is usually necessary in an attempt to revitalize the necrotic bone at the base of the lesion. It is generally recommended that at least 4 months be allowed between the marrow stimulation and chondrocyte implantation.

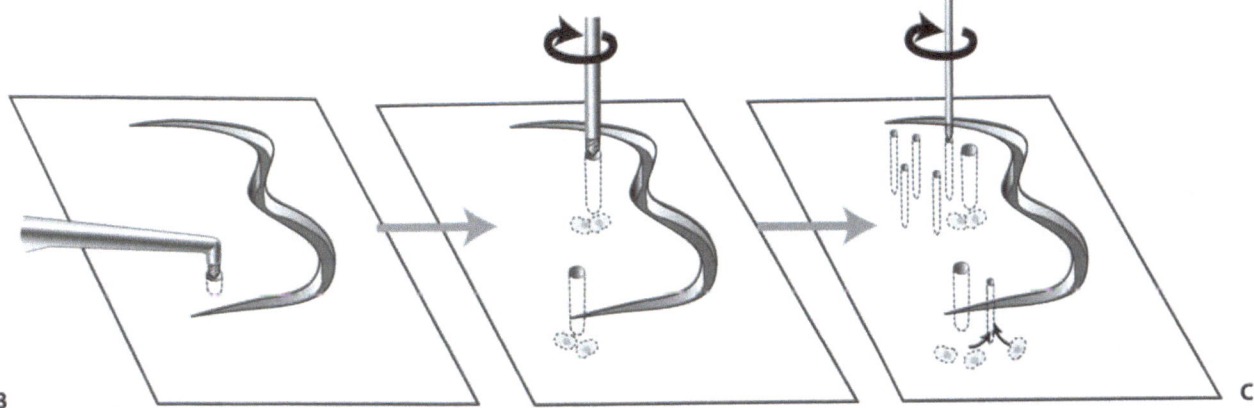

A,B   C

FIGURE 12.11 Conceptual illustration of in situ fixation of unstable osteochondral fragment. Antegrade transarticular drilling is used as a marrow stimulation adjunct. **A.** Probing of defect in situ and definition of fragment borders. **B.** In situ fixation with Herbert screws.

C. Antegrade transarticular drilling for marrow stimulation with ingress of pluripotent marrow cells into defect through subchondral plate.

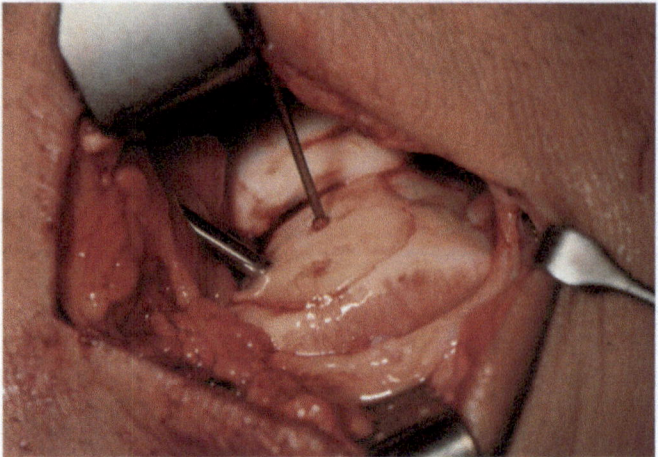

FIGURE 12.12 Intraoperative photo of antegrade drilling and Herbert screw fixation of large OCD fragment. Open arthrotomy was used to obtain adequate exposure for fixation of this large fragment.

At the time of cell implantation, depending on the location of the lesion, the appropriate arthrotomy is performed. A standard medial or lateral parapatellar arthrotomy provides adequate exposure in the knee (Figure 12.15). A medial parapatellar arthrotomy is preferred for multiple lesions. Access to posteromedial or posterolateral lesions of the talus may require a medial malleolar or fibular osteotomy, respectively. Defect preparation consists of sharp debridement all fissured or unstable cartilage down to but not penetrating subchondral bone. The resulting defect should ideally be contained, bound by vertically oriented shoulders of healthy articular cartilage (Figure 12.16).

If one must choose between leaving damaged cartilage behind and producing an uncontained lesion, however, one should choose the latter, as surrounding synovium or drill holes through bone can serve as anchors for the overlying periosteal flap. The steps following defect preparation are no different than that described in previous chapters. Once the integrity of the flap has been confirmed, the prepared culture chondrocytes are injected and the remaining sutures placed to complete the seal (Figure 12.17). A fibrin sealant may be employed to supplement the integrity of the flap. Note that if the patient desires autologous fibrin sealant to be used, this must be prepared well in advance of the implantation procedure and necessitates at least 1 unit of autologous blood. Suction drains are not used, as they may subsequently disrupt the periosteal patch and drain the implanted chondrocytes. If a drain must be used, it should be without suction (Figure 12.18).

As mentioned, problems such as instability from anterior cruciate ligament (ACL) deficiency, patellar maltracking, and mechanical malalignment must be addressed before undertaking autologous cultured chondrocyte implantation. If, for example, ACL reconstruction is to be undertaken concomitantly, it should be performed prior to chondrocyte implantation to avoid disruption of the periosteal graft. The lesions of OCD characteristically involve some degree of bony loss, and if greater than 1 cm in depth, this deficiency should be corrected through autologous cancellous bone grafting. An interval of 6 to 9 months between bone grafting and implantation

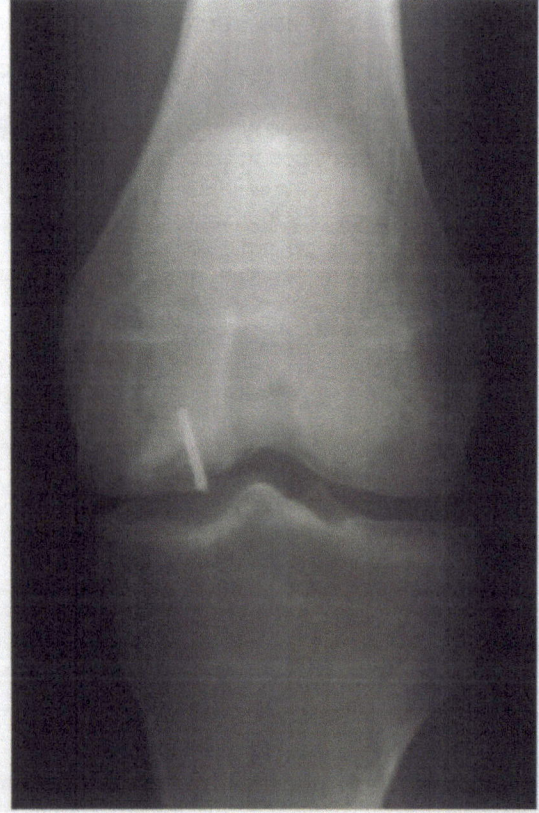

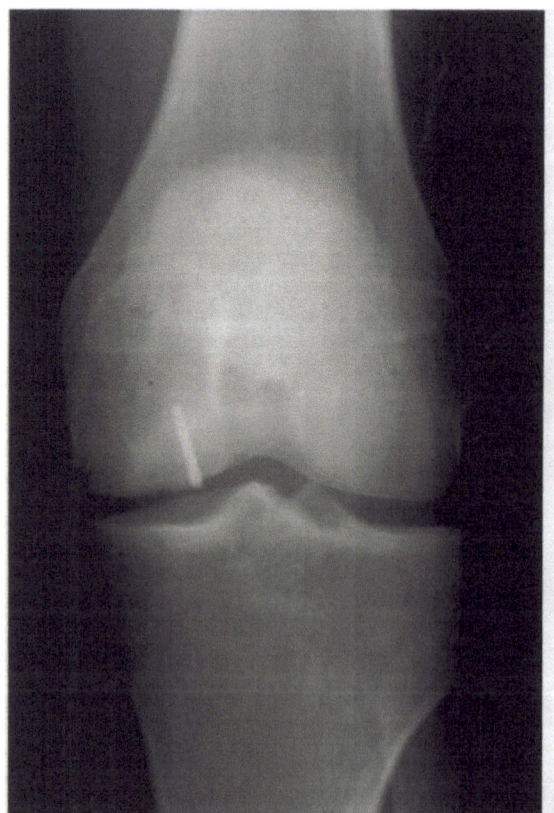

FIGURE 12.13 Two AP radiographs of the knee, the first demonstrating fixation of a large OCD lesion using a Herbert screw. The second image, at one year post-op, shows healing of the lesion.

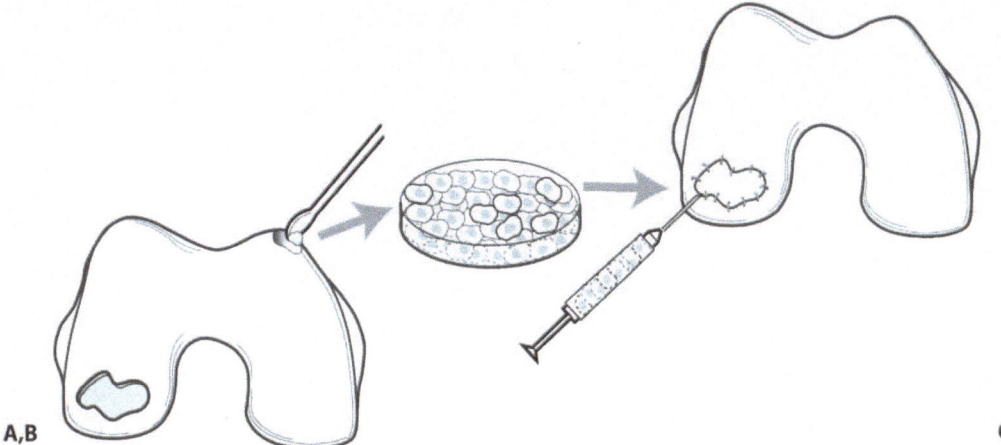

FIGURE 12.14 Conceptual illustration of ACI technique. **A.** Characterization of full-thickness articular defect left by detached osteochondral fragment and harvesting of chondrocytes. **B.** Chondrocytes cultured and multiplied in vitro. **C.** Reimplantation of cultured chondrocytes beneath suture periosteal graft.

will permit reconstitution of the subchondral plate. If a staged procedure is not possible for reconstitution of the subchondral plate in deep defects, a "sandwich" strategy can be employed in which bone grafting and chondrocyte implantation take place simultaneously (Figure 12.19). In brief, the technique involves using autologous bone graft to fill the defect. The bone graft is then covered with an appropriately sized periosteal graft with the cambium layer facing away from the articular surface. This periosteal graft will serve as the floor of the chondrocyte recipient site. A second periosteal graft is then sewn in place with its cambium layer facing toward the articular surface to serve as the ceiling of the recipient site. The chondrocytes are implanted as already described.

AUTOLOGOUS OSTEOCHONDRAL TRANSFER

Autologous osteochondral transfer entails the harvesting of osteochondral plugs varying in dimension from minimally weight bearing portions of the knee, followed by implantation into recipient osteochondral defects. It may be possible to perform osteochondral transfer to lesions involving the femoral condyles using arthroscopic technique only, whereas lesions involving the talus require open arthrotomy and or osteotomy for exposure. Lesions of the capitellum necessitate open arthrotomy. Recipient sites are first identified by probing and visual inspection (typically arthroscopically, Figure 12.20) and are debrided sharply back to a stable shoulder.

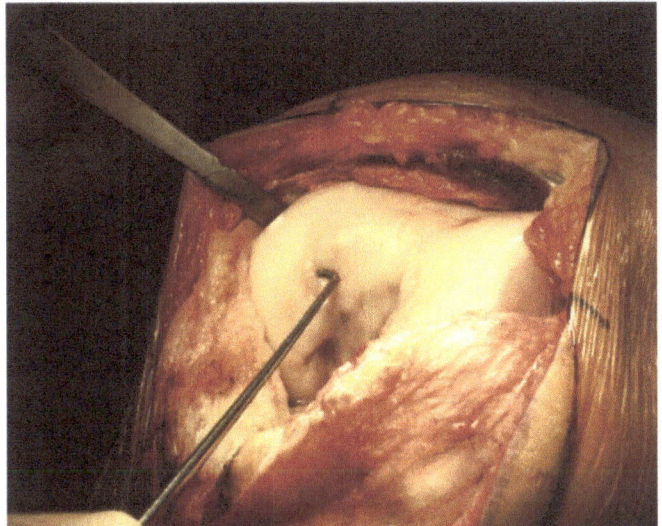

FIGURE 12.15 Intraoperative photo demonstrating a large OCD lesion located on the femoral condyle. Wide exposure was gained through a medial parapatellar arthrotomy. The extent of the lesion is determined by direct visualization and by probing to detect softened, diseased cartilage. (Reproduction of image by permission of Prof. Lars Peterson MD, Gothenburg Medical Center, Vastra Frolundra, Sweden.)

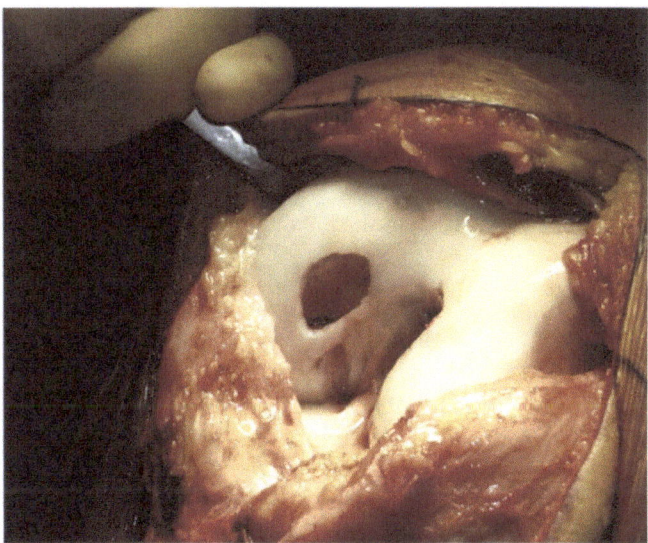

FIGURE 12.16 The lesion is sharply debrided back to previously determined margins, leaving a well-defined shoulder surrounding the defect. (Reproduction of image by permission of Prof. Lars Peterson MD, Gothenburg Medical Center, Vastra Frolundra, Sweden.)

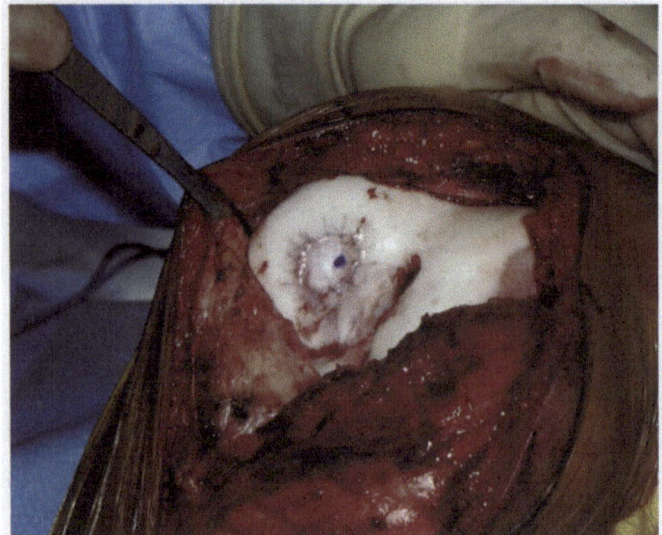

FIGURE 12.17 Previously illustrated OCD lesion of the femoral condyle following debridement, injection of cultured chondrocytes and suturing of the periosteal graft in place. (Reproduction of image by permission of Prof. Lars Peterson MD, Gothenburg Medical Center, Vastra Frolundra, Sweden.)

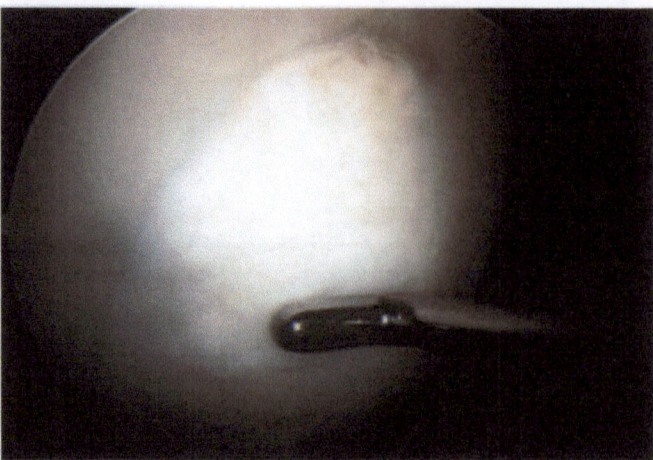

FIGURE 12.18 Intraoperative, arthroscopic look at repaired defect 24 months post-operatively. The defect has filled completely with firm, hyaline-like cartilage. (Reproduction of image by permission of Prof. Lars Peterson MD, Gothenburg Medical Center, Vastra Frolundra, Sweden.)

An elliptical shape to the recipient site may be the preferred geometry, given the findings of Gautier et al.[36] in grafting talar defects. This study reported that the mean percentage of rectangular area filled was only 76.1%, whereas the mean percentage of elliptical area filled was 96.9%. At least 75% fill is recommended to minimize the surface area between hyaline plugs that must be filled with fibrocartilage. After debridement, the defect is templated using a special graft guide. Once the number and sizes of grafts needed has been decided, harvesting of the plugs can proceed from either the superior lateral edge of the lateral femoral condyle above the sulcus terminalis, the superior medial aspect of the medial femoral condyle, or the superior lateral margin of the intercondylar notch. Meticulous attention should be given to achieving perpendicular access to the harvest site when taking donor plugs. Furthermore, plugs should be harvested manually rather then under power to avoid thermal injury to harvested chondrocytes. Following harvest of donor plugs, recipient sites are grafted in the base of the debrided defect by sequentially drilling with the appropriate-size drill (matching the intended plug) to the appropriate depth followed by dilating and graft seating. Each transfer should take place in serial fashion, as seating of each graft will slightly change the geometry of the recipient site. Each graft can be expected to expand by 0.1 to 0.2 mm in diameter after harvesting and the use of a dilator is generally recommended to avoid damage to the graft during insertion. There is biomechanical evidence that an "expansion-fit" technique for seating osteochondral plug necessitates higher loads to produce displacement from the graft site (Figure 12.21).[56]

It is paramount that the recipient area is prepared with the drill perpendicular to the plane of articular cartilage at that site. An attempt should be made to seat the cartilaginous cap of the graft flush with the surrounding articular cartilage

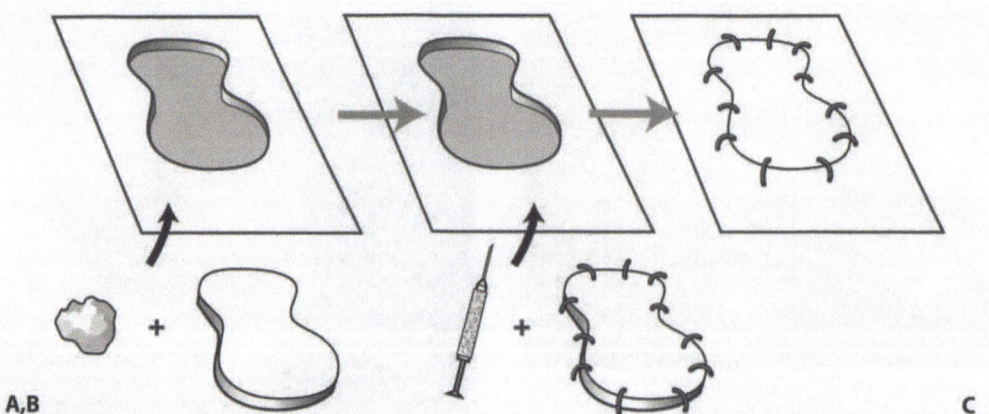

FIGURE 12.19 Conceptual illustration of "sandwich" technique. **A.** A deep defect is produced from detachment of an unstable osteochondral fragment. Autograft cancellous bone and periosteal graft (cambium layer facing into joint) are placed into defect. **B.** A second periosteal graft is sutured onto surrounding shoulder of healthy cartilage in standard fashion, with cambium layer facing away from joint. Autologous cultured chondrocytes are then injected into the space between two periostal grafts. **C.** Completed "sandwich" with (from *bottom* to *top*), cancellous autograft, first periosteal patch, cultured chondrocytes, and second periosteal patch.

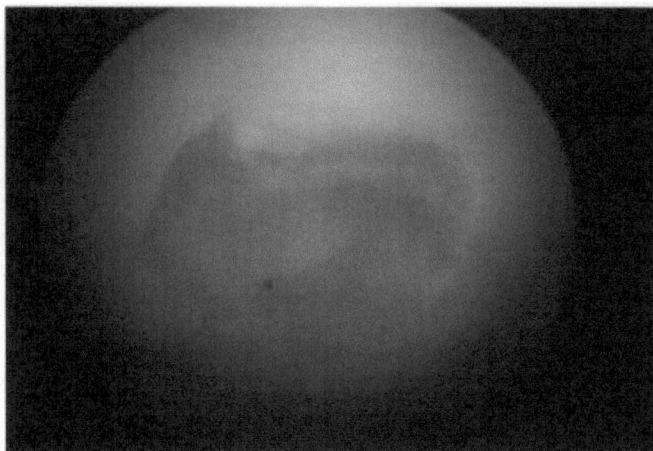

FIGURE 12.20 Intraoperative, arthroscopic view of a moderate sized, well-contained OCD lesion of the medial femoral condyle. (Reproduction of image by permission of Brian Cole MD, Midwest Orthopaedics, Chicago, Illinois.)

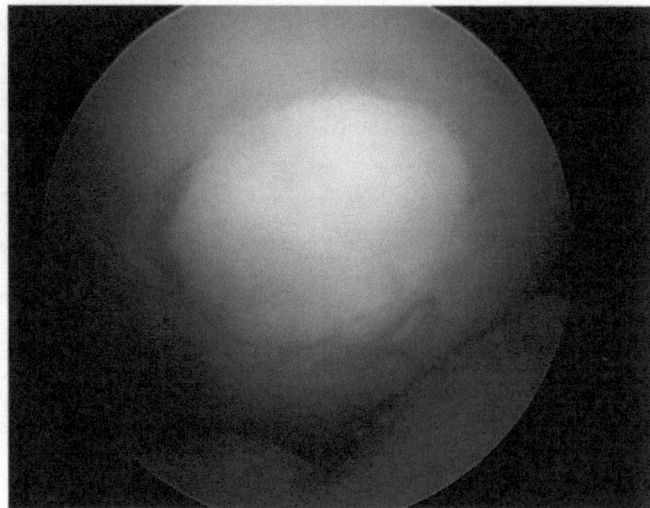

FIGURE 12.21 Intraoperative, arthroscopic view of previous lesion after transfer of single, autologous osteochondral plug. (Reproduction of image by permission of Brian Cole MD, Midwest Orthopaedics, Chicago, Illinois.)

as there is recent biomechanical evidence that elevation or depression of the graft by as little as 0.5 mm results in significantly increased peak joint contact pressures.[57] Donor sites are left open and typically can be expected to fill with cancellous bone and fibrocartilage by 12 weeks from the time of harvest. The knee is closed in a layered fashion over suction drainage which is removed 24 hours postoperatively. In the case of a medial malleolar osteotomy performed to gain access to the posteromedial aspect of the talus, it is typically reduced and fixed with several cannulated screws. A fibular osteotomy, if necessary, can be fixed with a one-third tubular or other small plate.

Concomitant instability or mechanical malalignment of the knee joint should be addressed either before or simultaneously with grafting of the defect. Most additional procedures should be performed after graft transfer, however, to avoid the loss of exposure that might result from the dynamic constraints that ACL reconstruction might impose upon the joint, for example. Figure 12.21 illustrates use of this technique to address a single, contained lesion of the medial femoral condyle.

FRESH OSTEOCHONDRAL ALLOGRAFT IMPLANTATION

This technique requires access to fresh donor material that has been retrieved, handled, and processed in strict accordance with criteria established by the American Association of Tissue Banks.[58] Preoperatively, donors and recipients are matched for size. When dealing with lesions of the femoral condyles, size is based upon the mediolateral dimension of the tibia at a point 5 mm distal to the articular surface on a standard PA film of the knee with the ray tube distanced 100 cm from the extremity and 15% magnification taken into consideration. Matches within 3 mm are considered to be acceptable. Grafting is typically performed 2 to 6 days following harvest. For the implantation procedure, a medial or lateral parapatellar arthrotomy is used to gain exposure of the lesion. Once exposed, all fissured or undermined cartilage is debrided sharply back to healthy borders, with the end result being a geometrically (typically rectangular) shaped defect

that can be matched by donor material. Subchondral bone in the base of the defect is debrided to a depth of 3 to 5 mm. The lesion is templated and a matching graft is cut from the donor stock. The graft is lavaged using pulsatile irrigation to remove remaining marrow. The graft is implanted and fixation typically achieved through press fit. Biodegradable pins can be used to supplement fixation, and particularly in the case of a massive allograft, interfragmentary screws can be used necessitating a second procedure for screw removal. The final graft thickness should range from 5 to 10 mm. The articular surface of the allograft should rest approximately 1 mm proud of the native articular surface to allow for subsidence (Figure 12.22). Deep bony defects should not be reconstituted with allograft bone, but rather with autograft to minimize exposure to allograft and possibility for transmission of infectious agents. Host immune reaction, although present following implantation of allograft bone, does not seem to present as a clinically significant problem and pharmacologic immunosuppression is not indicated.

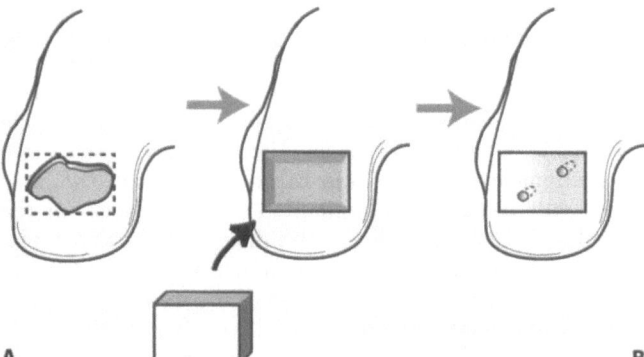

FIGURE 12.22 Conceptual illustration of allograft technique. **A.** A full-thickness articular defect is encountered on the distal femoral articular surface is trimmed to a rectangular shape. **B.** A matching osteochondral allograft is cut and sized to defect. **C.** The allograft is secured with bioabsorbable rods or other type of fixation as needed. The graft can be left 1 mm proud to allow for subsidence.

TABLE 12.3   Pearls and pitfalls of procedures for treating osteochondritis dissecans (OCD).

Technique	Pearl	Pitfall
Arthroscopic lavage and debridement	Lesion ≤1 cm diameter	Inadequate debridement can lead to further delamination
Arthroscopic marrow stimulation techniques	Ensure adequate depth of penetration Include periphery of lesion	Do not use suction drain
In situ fixation	Meticulous sculpting is needed to ensure anatomic reduction Bioabsorbable or buried fixation to avoid second operation	May need to further trim seated fragment to obtain congruent articular surface
Autologous chondrocyte implantation	Ensure watertight integrity of periosteal graft	Obtain viable subchondral plate before implantation
Autologous osteochondral graft	Achieve flush press-fit with surrounding cartilage	Plugs of small diameter have tendency to loose cartilage caps
Allograft	Anatomic reduction Autologous bone graft for deep defects	Avoid need for second operation for removal of fixation

SURGICAL PEARLS AND PITFALLS

Nonoperative Treatment

Nonoperative treatment is most commonly used for JOCD. Avoid prolonged immobilization of affected joints. In particular, strict immobilization of the knee in place of activity modification and restricted weight bearing is to be discouraged in the compliant patient. Relative immobilization, for example, in an air cast boot, might be continued for slightly longer periods, particularly when treating lesions of the talar dome. Lesions that show no clinical or radiologic signs of healing after more than 6 months should proceed to operative treatment.

Operative Treatment: General

Malalignment and instability are treated before or simultaneous with treatment for OCD defects. A thorough evaluation of the patient's willingness to comply with the postoperative rehabilitation program before undertaking any reparative procedure is required (Table 12.3).

Arthroscopic Lavage and Debridement

This technique may be more successful when used for lesions smaller than 1 cm in diameter. Defects greater than 1 cm in diameter should prompt serious consideration of alternate treatment strategies. Identification of coexisting pathology, such as unstable meniscal tears, is essential. Remove all loose bodies and perform thorough sharp debridement of unstable cartilage back to a healthy stable shoulder. Leaving cartilage of questionable quality because of a hesitancy to debride will only result in further delamination and destruction of the articular surface. Recognize that simple lavage and debridement has a marginal affect on stimulating repair processes and may not result in the formation of any meaningful repair cartilage in defects being treated.

Microfracture

Make sure extent of lesion is well defined. With the exception of ligament reconstruction, perform other intraarticular procedures (meniscal debridement, plica excision, etc.) before performing microfracture. Make sure that the defect is debrided back to a stable shoulder as this will serve to contain the "superclot" essential to the repair process. Include the periphery of the lesion when performing microfracture. Ensure adequate depth of penetration by visualization of efflux of fat and blood from holes. Do not use intraarticular drains.

Drilling

Make sure extent of lesion is well defined. Use a 1.6-mm smooth Kirschner wire for the knee, and a 1- to 1.2-mm wire for the talus or capitellum. Include periphery of lesion in procedure. Ensure adequate depth of penetration by visualization of efflux of fat and blood from holes. This technique may be preferred over other marrow stimulation techniques when treating stable lesions.

In Situ Fixation of Native Osteochondral Fragments

Make sure extent of lesion is well defined. Trim the fragment as needed to achieve anatomic reduction. Use autologous bone graft beneath fragment if necessary. Use either biodegradable or buried screws to avoid a second operation for hardware removal. Use antegrade drilling as marrow stimulation adjunct.

Autologous Cultured Chondrocyte Implantation

Use staged or "sandwich" procedure to restore viable subchondral plate in the case of deep OCD defects. Ensure watertight integrity of the periosteal patch. Use marrow stimulation technique at the time of cartilage harvest in attempt to revitalize subchondral plate at base of crater. Avoid suction drains.

Autologous Osteochondral Grafting

Be careful to both harvest donor plugs and prepare recipient sites perpendicular to the articular surface. Achieve flush fit with surrounding articular cartilage when seating graft. Consider preparing recipient site with elliptical geometry if possible to achieve optimal percentage fill. Be particularly careful with plugs of very small diameter as they have a greater tendency to lose their cartilage caps during handling.

Achieve press-fit with graft or fix with bioabsorbable pins to avoid second operation for screw removal.

REHABILITATION

Recovery requires a highly motivated and compliant patient, as well as a physical therapist educated about appropriate therapy regimens. This provision is particularly important following ACI, autologous osteochondral grafting, and use of osteochondral allografts. Concepts such as protected weight bearing, continuous passive motion (demonstrated to facilitate cartilage healing), and early active range of motion to optimize postoperative joint function are vital to the success of the aforementioned techniques.[59] Concomitant ACL reconstruction to restore ligamentous stability of the knee, osteotomy for malalignment, or other procedure may require modification of the following rehabilitation protocols (Table 12.4).

Arthroscopic Lavage and Debridement

Postoperatively, most patients undergoing arthroscopic lavage and debridement with or without removal of loose bodies can be discharged from the hospital or surgical care center on the same day as the procedure. A simple elastic, compression-type dressing suffices. One should initiate active range of motion to the limits of tolerance as well as quadriceps-strengthening exercises on the first postoperative day. Depending upon the size and location of the lesion (i.e., weight-bearing area versus minimally weight bearing area),

one may wish to restrict weight bearing for 6 to 8 weeks postoperatively. Patients may return to unrestricted athletic activity typically 4 to 6 months postoperatively after symptoms have resolved and strength and range of motion approaches that of the contralateral extremity. Note that defects treated in the patellofemoral compartment may benefit from initial restriction of active range of motion via a hinged knee brace with a 30° flexion stop since it is at 30° of flexion that the patella engages the trochlea.

Microfracture and Drilling

For procedures involving microfracture of the knee,[60,61] patients are typically discharged home on the day of the procedure with an elastic compression-type dressing and a hinged knee brace. Cold therapy as provided by commercially available reusable wraps may be an effective adjunct to pharmacologic analgesia postoperatively, especially during the first week. Continuous passive motion (CPM) with a home machine is initiated on the first postoperative day and is continued for 8 weeks. CPM is advanced as tolerated. If a home machine is not available, patients are counseled to put their knee through a full range of motion (as tolerated) for as many cycles as possible throughout each day. Postoperative weight bearing is restricted to touchdown for 6 to 8 weeks for lesions along the weight-bearing portions of the femoral condyles. Patellofemoral lesions are permitted to weight bear as tolerated with the knee in a hinged brace limited by a 30° flexion stop. After 6 to 8 weeks, patients are advanced to active range of motion and strengthening exercises using elastic resistance bands, and weight bearing is advanced gradually, with the eventual incorporation of more aggressive strengthening regimens. By 4 to 6 months postoperatively, unrestricted activity is permitted. Lesions treated with antegrade drilling may receive a shorter period of protected weight bearing,[33] 4 weeks, followed by initiation of active range of

TABLE 12.4 Summary of rehabilitation for procedures for OCD.

Technique	Summary
Arthroscopic lavage and debridement	1. AROM to limits of tolerance starting POD1 2. Isometric quad strengthening exercises starting POD1 3. Limited WB depending upon size/location of defect (6–8 weeks) 4. Limited AROM for patellofemoral defects (no more than 4 weeks) 5. Return to unrestricted activity 4–6 months
Microfracture/drilling	1. CPM starting POD1, 8h/day for 8 weeks 2. Touch-down weight bearing 6–8 weeks; WBAT for trochlear lesions with hinged knee brace 0°–30° 3. Return to unrestricted activity 4–6 months
In situ fixation	1. AROM and/or CPM starting POD1 2. Touch-down weight bearing minimum of 6–8 weeks 3. Return to unrestricted activity predicated upon radiographic union
Autologous chondrocyte implantation (ACI)	1. CPM starting POD1, advanced as tolerated; 6–8 h/day for 6 weeks; limit 0°–40° for trochlear defects 2. Touch-down weight bearing 6 weeks; WB advanced stepwise to WBAT weeks 6–12 3. Return to unrestricted activity 12–18 months
Autologous osteochondral grafting	1. CPM and/or AROM starting POD1, advancing as tolerated 2. Touch-down weight bearing for 2 weeks, followed by stepwise progression to WBAT over weeks 3–8 3. Return to unrestricted activity by 12 months
Allograft	1. CPM starting POD1; AROM starting when comfortable and advancing as tolerated 2. Touch-down weight bearing 6–12 weeks 3. Return to unrestricted activity with resolution of symptoms and radiographic incorporation of graft

AROM, active range of motion; POD, postoperative day; WB, weight bearing; CPM, continuous passive motion; WBAT, Weight Bearing As Tolerated.

motion, isometric strengthening, and closed-chain exercises and progression to weight bearing as tolerated over 1 week's time. It should be emphasized to patients having undergone microfracture of unstable OCD defects, that is, full-thickness cartilage lesions, that they may not appreciate improvement in knee function until 6 months postoperatively and that improvement can continue for up to 2 years.

Rehabilitation of talar lesions treated with antegrade drilling entails immediate active range of motion exercises and restricted weight bearing for 4 to 6 weeks. Return to unrestricted activity may be possible by 2 to 4 months postoperatively. Capitellar lesions treated in this manner should be rehabilitated with early range of motion.[15]

In Situ Fixation of Native Osteochondral Fragments

In situ fixation of native osteochondral fragments may involve open arthrotomy of the joint affected, and therefore may not be possible as a day surgery procedure. Postoperatively, patients are treated with immediate range of motion and touchdown weight bearing for 6 to 8 weeks. Return to unrestricted activity is predicated upon clinical and radiographic signs of fragment union.

Autologous Cultured Chondrocyte Implantation

In considering postoperative rehabilitation following autologous chondrocyte implantation, it is important to understand the time course of healing.[55] During the initial 6 weeks postoperatively, there is a rapid fill of the defect with a primitive repair tissue, followed over the next 7 to 26 weeks by matrix production and a "firming up" of the repair tissue. From approximately 27 weeks forward, the repair tissue continues to remodel, with further matrix production and undergoes a process of mechanical hardening. By 6 to 7 months post operatively the repair tissue has reached a putty-like consistency.

Autologous chondrocyte implantation involves open arthrotomy (and osteotomy for talar lesions) of the affected joint and a several-day hospital course is often required. CPM is initiated on postoperative day one, but not before 6 to 8 hours postoperatively, allowing sufficient time for cell attachment to occur. For lesions of the femoral condyles, CPM is then used for 6 to 8 hours daily over a period of 6 weeks postoperatively. CPM for trochlear lesions is restricted to 40° flexion to avoid peak patellofemoral contact pressures. Weight bearing is restricted to touchdown for 6 weeks postoperatively, and is advanced to full weight bearing over the ensuing 6 weeks. By 4 to 5 months postoperatively, most patients have discarded assistive devices for ambulation. By 9 to 12 months patients are permitted to start running. Activities such as kneeling and squatting are disallowed for 12 to 18 months postoperatively. Larger lesions, and in particular defects resulting from OCD, may take up to 24 months to heal.

Similar time-line and protocol are followed for procedures involving the talus.

Autologous Osteochondral Grafting

This technique may necessitate open arthrotomy (and osteotomy for talar lesions), and a several-day hospital course can be required. CPM and/or active range-of-motion exer-

cises begin immediately postoperatively. Partial joint loading has been shown to have a positive effect upon graft incorporation as well as on the formation of fibrocartilage in donor sites and between plugs in recipient sites. A more aggressive weight-bearing regimen is therefore used than, for example, in autologous chondrocyte implantation. Patients are restricted to touch-down weight bearing for 2 weeks postoperatively. Over the next 2 to 8 weeks, weight bearing is advanced at a rate dependent upon the size and number of defects treated. By 8 weeks, most patients are full weight bearing. By 3 months postoperatively, most patients are able to perform activities of daily living with minimal discomfort. At 6 months postoperatively, patients can begin a gradual return to running activities, with unrestricted activity beginning at 12 months postoperatively.

Fresh Osteochondral Allograft Implantation

This procedure involves open arthrotomy and necessitates a several-day hospital course. CPM is typically initiated on the first postoperative day and is advanced as tolerated. Active range of motion is begun in the first several weeks postoperatively. Touch-down weight bearing is continued for 6 to 12 weeks. Patients typically tolerate activities of daily living with minimal discomfort by 4 months. Provided there is clear radiologic evidence of graft incorporation and the patient has demonstrated muscular control, strength, and range of motion approaching that of the contralateral extremity, unrestricted activity may commence as early as 6 months postoperatively.

COMPLICATIONS

Arthroscopic Lavage and Debridement

Aside from failure of symptom resolution and subsequent need for further procedures, surgical complications are rarely encountered with simple arthroscopic lavage and debridement. Those encountered, such as superficial wound infection, septic arthritis, and deep venous thrombosis, are treated no differently than they would be in other settings.

Microfracture and Drilling

As with simple arthroscopic lavage and debridement, marrow stimulation techniques are most commonly performed arthroscopically, and complications such as superficial wound infection, septic arthritis, and deep venous thrombosis are treated no differently than they would be in other settings. Techniques such as transmalleolar and retrograde drilling of the talar dome, although theoretically could lead to pathologic fracture of the osseous pathway, have not been seen to produce such complications. Microfracture of lesions involving the trochlear groove may lead to a rough sensation in the patellofemoral joint after a patient has discontinued use of the hinged knee brace and has begun unrestricted active range of motion. Additionally, following microfracture of trochlear lesions, some patients experience catching during range of motion. Finally, it has been noted that some patients develop a recurrent, painless effusion approximately 6 to 8 weeks status postmicrofracture.[61] All the aforementioned developments typically resolve spontaneously and can be treated symptomatically. The most obvious and common complication of treating osteochondral fragments with antegrade drilling is subsequent fragment destabilization. In cases where the lesion remains ununited or becomes unstable, in situ fixation may be required.

In Situ Fixation of Native Osteochondral Fragments

Nonunion of fixed fragments is the most commonly encountered complication in this scenario and typically mandates fragment excision, repeat fixation, or progression to a resurfacing strategy such as autologous chondrocyte implantation, autologous osteochondral transfer, or fresh allograft implantation. The use of biodegradable pins for in situ fixation can be complicated by synovitis and recurrent effusion, a development best managed symptomatically at first. Persistent synovitis may necessitate arthroscopic synovial debridement. Loosening or backing out of screws has also been encountered, with subsequent damage to articular cartilage. Catching or clicking postoperatively should be evaluated radiographically, and loosened or disengaged hardware should be removed or replaced without delay.

Autologous Cultured Chondrocyte Implantation

Superficial wound infections, joint sepsis, and other general postoperative complications should be managed in the same aggressive manner as they would be in other scenarios. Delamination of the periosteal graft from surrounding host cartilage may occur within the first 6 months postoperatively, and typically presents with painful catching or locking of the knee. Management includes arthroscopic sharp excision of the delaminated flap. Large areas of delamination may necessitate repeat ACI, as attempts at resuturing have been uniformly unsuccessful. Catastrophic graft delamination represents the most common mode of ACI failure to date. An additional complication, seen in 10% to 15% of patients,[55] is hypertrophy of the periosteal graft (Figure 12.23).

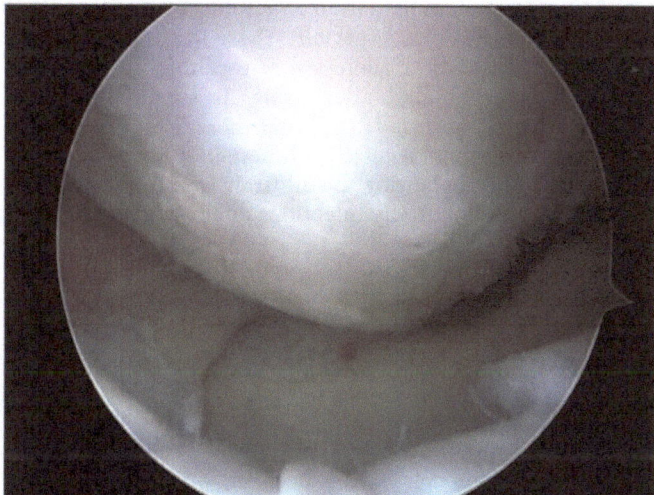

FIGURE 12.23 Graft hypertrophy in a patient 28 months status post autologous chondrocyte implantation into a femoral condylar lesion. (Reproduction of image by permission of Tom Minas MD, MS, Brigham and Women's Hospital, Boston, MA.)

Graft hypertrophy presents with new onstet of pain, effusion, and catching in a previously well functioning joint. If suspected, arthroscopic examination of the joint should be performed, with assessment of flap stability and debridment of the hypertrophic area using an arthroscopic shaver. Finally, as with any procedure requiring open arthrotomy, intraarticular adhesions can form postoperatively with resultant decrease in range of motion. When unresponsive to physical therapy, management consists of arthroscopic release using electrocautery and/or shaving followed by gentle manipulation under anesthesia. Care should be taken to avoid iatrogenic delamination of the periosteal graft during manipulation.

Autologous Osteochondral Grafting

General complications such as hemarthrosis, effusion, wound infections, and joint sepsis should be managed in the same aggressive manner as they would be in other settings. Subsidence of grafts in relation to surrounding host cartilage may be treated with observation if asymptomatic. If symptomatic, one should consider repeat osteochondral grafting, ACI, or other restorative technique. Loose bodies generated during or following graft placement that present during the postoperative course with painful catching and/or locking of the joint should be treated with arthroscopic excision. Donor site pain should be treated symptomatically, and patients can be counseled that it typically improves with time, although this may require many months.

Fresh Osteochondral Allograft Implantation

General complications such as wound infections and joint sepsis should be managed in the same aggressive manner as they would be in other scenarios. Loose bodies may be inadvertently generated during the implantation process and later become symptomatic with painful catching and clicking. Management consists of arthroscopic removal. Graft resorption with collapse of the allogenic articular surface may necessitate salvage procedures such as total joint arthroplasty. Depending on the size of the lesion and the age and demands of the patient in question, one might also entertain repeat allograft, autologous chondrocyte implantation, or autologous osteochondral grafting.

RESULTS

Although William Hunter's comment does not target OCD exclusively, it is poignantly applicable to the end result of subchondral necrosis: fragmentation, permanent destruction of overlying hyaline articular cartilage, loss of joint congruity, and finally, development of a painful, nonfunctional arthritic joint. The disease process of OCD—destabilization of the subchondral base underlying a given area of articular cartilage—must be kept in mind when entertaining the efficacy of various treatment options. Treatments that produce union of the native fragment to underlying bone should theoretically provide the best outcome, as destabilization is arrested, native hyaline cartilage is preserved, and joint congruity is maintained. Clearly, timely diagnosis and accurate characterization of the defect in question are essential to permit nonoperative strategies such as activity modification, joint immobilization, or operative techniques such as marrow stimulation or in situ fixation to succeed. The production of fibrocartilage through marrow stimulation techniques should almost be an afterthought in the context of early stable OCD as the true hope is that enhancement of blood supply to the fragment will result in osseous union with preservation of native hyaline cartilage. Implementation of strategies such as autologous chondrocyte implantation, autologous osteochondral grafting, and fresh allograft implantation reflects a failure to capture OCD in its early stages. They represent attempts to salvage the articular surface and stave off the potentially severe limitations in functionality imposed by nonbiologic resurfacing arthroplasty.

Although it appears to be more successful in the treatment of talar than capitellar or femoral condylar lesions, simple arthroscopic lavage with debridment and excision of loose bodies has not enjoyed consistent success in either juvenile or adult populations. One might consider the presence of loose bodies to represent a relative contraindication to simple arthroscopic lavage and debridement, as the presence of loose bodies indicates the existence of a previously unstable OCD defect that has failed to unite. By necessity, therefore, there also exists a full-thickness articular defect that must be addressed by means other than simple arthroscopic lavage. Marrow stimulation techniques such as microfracture and drilling can stimulate osseous union of an osteochondral fragment if the defect is detected at an early stage. When marrow stimulation affects osseous union, there is every reason to believe that treatment will be lasting as hyaline cartilage and joint congruity are preserved. Successful management of unstable lesions with full-thickness cartilage defects with this technique requires the formation of a stable and integrated layer of fibrocartilage to replace the destroyed hyaline cartilage. Fibrocartilage has been shown to have wear characteristics that are inferior to those of native hyaline cartilage,[19,21] and one can therefore expect that this type of repair will eventually degenerate and require further attention. In situ fixation of osteochondral fragments with buried or bioabsorbable types of implants, similar to marrow stimulation techniques used in the context of early-stage lesions, attempts to achieve osseous union and preserve native hyaline cartilage. Autologous chondrocyte implantation, autologous osteochondral grafting, and implantation of fresh allografts, when successful, result in restoration of hyaline articular cartilage and a congruent joint surface.

Multiple studies have provided long-term follow-up that clearly demonstrates the consequences of treatment failure that typically leads to arthrosis. Linden[8] reported on 67 joints in 58 patients with an average follow-up of 33 years. Twenty-three of these cases were diagnosed before epiphyseal closure representing JOCD. In 79% of adult cases, radiographic changes were consistent with arthrosis, whereas none of the JOCD cases demonstrated significant arthritic changes. Of note, this discrepancy has not been borne out in more recent literature. One possible explanation of Linden's findings is that in only 1 of 23 cases of JOCD did the patient have a loose body, and in 2 other cases a fragment was considered to be loose but nondisplaced. This finding contrasted to the finding that 25 of 44 adult cases had loose bodies present and an additional 15 had fragments considered to be loose but nondisplaced. Thus, it would appear that JOCD cases were

diagnosed at a significantly earlier stage in their disease than adult cases. Twyman et al.[18] followed 22 knees in 18 patients for an average of 33.6 years, all diagnosed before epiphyseal closure, and found that 32% had clear evidence of moderate or severe arthrosis. Only 50% had good or excellent clinical outcomes as judged by Hughston's score.[48] Furthermore, articular degeneration following treatment failure is not limited to the knee. Takahara et al.[17] presented data on 57 cases of OCD of the humeral capitellum with an average follow-up of 12.6 years. A poor clinical outcome was found in 50% of patients treated. Bauer et al.[14] followed 31 capitellum humeri for an average of 23 years: 23 of 31 had been treated surgically with open arthrotomy and removal of loose bodies, Thirteen of 30 elbows available for clinical examination reported significant symptoms, and 19 of 31 showed radiographic signs of degenerative disease at the time of follow-up. Table 12.5 provides a comprehensive summary of the results of various treatment modalities addressing OCD of the femoral condyles, talus and or humeral capitellum.

The foregoing results suggest several trends. JOCD typically presents in early stages, and a trial of conservative therapy consisting of activity modification may be used for a period of 6 months. Restricted weight bearing may be included in this regimen, but this may be difficult to enforce in a younger pediatric population without concomitant cast immobilization of the extremity. Most JOCD lesions that fail conservative treatment can be addressed successfully with marrow stimulation techniques, such as antegrade transarticular drilling of defects to stimulate revitalization of subchondral bone. Perforation of articular cartilage with small-gauge smooth Kirschner wires does not appear to cause long-term problems, and an antegrade approach is technically easier and obviates the risk of fragment displacement incurred by a retrograde approach. Lesions not amenable to marrow stimulation should be fixed in situ with buried (Herbert or equivalent type screws, or biodegradable fixation). Adult OCD tends to present in more advanced stages, and consequently a more aggressive approach is indicated. Stable lesions can be treated arthroscopically with a combination of marrow stimulation and in situ fixation with biodegradable or buried implants. Unstable detached lesions, if small, can be treated with autologous chondrocyte implantation or autologous osteochondral grafting. Larger lesions, especially those with concomitant bone loss, may be best addressed with either autogenic or allogeneic osteochondral allografting. It should be noted, however, that in the case of the latter therapy, it is preferable to replace more than several millimeters of bone loss with autograft before implanting the allograft to minimize recipient exposure to potentially infectious donor material.

SUMMARY

Modalities such as autologous chondrocyte transplantation have produced exciting results, but remain limited to specialized centers and incur significant expense. The use of biologic scaffolds and multipotent stem cells to regenerate hyaline cartilage remains on the horizon, providing enticing directions for further research,[35,56] and promises to eliminate problems such as donor site morbidity. Regardless of the modality employed, however, the successful operative treatment of OCD is linked inexorably to timely diagnosis. If

TABLE 12.5   Results of procedures used to address OCD lesions.

Technique	Author	Results	Comments
Nonoperative treatment	Hefti et al. (1999)[6]	154 patients; mean follow-up 3 years, 11 months 25.3% "normal" knees, 46.8% "nearly normal" knees, 27.9% "abnormal" knees	Statistically significant correlation between age and outcome
	Yoshida et al. (1998)[9]	51 knees in 38 patients; mean follow-up 11.5 years 81% overall rate of good clinical outcome with conservative treatment; 55% intercondylar medial condyle, 89% lateral condyle, 100% inferocentral medial condyle.	All patients diagnosed and treatment instituted before epiphyseal closure. Mean time to healing 12–18 months. Treatment consisted of complete restriction of all sporting activities without immobilization or change in weight-bearing status.
	Cahill et al. (1989)[3]	92 knees in 76 patients; mean follow-up 4.3 years 50% good clinical outcome	All patients diagnosed and treatment instituted before epiphyseal closure Moderate correlation between larger lesion size and failure
	Crawfurd et al. (1990)[62]	21 knees; mean follow-up 7.5 years (8–22) 62% healed overall; 30% (3/10) classical location (lateral medial condyle) healed	All patients diagnosed and treatment instituted before epiphyseal closure Rates of spontaneous healing varied with location of lesion
	De Smet et al. (1997)[47]	14 knees in 14 patients; 5 JOCD and 9 adults; mean follow-up 3.6 years 29% good clinical outcome overall 60% in JOCD group 11% in adult	Study demonstrated that instability as determined by MRI is predictor of poor outcome Also showed inverse correlation between size of lesion and rate of spontaneous recovery
	Hughston et al. (1984)[48]	22 knees in 18 patients; mean follow-up 9.4 years 82% rated good or excellent	Inverse correlation found between size of lesion and rate of recovery
	Green et al. (1953)[5]	18 knees, all JOCD; mean follow-up 4.5 years 17/18 rated "excellent"	Lesions treated conservatively with restricted weight bearing and/or cast immobilization
	Takahara et al. (1999)[46]	24 capitellum humeri; mean follow-up 5.2 years 54% significant pain with ADLs	Treatment consisted of activity modification only without immobilization Trend (not statistically significant) toward positive correlation between radiographic stage at diagnosis and clinical outcome
	Canale et al. (1980)[63]	16 osteochondral lesions of talus; mean follow-up 11.2 years 69% good clinical outcome 38% radiographic evidence of degenerative arthritis	Nonoperative treatment consisted of cast immobilization, patellar tendon weight-bearing brace, ankle corset, or arch supports
Arthroscopic/open lavage and debridement with fragment excision	Anderson and Pagnani (1997)[12]	19 knees; mean follow-up 9 years 9 treated with miniopen arthrotomy; 11 treated arthroscopically 11 JOCD 26% good or excellent by Hughston scale	Concluded that lavage and fragment excision is unsatisfactory, whether in JOCD or adult cases Recommended in situ fixation of fragment when possible
	Aglietti et al. (2001)[64]	20 knees; mean follow-up 9 years All treated with arthroscopic fragment excision, curettage and debridement of crater 85% satisfactory outcome by ICRS scale	6 lesions stage III and 14 lesions stage IV by Guhl criteria Lesion size >2 cm² on PA view statistically correlated with accelerated radiographic deterioration
	Ogilvie-Harris et al. (1999)[65]	33 tali; mean follow-up 7.4 years 100% good or excellent clinical outcome	Base of lesion debrided to cancellous bone using power burr
	Takahara et al. (1999)[17]	39 capitellum humeri; mean follow-up 12.6 years 26% good clinical outcome	Treatment comprised fragment excision alone; poor outcome correlated with increasing size of lesion
	Ruch and Poehling (1998)[66]	12 capitellum humeri: mean follow-up 3.2 years 91% good clinical outcome	Worse outcome statistically correlated with presence of triangular avulsion fragment off lateral capsule
	Byrd and Jones (2002)[67]	10 capitellum humeri in 10 baseball players; mean follow-up 3.9 years 100% excellent outcome, but only 4/10 returned to competitive baseball at previous level	Treatment included synovectomy, chondroplasty, abrasion arthroplasty, and/or loose body excision depending upon arthroscopic status of lesion
Microfracture	Gill (2000)[60]	100 knees 86% normal to near normal	2–3 years required for maximum functional improvement
Drilling	Kocher et al. (2001)[7]	30 knees in 23 patients; mean follow-up 3.9 years 100% improved Lysholm score (mean 34.2) 100% radiographic healing	All stable lesions in skeletally immature individuals, having failed nonoperative treatment for mean 6 months Treatment comprised arthroscopic, transarticular drilling of lesions

TABLE 12.5   (Continued)

Technique	Author	Results	Comments
	Anderson et al. (1997)[68]	24 knees; mean follow-up 5 years 22/24 good or excellent by Hughston scale 20/24 normal or nearly normal by IDKC scale; 20/24 radiographic healing 2/4 healing in adult versus adolescent patients	Trend toward higher success rate in JOCD
	Aglietti et al. (1994)[69]	16 knees in 14 patients; mean follow-up 56 months 95% radiographic healing	All stable lesions in skeletally immature individuals, having failed nonoperative treatment for mean 16 months Do not recommend for Guhl stage II or higher lesions Drilling antegrade, transarticular
	Bradley and Dandy (1989)[70]	11 knees in 10 patients; mean follow-up 1 year 82% radiographic and clinical healing	All stable lesions in skeletally immature individuals, having failed nonoperative treatment
	Kumai et al. (1999)[71]	18 ankles in 17 patients; mean follow-up 4.6 years 72% good clinical outcome	All lesions medial Treatment comprised arthroscopic drilling, percutaneous and transmalleolar without osteotomy Outcome improved in younger patients (30 years)
	Angermann and Jensen (1989)[13]	20 ankles; mean follow-up 12 years 85% satisfactory early results >50% pain during activity at long-term follow-up	Treatment comprised open arthrotomy without osteotomy for medial lesions and transarticular drilling; results deteriorated with time
	Schuman et al. (2002)[16]	38 ankles in 38 patients; mean follow-up 4.8 years 82% excellent or good outcome by Olgilvie–Harris score	Treatment comprised arthroscopic drilling and curettage of lesions; no osteotomies were performed; weight bearing as tolerated at 3–5 days postoperatively
In situ fixation	Anderson et al. (1990)[72]	17 knees; mean follow-up range 5–7 years 16/17 radiographic union 11/17 excellent or good by Hughston scale 57% smooth articular cartilage by MRI	Treatment comprised open arthrotomy, curettage of fragment base with autologous bone grafting and fragment fixation using Kirschner wires
	Dervin et al. (1998)[26]	9 knees; mean follow-up 33 months 7/9 excellent or good by Hughston scale 8/9 radiographic union	All skeletally mature at time of treatment Biodegradable, 2-mm polylactic pins used for fixation Drilling or crater used as adjunct
	Cugat et al. (1993)[25]	15 knees in 14 patients; mean follow-up 43 months 93% excellent or good results	Treatment comprised arthroscopic fixation via cannulated screws; second operation for screw removal required
	Zuniga et al. (1993)[73]	11 knees; mean follow-up 16.3 months 82% excellent or good results	Treatment comprised arthroscopic Herbert screw fixation, with additional use of absorbable poly (p-dioxanone) needles in 4/11 cases for rotational control
	Yoshizumi et al. (2002)[41]	3 knees 100% healing	Limited case report; treatment consisted of "biologic fixation" using a 2-mm oversized osteochondral allograft
	Kumai et al. (2002)[27]	27 ankles; mean follow-up 7 years 89% good clinical outcome 89% radiographic improvement	Treatment comprised fixation of osteochondral fragments with autologous cortical bone pegs taken from distal tibia Drilling of crater used as adjunct
	Kuwahata and Inoue (1998)[28]	8 capitellum humeri in 7 patients; mean follow-up 32 months 100% radiographic healing	Treatment comprised cannulated Herbert screw fixation with cancellous autografting of crater; motion started at 2 weeks
ACI	Brittberg et al. (1994)[31]	23 knees in 23 patients; mean follow-up 39 months 14/16 excellent or good for femoral condylar lesions 2/7 excellent or good for patellar lesions	Analysis of cartilage repair material revealed hyaline-like substance Study group not substratified into OCD patients
	Peterson et al. (2000)[34]	18 patients with OCD affecting knee joint; mean follow-up 3.1 years 89% good to excellent clinical results	Mean size of defect 4.7 cm²
	Koulalis et al. (2002)[33]	8 ankles; mean follow-up 17.6 months 100% excellent to good results	Mean size of defect 1.84 cm²
Mosaicplasty	Gautier et al. (2002)[36]	11 ankles; mean follow-up 24 months 82% excellent and 18% good results by Hannover ankle assessment	9/11 patients returned to premorbid level of sporting activity; concluded ideal candidate for procedure is patient with OCD, <45 years nonsmoker, otherwise healthy and reliable
	Hangody et al. (2001)[37]	36 ankles; mean follow-up 4.2 years 28/36 excellent, 6/36 good by Hannover ankle assessment	Mean size of defect 1 cm², diameter of plugs 3.5–6.5 mm

TABLE 12.5   (Continued)

Technique	Author	Results	Comments
Allograft	Nakagawa et al. (2001)[39]	1 capitellum (case report); no restrictions in activity at 35-month follow-up	Autologous osteochondral grafting combined with wedge osteotomy of lateral condyle
	Bugbee et al. (1999)[42]	61 knees; mean follow-up 50 months (24–128) 86% success rate	Mixed etiologies in patient population
	Ghazavi et al. (1997)[45]	126 knees in 123 patients; mean follow-up 7.5 years 85% success	Mixed etiologies in patient population
	Convery et al. (1991)[43]	9 knees in 8 patients; mean follow-up 66 months 8/9 success	Mixed etiologies in patient population
	Garret (1994)[44]	17 knees; mean follow-up 3.5 years 16/17 success	Mixed etiologies of patients; one patient failed with fragmentation of graft
	Meyers et al. (1989)[23]	40 knees in 39 patients; mean follow-up 3.2 years 77.5% success	Mixed etiologies of patients; patients with unicompartmental traumatic arthritis had 70% failure rate

JOCD, juvenile-onset osteochondritis dissecans; ADL, activities of daily lining; ICRS, International Cartilage Repair Society.

the pathology can be arrested at an early stage, before destruction of overlying articular cartilage, then a congruent, native joint surface can be maintained. As with many other conditions, therefore, the true challenge may lie in early detection. As a brief but not insignificant aside, orthopaedics, as a referral-driven subspecialty, cannot and indeed should not shoulder the sole responsibility in this matter. Rather, orthopaedists should assist their primary care colleagues— pediatricians, family physicians, and internists seeing knee pain on a daily basis—in formulating more sensitive and specific screening algorithms. Although rare, representing less than 1.2% of all knee problems, the diagnosis of OCD is not one to miss.[32] MRI and other imaging studies play vital roles in influencing outcome by serving as a noninvasive means of defining fragment stability, and thereby determining need for early operative intervention. Future directions in the treatment of osteochondritis dissecans, therefore, should be focused not only upon the development of techniques to salvage joint surfaces once full-thickness lesions have developed, but should perhaps above all target education, thereby affecting early diagnosis, accurate characterization, and timely intervention.

References

1. Stone JW. Osteochondral lesions of the talar dome. J Am Acad Orthop Surg 1996;4(2):63–73.
2. Schenck R, Goodnight JM. Current concepts review: osteochondritis dissecans. J Bone Joint Surg 1996;78A:439–456.
3. Cahill BR, Phillips MR, Navarro R. The results of conservative management of juvenile osteochondritis dissecans using joint scintigraphy. Am J Sports Med 1989;17(5):601–605.
4. Cahill BR:.Osteochondritis dissecans of the knee: treatment of juvenile and adult forms. J Am Acad Orthop Surg 1995;3(4). 237–247.
5. Green WT, Banks HH. Osteochondritis dissecans in children. J Bone Joint Surg 1953;35A(1):26–47.
6. Hefti F, Beguiristain J, Krauspe R, et al. Osteochondritis dissecans: a multicenter study of the European Pediatric Orthopedic Society. J Pediatr Orthop B 1999;8(4):231–245.
7. Kocher MS, Micheli LJ, Yaniv M, Zurakowski D, Ames AA, Adrignolo AA. Functional and radiographic outcome of the juvenile osteochondritis dissecans of the knee treated with transarticular arthroscopic drilling. Am J Sports Med 2001; 29(5):562–566.
8. Linden B. Osteochondritis dissecans of the femoral condyles. J Bone Joint Surg 1977;69A:769–776.
9. Yoshida S, Ikata T, Takai H, Kashiwaguchi S, Katoh S, Takeda Y. Osteochondritis dissecans of the femoral condyle in the growth stage. Clin Orthop 1998;346:162–170.
10. Radin EL, Ehrlich MG, Chernack R, Abernathy P, Paul I, Rose RM. Effect of repetitive impulsive loading on the knee joints of rabbits. Clin Orthop 1978;131:288–293.
11. Konig, F. Uber freie korper in den gelenken. Zeitschr Chir 1888;27:90–109.
12. Anderson AF, Pagnani MJ. Osteochondritis dissecans of the femoral condyles: long-term results of excision of the fragment. Am JSports Med 1997;25(6):830–834.
13. Angermann P, Jensen P. Osteochondritis dissecans of the talus: long-term results of surgical treatment. Foot Ankle 1989;10(3): 161–163.
14. Bauer M, Jonsson K, Josefsson PO, Linden B. Osteochondritis dissecans of the elbow: a long-term follow-up study. Clin Orthop 1992;284:156–160.
15. Bradley JP, Petrie RS. Osteochondritis dissecans of the humeral capitellum: diagnosis and treatment. Clin Sports Med 2001; 20(3):565–590.
16. Schuman L, Struijs PAA, Dijk CN. Arthroscopic treatment for osteochondral defects of the talus: results at follow-up at 2 to 11 years. J Bone Joint Surg 2002;84B(3):363–368.
17. Takahara M, Ogino T, Isao S, Kato H, Minami A, Kaneda K. Long term outcome of osteochondritis dissecans of the humeral capitellum. Clin Orthop 1999;363:108–115.
18. Twyman RS, Desai K, Aichroth PM. Osteochondritis dissecans of the knee: a long-term study. JBone Joint Surg 1991;73B: 461–464.
19. Mankin HJ. The response of articular cartilage to mechanical injury. J Bone Joint Surg 1982;64A(3):460–466.
20. Hunter, W. Of the structure and disease of articulating cartilages. Philos Trans R Soc Lond 42:514–521, 1743.
21. O'Driscoll S. Current concepts review: the healing and regeneration of articular cartilage. J Bone Joint Surg 1998;80A: 1795–1812.
22. Paré A, Oeuvres completes. Paris: JB Bailliere; 1840;32.
23. Meyers MH, Akeson W, Convery R. Resurfacing of the knee with fresh osteochondral allograft. J Bone Joint Surg 1989;71A: 704–713.

24. Browne JE, Branch TP. Surgical alternatives for treatment of articular cartilage lesions. J Am Acad Orthop Surg 2000;8(3): 180–189.

25. Cugat R, Garcia M, Cusco X, et al. Osteochondritis dissecans: a historical review and its treatment with cannulated screws. Arthroscopy 1993;9(6):675–684.

26. Dervin GF, Keene GCR, Chissell HR. Biodegradable rods in adult osteochondritis dissecans of the knee. Clin Orthop 1998; 356:213–221.

27. Kumai T, Takakura Y, Kitada C, Tanaka Y, Hayashi K. Fixation of osteochondral lesions of the talus using cortical bone pegs. J Bone Joint Surg 2002;84B(3):369–374.

28. Kuwahata Y, Inoue G. Osteochondritis dissecans of the elbow managed by Herbert screw fixation. Orthopedics 1998;21(4): 449–451.

29. Mackie IG, Pemberton DJ, Maheson M. Arthroscopic use of the Herbert screw in osteochondritis dissecans. J Bone Joint Surg 1990;72B:1076.

30. Smillie S: Treatment of osteochondritis dissecans. J Bone Joint Surg 1957;39B:248–260.

31. Brittberg M, Lindahl A, Nilsson A, Ohlsson C, Isaksson O, Peterson L. Treatment of deep cartilage defects in the knee with autologous chondrocyte transplantation. N Engl J Med 1994; 331(14):889–895.

32. Peterson L, Brittberg M, Kiviranta I, Akerlund E, Lindahl A. Autologous chondrocyte transplantation: biomechanics and long-term durability. Am J Sports Med 2002;30(1):2–12.

33. Koulalis D, Schultz W, Heyden M. Autologous chondrocyte transplantation for osteochondritis dissecans of the talus. Clin Orthop 2002;395:186–192.

34. Peterson L, Minas T, Brittberg M, Nilsson A, Sjogren-Jansson E, Lindahl A. Two- to 9-year outcome after autologous chondrocyte transplantation of the knee. Clin Orthop 2000;374:212–234.

35. Bobic V, Morgan CD, Carter T. Osteochondral autologous graft transfer. Oper Tech Sports Med 2000;8(2):168–178.

36. Gautier E, Kolker D, Jakob RP. Treatment of cartilage defects of the talus by autologous osteochondral grafts. J Bone Joint Surg 2002;84B:237–244.

37. Hangody L, Kish G, Modis L, et al. Mosaicplasty for the treatment of osteochondritis dissecans of the talus: Two- to seven-year results in 36 patients. Foot Ankle Int 2001;22(7):552–558.

38. Kish G, Modis L, Hangody L. Osteochondral mosaicplasty for the treatment of focal chondral and osteochondral lesions of the knee and talus in the athlete, rationale, indications, techniques and results. Clin Sports Med 1999;18(1):45–65.

39. Nakagawa Y, Matsusue Y, Ikeda N, Asada Y, Nakamura T. Osteochondral grafting and arthroplasty for end-stage osteochondritis dissecans of the capitellum. Am J Sports Med 2001; 29(5):650–655.

40. Scranton PE. Management of osteochondral lesions of the talus. Presented at AAOS Annual Meeting; 2002.

41. Yoshizumi Y, Sugita T, Kawamata T, Ohnuma M, Maeda S. Cylindrical osteochondral graft for osteochondritis dissecans of the knee. Am J Sports Med 2002;30(3):441–445.

42. Bugbee WD, Convery FR. Osteochondral allograft transplantation. Clin Sports Med 1999;18(1):67–75.

43. Convery FR, Meyers MH, Akeson WH. Fresh osteochondral allografting of the femoral condyle. Clin Orthop 1991;273:139–145.

44. Garrett JC. Fresh osteochondral allografts for treatment of articular defects in osteochondritis dissecans of the lateral femoral condyle in adults. Clin Orthop 1994;303:33–37.

45. Ghazavi MT, Pritzker KP, Davis AM, Gross AE Fresh osteochondral allografts for post-traumatic osteochondral defects of the knee. J Bone Joint Surg 1997;79B:1008–1013.

46. Takahara M, Ogino T, Fukushima S, Tsuchida H, Kaneda K. Nonoperative treatment of osteochondritis dissecans of the humeral capitellum. Am J Sports Med 1999;27(6):728–732.

47. De Smet AA, Ilahi OA, Graf BK. Untreated osteochondritis dissecans of the femoral condyles: prediction of patient outcome using radiographic and MR findings. Skeletal Radiol 1997;26: 463–467.

48. Hughston JC, Hergenroeder PT, Courtenay BG. Osteochondritis dissecans of the femoral condyles. J Bone Joint Surg 1984; 66A:1340–1348.

49. Mandelbaum BR, Browne JE, Fu F, et al. Articular cartilage lesions of the knee. Am J Sports Med 1998;26(6):853–861.

50. Minas T. A practical algorithm for cartilage repair. Oper Tech Sports Med 2000;8(2):141–143.

51. DeSmet AA, Iliahi OA, Graf BK. Reassessment of the MR criteria for stability of osteochondritis dissecans in the knee and ankle. Skeletal Radiol 1996;25:159–163.

52. Mesgarzadeh M, Sapega AA, Bonakdarpour A. Osteochondritis dissecans: analysis of mechanical stability with radiography, scinitigraphy, and MR imaging. Radiology 1987;165:775–780.

53. O'Connor MA, Palaniappanm M, Khan N, Bruce CE. Osteochondritis dissecans of the knee in children: a comparison of MRI and arthroscopic findings. JBone Joint Surg 2002;84B: 258–262.

54. Jackson DW, Scheer MJ, Simon TM. Cartilage substitutes: overview of basic science and treatment options. J Am Acad Orthop Surg 2001;9(1):37–52.

55. Minas T, Peterson L. Advanced techniques in autologous chondrocyte transplantation. Clin Sports Med 1999;18(1):13–44.

56. Martin DS, Martin TL, Shu H, Spector M. Push out strength of expansion-fit versus exact-fit osteochondral plugs. Presented at AAOS Annual Meeting; 2001.

57. Koh JL, Wirsing KM, Lautenschlager E, Zang L. The effect of graft height mismatch on contact pressure following osteochondral grafting: a biomechanical study. Presented at AAOS Annual Meeting; 2002.

58. Standards for tissue banking. McLean VA:American Association of Tissue Banks; 1984–1989.

59. Salter RB, Simmonds DF, Malcolm BW, et al. The biological effect of continuous passive motion on the healing of full-thickness defects in articular cartilage. An experimental investigation in the rabbit. Bone Joint Surg 1980;62A:1232–1251.

60. Gill TJ. The role of the microfracture technique in the treatment of full-thickness chondral injuries. Oper Tech Sports Med 2000;8(2):138–140.

61. Steadman JR, Rodkey WG, Rodrigo JJ. Microfracture: surgical technique and rehabilitation to treat chondral defects. Clin Orthop 2001;391S:362–369.

62. Crawfurd EJP, Emery RJH, Aichroth PM. Stable osteochondritis dissecans—does the lesion unite? J Bone Joint Surg 1990;72B: 320.

63. Canale T, Belding R. Osteochondral lesions of the talus. J Bone Joint Surg 1980;62A(1):97–102.

64. Aglietti P, Ciardullow A, Giron F, Ponteggia F. Results of arthroscopic excision of the fragment in the treatment of osteochondritis dissecans of the knee. Arthroscopy 2001;17(7):741–746.

65. Ogilvie-Harris JJ, Sarrosa EA. Arthroscopic treatment of osteochondritis dissecans of the talus. Arthroscopy 1999;15(8): 805–808.

66. Ruch DS, Poehling GG. The arthroscopic management of osteochondritis dissecans of the adolescent elbow. Arthroscopy 1998;14(8):797–803.

67. Byrd JW, Jones Kay S. Arthroscopic surgery for isolated capitellar osteochondritis dissecans in adolescent baseball players. Am J Sports Med 2002;30(4):474–478.

68. Anderson AF, Richards DB, Pagnani MJ, Hovis WD. Antegrade drilling for osteochondritis dissecans of the knee. Arthroscopy 1997;13(3):319–324.

69. Aglietti P, Buzzi R, Bassi PB, Forti M. Arthroscopic drilling in juvenile osteochondritis dissecans of the medial femoral condyle. Arthroscopy 1994;10(3):286–291.

70. Bradley JP, Dandy DJ. Results of drilling osteochondritis dissecans before skeletal maturity. J Bone Joint Surg 1989;71B:642–644.

71. Kumai T, Takakura Y, Higashiyama I, Tamai S. Arthroscopic drilling for the treatment of osteochondral lesions of the talus. J Bone Joint Surg 1999;81A(9):1229–1235.

72. Anderson AF, Lipscomb AB, Coulam C. Antegrade curettement, bone grafting and pinning of osteochondritis dissecans in the skeletally mature knee. Am J Sports Med 1990;18(3):254–261.

73. Zuniga JJR, Sagastibelza J, Blasco JJL, Grande MM. Arthroscopic use of the Herbert screw in osteochondritis dissecans of the knee. Arthroscopy 1993;9(6):668–670.

13

Meniscal Transplantation

Jack Farr and Wayne K. Gersoff

BACKGROUND

The knee is a complex joint. Optimal function requires the integrity of its structural components. Appreciation of the structural and functional importance of the meniscus has undergone a great evolution. The meniscus is no longer viewed as an accessory structure that can be removed without consequence. The functions of the meniscus include shock absorption, optimizing contact areas, pressure transduction, stabilization, and nutrition. All are essential to normal knee function. Although total meniscectomy is avoided whenever possible, unfortunately there are situations where the tear type dictates a partial meniscectomy. Although casually thought of as a "partial meniscectomy," the common loss of the majority of the posterior horn increases stress to the point, suggesting, in these circumstances, that a better term would be "biomechanical absence of the meniscus." The concept of meniscal transplantation was developed to attempt to restore normal structure and function of the knee in an effort to decrease pain and the likelihood of arthrosis developing in the affected compartments.

BASIC SCIENCE CONSIDERATIONS

The utilization of meniscal allografts in the clinical setting is strongly based on basic science considerations. These considerations are not unlike those associated with the use of other soft tissue allograft: immunology, tissue preservation, chondroprotective potential, and healing potential. Meniscal allograft has been described as "immunologically privileged."[1,2] The unique fibrocartilaginous tissue of the meniscus is relatively acellular. These cellular components (which have the greatest number of histocompatibility antigens) are shielded by the extracellular matrix the cells maintain. As a result, systemic rejection rarely occurs. Nevertheless, there is evidence that some form of immune response does occur.[3–5] The potential for a localized immune response certainly exists: (1) even after deep freezing, histocompatability antigens can be expressed on the cells of a meniscal allograft[6]; (2) the bone and synovial attachments to the meniscal allograft remain antigenic; and (3) the existence of immunoreactive cells in fresh-frozen meniscal allograft has been demonstrated.[7] The localized response most likely has an effect on graft revascularization, repopulation, incorporation, and healing response.[8–10] Clinically, it appears that results have not been compromised by a localized immune response. As research continues, the goal will be to minimize any negative immunologic response and to maximize the positive healing, incorporation, and remodeling process.

The meniscal allograft is usually processed by one of four techniques: fresh, cryopreserved, fresh-frozen, or freeze-dried. The tissue itself is obtained only from a tissue banking resource that is compliant with all standards equivalent to those set by the American Association of Tissue Banks. The U.S Food and Drug Administration (FDA) continues to take an active role in monitoring the transplant tissue process, which provides the best opportunity to utilize disease-free and uncompromised (no evidence of degenerative change) allograft tissue. Fresh allograft tissue offers some advantages for cell viability but is logistically not practical for most surgeons. The process of freeze-drying or lyophilization causes cell death, yet the major disadvantage of this process is the effect it has on the structural properties of the meniscal allograft, such as graft shrinkage and potential damage to the collagen fibers.[11–13]

Cryopreserved and fresh-frozen tissue avoid the structural damage seen with lyophilization. Specifically, cryopreservation involves a slow freezing rate of the allograft tissue utilizing a chemical cryoprotectant such as dimethyl sulfoxide (DMSO). This method allows for a slight increase in cell viability and preservation of some degree of cell membrane integrity. Both cryopreserved and fresh-frozen tissue allow for prolonged storage; this allows not only complete appropriate serologic testing, but also creates a "bank" of multiple sizes.[14,15] Meniscal allografts that are fresh frozen undergo a more rapid freezing process that ultimately results in cell death but without adversely affecting the structural properties of the graft. Cell viability may not be an important issue, as experimental studies have suggested that there are no significant outcome differences between cryopreserved and deep frozen grafts.[2,16,17]

Animal studies by Arnozocky et al.[18] and Jackson et al.[2] have demonstrated the repopulation of meniscal allograft tis-

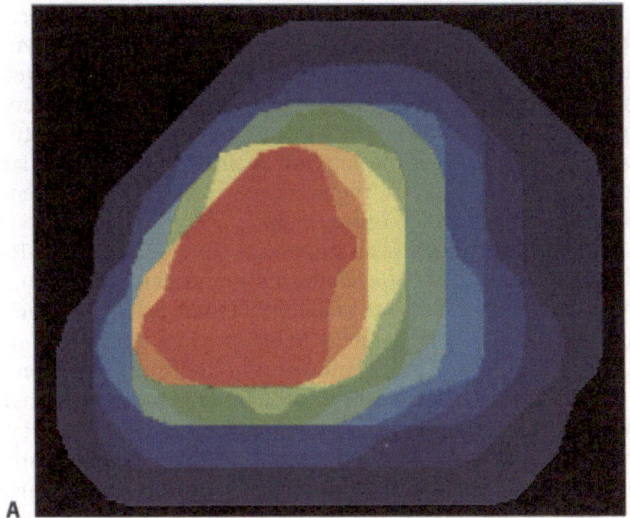

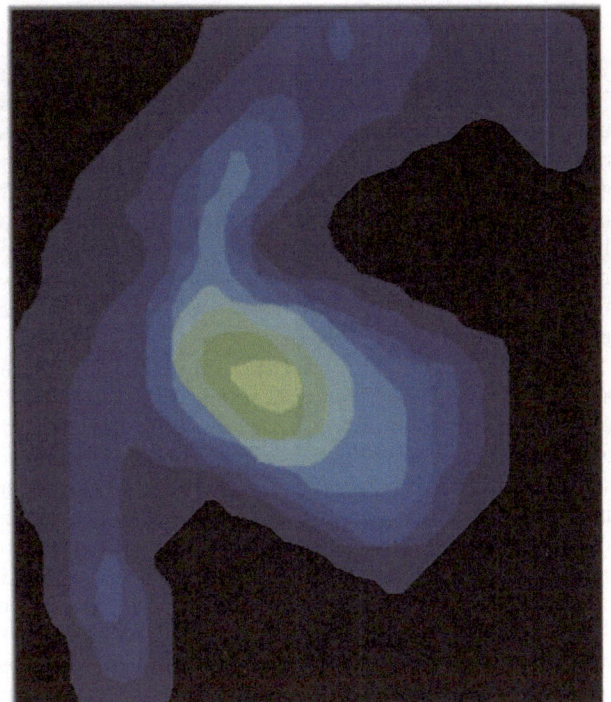

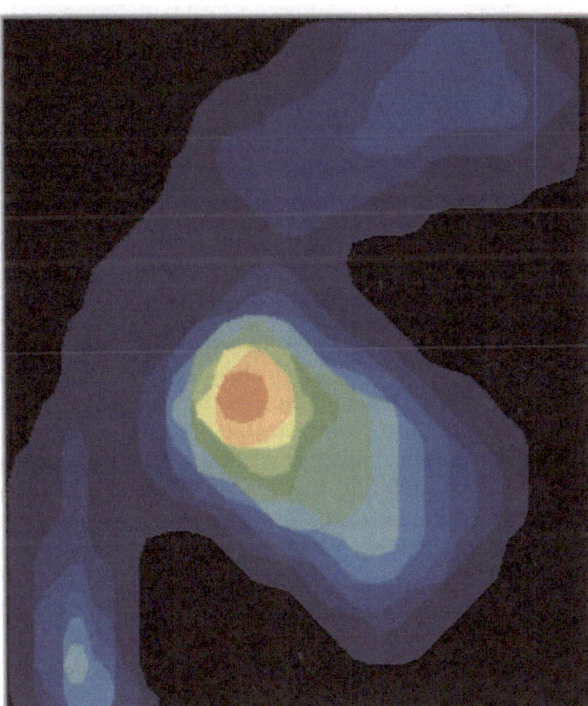

FIGURE 13.1 Tekscan measurements. **A.** Without meniscus. **B.** With meniscus. **C.** With bridge allograft. Red and orange color denotes increased contact force, which is reduced in the intact state and transplantal state. (Data from Cole et al.)

sue by host-derived cells whose origin is most likely the synovial membrane. Biopsies retrieved from human specimens have also supported these findings.[7] Although future research will provide insight into the enhancement of the process of repopulation and incorporation, at present the utilization of fresh-frozen tissue compared to either fresh or cryopreserved is simpler, less costly, and still provides the essential biologic scaffolding for successful function and incorporation.

Although it is apparent that the meniscal allograft will heal, gradually repopulate, and not be systemically rejected,

the final important consideration is its function. Animal studies performed by Szomor et al.,[19] Cole and Harner,[20] and Alhalki et al.[21,22] have all demonstrated chondroprotective effects of meniscal transplantation tissue. The chondroprotective benefits of the meniscus transplant are also better as compared to a total meniscectomy, but they are not identical to that of a normal meniscus.[23–26] Similar improvements in contact/stress in a cadaver model were shown by Cole and Farr (Unpublished data) using Tekscan contact pressure measurements (Figure 13.1).

ANATOMIC CONSIDERATIONS

The efficiency of the human body dictates that form follows function. The meniscus is no exception. Although there are many subsets of meniscal function, the primary role is to optimize the environment for the articular cartilage. The meniscal anatomy is based on these functions. As gait and the knee have evolved, the meniscus plays a different role in the knee for each animal. The ultimate goal of meniscal transplantation is restoring anatomy to restore function and relieve symptoms.

It is well known that each of the semilunar shaped menisci is unique in form. This macroscopic form is dictated by function in both compartments, appreciating the dynamics during the "screw-home" mechanism. The medial meniscus is longer anterior to posterior than medial to lateral whereas the lateral meniscus is more equal in these measurements. Although both menisci have meniscal capsular attachments (coronary ligaments), the medial meniscus has less excursion during flexion extension (4–6 mm) than the lateral meniscus (8–14 mm),[27] partly because of the firm attachment of the medial meniscus to the deep fibers of the medial collateral ligament. In addition, the lateral meniscus has a less rigid attachment in the region of the popliteal hiatus. The attachment in this region has somewhat variable anatomy with the meniscofemoral ligaments of Humphrey and Wrisberg and the popliteomeniscal fasiculi. The ligaments of Humphrey and Wrisberg are associated with the posterior cruciate ligament (PCL) and run from the PCL femoral attachment region of the femur to the posterior horn of the lateral meniscus medial to the popliteal hiatus.

In the region of the popliteal hiatus, the posterosuperior and anteroinferior popliteomeniscal fasiculi stabilize the lateral meniscus.[28] The circular form of the lateral meniscus places both horns in close approximation, whereas the attachments sites of the medial meniscus are at the anteroposterior (AP) extremes of the plateau. In fact, the medial meniscus anterior horn is attached on the anterior slope/margin of the medial tibial plateau. The attachment site of the medial meniscus is variable, and it may not attach to bone in some individuals.[29] In addition, there is considerable variation in the site of attachment of the "intermeniscal" ligament. This ligament more typically is firmly attached to the medial meniscus anterior horn (at times, covering the horn when viewed arthroscopically) and extends to the synovium/capsular tissue anterior to the lateral meniscus anterior horn. Further complicating anterior horn anatomy is the patellomeniscal ligament, inserting anteromedially at the periphery of the medial meniscus. When this anatomy is considered in meniscal transplantation, it is obvious that certain structures will not be reestablished at the time of surgery, especially the unique structures stabilizing the posterior horn of the lateral meniscus.

The microscopic anatomy underlying this gross anatomy must also be considered when transplanting menisci. The microscopic anatomy may be subdivided into structure, vascular supply, and innervation. The structure is composed of a cellular component and an extracellular matrix. The cells are unique fibromeniscochondrocytes, exhibiting different characteristics in different regions of the meniscus. For example,

elongated cells are located superficially and are more fibrocytic in nature whereas deep cells are more ovoid and synthesize complex proteoglycans (more fibrocartilage in nature). The cells in certain regions may use anaerobic metabolism, explaining function in areas of low or absent vascular profusion.[30] These cells synthesize and maintain the extracellar matrix. Without the cells, the meniscus will gradually degenerate, become torn and nonfunctional.

The microstructure is an important component in meniscal function as this collagen forms circumferential fibers, which are then linked by radially oriented collagen fibers. Together this network of fibers helps to resist tension, compression, and shear. The circumferential fibers run from bony horn attachment to bony horn attachment and resist axial load/compression loads by converting radial forces to tension forces, which are termed hoop stress; this not only transforms the axial load, but also maintains the shape of the meniscus, thus maintaining contact areas. As stress is defined as force per unit area, it is apparent the meniscus can reduce stress to the articular cartilage both by redirecting force (through hoop stress) and by increasing the surface contact area (compared with isolated femoral tibial articular cartilage loading in the absence of a meniscus) where force transmission occurs. This understanding emphasizes the importance of reestablishing these functions both micro- and macroscopically.

The molecular structure of the matrix allows the meniscus to transmit as much as 50% of joint load in the medial compartment and 70% in the lateral compartment.[31] This load sharing varies with range of motion and gradually increases with increased flexion. Upon meniscal removal, the stress greatly increases, and the lateral meniscus loss results in higher ipsilateral compartment articular stress than medial meniscus loss. Note that compartment contact area decreases rapidly and stresses rapidly increase with even small amounts of meniscal loss; this is important when considering the effect of what would appear to be a "minor" partial meniscectomy.

When a common posterior horn flap tear violates the majority of the hoop-stress bearing circumferential fibers, this "standard" partial meniscectomy may more closely resemble a total meniscectomy from a biomechanical or stress aspect than might be casually assumed. The maintenance of form is also important in the medial compartment in regards to stability. The posterior horn of the medial meniscus provides some decrease to anterior tibial translation.[32] This interdependence underlines the concern for the anterior cruciate ligament-(ACL) deficient and medial meniscus-deficient knee: higher than normal forces will be present in either structure if only one is reconstructed.

The vascular network has received attention as it has been shown to be a strong predictor of meniscal tear healing potential. This factor is also important for the meniscal transplant as the peripheral soft tissue healing can be closely compared with a very peripheral (meniscocapsular junction) "bucket-handle" meniscal tear repair. The majority of the meniscus is poorly vascular or avascular. At the periphery (the meniscocapsular junction), branches of the medial and lateral geniculate superior and inferior branches supply the meniscus. The vascular penetration varies by study type, but is usually accepted at between 10% and 30% of the width of the medial meniscus and 10%–25% of the lateral meniscus, noting additional perfusion is present at the horn attachments.[30] This rich peripheral vascular network allows early peripheral attachment of the meniscal transplant and serves as one potential source of host cells to repopulate the meniscal transplant tissue.

The majority of the meniscus is not innervated, and the present known nerve fiber distribution follows somewhat the pattern of the vascularity. The horns and meniscocapsular junctions are most heavily innervated. A variety of nerve endings are present and may represent both mechanoreceptors and proprioceptive functions.[30] The extent and importance of ingrowth of host innervation are unknown.

When transferring this basic science knowledge to the clinical setting, it is important to understand and respect both the micro- and macroanatomy as it relates to physiologic maturation. The concepts of cyclic loading and graft protection are important in the development stages. Fixation must take into account the microarchitecture. The current standard for pullout strength comparison is the vertical mattress suture, which captures the circumferential fibers. Respect for the biology of the transplant and the concept of initial healing responses, remodeling, and maturation cannot be overemphasized.

SURGICAL PROCEDURES

Indications and Contraindications

The indications for meniscal transplantation continue to evolve within the entire spectrum of cartilage and knee restoration. At present, the indication is for pain relief in symptomatic patients. It is important that the pain is well localized to the meniscal-deficient compartment and that the pain is not secondary to incomplete conservative management and rehabilitation. Longer-term studies are necessary to comment on the effect of articular cartilage "protection" and, specifically for the medial meniscus, whether the added stability of the meniscal transplant places less strain on an ACL reconstruction, allowing a more physiologic result. Age indications are relative, with more focus placed on biologic age, taking into account activity level and ability to fully and actively follow the postoperative course and rehabilitation. The chronologic age for most sites is below the age of 50. When pain is not a major concern of the patient, in some cases an assessment of ipsilateral subchondral bone overload evaluated by bone scan or magnetic resonance imaging (MRI) may be useful in deciding for or against meniscal transplant.

There are some special contraindications that are provisional and reversible. Certainly, the work of Noyes and Barber-Weston[33] pointed out the relative contraindication of meniscal transplantation when grade III or IV chondrosis is present, but transplantation may be performed if these lesions are treated with cartilage restoration. This condition obviously eliminates patients with advanced radiographic classic "primary" arthritis with marked joint space narrowing and osteophytic change. Nevertheless, primary osteoarthritis must not be confused with the early changes brought on by the biologic or biomechanical absence of the meniscus in question. These postmeniscectomy articular cartilage changes must be carefully analyzed for potential for restoration. Tibiofemoral malalignment, which leads to overloading of the ipsilateral compartment, is a contraindication, yet this may be reversed with the appropriate corrective osteotomy before or concomitant with meniscal transplantation. Likewise, instability is a contraindication but can be corrected before or concomitant with the transplantation. Controversy exists as to what body mass index (BMI) is too high for transplantation, but clearly obesity compromises even a normal knee joint. The weight limit should be considered in light of articular cartilage studies suggesting a BMI greater than 35. Active infection, inflammatory arthritis, and crystal arthritis are also usually considered contraindications.

Surgical Techniques

Though there are multiple variations for accomplishing meniscal transplantation, several common themes are present. For a detailed explanation of each technique, the various authors' original work should be consulted.[34] Macroscopic considerations focus on correct position of the meniscal transplant to allow it to function as closely as possible to the native meniscus. There are multiple nuances for each technique, and their relative importance is not fully known at present. Nevertheless, in vitro testing by Howell et al.[21,22] has demonstrated the importance of bone attachment and precise horn attachment site. Thus, it stands to reason that each point in a technique be adhered to as closely as possible so as to not create additive error. It must be kept in mind that the goal is normalization of contract area with resultant stress reduction to a physiologic level and that this must be accomplished with the meniscal tissue functioning throughout a physiologic range of motion.

There are technique differences for the host and the donor tissue. As is evident, the transplant size should closely mimic the host size. To accomplish this the surgeon must work closely with the providing tissue bank. Before ordering the transplant, sizing studies are performed. Although MRI and computed tomography (CT) have been used, plain radiographs of the host have been shown by Pollard et al.[35] to allow acceptable matching. True AP and true lateral radiographs are obtained with appropriate magnification markers. The original Pollard paper noted some confusion about magnification marker placement. The marker should be attached to the knee (skin) at the same height above the film plate (not on the film plate) as the tibia in that plane; therefore, this requires changing from an AP to a lateral view. Direct sizing measurements are made on the AP film for the medial to lateral dimension, using the center of the involved compartment's tibial spine to the margin edge of that compartment.

On lateral films, longitudinal lines are extended from the anterior and posterior proximal tibia adjacent to the joint. The lines are connected with an anterior-to-posterior line. This anterior-to-posterior line measurement is used for the AP meniscal sizing after using a percentage magnification multiplier that corrects for image magnification on the radiograph. These initial numbers are corrected for magnification (typical magnification is 105%–120%). For the anterior-to-posterior dimension of the desired allograft, the corrected for magnification anterior-to-posterior measurement is taken from the lateral radiograph and then multiplied by 0.8 for the medial meniscus and 0.7 for the lateral meniscal measure-

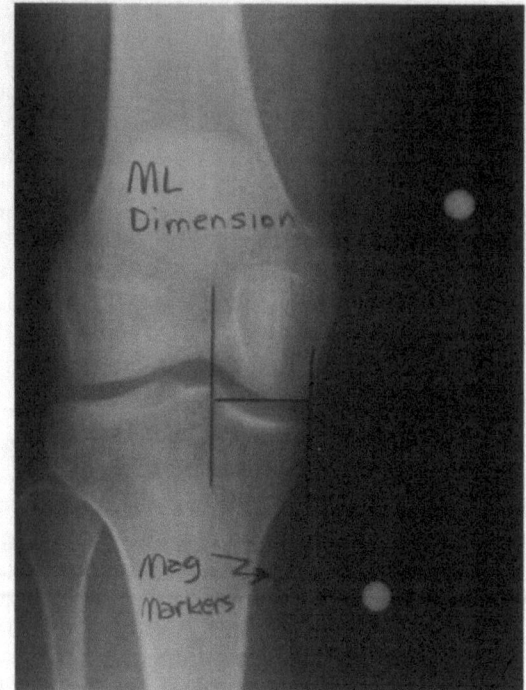

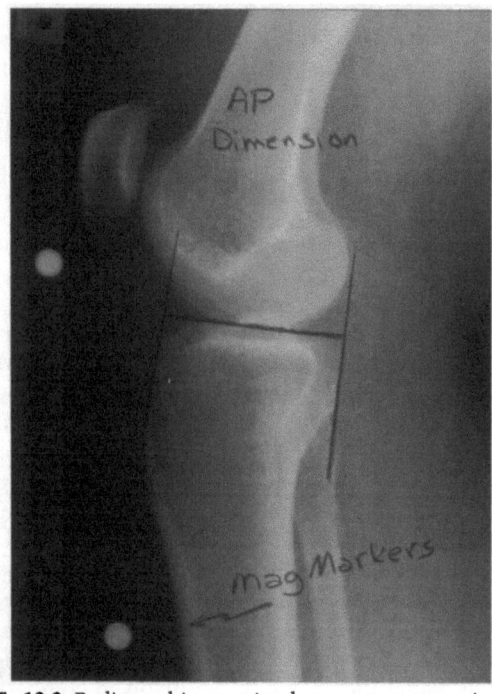

FIGURE 13.2 Radiographic meniscal measurements. **A.** Lateral. **B.** Anterior posterior.

ment (Figure 13.2). The surgeon and or the supplier may interpret these "marker films," but the surgeon is ultimately responsible and is best able to comment on whether a margin is falsely enlarged (for example, by an osteophyte).

With the history of poor results with freeze-dried transplants, current technique calls for fresh-frozen or cyropreserved specimens appropriately tested and screened for disease agents. These tissues are delivered to the operating room frozen, where size, side and and right versus left should be checked before the patient is anesthetized.

Once the tissue is confirmed, it is thawed per the specifications of the supplying tissue bank and then thoroughly washed, with special attention to the cancellous bone to remove residual soft tissue and marrow elements.

Before thawing of the meniscal tissue, the patient undergoes arthroscopy to be sure all indications are met and contraindications are recognized and managed as already described. Alternatively, the procedure may be performed as an open procedure, which is often the case if performed with major cartilage restoration. Even in these cases, however, it is often easier to perform the transplant first arthroscopically assisted as posterior horn access and visualization may be superior to open access. Full visualization is necessary to accurately identify the center of attachment for each horn. Usually the remnant guides positioning, but in cases of complete absence, adjacent landmarks are identified using prior studies in which the horn attachment sites have been documented.

In most techniques, bony attachment is used in light of the biomechanical studies of Howell et al.[21,22] Some surgeons continue to utilize soft tissue fixation alone, but these techniques need to be critically reviewed before use as a first choice. With all techniques, the goal is to place the horns in the anatomic position in an attempt to duplicate the native absent meniscus. Each technique achieves this with some variation on a theme. The two main categories are bone plugs and bone bridges. Each technique is described in the literature, which should be consulted directly.[34]

Preparation of the knee is very important. Full access to the horns and periphery are essential. In tight compartments, it may be necessary to perform relaxing incisions to adequately visualize the posterior horns. The meniscal remnant is resected to a firm 1- to 2-mm peripheral meniscocapsular junction with attention to creating a bleeding synovial bed; this may be further stimulated for a healing response with use of perimeniscal synovial abrasion and trephination. Trimming the notch side of the condyle and adjacent tibial spine may further enhance posterior horn visualization; this is routinely mentioned and used, yet immediately eliminates load bearing of the spine–condyle interface. This "standard" preparation thus negates one criticism of the bone bridge used medially, which obviously removes a significant portion of the host medial spine. Classically, however, the plug technique (Figure 13.3) is used medially to avoid this spine debridement while the bone bridge technique is used laterally, as it is difficult to have the tunnels as close together as would be called for by the anatomy of the lateral meniscal horn attachments. If bone plugs are used medially, their proponents acknowledge the ability to modify the anterior horn attachment site intraoperatively as needed.

The optimal site of plug placement and tunnel position has been demonstrated radiographically.[36] Appropriate positioning of both anterior and posterior plugs is critical to obtain the anatomic positioning of the meniscal tissue and allow for biomechanical efficiency. Therefore, the anterior horn bone plug should not be selected on the basis of ease of placement. The bone plugs can be reduced first and then the meniscal tissue reduced as in a bucket-handle tear. Alternatively, the posterior bone plug can be reduced first with the meniscal tissue, then placed, and finally the anterior horn bone plug reduced. Although the posterior tun-

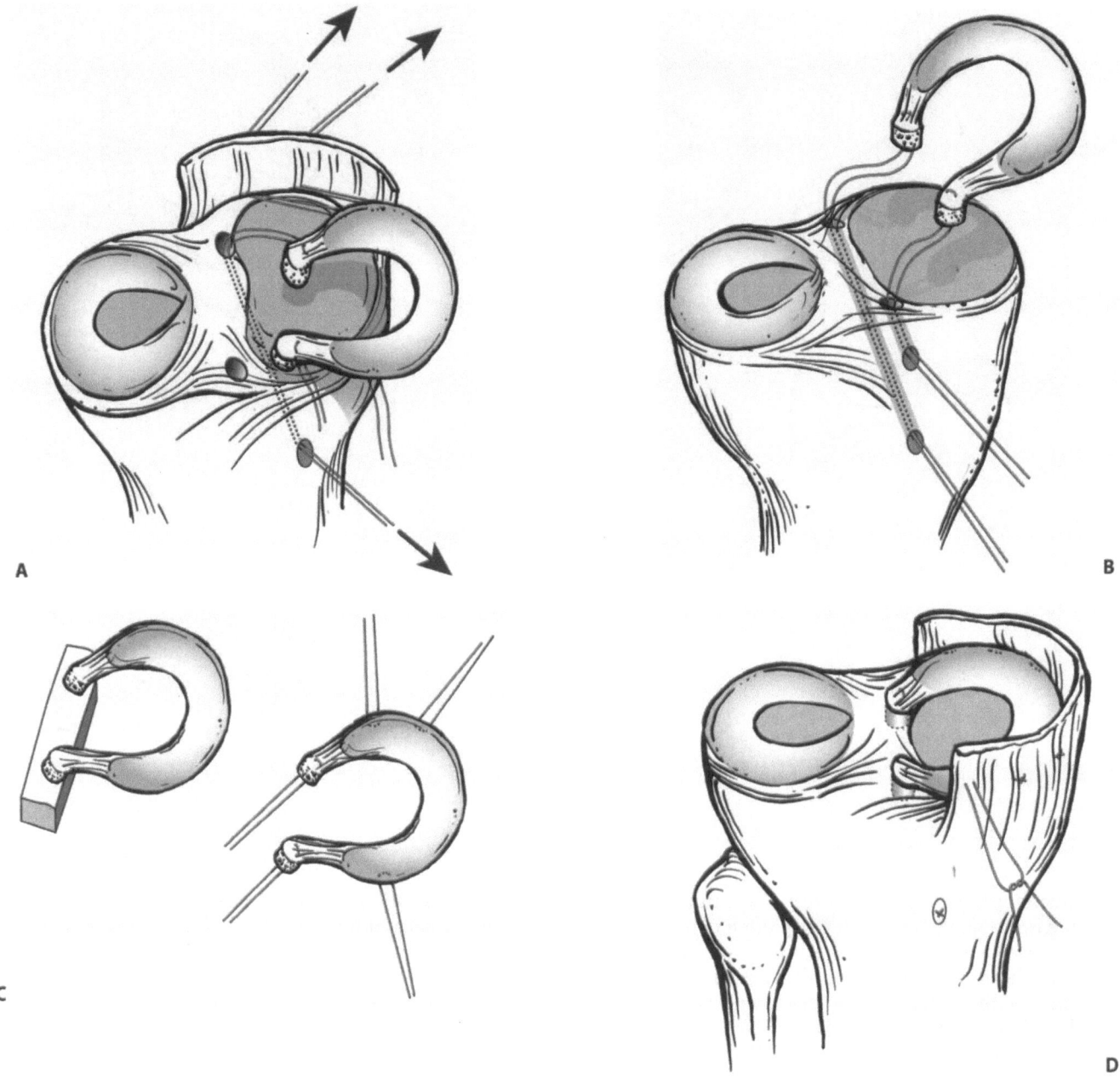

A

B

C

D

FIGURE 13.3A–D Bone plug technique.

nel is typically placed with a guide from the tibia anteriorly to the posterior horn attachment, the anterior tunnel is usually placed under direct visualization. The plugs are fixed typically with suture through bone, buttons or soft tissue.

Bone bridge techniques are described as the keyhole method, the trough, and slot techniques.[34] The keyhole technique is technically demanding (Figure 13.4). After the keyhole is made between the horn attachment sites, measurements are transferred to the meniscal transplant bone. At times, the bone portion of the transplant may be insufficient to form a complete "key" and thus the technique is converted to trough or slot. The trough uses a box chisel to cut free hand a trough: like the keyhole this then allows press-fit fixation of the bridge in the keyhole or trough (Figure 13.5).

The trough meniscal transplant bone is rectangular. In both techniques, the bone bridge then uses press-fit fixation of the bridge in the keyhole or trough. The slot technique uses a standard 8-mm rectangular slot with 7-mm bridge (Figure 13.6. The 7-mm bridge is inserted and fined tuned in the AP direction by capture of the meniscus by the femoral condyle with hoop stress in the development in the construct. The bone bridge is fixed in the slot, typically using an interference fit screw, thus separating the fixation and the fine tuning of anterior to posterior fit.[37] Disadvantage of the press-fit is that if fit occurs prematurely, then full posterior positioning may not be achieved. If fit is secured and the position is too anterior, extraction is difficult, and further impaction may result in fracture of the anterior horn bony attachment.

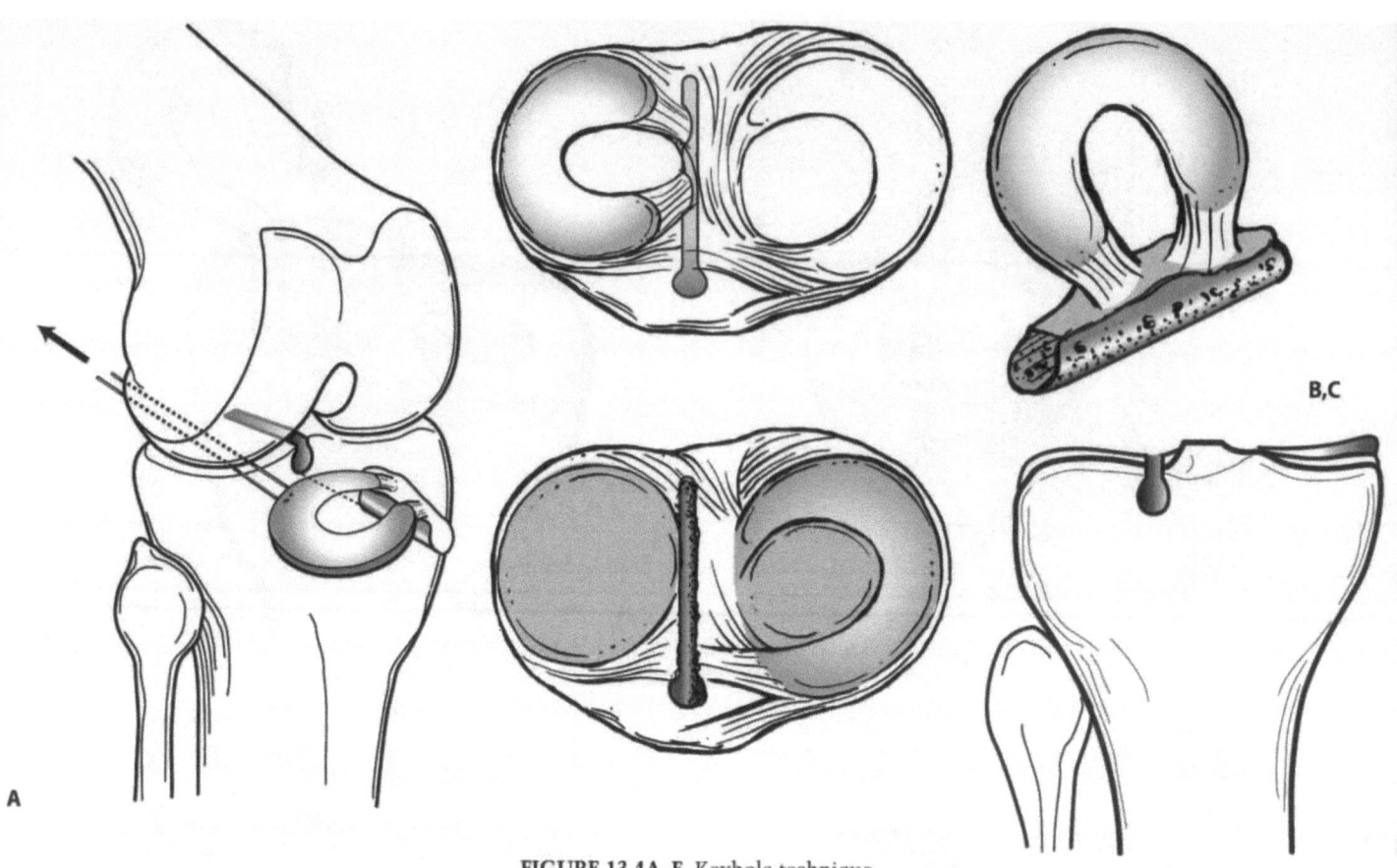

FIGURE 13.4A–E Keyhole technique.

Regardless of the bony fixation technique, full posterior positioning is essential. The soft tissue portion of the graft is pulled into place with a positioning suture at the junction of the posterior horn and middle one third. A nitenol suture passer may facilitate this suture placement through the meniscal capsular junction and "inside-out" into a previously prepared posterior medial or lateral accessory incision, as for medial and lateral meniscal repairs. After reduction, the knee is cycled to document anatomic-appearing positioning of the meniscus. With proper sizing and placement, the transplant typically tracks smoothly without displacement or subluxation. In light of the marked healing response, fewer sutures may be placed than for a white or red bucket-handle tear. Typically 6 to 10 2-0 nonabsorbable vertical mattress sutures are placed, occasionally supplemented with all-inside bioabsorbable devices at the extremes of the posterior horn. As with any meniscal repair, care is taken to avoid neurovascular compromise.

Complications

Complications may be divided into logical groupings for meniscal allografts. It is assumed that surgeons undertaking these advanced surgeries are familiar with complications that may occur with meniscal repair using the commonly accepted methods of inside-out fixation, outside-in fixation, and all-inside fixation. These "standard" complications associated with meniscal repair include infection, failure to heal, late retearing, tearing at a new site, neurovascular compromise, arthrofibrosis, sympathetically mediated pain, and injury to ligamentous and articular cartilage tissue. Furthermore, the time to healing may occur in a staged manner. The stages are yet to be defined, yet we may project from musculoskeletal healing in general that there will be an early "healing response," followed by intermediate repopulation and creeping with an equivalent to substitution and then maturation/remodeling phases. Each phase has a unique complication profile.

For meniscal transplantation, particularly, close cooperation with one's tissue source is essential. Historically, cases have been reported in which a surgeon received a right meniscus or a lateral meniscus when the opposite was required. Rather than subjecting the patient to a clearly suboptimal result, delaying the case is best in those rare circumstances. Even with the use of precise sizing techniques, occasionally a meniscus transplant tissue is improperly sized. Incorrectly sized meniscal transplants will create nonphysiologic stress transfer. Minor modifications may be attempted to optimize a suboptimal set of circumstances, and the potential for early revision must be discussed with the patient. On the other hand, revision is less common for minor perceived mismatches. The various surgical techniques allow for minor

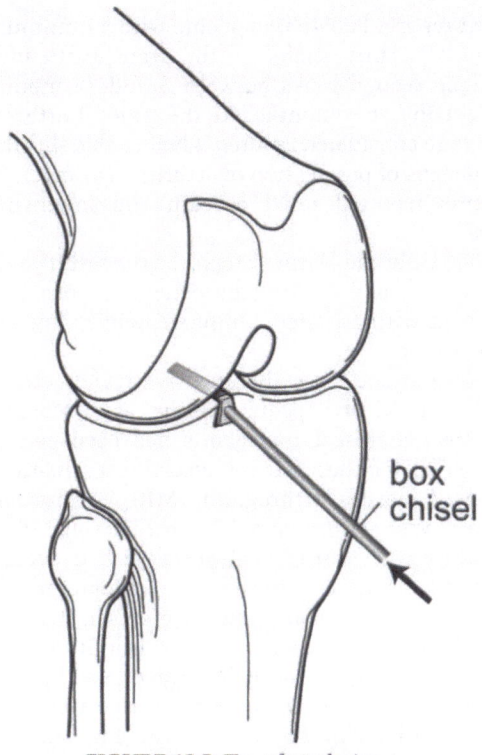

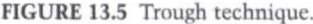

FIGURE 13.5 Trough technique.

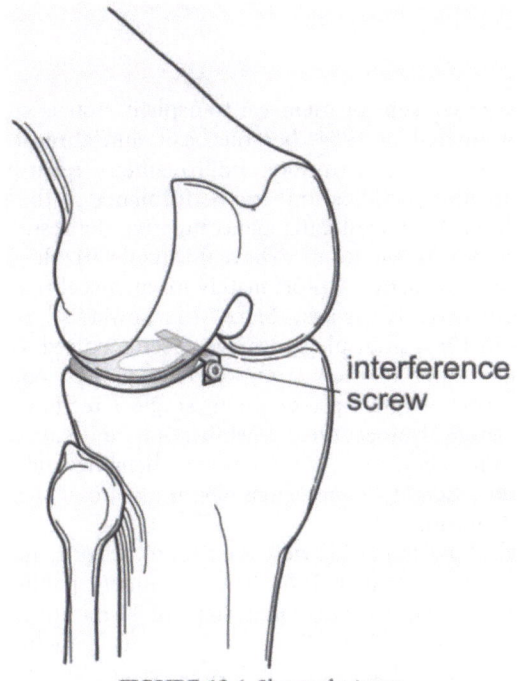

FIGURE 13.6 Slot technique.

modifications and adjustments, but these should not be considered as routine for every transplantation. During implantation, the bone plug may avulse from the meniscal attachment or, with the bone bridge technique, the bridge may fracture or avulse from the soft tissue. If fixation is press-fit, then this may fail during cyclic loading depending on the position and extent of bone damage.

Theoretical complications will evolve and are beyond the scope of this chapter. Such considerations include sensitization, with histocompatibility antigen–antibody formation and how this could affect future transplantations remote from the knee (heart, pancreatic islet cells, etc.). It is important for the tissue bank, in the case of transplants, and the manufacturing company, in the case of tissue-engineered constructs, to inform the patient and surgeon of associated materials, methods, and nutrients used in the process of manufacturing, preserving, providing nutrition, and transporting the tissues.

During the initial postoperative phase, there are the normal concerns for bacterial infection, thromboembolic disease, and arthrofibrosis. Unique concerns are failure to heal and thus the use of limited protected motion. Late complications include failure of the biologic process with gradual degeneration of the graft and degenerative tears. Shrinkage of the meniscal allograft is a concern when using freeze-dried tissue. Once healed and functioning, the transplanted meniscus can be injured in a similar fashion as a "normal" meniscus. The long-term effect on the articular cartilage is under study. If the articular cartilage is damaged, this condition should be addressed at the time of meniscal transplant.

REHABILITATION

The goal of rehabilitation is to allow early return to painfree normal function without compromising the healing and remodeling process.[38,39] If the surgeon is confident about the bony and soft tissue repair and fixation, then early motion is beneficial to the transplant healing process and nutrition of the opposing articular surface and aids to decrease arthrofibrosis. During this early phase, motion is protected in a range-of-motion brace, which is set to allow full extension and limited to 60° to 90° of flexion as there is limited meniscal soft tissue excursion within this range.[27] Continous passive motion (CPM) is used at the discretion of the surgeon and is usually reserved for advanced cases with performed with concomitant procedures. Weight bearing is initially minimal for the first 4 to 6 weeks during the ingrowth and repopulation phase of healing on an empiric basis. Quadriceps isometrics are begun immediately and, as weight bearing is allowed, gradual addition of 30° closed-chain dips (limited squats) are added. At 6 weeks the brace is discontinued and full motion is allowed and encouraged, but without loading. Protocols are in a state of flux as the goal is both a good short- and long-term result. In general, activity is gradually increased at 4 to 6 months, and light recreational activities may be added when strength, proprioception, agility, and motion are near normal. Squatting and hyperflexion are discouraged, as are high-load, high-impact repetitive activities, although in the young patient, noncompliance with these recommendations is common without short-term effects. Once again, this is a salvage procedure, with long-term success the goal, not a short-term return to sport.

CLINICAL RESULTS

The basic concept of meniscal transplantation is similar to that originated in 1984, but the basic and clinical science has undergone continuous improvement regarding our understanding, application, and performance of the surgical procedure. When analyzing and comparing the results of any procedure, it is important to have minimal variables between the individual series. Unfortunately for meniscal transplantation, this is rarely the case. Since Milachowski's[11] first publication in 1989, multiple series have been reported. However, variables differ in each study, such as patient population, knee arthrosis, graft preservation, surgical technique, additional surgical procedures, rehabilitation, and parameters of follow-up. Therefore, it becomes challenging and difficult to make accurate conclusions about the role of meniscal transplantation.

Milachowski et al.[11] were the first to perform an isolated meniscal transplant in 1984. The subsequent publication in 1989 on 22 patients with an average of 14-month follow-up demonstrated healing of 15 of 18 grafts peripherally by arthroscopic evaluation. Milachowski et al.[11] had used both fresh-frozen and freeze dried grafts, with the fresh-frozen tissue appearing more normal microscopically.

Garrett[40] reported 2- to 7-year follow-up of 43 patients in 1993. The patient population in this study was certainly complex, consisting of the salvage type of patient. Only 6 patients had an isolated meniscal transplant, and 28 patients underwent second-look arthroscopies, with 20 patients demonstrating healing of the meniscus allograft. The 8 failures were attributed to grade IV chondromalacia. The remaining 15 patients were asymptomatic and considered to have a good outcome.

Noyes and Barber-Westin[33] evaluated a large series of patients in 1995, reviewing 96 fresh-frozen irradiated grafts in 82 patients. The results were extremely poor. Of the total 96 implants, 58% failed completely, 31% were partially healed, and 9% healed. Twenty-nine menisci had to be removed less than 2 years after surgery. The surgical technique involved attachment only of the posterior horn with bone plugs. No transplant was attached with bone both anteriorly and posteriorly. All grafts were irradiated. The presence of grade IV arthrosis was associated with a 50% failure rate.

In contrast, Cameron and Seha[41] reported their results on 67 irradiated menisci without bone anchors in patients with generally advanced unicompartmental arthritis. These patients also underwent an osteotomy to unload that compartment at the time of surgery. At an average of 31 months follow-up, 87% demonstrated a good or excellent result.

Von Arkel and de Boer[42] reported on 23 patients with a minimum of 2-year follow-up who underwent isolated meniscal transplantation. There were 3 failures at less than 24 months with uncorrected malalignment. The remaining 20 patients were thought to have a satisfactory result.

Stollesteimer et al.[43] reported a series of 22 patients with 23 cryopreserved allografts. Implantation was done arthroscopically, assisted with bone plugs. The patients were followed for an average of 40 months. The most significant finding in their study was pain reduction in all patients. Although not associated with an adverse outcome, the allograft demonstrated a 37% shrinkage on MRI studies.

Carter reported on 46 transplants with a minimum 2-year follow-up.[44,45] Thirty-eight of the transplants underwent arthroscopic second looks between 3 and 48 months, with most occurring at 6 months. At the time of arthroscopy, 4 patients were considered failures, 4 had visible shrinkage, and 2 showed signs of progression of arthritis. However, 32 of the 38 patients reported relief of pain and improvement in activities.

In 1999, Cole and Harner[20] reported the results of 22 fresh-frozen menisci, and 88% of the patients reported improvement of pain with associated improvement in knee function in all but 1 case.

Rodeo[46] presented a comprehensive review of the literature at a national orthopedic meeting; as of March 2001, a total of 1599 meniscal transplants had been performed in 1551 patients. Of these, direct objective evaluation of the transplanted tissue (arthrogram, MRI, arthroscopy, and arthrotomy) was performed for 366 menisci in 338 patients. The age range was from 10 to 68 years, with an average of 33. The series included fresh, fresh frozen, cryopreserved, freeze-dried, irradiated, and nonirradiated menisci. The meniscus was implanted both with and without bone plugs. Concomitant procedures were performed in all but 136 cases. The degree of arthrosis in the knee varied from grade I to grade IV (modified Outerbridge), and there was no consistent rehabilitation.

The author's (W.K.G) personal experience (unpublished data) began in 1991. The current series consists of 80 meniscal transplants in 80 patients. During the time of this series, there have been subtle changes in the surgical procedure, rehabilitation, and understanding of the associated basic science. Of these 80 patients, 28 had undergone concomitant procedures consisting of ACL reconstruction, autologous cultured chondrocyte implantation, or tibial osteotomy. Of the patients, 52 have been followed for more than two years, 40 can be considered to have a good or excellent result with improvement in pain and function, 8 patients would be considered failures, with the remaining 4 having a fair result. The 8 failures, 6 of which were more than five years postimplantation, are attributed to preexisting grade IV arthritic changes or uncorrected malalignment, and these surgeries were performed early in the series before these factors were known to be deleterious to the outcome of meniscal transplantation.

Present indications, techniques, and graft selection are based on the results of these earlier studies. Certain principles have achieved somewhat uniform acceptance. The grafts should be cryopreserved or fresh frozen. The procedure may be performed either open or arthroscopically assisted with the use of bone fixation, both anteriorly and posteriorly. The patient should have a prior subtotal meniscectomy with normal or correctable alignment, a ligamentously stable or correctable joint, and grade II changes or less chondrosis or restorable chondral defects in the affected compartment.

CONCOMITANT PROCEDURES

Ligamentous Reconstruction

The ACL is the ligament most commonly requiring reconstruction at the time of meniscal transplantation. In a clinically unstable knee, a transplanted meniscus is subjected to the same abnormal forces that often result in a native meniscal tear. Therefore, if the knee is unstable, stability must be achieved at or before the time of meniscal transplantation. This philosophy applies to instability of the PCL, the collateral ligaments, or the posterior corners.

Ligament reconstruction and meniscal transplantation may be done as a single-stage procedure. Placement of the tibial tunnel for the ACL need be only minimally altered, depending upon the choice of technique for the meniscal transplantation procedure. The authors have found that the bone bridge or slot technique allows for accurate placement of the bone trough with minimal adjustment and without compromise of the tibial tunnel. The area of intersection of the slot and tunnel, if any, will be between the bone of the allograft bone bridge and the tendon of the ACL graft (hamstring or patellar tendon); this is actually technically easier than performing the ACL reconstruction first. If the ACL has previously been reconstructed, then extreme care must be taken to not harm the soft tissue portion, which will intersect the slot on the medial side.

In performing the combined procedure, either slot or ACL tunnel may be prepared first, but keeping in mind the position of the ensuing bony cut; that is, neither should allow the second procedure guides to "fall into" the created tibia defect. When passing the graft materials, first pass the ACL graft, but fixate only on the femoral side. After it is secure, then pass the bone bridge into the trough. If there is impingement, push the graft to the opposite side of the tunnel with a probe to allow for passage of the bone bridge. Alternatively, a ronguer can nibble away a small portion of the bone bridge at the site of impingement. Once the bone bridge is in place, the meniscus is fixed, followed by tightening and fixing of the tibial side of the ACL graft.

Malalignment

The importance of alignment has been previously underestimated.[41,42] Weight-bearing X-rays must be taken as part of the preoperative evaluation. If there is malalignment of even a few degrees as compared to the normal extremity, realignment osteotomy should be considered; this is especially true on the medial side, which has greater stress even in "normally" aligned extremities. With newer techniques allowing for more distally placed osteotomies, intersection with the tunnels, trough, or slot for the meniscal allograft can be avoided with planning. The procedures can be done at a single-stage surgery. The osteotomy should be performed first, obtaining good rigid fixation. The meniscal transplant can then be performed with care to not disrupt the osteotomy. If there is concern for a fracture to propagate from the slot to the osteotomy, a prophylactic screw may be placed in the proximal tibia transversely.

Chondral Defects

The presence of a chondral defect has previously been a contraindication for meniscal transplantation in light of the study in which Noyes demonstrated poor results in knees with grade III to IV chondrosis. With the ability to restore articular cartilage by either osteochondral grafting or autologous cultured chondrocyte implantation, the number of treatable patients can be expanded. The choice for cartilage restoration should follow guidelines based on size and location as highlighted in different publications.

Regardless of the technique applied for articular cartilage restoration, the meniscal allograft should be placed and sutured before the full osteochondral plug placement or periosteal fixation. This step avoids damage to the graft or periosteum during reduction of the meniscus and suturing of the meniscal allograft peripherally. The experience with autologous chondrocyte implantation and meniscal transplantation has been presented to the International Cartilage Repair Society (Toronto, Ontario, 2002) by the author (W.K.G). Twenty-two patients with an average of 28 months follow-up were reviewed who demonstrated an improvement in the Cincinnati knee rating score of 2.4 preoperatively to 7.6 postoperatively. The most common complication was arthrofibrosis (13%), and 2 (9%) were considered clinical failures.

ASYMPTOMATIC POSTMENISCECTOMY KNEE

The natural history of the meniscus-deficient knee is well documented. Nevertheless, not every postmeniscectomy patient develops degenerative arthrosis. There are several factors that are important in this treatment algorithm. Certainly these patients must undergo rigorous education about the signs and symptoms associated with knee degeneration. They should also be followed closely with standing 45° PA radiographs. The measurement of articular cartilage degradation products is currently changing from a laboratory setting to the clinical realm and may play an added role in early detection of postmeniscectomy articular cartilage damage. The breakdown of articular cartilage can progress very rapidly in the meniscally-deficient joint. The factors that need to be considered are activity level, physiologic age, rehabilitative potential, goals, and expectations.

The authors suggest that, in select postmeniscectomy individuals who have higher demands on their knee, who have rehabilitation potential, and who have realistic goals, there is a role for early consideration of meniscal allograft transplantation. The potential for articular cartilage breakdown in the younger patient and creation of a negative knee environment is too high to ignore. By the time the patient is symptomatic, and has positive X-rays or a positive bone scan, the articular cartilage has already been damaged.

SUMMARY

Meniscal transplantation has evolved as a successful procedure for the reconstruction of the meniscally deficient knee, although success will be further enhanced and improved by collaboration with basic science research. While early results were promising, the further understanding and development of the technique in more recent studies demonstrates improved results. As meniscal repair and preservation techniques continue to advance, the meniscus-deficient knee will become less common. However, the technology of meniscal transplantation will continue to be an integral procedure for the preservation of knee function.

References

1. Arnoczky SP, Milachowski, KA. Meniscal allografts: where do we stand? In: Ewing JW (ed). Articular Cartilage and Knee Joint Function: Basic Science and Arthroscopy. New York: Raven, 1990:129–136.

2. Jackson DW, Whelan J, Simon TM. Cell survival after transplantation of fresh meniscal allografts. DNA probe analysis in a goat model. Am J Sports Med 1993;21:540–550.

3. Nemzek JA, Arnoczky SP, Swenson CL. Retroviral transmission by the transplantation of connective-tissue allografts. An experimental study. J Bone Joint Surg Am 1994;76:1036–1041.

4. Ochi M, Ikuta Y, Ishida O, et al. Cellular and humoral immune responses after fresh meniscal allografts in mice: a preliminary report. Arch Orthop Trauma Surg 1993;112:163.

5. Ochi M, Ishida O, Daisaku H, Ikuta Y, Akiyama M. Immune response to fresh meniscal allografts in mice. J Surg Res 1995; 58:478–484.

6. Khoury MA, Goldberg VM, Stevenson S. Demonstration of HLA and ABH antigens in fresh and frozen human menisci by immunohistochemistry. J Orthop Res 1994;12:751–757.

7. Rodeo SA, Seneviratne A, Suzuki K, Felker K, Wickiewicz TL, Warren RF. Histological analysis of human meniscal allografts. A preliminary report. J Bone Joint Surg Am 2000;82:1071–1082.

8. DeBoer HH, Koudstall J. The fate of the meniscus cartilage after transplantation of cryopreserved nontissue-antigen-matched allograft: a case report. Clin Orthop 1991;266:145–151.

9. DeBoer HH, Koudstaal J. Failed meniscus transplantation. A report of three cases. Clin Orthop 1994;306:155–162.

10. Gao J, Wei X, Messner H. Healing of the anterior attachment of the rabbit meniscus to bone. Clin Orthop 1998;348:246–258.

11. Milachowski KA, Weismeier K, Wirth CJ. Homologous meniscus transplantation. Experimental and clinical results. Int Orthop 1989;13:1–11.

12. Yahia LH, Drouin G, Zukor D. The irradiation effect on the initial mechanical properties of meniscal grafts. Biomed Mater Eng 1993;3:211–221.

13. Yahia L, Zukor D. Irradiated meniscal allotransplants of rabbits: study of the mechanical properties at six-months postoperation. Acta Orthop Belg 1994;60:210–215.

14. Arnoczky SP, McDevitt CA, Schmidt MB, Mow VC, Warner RE. The effect of cryopreservation on canine menisci: a biochemical, morphologic, and biomechanical evaluation. J Orthop Res 1988;6:1–12.

15. Shibuya S. Meniscus transplantation using a cryopreserved allograft. Histological and ultrastructural study of the transplanted meniscus. J Orthop Sci 1999;4:135–141.

16. Fabbriciani C, Lucania L, Milano G, et al. Meniscal allografts: cryopreservation vs deep-frozen technique. An experimental study in goats. Knee Surg Sports Traumatol Arthrosc 1997; 5:124–134.

17. Jackson DW, McDevitt CA, Simon TM, et al. Meniscal transplantation using fresh and cryopreserved allografts. An experimental study in goats. Am J Sports Med 1992;20:644–656.

18. Arnoczky SP, DiCarlo EF, O'Brien SJ, Warren RF. Cellular repopulation of deep-frozen meniscal autografts: an experimental study in the dog. Arthroscopy 1992;8:428–436.

19. Szomor ZL, Martin TE, Bonar F, Murrell GA. The protective effects of meniscal transplantation on cartilage. An experimental study in sheep. J Bone Joint Surg Am 2000;82:80–88.

20. Cole JB, Harner CD. Degenerative arthritis of the knee in active patients: evaluation and management. J Am Acad Ortho Surg 1999;7:389–402.

21. Alhalki MM, Howell SM, Hull ML. How three methods for fixing a medial meniscal autograft affect tibial contact mechanics. Am J Sports Med 1999;27:320–328.

22. Alhalki MM, Hull ML, Howell SM. Contact mechanics of the medial tibial plateau after implantation of a medial meniscus allograft. A human cadaveric study. Am J Sports Med 2000; 28:370–376.

23. Aagaard H, Jorgenson U, Bojaen-Moller F. Reduced degenerative articular changes after meniscal allograft transplantation in sheep. Knee Surg Sports Traumatol Arthrosc 1999;7:184–191.

24. Bylski-Austrow DI, Meade T, Malturned J, Noyes FB. Irradiated meniscal allografts: mechanical and histological studies in the goat. Trans Orthop Res Soc 1992;17:175.

25. Cummings JF, Mansour JN, Howe Z, et al. Meniscal transplantation and degenerative articular change: an experimental study in the rabbit. Arthroscopy 1997;13:485–491.

26. Palette GA, Manning T, Snell E, et al. The effect of allograft meniscal replacement on intraarticular contact area and pressures in the human knee: a biomechanical study. Am J Sports Med 1997;25:692–698.

27. Thompson WO, Thaete FL, Fu FH, Dye SF. Tibial meniscal dynamics using three-dimensional reconstruction of magnetic resonance images. Am J Sports Med 1991;19:210–216.

28. Simonian PT, Sussmann PS, van Trommel M, Wickiewicz TL, Warren RF. Popliteomeniscal fasciculi and lateral meniscal stability. Am J Sports Med 1997;25:849–853.

29. Berlet GC, Fowler PJ. The anterior horn of the medial meniscus. An anatomic study of its insertion. Am J Sports Med 1998; 26(4):540–543.

30. Arnoczky SP, McDevitt CA. The meniscus: structure, function, repair, and replacement. In: Buckwalter JA, Einhorn TA, Simon SR (eds.) Orthopaedic Basic Science: Biology and Biomechanics of the Musculoskeletal System. Rosemont, IL: American Academy of Orthopaedic Surgeons, 2000:531–545.

31. Walker PS, Erkman MJ. The role of the menisci in force transmission across the knee. Clin Orthop 1975;109:184–192.

32. Levy IM, Torzilli PA, Warren RF. The effect of medical meniscectomy on anterior-posterior motion of the knee. J Bone Joint Surg Am 1982;64:883–888.

33. Noyes FR, Barber-Westin SD. Irradiated meniscus allografts in the human knee. A two- to five-year follow-up study. Orthop Trans 1995;19:417.

34. Cole BJ, Carter TR, Rodeo SA. Allograft meniscal transplantation background, techniques and results. J Bone Joint Surg 2002; 84A(7):1236–1250.

35. Pollard ME, Knag Q, Berg EE. Radiographic sizing for meniscal transplantation. Arthroscopy 1995;11:684–687.

36. Urban WP, Nyland J, Caborn DN, Johnson DL. The radiographic position of medial and lateral meniscal horns as a basis for meniscal reconstruction. Arthroscopy 1999;15(2):147–154.

37. Farr J, Cole BJ. Meniscus transplantation: bone bridge in slot technique. Oper Tech Sports Med 2002;10(3).

38. Fritz JM, Irrgang JJ, Harner CD. Rehabilitation following allograft meniscal transplantation: a review of the literature and case study. J Orthop Sports Phys Ther 1996;24:98–106.

39. Kohn D, Moreno B. Meniscus insertion anatomy as a basis for meniscal replacement: a morphological cadaveric study Arthroscopy 1995;11:96–103.

40. Garrett JC. Meniscal transplantation: a review of 43 cases with two- to seven-year follow-up. Sports Med Arthrosc Rev 1993;1:164–167.

41. Cameron JC, Seha S. Meniscal allograft transplantation for unicompartmental arthritis of the knee. Clin Orthop 1997;337: 164–171.

42. Van Arkel ER, de Boer HH. Human meniscal transplantation. Preliminary results at 2- to 5-year follow-up. J Bone Joint Surg Br 1995;77:589–595.

43. Stollsteimer GT, Shelton WR, Dukes A. Meniscal allograft transplantation: a one- to five-year follow-up of 22 patients. Arthroscopy 2000;16:343–347.
44. Carter TR. Meniscal allograft transplantation. Read at the Annual Meeting of the American Orthopaedic Society for Sports Medicine; June 22–25, 1997; Sun Valley, ID.
45. Carter TR. Meniscal allograft transplantation. Sports Med Arthosc Rev 1999;7:51–62.
46. Rodeo SA. Meniscal allografts-where do we stand? Am J Sports Med 2001;29:246–261.

14

Realignment of the Femur and Tibia

Justin P. Roe and Peter J. Fowler

BACKGROUND

Realignment procedures or osteotomy about the knee performed either alone or in combination with articular cartilage-restoring surgeries are a viable and effective option in the treatment of articular cartilage lesions. It is generally agreed that in the lower limb, articular cartilage disease is frequently associated with malalignment. The load through the knee joint is a function of alignment. Changes in the axial alignment of the femur or tibia in either the coronal or sagittal plane will influence the distribution of this load and result in abnormal stresses on articular cartilage.[1] It follows that surgical treatment for articular cartilage disease that does not include the correction of malalignment will have less chance of success. Therefore, the assessment and correction malalignment must be at the forefront in the treatment algorithm when considering the management of unicompartmental articular cartilage disease.

A primary goal of osteotomy, whether tibial or femoral, opening or closing wedge with either internal or external fixation methods, is to reposition the weight-bearing line so that the load distribution through the knee is normal or as close to normal as possible, minimizing stresses on the affected compartment.[2,3] Although "appropriate" postoperative alignment has been studied extensively,[4,5] there is no clear consensus on the correction angle when performing an osteotomy in the younger patient with a cartilage defect.[6]

It has been recently suggested that, in valgus tibial osteotomy, the weight-bearing line should be relocated to the middle to outer third of the lateral compartment.[7] We would argue that this amount of correction is excessive and, based on the work of Dugdale et al.,[5] in the patient with arthrosis we prefer a weight-bearing line that intersects at a point 62% of the tibial width from the edge of the medial plateau to produce a mechanical axis of 3° to 5°. One should be cautioned against the recommendations of Coventry,[8] Cass and Bryan,[9] and Rudan and Simurda[10] to accept an anatomic valgus of greater than 10°. In the younger patient with malalignment and articular cartilage lesions, an excessively large correction angle may not be required, and repositioning the weight-bearing line to neutral or just beyond, medially or laterally, is frequently desirable.

INDICATIONS AND CONTRAINDICATIONS

The indications for knee osteotomy (Table 14.1) are not confined to a deviation in mechanical axis (malalignment) with arthrosis. When knee instability is associated with malalignment, osteotomy may help restore stability, improve symptoms, and possibly delay the progression of arthrosis.[11] Sagittal imbalance can be of particular interest in instability, and in these situations the role of the tibial slope must be taken into consideration and addressed when corrective osteotomy is planned. Malalignment in the setting of any articular cartilage restoration procedure is a clear indication for an osteotomy before or combined with the cartilage restoration or "protection" procedure such as osteochondral autograft or meniscal allograft.

When considering the younger patient, Morrey[12] reported that valgus osteotomy can be offered with confidence in those with secondary degenerative arthritis, a varus knee, and localized medial joint pain, but should be avoided in those who have previously undergone a lateral meniscectomy. The range of treatment options for younger patients with isolated cartilage lesions is limited. Consequently, the list of contraindications to knee osteotomy in this group is relatively short. However, severe degeneration in the opposite tibiofemoral compartment and gross loss of range of motion will certainly affect the outcome of osteotomy and may be considered as contraindications.[7]

SURGICAL TECHNIQUES

Alignment is determined by the line extending from the center of the hip to the center of the ankle, that is, the mechanical axis of the limb.[13] This line typically passes immediately medial to the center of the knee, and by definition, malalignment occurs when this line does not lie close to the center of the knee.[14,15] Sagittal plane alignment, which should also be considered, involves evaluation of the posterior tibial slope angle (PTSA) on a lateral radiograph (Figure 14.1).

TABLE 14.1   Indications for knee osteotomy.

Malalignment and arthrosis
Malalignment and instability
Malalignment and arthrosis and/or instability
Malalignment and articular cartilage procedure and/or instability

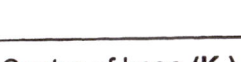

Center of femoral head
(H)

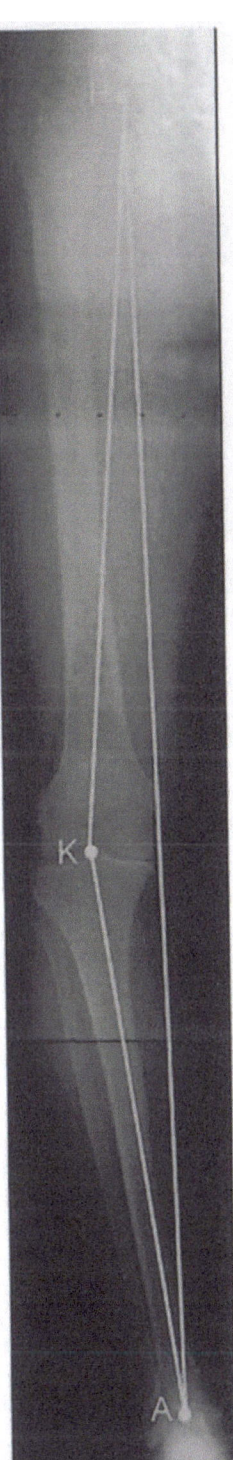

Center of knee (K)

Center of ankle
(A)

A

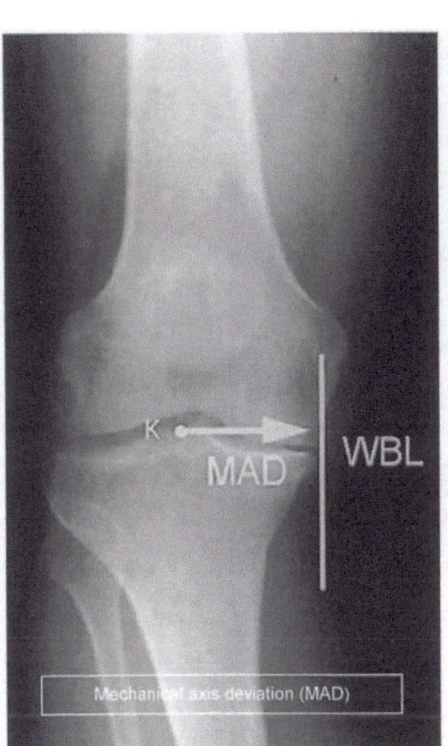

B

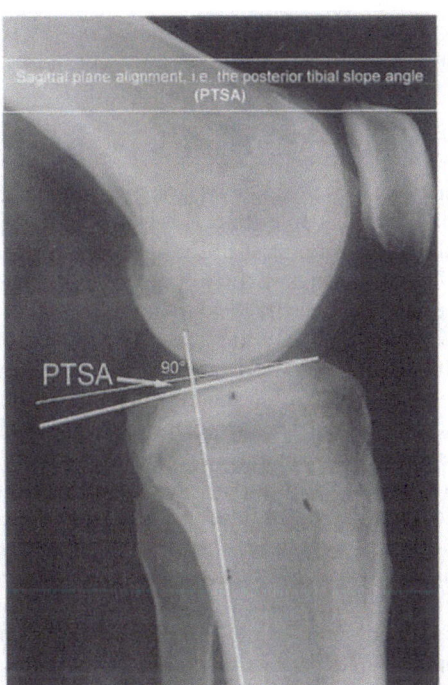

C

FIGURE 14.1 A. In this malaligned (varus) limb the weight bearing line (WBL) falls just medial to the medial tibial plateau. *HK*, femoral mechanical axis; *KA*, tibial anatomic and mechanical axis; *HKA*, angular measurement of the mechanical axis of the limb. **B.** MAD, distance from the center of the knee to the WBL. **C.** A *perpendicular* is made from the line drawn along the longitudinal axis of the tibia. A *line* is then drawn along the bony slope of the tibial plateau. The *PTSA* is the acute angle formed by the intersection of these two lines.

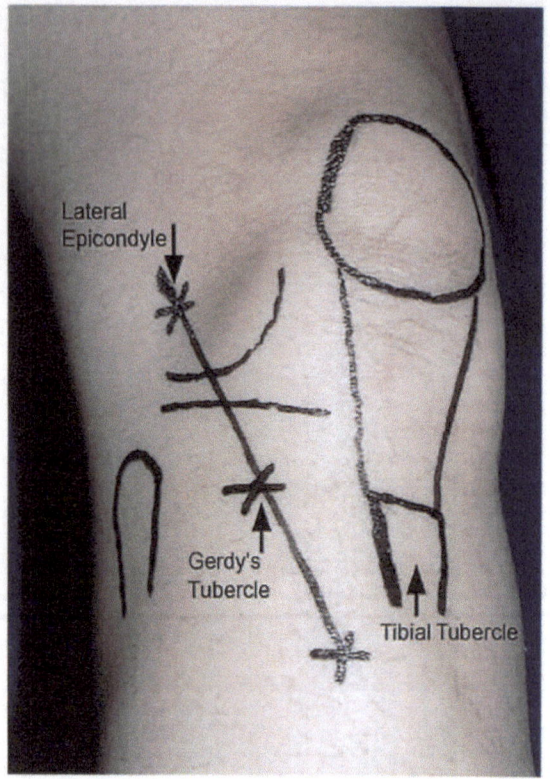
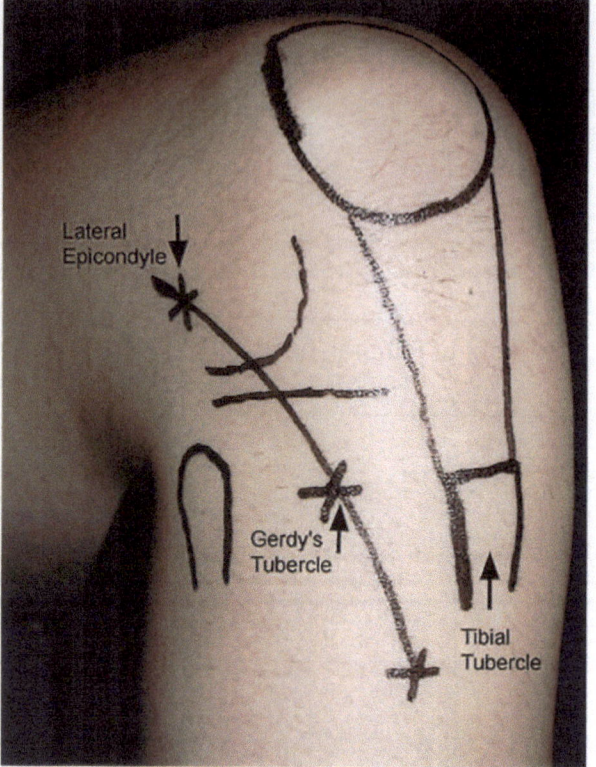

FIGURE 14.2 Skin incision for a lateral approach to the proximal tibia. Note that the incision, made along a line extending distally from the lateral femoral epicondyle, over Gerdy's tubercle, and end-ing just lateral to the tibial tubercle, is straight with the knee extended (**A**) and slightly curved with the knee flexed to 90° (**B**).

Varus Knee

Techniques to realign the varus knee include the classic lateral closing-wedge osteotomy, the adaptable medial opening-wedge osteotomy (preferred in most situations by the senior author), and the more flexible osteotomy with external fixation.

LATERAL CLOSING WEDGE HIGH TIBIAL OSTEOTOMY

The Coventry lateral closing wedge is performed through an incision made along a line from the lateral epicondyle over Gerdy's tubercle extending distally just lateral to the tibial tubercle.[3] This incision is slightly curved if the knee is flexed at 90° and straight when the knee is in the extended position (Figure 14.2). The iliotibial band is identified distally anterior to the fibular collateral ligament and partially elevated by sharp dissection off Gerdy's tubercle. The common peroneal nerve is identified by palpation posterior to the fibular head. The fibular head is not routinely osteotomized, but if required to close the osteotomy, the proximal tibiofibular joint is released. Soft tissues are released from the posterior aspect of the tibia. A retractor placed on the bone posteriorly protects the neurovascular structures and facilitates carrying out the osteotomy under direct vision. The upper limb of the osteotomy is made 2 cm below and parallel to the joint line. The appropriate-sized wedge is then marked out, cut, and removed. Using bone rongeurs, small curettes, and up-cutting Kerrison rongeurs, cortical bone posteriorly and cancellous bone medially are removed across the osteotomy site. The osteotomy is closed with the knee in extension and fixed with a single-step staple. Care is taken to ensure that the pos-terior tibial slope has not been decreased due to failure to complete the osteotomy posteriorly, to remove cortical bone from the osteotomy site or to adequately release the proximal tibiofibular joint (Figure 14.3).

PEARLS AND PITFALLS
Complete exposure and mobilization of the proximal tibiofibular joint, visualization anteriorly beneath the patellar tendon, exposure of the posterior tibia, and protection of the neurovascular structures with a curved, blunt retractor placed directly on bone are essential steps in performing the lateral closing-wedge osteotomy. Making the osteotomy 2 cm distal to the lateral joint line will ensure that the proximal fragment is sufficiently large to avoid the risk of avascularity and will avoid violation of the tibial tubercle (Table 14.2).

As with all osteotomies of the proximal tibia, the osteotomy cut must match the posterior slope of the tibial plateau to reduce the likelihood of altering the tibial slope. As mentioned, completion of the posterior cortical bone resection with pituitary and Kerrison rongeurs or small bone curettes will prevent risk of damage to the posterior neurovascular structures. An unstable osteotomy can be avoided with the use of fluoroscopy to confirm that the osteotomy has been completed and that the medial tibial cortex has not been compromised.

MEDIAL OPENING WEDGE HIGH TIBIAL OSTEOTOMY

The authors' preferred technique of medial opening wedge high tibial osteotomy (HTO) is a modification of the technique described by Puddu et al.[16] This method allows

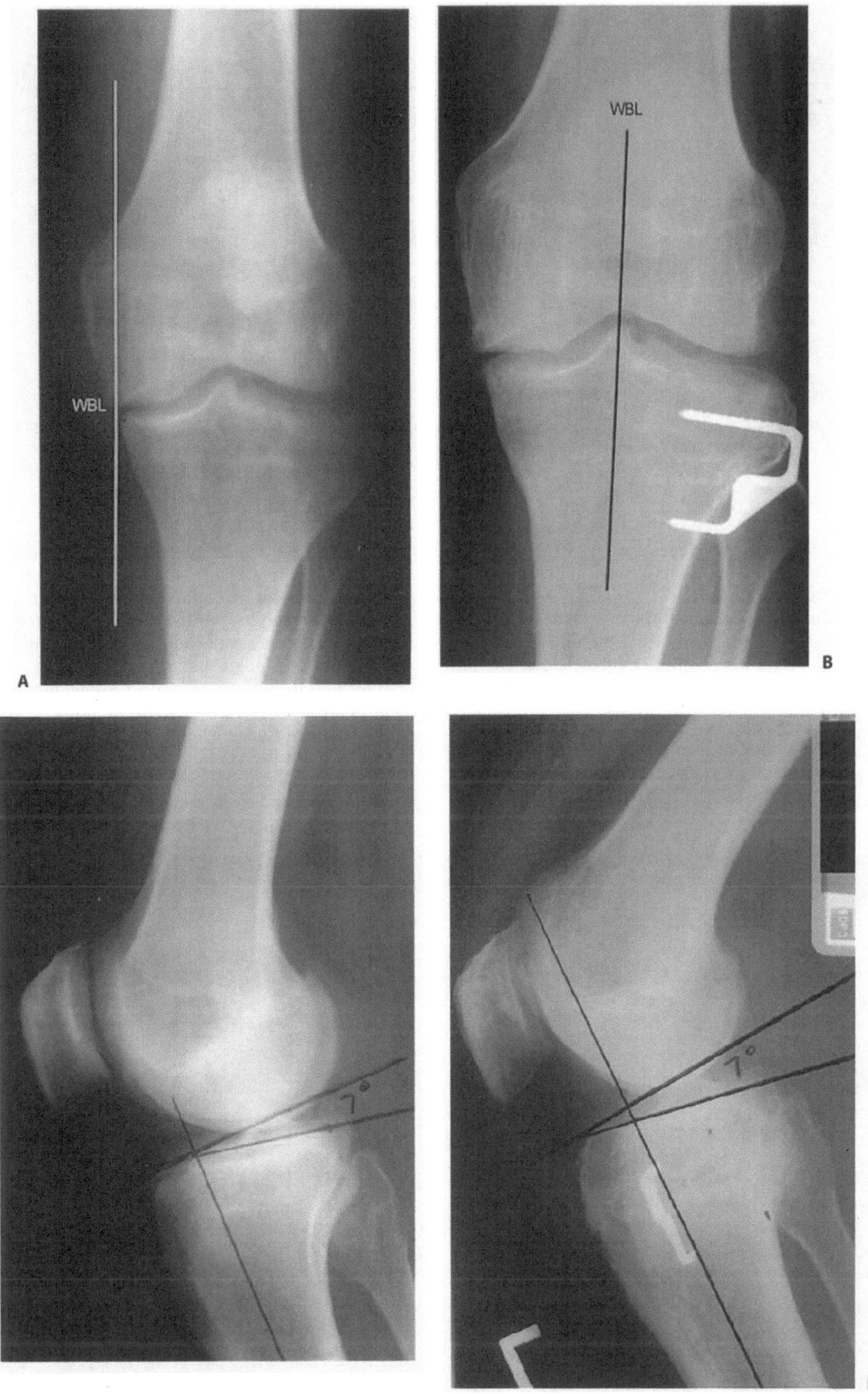

FIGURE 14.3 Case: 39 year old man with varus deformity and medial compartment arthrosis. **A.** Before lateral closing-wedge HTO, the WBL is just medial to the medial tibial plateau. **B.** 5-year follow-up anteroposterior (AP) radiograph shows the WBL through the center of the knee, a well united osteotomy, and minimal progression of arthrosis. **C.** The preoperative PTSA is 7°. **D.** The PTSA is unchanged on the 5-year follow-up lateral view.

TABLE 14.2   Pearls and pitfalls.

Procedure	Pearls	Pitfalls
All osteotomies	Adequate exposure	Violation of opposite cortex
	Use of intraoperative fluoroscopy and guide pins	Making asymmetric bone cuts in sagittal plane
	Accurate preoperative planning and radiographic evaluation	Opening the osteotomy before the anterior and posterior cortices are osteotomized
High tibial lateral closing	Make osteotomy 2 cm distal to lateral joint line	Decreasing tibial slope inadvertently
	Complete posterior cortical resection in piecemeal fashion with Kerrison rongeurs	
High tibial medial opening	Use oscillating saw to breach cortex only	Suboptimal guide pin positioning
	Make osteotomy below the guide pin	Neglecting the posterior tibial slope when making the osteotomy
	Pay particular attention when securing osteotomy plate	Violation of opposite cortex and destabilizing osteotomy
Distal femoral varus lateral opening	Slight flexion of knee facilitates exposure	
	Make osteotomy above the guide pin	
	Use oscillating saw to breach lateral cortex only	
Distal femoral varus medial closing	Make osteotomy proximal to the patellofemoral articular surface	Removal of too large a wedge of bone
	Identify the medial and lateral tibiofemoral joint using guide pins	

correction of deformity in all planes and, in particular, allows more precise attention to be paid to planned alterations to tibial slope in the sagittal direction.

The procedure is carried out through a vertical skin incision, which extends 5 cm distally from the medial joint line and is centered between the anterior tubercle and the posteromedial border of the tibia. The gracilis and semitendinosus tendons and the superficial medial collateral ligament are preserved and retracted medially to expose the posteromedial border of the proximal tibia (Figure 14.4). A guide pin is inserted obliquely along a line proximal to the tibial tubercle starting approximately 4 cm below the medial joint line and extending to a point 1 cm distal to the lateral joint line. The osteotomy is made below the guide pin using a small oscillating saw to broach the medial, anteromedial, and posteromedial cortices followed by narrow, sharp, thin, flexible osteotomes to a point just 1 cm short of the lateral cortex. Throughout the procedure, a mobile, low-dose ionizing radiation fluoroscope is used liberally to monitor the cut (Figure 14.5). Frequent imaging helps prevent violation of the lateral cortex and misdirection of the osteotome. The osteotomy is opened gradually to the desired correction angle with a cali-

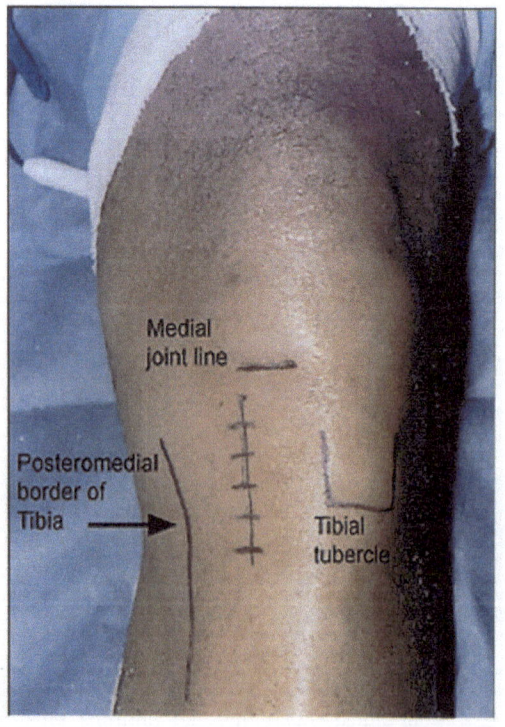

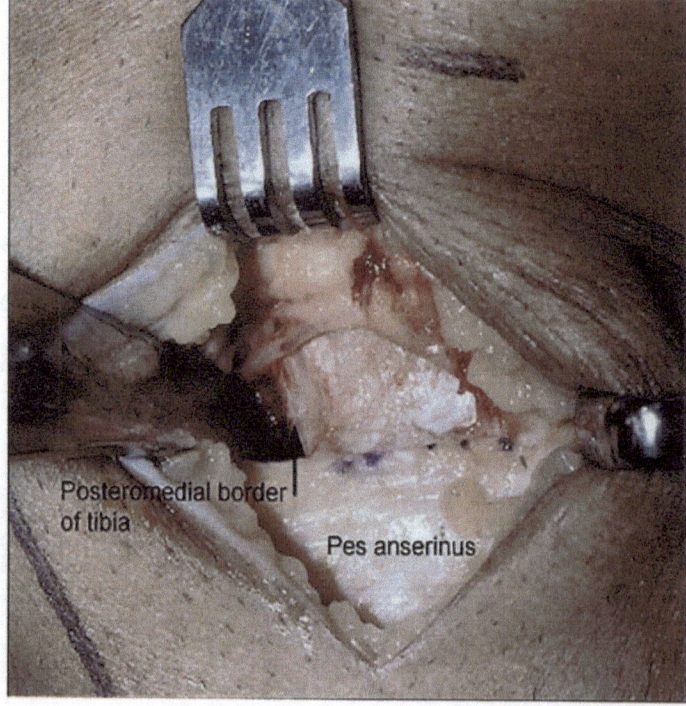

FIGURE 14.4 The surgical approach to medial opening-wedge HTO. **A.** The skin incision is centered between the posteromedial border of the tibia and the tibial tubercle and extends distally from the medial joint line. **B.** The posteromedial border of the tibia is exposed with a blunt retractor placed deep to the superficial MCL. The pes anserinus is left intact.

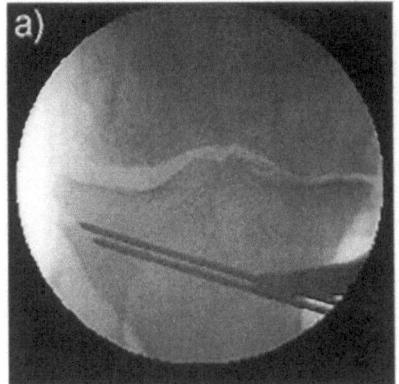 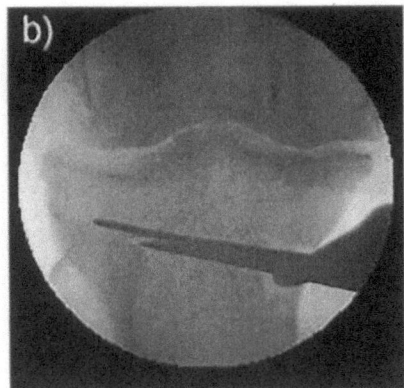 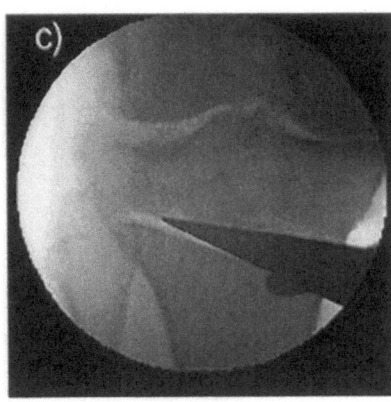

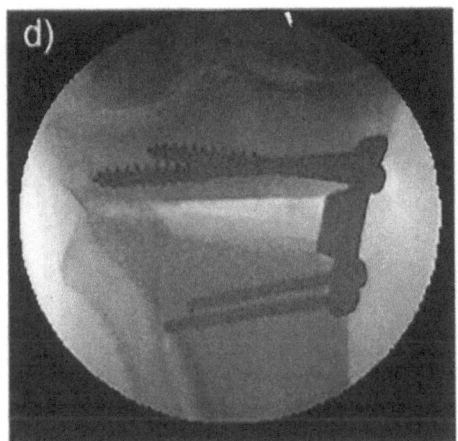 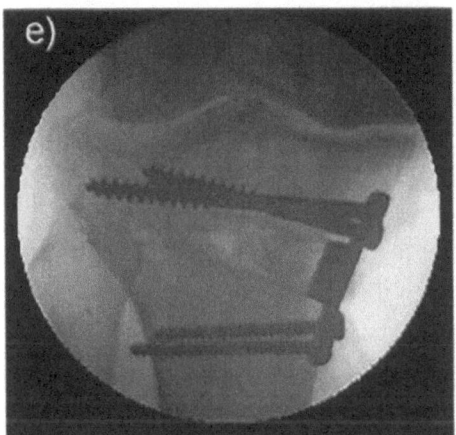

FIGURE 14.5 Use of intraoperative fluoroscopy during medial opening-wedge HTO. **A.** The guide pin is directed toward the tip of the fibular head and from a point 4 cm distal to the medial joint line. Placement should be optimal before proceeding. **B.** The osteotomy is made *below* the guide pin. **C.** The osteotomy is gradually opened to the desired width using a calibrated wedge. **D.** Fixation is achieved with a four-hole Puddu plate. Care is taken to avoid intraarticular or intraosteotomy screw placement. **E.** Defect has been filled with tricortical bone graft.

brated wedge and fixed with a four-hole Puddu plate (Arthrex, Inc., Naples, FL) secured with two 6.5-mm cancellous screws proximally and two 4.5-mm cortical screws distally. A trapezoid-shaped plate may be used to achieve or prevent a change in tibial slope (Figure 14.6). Bone grafting is recommended in all opening-wedge osteotomies greater than 7.5 mm. Allograft cancellous bone chips or tricortical wedges may be used unless there is an expressed desire by the patient for autograft bone. In our practice, osteotomies less than 7.5 mm are rarely grafted.

PEARLS AND PITFALLS
Dissection of the most superior fibers of the patellar tendon insertion on the tibial tubercle improves exposure. The use of a low-dose ionizing radiation fluoroscope throughout the procedure is critical for proper guide-pin placement, for prevention of lateral cortex violation, and misdirection of the osteotome, to avoid intraarticular screw placement, and to confirm adequate seating of the bone graft and filling of the defect (see Table 14.2).

The tip of the fibular head is a helpful reference when aiming the guide pin. Guide-pin placement should be optimal before proceeding and repeated as necessary to achieve correct obliquity of the osteotomy. For larger corrections, placement should be more horizontal. Greater obliquity increases the risk of fixation failure but, on the other hand, provides increased depth, which may be appropriate for smaller corrections. The osteotomy should always be carried out parallel to the joint line in the sagittal plane and below the guide pin to help prevent intraarticular fracture. The use of thick, traditional osteotomes carries an inherent risk of creating an extraarticular or intraarticular fracture. This risk is considerably minimized with thin, flexible osteotomes.

The tibial tubercle is the most anterior point and just lateral to the midpoint of the tibia. Therefore, to avoid altering the posterior tibial slope, the distraction of the osteotomy anteriorly (at the tibial tubercle) should be one-half its distraction posteromedially. Tension of the medial collateral ligament (MCL) should be assessed during distraction of the osteotomy, and lengthening by fenestration (of the MCL) may assist in achieving larger corrections. Finally, strict attention to detail is necessary to avoid intraarticular or intraosteotomy screw penetration during fixation of the plate and to

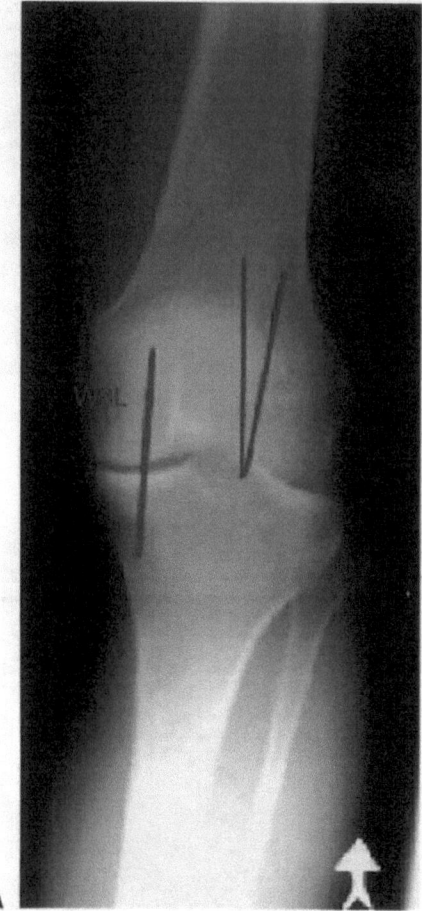
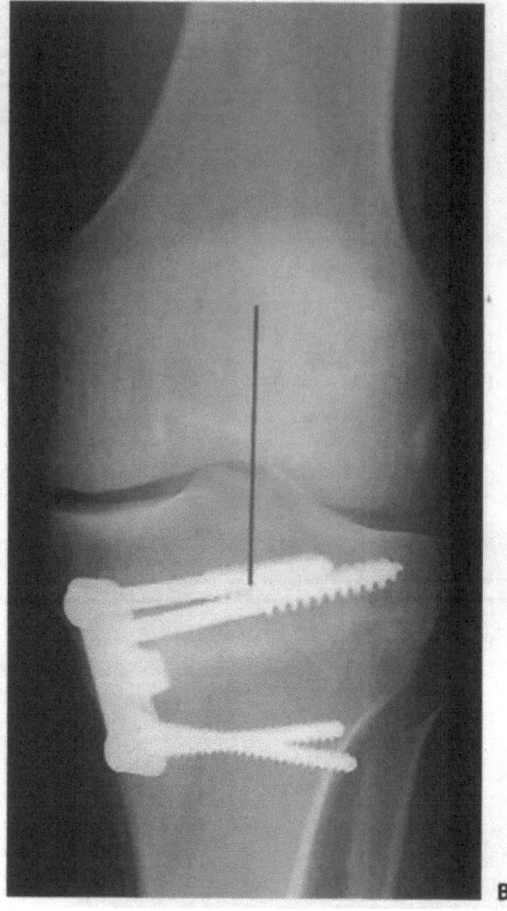

FIGURE 14.6 Case: 31-year-old man with isolated medial compartment articular cartilage disease, varus malalignment, and intact ACL and PCL. **A.** The AP view shows the WBL through the center of the medial compartment and the predicted correction angle. **B.** Postoperatively, the mechanical axis of the limb is normalized.

ensure that the defect is completely obliterated with bone graft or a substitute.

OSTEOTOMY WITH EXTERNAL FIXATION SYSTEMS

Various external fixation devices may be employed to address large or multiplanar deformities. As described by Catagni et al.,[17] the Ilizarov frame in the treatment of genu varum addresses both the bony and soft tissue components of the deformity. According to these authors, osteotomy distal to the tibial tuberosity allows slight lateral translation of the tibia for correction of the tension on the ligamentous and capsular structures. Althought medial compartment arthritis and posttraumatic deformity are most amenable to acute correction, skeletally mature patients with residual Blount's disease deformity and the younger population with idiopathic genu varum are best treated with gradual correction. External frames are recommended for deformities greater than 20° to 25° of mechanical varus requiring gradual correction.

Valgus Knee

Realignment of the valgus knee may be approached from the femoral or tibial side. Each, according to some authors, may have a negative mechanical consequence.[18] All techniques, femoral or tibial, opening or closing, have a place in the treatment of the valgus deformity. Varus-producing proximal tibial osteotomy in patients with lateral compartment arthrosis has been regarded as controversial because of the tendency to result in joint line obliquity.[8,19]

Coventry,[8] taking both the anatomic axis and the tilt of the plateau into consideration, recommended a supracondylar femoral varus osteotomy if the valgus deformity is more than 12° or if the postoperative tilt of the tibiofemoral joint surface exceeds 10°.[8] Chambatet et al.,[18] on the other hand, advocates that all valgus deformities be corrected from the tibial side. Here too, although opinions are more uniform than in proximal tibial valgus osteotomy, the degree of correction suggested varies. Several authors recommend correcting the valgus knee to a 0° tibiofemoral angle.[19,20] According to Morrey and Edgerton,[21] in the valgus knee, the mechanical axis should be repositioned medial to the medial spine. Phillips and Krakow recommend a mechanical axis of 4° varus.[22]

PROXIMAL TIBIAL VARUS OSTEOTOMY

A proximal tibial varus osteotomy is recommended for smaller valgus deformities or those localized to the tibia (which can occur especially after trauma or lateral meniscectomy).[23] One can perform a lateral opening wedge rather than the medial closing wedge of Coventry,[8] Shoji et al.,[24] or Chambat and Dejour.[18]

LATERAL OPENING

This opening is carried out through a straight skin incision similar to that for the lateral closing wedge, made with the knee extended. The osteotomy is oblique, starting 4 cm distal to the lateral joint line and ending 1 to 2 cm distal to the medial articular surface. The fibula is not osteotomized. Residual medial laxity secondary to lengthening of the MCL is less commonly encountered with this technique. The medial structures are not weakened as they are with a medial closing-wedge procedure and dissection around the pes anserinus is avoided (Figure 14.7)

MEDIAL CLOSING

The approach for the medial closing-wedge osteotomy is similar to medial opening wedge, with posterior retraction of the pes anserinus tendons and the superficial MCL. The osteotomy is made 2 cm distal to the joint line, and then a wedge of predetermined size is removed. The superficial MCL is not violated, and reefing or plication of the ligament is not required. Fixation is achieved with one or two osteotomy staples. With respect to alignment, Coventry states that overcorrection is undesirable and that one should aim for a postoperative weight-bearing line that passes through the center of the knee.[8]

DISTAL FEMORAL VARUS OSTEOTOMY

Distal femoral varus osteotomy (DFVO) has been successful in the surgical management of valgus knee deformi-

ties.[19,20,25,26] In addition to mechanical axis corrections, any valgus tilt of the joint line can be addressed more effectively than with proximal tibial varus osteotomy. Internal fixation of supracondylar femoral closing-wedge varus osteotomy may be accomplished with medially or laterally placed devices. Laterally based approaches are based on tension-band principles, with fixation on the lateral, tension side of the femur.[27]

MEDIAL CLOSING DVFO

The technical effectiveness of medial approaches depends on an intact lateral cortex and closure of the osteotomy with a 90° blade-plate.[19,20,26] According to Marti et al.,[28] the medially held varus osteotomy creates an unstable situation and requires a much more rigid fixation. This technique is suitable for larger corrections and requires that only a small wedge of bone be removed. Fixation of the diaphysis into the cancellous metaphysis results in an extremely stable construct (Figure 14.8).

PEARLS AND PITFALLS

Accurate identification of the medial and lateral tibiofemoral joint using the guide pins placed under fluoroscopic control will help establish a reference point. The patellofemoral joint may also be identified with a guide pin to mark the anterior part of the femoral articular surface and its inclination. A guide pin can then be placed through the distal medial femoral condyle (parallel to the tibiofemoral joint) 2 cm proximal to the articular surface (see Table 14.2).

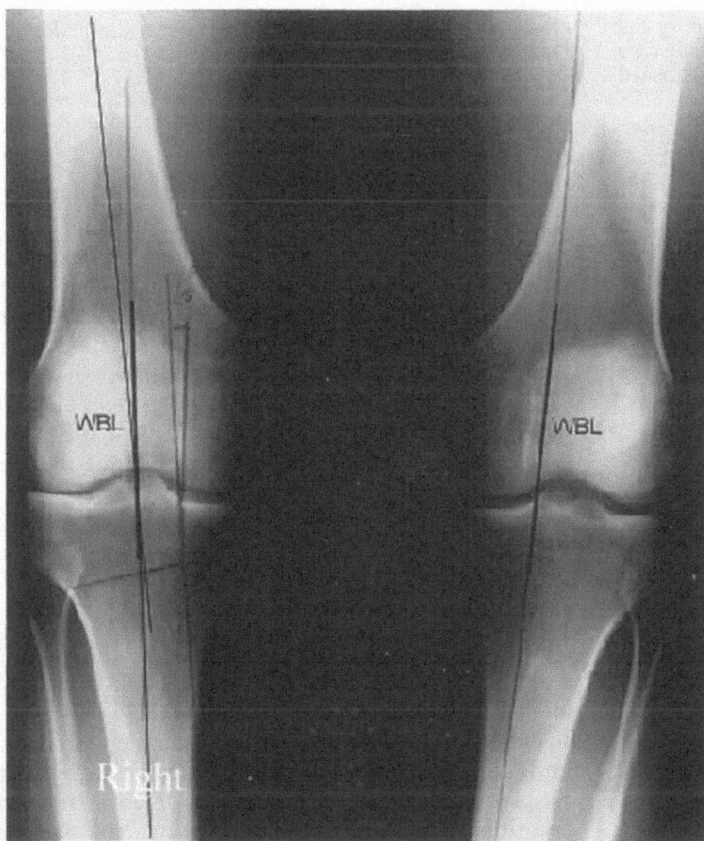
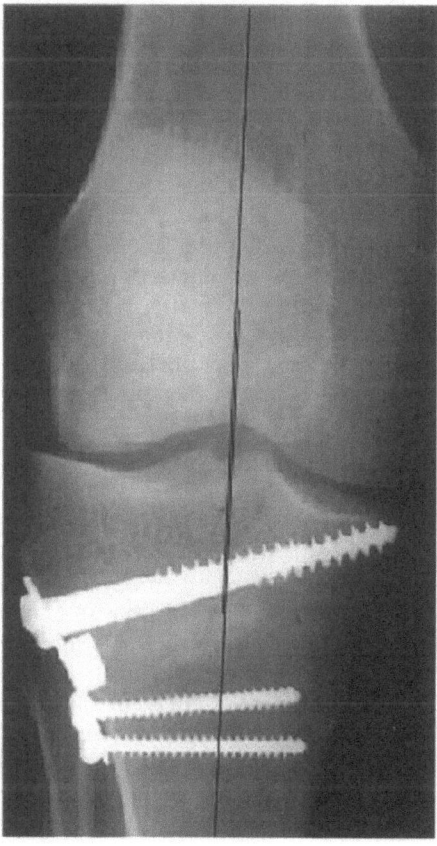

FIGURE 14.7 Case: 37-year-old elite athlete with lateral compartment arthrosis and a PCL-deficient right knee. **A.** Preoperative bilateral standing AP views reveal WBL passing directly through the center of the right knee, but more laterally than in the normal contralateral knee. **B.** A varus producing (tibiofemoral angle, 0°) lateral opening-wedge HTO was carried out to off-load the diseased lateral compartment.

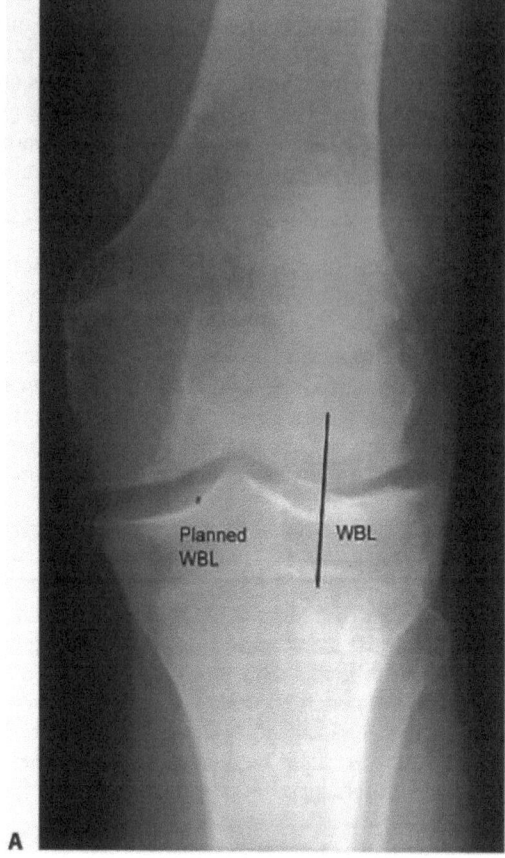
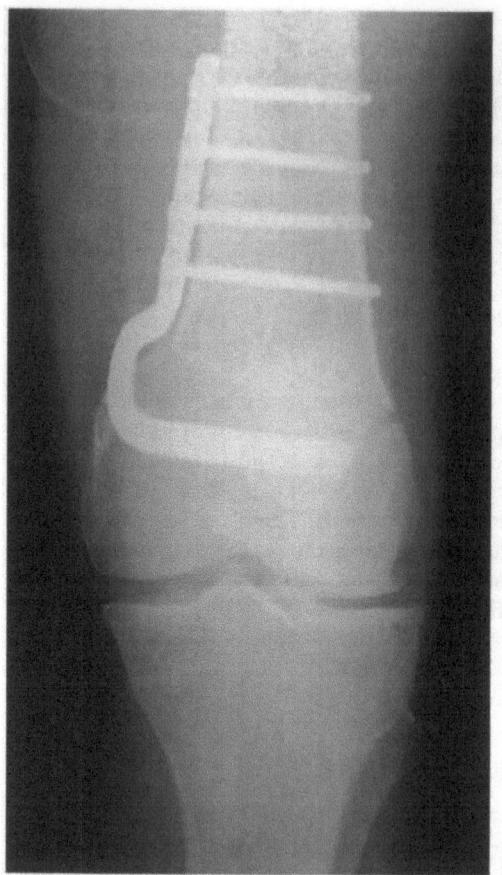

FIGURE 14.8 Case: **A.** 41-year-old man with a valgus deformity and lateral compartment arthrosis secondary to osteochondritis dissecans treated 20 years earlier with arthroscopic debridement. **B.** A medial closing-wedge distal femoral varus osteotomy was performed to "off-load" the lateral compartment.

The osteotomy is made just proximal to the patellofemoral articular surface. Because the proximal cortical fragment can be impacted into the cancellous bone of the distal fragment without difficulty, removal of only a small wedge of bone is sufficient regardless of the amount of correction desired. Perforation of the lateral cortical bridge using a 2-mm drill may facilitate easier closure of the osteotomy.

LATERAL OPENING DFVO

Some authors report that better and more reproducible results with fewer technical difficulties can be achieved with distal femoral varus opening-wedge osteotomy.[29,3] The lateral aspect of the distal femur is exposed through a standard straight 15 cm incision that starts 2.5 cm from the lateral joint line. The osteotomy is made with the knee in extension, under fluoroscopic guidance, using a guide pin directed slightly obliquely from a proximal point 4 cm above the lateral epicondyle to a distal point on the medial cortex. A medial hinge of approximately 0.5 cm of intact bone is preserved. Fixation is achieved with a T-shaped tooth-plate (Arthrex, Inc, Naples, FL) (Figures 14.9, 14.10).

PEARLS AND PITFALLS

Retraction of the vastus lateralis from the lateral intermuscular septum and slight flexion of the knee facilitates good exposure. Continual use of fluoroscopy when drilling the guide pin at an oblique angle of 20° from the perpendicular to the lateral femoral cortex directed distally and three finger-breadths above the epicondyle ensures that the trochlear groove is avoided. The oscillating saw and osteotome must be kept proximal to the guide pin and the osteotomy must be made 90° to the long axis of femur to prevent an intraarticular fracture. It is important to preserve a medial hinge of 0.5 cm of intact bone to prevent destabilizing the osteotomy (see Figure 14.9).

TIBIAL DEFLEXION OSTEOTOMY FOR INCREASED POSTERIOR TIBIAL SLOPE

Sagittal plane balance is dependent on the anterior cruciate ligament (ACL), the medial meniscus, and the posterior tibial slope. In situations of chronic anterior laxity with underlying meniscal and chondral deficiency, tibial slope must be considered as a potential factor for correction of the sagittal plane imbalance.[31] Dejour and Bonnin[32] found a highly significant correlation between the mean anterior tibial translation and the tibial slope angle in both normal and ACL-deficient knees. For every 10° increase in posterior tibial slope, the anterior tibial translation increased 6 mm as shown on monopodal stance radiographs. There was greater anterior tibial translation in ACL injured subjects.

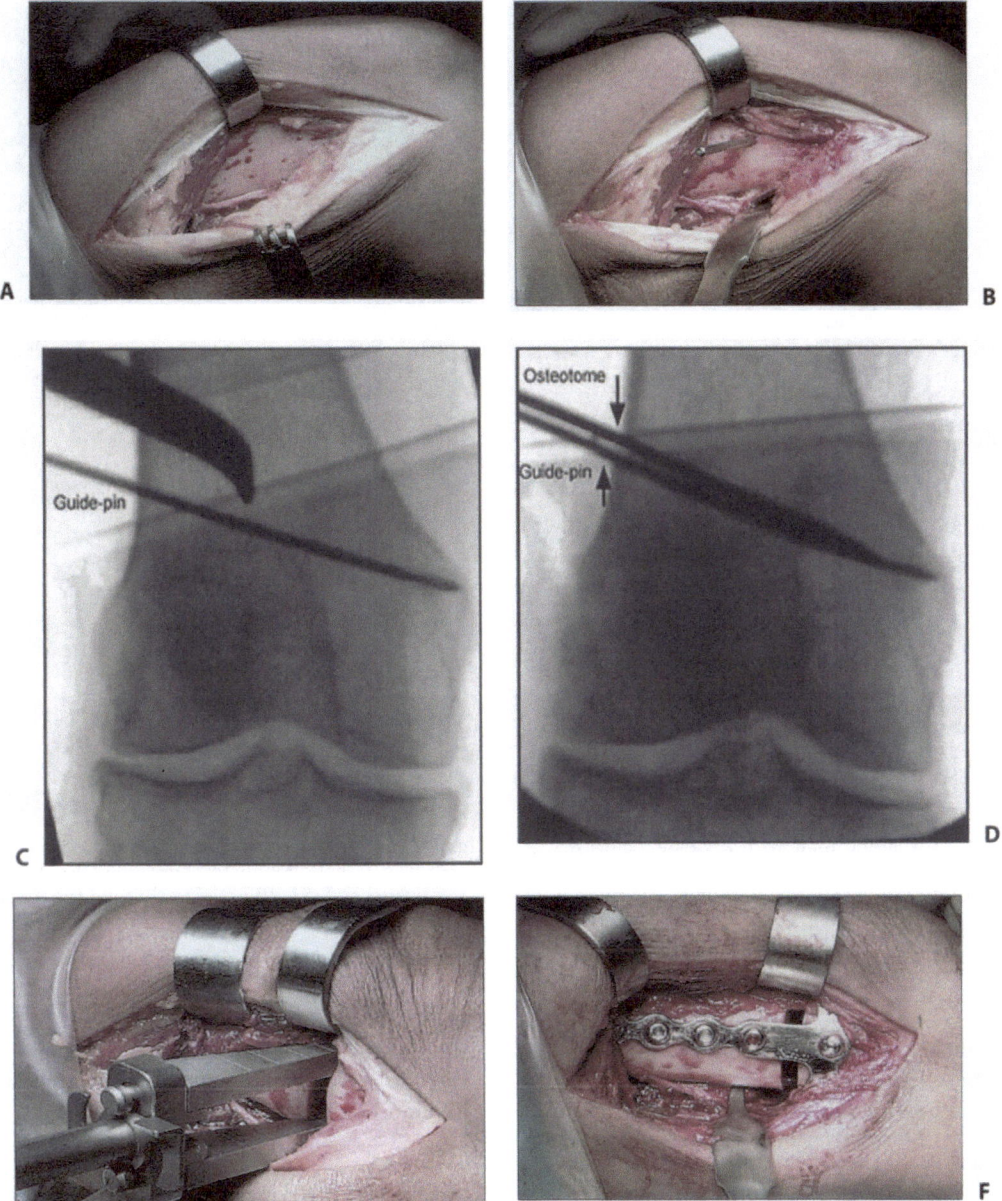

FIGURE 14.9 Surgical technique for lateral opening distal femoral varus osteotomy. **A.** Exposure of the lateral aspect of the distal femur with retraction of the vastus lateralis from the lateral intermuscular septum. Note the knee is slightly flexed. **B.** The guide pin is directed distally from a point 3 to 4 fingerbreadths above the lateral femoral epicondyle. **C.** Intraoperative fluoroscopy shows the position of the guide pin. **D.** The osteotomy is made *above* the guide pin. **E.** The osteotomy is opened gradually using a calibrated wedge opener. B Fixation is achieved with a T-shaped tooth-plate.

Anterior closing-wedge high tibial osteotomy at the time of or before ACL reconstruction should be considered in patients with a posterior tibial slope of greater than 10° combined with ACL deficiency.[31,33] Decreasing the tibial slope by anterior closing-wedge osteotomy can also reduce flexion contracture associated with fracture malunion or growth plate arrest.

TIBIAL ANTIRECURVATUM OSTEOTOMY FOR DECREASED POSTERIOR TIBIAL SLOPE

Symptomatic hyperextension deformity requiring corrective osteotomy is uncommon. A combined hyperextension varus deformity with or without a posterior cruciate ligament (PCL) or posterolateral complex deficiency may require corrective osteotomy to increase tibial slope in single or combined procedures (Figure 14.11). The approach may depend on the size of the correction required. An anteromedial opening-wedge osteotomy above the level of the tibial tubercle can achieve a reduction in the varus deformity as well as an increase in tibial slope. The size of the opening is limited by the effect on the extensor mechanism and the distalization of the tibial tubercle.

For pure sagittal deformities that require larger corrections, the tibial tubercle can be osteotomized as a 6-cm bone block and elevated, leaving the peripheral capsuloligamen-

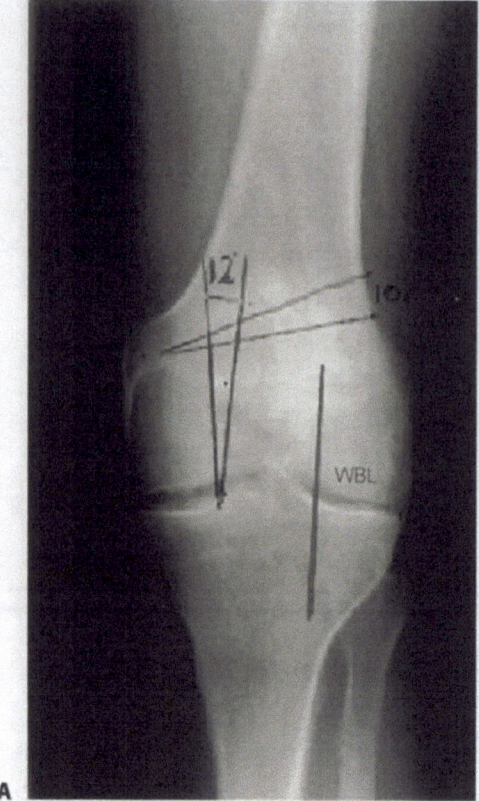
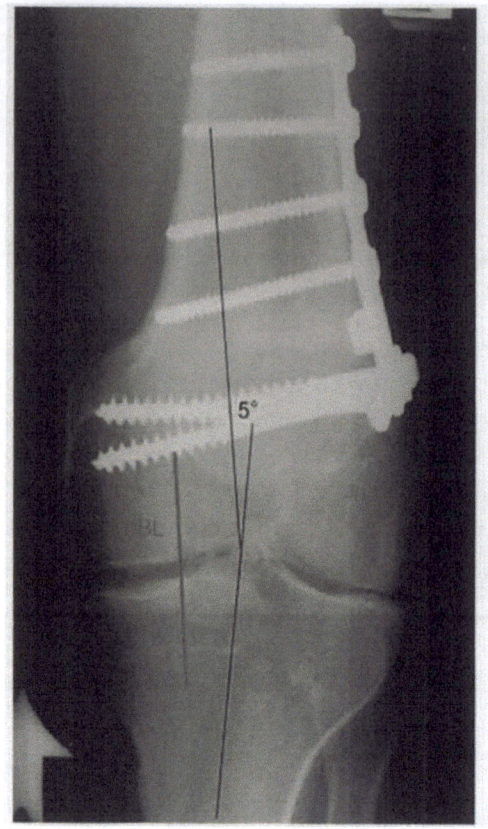

FIGURE 14.10 Case: 50-year-old man with a valgus deformity. **A.** Before lateral opening distal femoral varus osteotomy, AP radiograph shows the WBL well into the lateral compartment. The mechanical axis is 12° of valgus and there is evidence of lateral compartment arthrosis. **B.** Following lateral opening DFVO, the mechanical axis is 5° of varus and the WBL passes through the medial compartment.

tous structures attached. In our experience, which is similar to that of Moroni et al.,[34] bony recurvatum alone or in combination with secondary capsuloligamentous laxity are indications for surgery. Normalization of sagittal alignment should be a priority over a ligament reconstruction, and in chronic PCL deficiency or rotatory/posterior instability, it may be the only operative procedure required. In these cases, an opening-wedge osteotomy is performed through the bed of the osteotomy starting 4 cm distal to the joint line anteriorly, extending obliquely and posteriorly to a point 1 cm distal to the joint line, leaving a 0.5- to 1-cm posterior hinge. The tibial tubercle can then be replaced at the desired level. Screw fixation of the tubercle and the osteotomy is augmented with corticocancellous allograft or autograft (Figure 14.12). External fixation and graduated correction with osteotomy distal to the tibial tubercle is also a consideration in multiplanar deformities.

REHABILITATION

Early postoperative knee range-of-motion (ROM) exercises benefit joint healing and articular cartilage nourishment as well as lower limb neuromuscular function. In addition, the return to normal weight bearing is essential for healthy bone turnover and healing. Postoperative physical therapy programs should focus on these components while respecting the desired outcomes of the realignment procedure, which include union and restoring and maintaining alignment (Table 14.3).

Range of Motion

The restoration of full ROM is an important factor in the long-term success of the surgical procedure. Full extension should be achieved by postoperative week 6. If progress is behind schedule, active exercises with slight volitional overpressure are recommended.

Weight Bearing

Weight-bearing progression depends on the type of osteotomy and any other cartilage restoration procedure performed. After an opening-wedge osteotomy, patients are restricted to touch-down weight bearing, equivalent to 25 to 40 pounds for the first 6 weeks. If any osteocartilaginous procedure has been performed in combination, the opening-wedge protocol takes preference. Following closing-wedge osteotomy, patients are instructed to protected weight bearing for the first 6 weeks. If a cartilage restoration procedure has been performed as well, a partial weight-bearing protocol should take preference.

From the 6-week mark, progression of weight-bearing status depends on the radiographic appearance of the osteotomy.

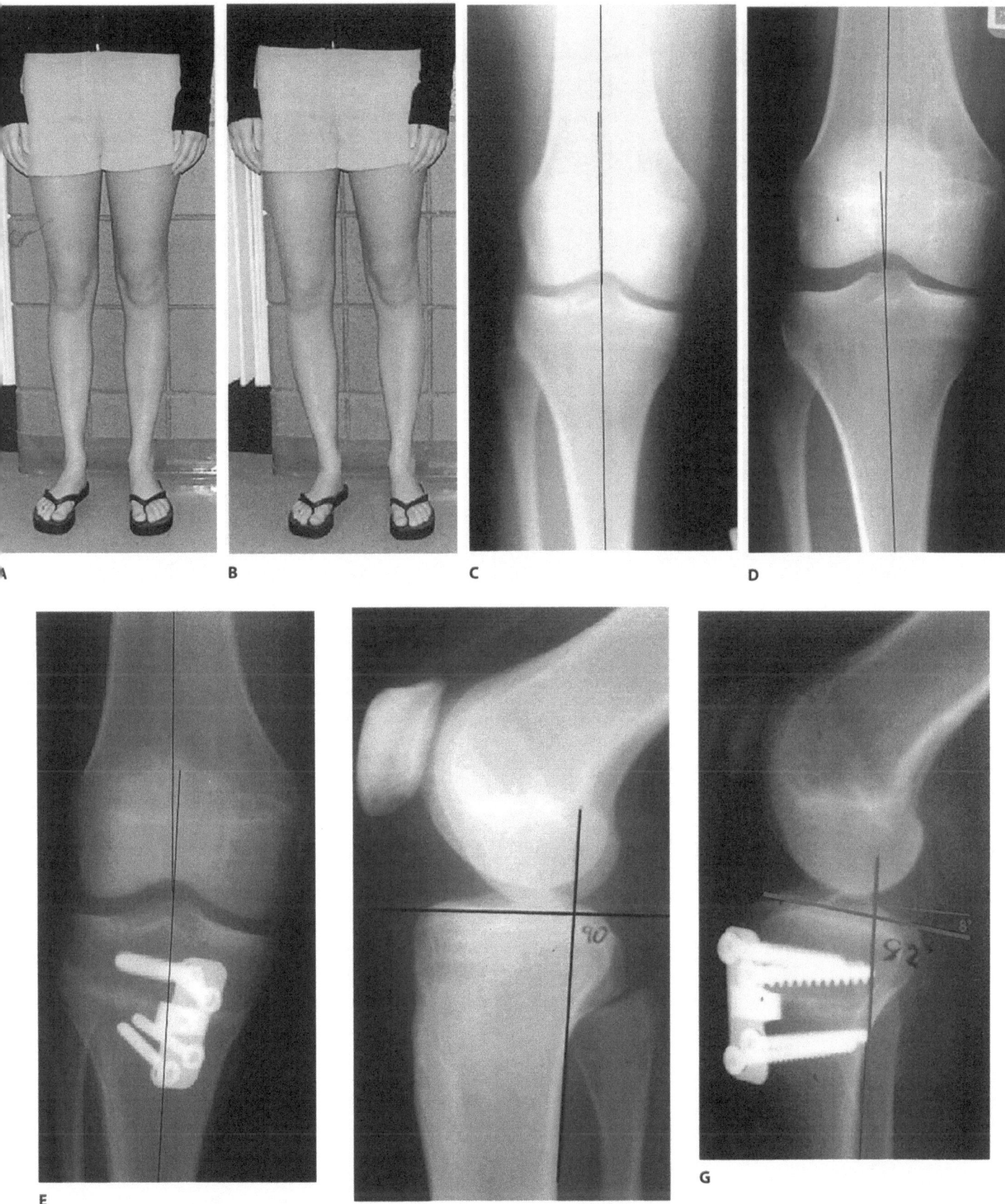

FIGURE 14.11 Case: 17-year-old girl with symptomatic varus hyper-extension thrust of the right knee, shown in the relaxed position (**A**) and in the symptomatic thrust position (**B**). Preoperative AP radiographs demonstrate the relaxed position (**C**) with varus alignment and the thrust position (**D**) with opening of the lateral joint space. **E.** Axial alignment has been improved. **F.** Preoperative PTSA of 0° has been increased to 8° (**G**) postoperatively.

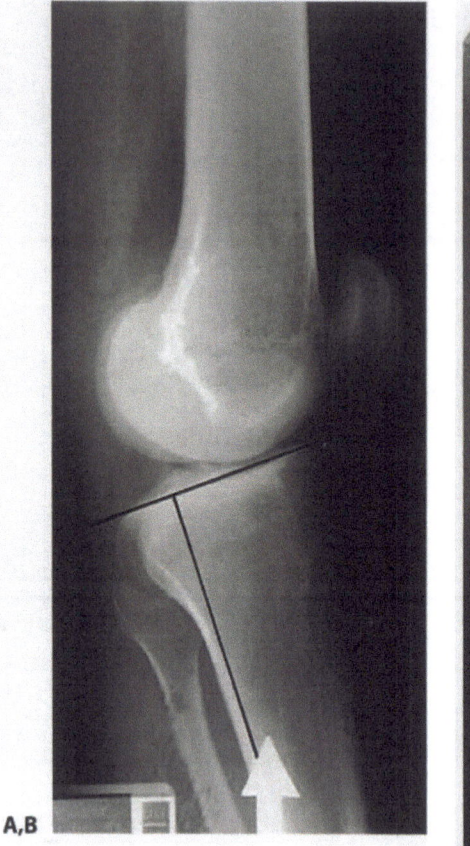
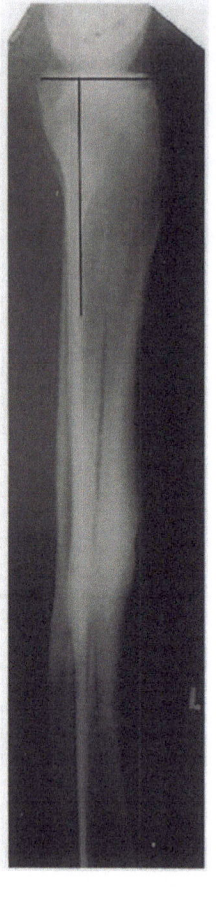
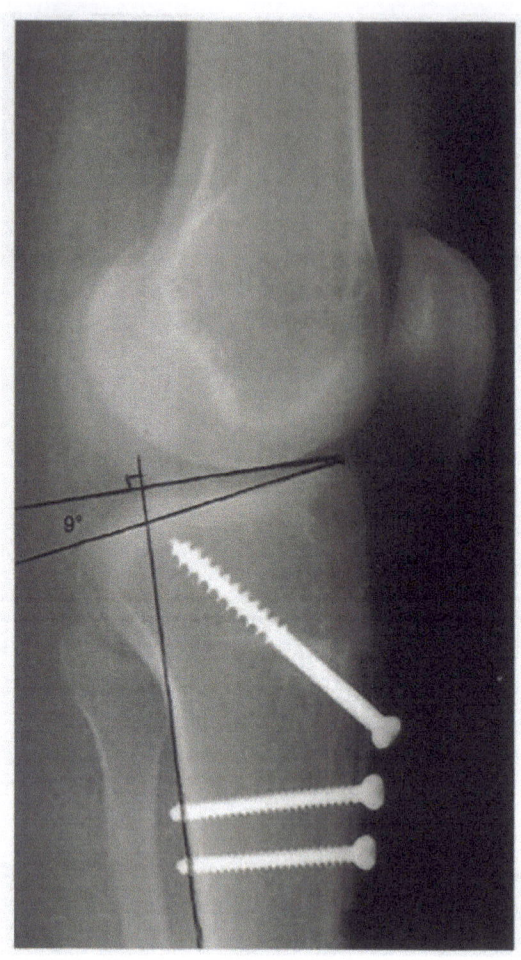

A,B

9°

C

FIGURE 14.12 Case: 31-year-old man with a recurvatum deformity of the knee as a result of a tibial diaphyseal malunion. Preoperative radiograph demonstrates decreased PTSA (**A**) and the tibial dia- physeal malunion (**B**) which exacerbated his symptoms. **C.** Following anterior opening-wedge osteotomy performed through the bed of a tibial tubercle osteotomy, the PTSA is increased.

TABLE 14.3   Postoperative rehabilitation guidelines.

Timeline	Exercise
0–3 weeks	• Passive range of motion (ROM) using slider board • Pedal rocking on bicycle • Isometric quadriceps setting
3–6 weeks	• Full-circle pedaling on bicycle, very light resistance • Active ROM • Side-lying gluteus medius strengthening • Hip ab/adduction, flexion and extension with resistance fixed above knee, i.e., pulley or resistance tubing • Pool exercises: hip ab/adduction, flexion and extension, knee flexion and extension • Gait pattern training with crutches focusing on proper heel strike/toe off • Pool: deep-water running or cycling • Leg press or squat with weight off-loaded to 24–40 pounds (watch ROM restriction associated with any cartilage/meniscus restoration/repair)
6–9 weeks	• Pool: shallow-water walking as weight-bearing restrictions allow • As a general guideline, when 60% of body is submerged, 60% of body weight is off-loaded • Standing/seated calf raise • Bilateral wobble-board balancing as weight-bearing status allows • Knee flexion/extension with very light resistance
Upon full weight bearing	• Gait training to restore normal gait • Step up and step down to work on alignment and eccentric control • Elliptical trainer and bicycle for cardiovascular conditioning

It is anticipated that patients with a closing-wedge osteotomy, if there is consolidation and progression to union, could be allowed to weight bear as tolerated with the use of a cane or a single crutch. An opening-wedge osteotomy should progress to partial weight bearing for 3 weeks and then to protected weight bearing for 3 weeks if there is radiographic consolidation and no evidence of hardware loosening (see Table 14.3).

Neuromuscular programs aimed at maintaining surrounding joint strength and muscle function should be employed along with pain management modalities during the initial postoperative 6 weeks. During weeks 6 to 12, a more functional program can be instituted and methods to improve muscular endurance can be instituted after postoperative week 12. Gait retraining and a return to a fully functional state should be additional goals throughout the rehabilitation process. Therapy directed to correct functional impairments in addition to those already mentioned should also take place after week 12.

COMPLICATIONS AND MANAGEMENT

The list of possible intraoperative, early postoperative, and late postoperative complications following any realignment procedure around the knee can be exhaustive. However, one would agree with Coventry[35] that the early complications of upper tibial osteotomy are those of any other surgery of the lower extremity. Outlined here are some of the common complications of osteotomy about the knee that may require supervised neglect or active intervention. Intraoperative complications include intraarticular fracture, intraarticular screw placement, and violation of the opposite cortex with resultant instability of the osteotomy. The use of fluoroscopy throughout is the best form of prevention of these problems. Otherwise, early recognition and immediate management are critical. Intraarticular fracture should be assessed intraoperatively with fluoroscopy, and interfragmentary screw stabilization carried out if required (Figure 14.13). A fracture detected postoperatively may require internal fixation with or without revision of the osteotomy, or a simple modification of the postoperative rehabilitation protocol with immobilization and nonweight bearing for a period of time, as well as radiographic monitoring of the fracture.

Violation of the opposite cortex during opening-wedge tibial osteotomy does not usually require any additional treatment. In closing-wedge tibial osteotomy and distal femoral osteotomy, the opposite cortex, if violated and unstable, may require additional fixation or modification of the postoperative protocol to prevent loss of correction.

Delayed union or nonunion can result in continuing pain, hardware failure, or loss of correction. In the latter two, revision osteotomy and bone grafting are indicated. If alignment has been maintained but is persistent pain, supplemental procedures to stimulate union may be instituted before revision. In this situation, revision may include bone grafting alone. Numerous authors have discussed overcorrection into valgus.[6,18,24,36,37] From the cosmetic point of view, a valgus deformity is not as well tolerated as a varus deformity. Critical assessment of alignment both intraoperatively and in the early postoperative period is essential. If there is "over-

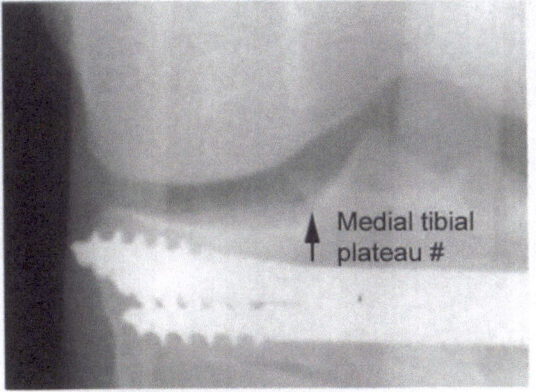

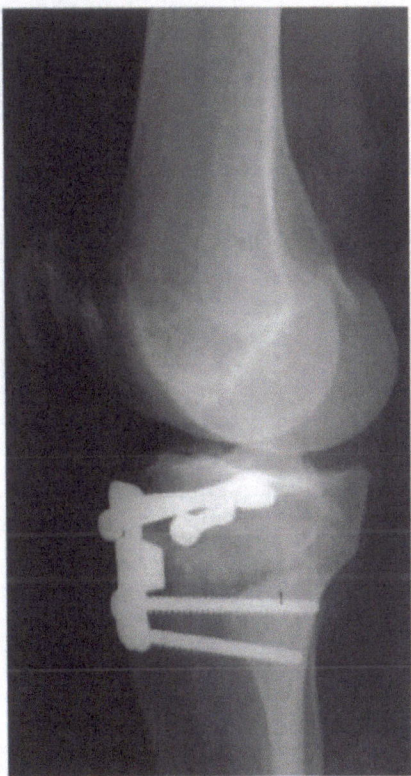

FIGURE 14.13 Postoperative radiographs of an anterolateral opening-wedge HTO that was complicated by an intraarticular fracture of the medial tibial plateau (**A**). The fracture was detected and stabilized at the time with an interfragmentary screw (**B**).

correction" or "excessive" varus or valgus, the osteotomy should be revised (Figure 14.14).

The frequency of thromboembolic disease is lower following osteotomy than total knee arthroplasty, and appropriate methods of prophylactic antithrombotic regimens are controversial.[7] In our practice, chemical prophylaxis is not routinely prescribed for patients undergoing knee osteotomy. Mobilization is encouraged on the first postoperative day. Patients with specific risk factors for deep venous thromboembolism (DVT) or pulmonary embolism (PE) are anticoagulated with low molecular weight heparin subcutaneously throughout the perioperative period and undergo lower limb venous studies before discharge from hospital. Patients with a past history of DVT or PE are anticoagulated with coumadin for 6 weeks.

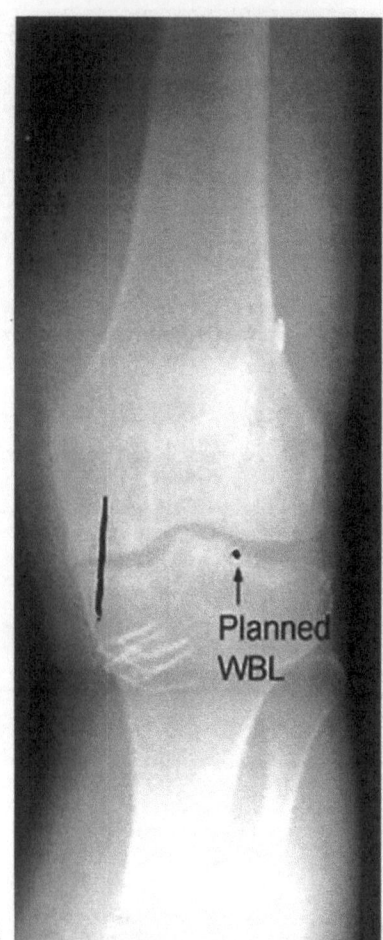
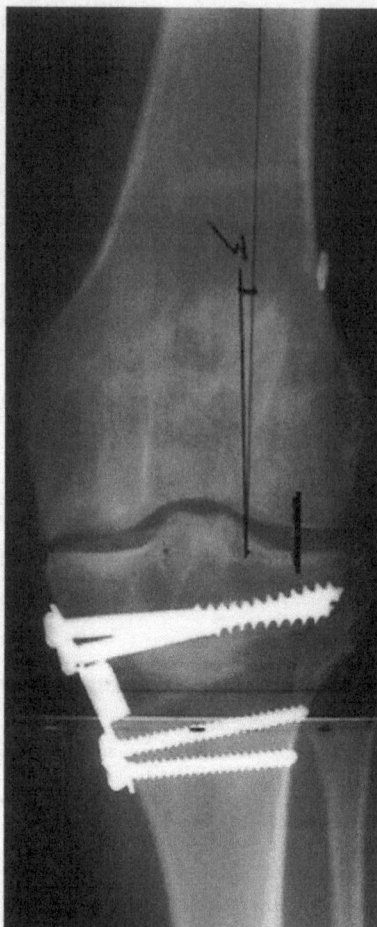
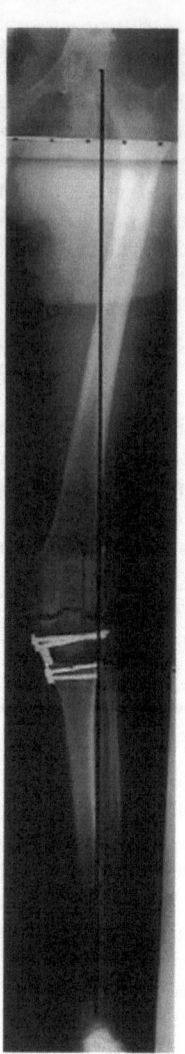

Planned
WBL

A,B

C

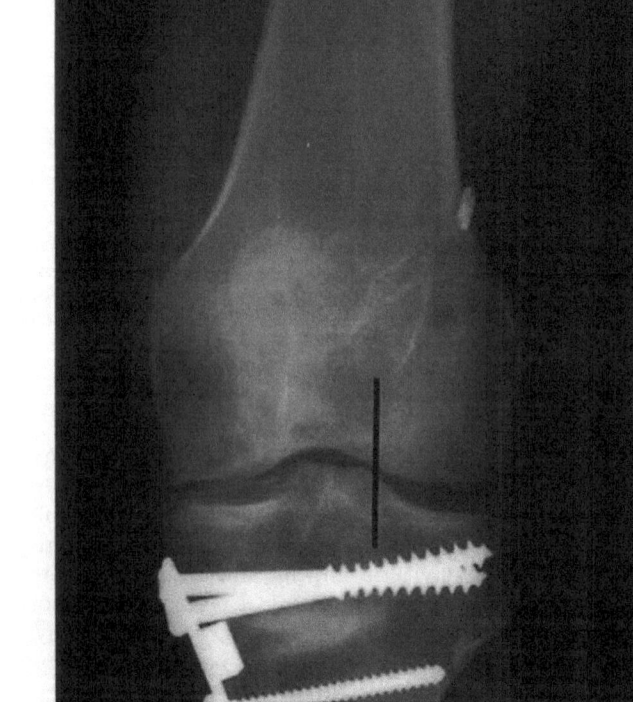

D

FIGURE 14.14 Case: 50-year-old woman with medial compartment arthrosis, varus malalignment of the left knee, previous ACL reconstruction, and partial medial meniscectomy. B Preoperative AP view demonstrates planned WBL to a point just lateral to the lateral tibial spine. **B.** Early postoperative and (**C**) weight-bearing radiographs at 3 weeks after valgus opening-wedge HTO show that her alignment was overcorrected well into the lateral compartment. At this time, revision HTO to decrease the patient's valgus alignment was carried out. **D.** Radiographs 6 months following revision HTO show the WBL just lateral to the lateral tibial spine and a united osteotomy.

RESULTS

Successful long-term results (Table 14.4) following realignment osteotomy are linked to careful patient selection, accurate surgical technique, and appropriate postoperative alignment.[7] The current literature reports on the results of series of patients treated with osteotomy for unicompartmental arthrosis. However, few authors have examined the results of knee osteotomy performed in combination with cartilage restoration procedures.

When evaluating many of the clinical series reporting on knee osteotomy, it is often difficult to ascertain the effects of patient selection and technical error on long-term outcome. In patients with more complicated knee problems, the objective of the osteotomy should be clear, as results of surgery will depend to a great extent on why the procedure was carried out. Review of the data, therefore, should be meticulous and questioning.

Valgus High Tibial Osteotomy

Hernigou and associates[6] found, at a mean follow-up of 11.5 years, that results in 93 knees treated with proximal tibial opening-wedge osteotomy for varus deformity and medial compartment osteoarthritis deteriorate with time at an average of 7 years following the procedure. They also found however, that alignment was a determinant of long-term results. There were good or excellent results in 90% after 5 years and in 45% after 10 years. In 20 knees with a postoperative hip-knee-ankle angle of 183° to 186°, there was no pain and no progression of arthrosis. In those that were undercorrected (an angle less than 183°), the results were less satisfactory and there was a tendency for a slow deterioration. All 5 knees that were overcorrected (angle more than 186°) had progressive degenerative changes in the lateral compartment.[6]

Morrey[12] reported on 34 consecutive lateral closing-wedge osteotomies in 33 patients with an average age of 31.3 years and with secondary arthritis. At an average follow-up of 7.5 years, 24 (73%) were satisfactory with improved pain and mean activity level, whereas 9 were failures, with 5 requiring total knee arthroplasty at a mean of 4.5 years after osteotomy (range 2–8 years).

Yasuda and associates[37] showed that overcorrection was, in their patients, associated not only with better long-term clinical results but also with a marked decrease in the loss of valgus correction between 1 and 10 years. They evaluated 56 of 86 knees, at an average follow-up of 11 years 3 months (only 45 knees had both clinical and radiographic assessments). They reported a survival rate of 88% at 6 years and 63% at 10 years.

In a recent paper, Coventry et al.[4] report on lateral closing-wedge proximal tibial osteotomy in 87 knees at a median of 10 years. Using moderate or severe pain or conversion to arthroplasty as a definition of failure, they found an 87% survival rate at 5 years and a 66% survival rate at 10 years. Relative weight and angular correction were the only risk factors associated with the duration of survival. If valgus angulation at 1 year was less than 8° in a patient whose weight was more than 1.32 times the ideal weight, the rate of survival decreased to 38% at 5 years and to 19% at 10 years. The number of patients in each subgroup, however, was not reported.

Billings and associates[38] reported the long-term results of 64 knees after valgus osteotomy using a calibrated osteotomy guide and rigid internal fixation at an average of 8.5 years. They found 21 knees (33%) had undergone a total knee arthroplasty at an average of 65 months, and the survivorship analysis showed an expected rate of survival, with conversion to a total knee arthroplasty as the end point, of 85% at 5 years and 53% at 10 years.

Varus High Tibial Osteotomy

Results of proximal tibial varus osteotomy are not comparable to those of proximal tibial valgus osteotomy. Shoji and associates reported "far inferior" results in retention of mobility, relief of pain, and achievement of stability in a group of 49 varus osteotomies compared to a previously published series of 63 valgus osteotomies.[24] Coventry reported that 24 (77%) of 31 knees had no pain or only occasional mild pain at an average of 9.4 years after a closing-wedge varus osteotomy for valgus deformity and with painful osteoarthritis of the lateral compartment; the remaining 7 continued to have moderate or severe pain.[8]

Recently, Marti and associates reported 88% good or excellent results at a mean follow-up of 11 years for lateral opening wedge varus osteotomy.[23] These late results are better than those previously described by Harding,[39] and certainly seem to reflect more favorably on lateral opening-wedge osteotomy for correction of valgus deformity less than 15°.

Distal Femoral Varus Osteotomy

As with high tibial osteotomy, success rates for distal femoral varus osteotomy (DFVO) have been variable.[7] McDermott and associates[19] reported a 92% successful result at 4 years, with 1 of 22 patients requiring a total knee arthroplasty at 3 years.[19] Healy and associates[26] had 93% good or excellent results at an average follow-up of 4 years in 15 knees with osteoarthritis, and an overall 83% good or excellent results on the Hospital for Special Surgery (HSS) knee score. They concluded that they could not recommend the procedure for patients with rheumatoid arthritis.

Miniaci and associates[29] reviewed 35 of 40 DFVOs at an average of 5.5 years and a minimum of 2 years follow-up. Eighty-six percent had a good or excellent results on the HSS knee score, with 25 of 26 with lateral compartment arthrosis having significant improvement of their pain. Aglietti and Menchetti[40] reported on 18 knees with valgus osteoarthritis that had a DFVO performed on patients with an average age of 54 years. The mean follow-up was 9 years, and 13 (77%) of 17 knees reviewed were found to be good or excellent according to the Knee Society rating system. Finkelstein and associates[25] reported on 21 knees in 20 patients with an average age of 56 years at a mean follow-up of 133 months after DFVO. They found that 13 of the osteotomies were still successful at the most recent follow-up, whereas 7 had failed and required total knee arthroplasty. Using the Kaplan–Meier method, the probability of survival at 10 years was 64%.

Anterior Opening-Wedge HTO

Moroni et al.[34] reported on 25 patients, average age 23 years, at an average follow-up of 14.5 years following 27 opening

TABLE 14.4 Results.

Author	Date	Type	Number of knees	Average follow-up (years)	Average age (years)	Type of study	Results (%)	Comments
Hernigou et al.[6]	1987	MO	93	11.5	60.3	R	Good or Excellent rating: 90% @ 5 yrs 45% @ 10 yrs	Time and alignment major determinants to long-term results Significant early complications
Cass et al.[9]	1988	LC	86	Minimum 5	60	R	Satisfactory: 94% @ 2 yrs 87% @ 5 yrs 69% @ 10 yrs 36% failed (TKA)	Increasing age and female gender not significant negative factors Recommended standing postoperative anatomic axial alignment of 10°–12° valgus
Morrey[12]	1989	LC	34	7.5	31.3	R	73% satisfactory 26% failures @ 4.5 yrs (avg.)	HTO can be offered with confidence to young patients Disparity between the functional results and radiographic appearance was common
Rudan and Simurda[10]	1991	LC	128	7.5	58.5	R	HSS scores 78% G/E @ 6–9 yrs 70% G/E @ 10+ yrs 10.9% revision rate	Equal prognosis for men and women in uncontrolled groups No significant difference in results in patients older than 60 years compared to younger than 60 years
Yasuda et al.[37]	1992	LC ex. Fix	56	11.25	59.8	R	Survival: 63% @ 6 yrs 18% @ 10+ yrs	11 knees evaluated by telephone interview at 10+ years and included only in the clinical analysis of knee function Knee joint function remained favourable for approx. 5–10 yrs but deteriorated gradually after 10 yrs
Coventry et al.[4]	1993	LC	87	10	63	R	Survival: 87% @ 5 yrs 66% @ 10 yrs	Relative weight (less than 1.7) and angular correction (>5° valgus) only risk factors associated with improved duration of survival
Billings et al.[38]	2000	LC*	64	8.5	49	R	33% failures @ 5.5 yrs (avg.) Survival: 87% @ 5 yrs 53% @ 10 yrs	
Shoji et al.[24]	1973	MC HTO	49	2.6	60.2	R	61% persistent instability 47% persistent pain 6% lacking desired mobility	Results compared to previously published series of HTO for varus deformity and found to be "far inferior"
Coventry[8]	1987	MC HTO	31	9.4	59	R	77% mild/no pain 20% failure (TKA) @ 9.8 yrs (avg.)	Tibiofemoral angle >12° or postoperative obliquity of joint line >10° may be indications for DFVO Correction to 0° anatomic tibiofemoral alignment is recommended
McDermott et al.[19]	1988	DFVO	22 (pts)	4	53	R	92% success @ 2 yrs 1 pt TKA @ 3 yrs	Short-term follow-up
Healy et al.[26]	1988	DFVO	15	4	56	R	93% G/E @ 4 yrs with OA 83% including RA pts	Not recommended for RA Relatively short follow-up
Miniaci et al.[27]	1990	DFVO	35	5.5		R	HS scores: 86% G/E	
Aglietti and Manchett[40]	2000	DFVO	17	9	54	R	KSS scores: 77% G/E	
Finklestein et al.[25]	1996	DFVO	21	11	56	R	7 failures (TKA) Survival: 64% @ 10 yrs	

yrs, years; avg., average; pts, patrents; LC, lateral closing; LC*, calibrated guide + rigid internal fixation; MC, medial closing; HTO, high tibial osteotomy; DFVO, distal femoral varus osteotomy; R, retrospective; TKA, total knee arthroplasty; HSS, Hospital for Special Surgery; KS, Knee Society; RA, rheumatoid arthritis; OA, osteoarthritrs; G/E, good/excellent.

wedge osteotomies of the proximal tibia for genu recurvatum. They found that when the osteotomy was performed proximal to the tibial tuberosity with detachment of the tuberosity (18 knees), 78% had good or excellent results. In the 5 procedures that were performed distal to the tuberosity, only 1 had a good result. They also found that in the 21 knees with an entirely or predominantly osseous deformity, results were good or excellent in 86%, whereas those in which the deformity was predominantly in the soft tissues results were fair or poor because of an increased obliquity of the tibial plateau (overcorrection).

Our experience is similar and, as discussed earlier, we would recommend an osteotomy proximal to the tibial tuberosity.

SUMMARY

The natural history of the focal chondral defect in the meniscectomized knee has not been precisely determined.[41] The prognosis, if left untreated, is guarded.

The approach of the orthopaedic surgeon in the treatment of articular cartilage lesions, therefore, should be comprehensive. Not only should it include realignment to "off-load" the diseased compartment, as has been discussed here, but also procedures to allow regeneration or replacement of articular cartilage. The future looks at restoring normal alignment and joint stability as the foundation for successful treatment of articular cartilage lesions. It is to be hoped that the combination of these procedures will enable improved results to be achieved in the treatment of articular cartilage lesions in the knee.

Reference List

1. Cooke TDV, Pichora DS. Knee dysplasia: an unusual but important problem associated with progressive arthritis. J Bone Joint Surg Br 1985;67

2. Maquet P. The biomechanics of the knee and surgical possibilities of healing osteoarthritic knee joints. Clin Orthop Res 1980;146:102–110.

3. Coventry MB. Upper tibial osteotomy for gonarthrosis. The evolution of the operation in the last 18 years and long term results. Orthop Clin N Am 1979;10:191–210.

4. Coventry MB, Ilstrup DM, Wallrich SL. Proximal tibial osteotomy: a critical long-term study of 87 cases. J Bone Joint Surg Am 1993;75:196.

5. Dugdale TW, Noyes FR, Styer D. Pre-operative planning for high tibial osteotomy. Clin Orthop 1992;274:248–264.

6. Hernigou P, Medevill D, Debeyre J, et al. Proximal tibial osteotomy with varus deformity: a ten- to thirteen-year follow-up study. J Bone Joint Surg Am 1987;69:332.

7. Hanssen AD, Stuart MJ, Scott RD, Scuderi GR. Surgical options for the middle-aged patient with osteoarthritis of the knee joint. Instr Course Lect 2001;50:499–511.

8. Coventry MB. Proximal tibial varus osteotomy for osteoarthritis of the lateral compartment of the knee. J Bone Joint Surg Am 1987;69:32–38.

9. Cass JR, Bryan RS. High tibial osteotomy. Clin Orthop 1988;230: 196–199.

10. Rudan JF, Simurda MA. Valgus high tibial osteotomy. A long-term follow-up study. Clin Orthop 1991;157–160.

11. Badhe NP, Forster IW. High tibial osteotomy in knee instability: the rationale of treatment and early results. Knee Surg Sports Traumatol Arthrosc 2002;10:38–43.

12. Morrey BF. Upper tibial osteotomy for secondary osteoarthritis of the knee. J Bone Joint Surg Br 1989;71:554–559.

13. Paley D, Herzenberg JE, Tetsworth K, McKie J, Bhave A. Deformity planning for frontal and sagittal plane corrective osteotomies. Orthop Clin N Am 1994;25:465.

14. Moreland JR, Bassett LW, Hanker GJ. Radiographic analysis of the axial alignment of the lower extremity. J Bone Joint Surg Am 1987;69:749.

15. Hsu RWW, Himeno S, Coventry MB, Chao EYS. Normal axial alignment of the lower extremity and load-bearing distribution of the knee. Clin Orthop 1990;215–217.

16. Puddu G, Cipolla M, Franco V. A plate for open wedge tibial and femoral osteotomies. Presented at The Congress of the International Society of Arthroscopy, Knee Surgery and Orthopaedic Sports Medicine; 1999; Washington, DC.

17. Catagni MA, Guerreschi F, Ahmas TS, Cattaneo, R. Treatment of genu varum in medial compartment osteoarthritis of the knee using the Ilizarov method. Orthop Clin N Am 1994;25:509–514.

18. Chambat P, Selmi TAS, Dejour D, Denoyers J. Varus tibial osteotomy. Oper Tech Orthop 2000;8:44–47.

19. McDermott GP, Finkelstein JA, Farine I, Boynton EL, MacIntosh D, Gross AE. Distal femoral varus osteotomy for valgus deformity of the knee. J Bone Joint Surg Am 1988;70:110–116.

20. Learmouth ID. A simple technique for varus supracondylar osteotomy in genu valgum. J Bone Joint Surg Br 1990;72:235–237.

21. Morrey BF, Edgerton BC. Distal femoral osteotomy for lateral gonarthrosis. Instr Course Lect 1992;41:77–85.

22. Phillips MJ, Krakow KA. Distal varus osteotomy: indications and surgical technique. Instr Course Lect 1999;48:129.

23. Marti RK, Verhagen RAW, Kerkhoffs GMMJ, Moore HA. Proximal tibial varus osteotomy: indications, technique and five- to twenty-one-year results. J Bone Joint Surg Am 2001;83: 164–170.

24. Shoji H, Insall J. High tibial osteotomy for osteoarthritis of the knee with valgus deformity. J Bone Joint Surg Am 1973;55: 963–973.

25. Finkelstein JA, Gross AE, Davies A. Varus osteotomy of the distal part of the femur. J Bone Joint Surg Am 1996;78:1348–1352.

26. Healy WL, Anglen JO, Wasilewski SA, Krakow KA. Distal femoral varus osteotomy. J Bone Joint Surg Am 1988;70: 102–109.

27. Miniaci A, Grossman SP, Jakob RP. Supracondylar femoral varus osteotomy for genu valgum. A prospective review. Am J Knee Surg 1990;2:65–73.

28. Marti RK, Schroder J, Witteveen A. The closed wedge supracondylar osteotomy. Oper Tech Orthop 2000;8:55.

29. Puddu G, Franco V. Femoral antivalgus opening wedge osteotomy. Oper Tech Orthop 2000;8:56–60.

30. Beaver RJ, Jinxiang-Yu, Sekyi-Otu A, et al. Distal femoral varus osteotomy for genu valgum. A prospective review. Am J Knee Surg 1991;1:17.

31. Neyret P, Zuppi G, Selmi TAS. Tibial deflexion osteotomy. Oper Tech Orthop 2000;8:61–66.

32. Dejour H, Bonnin M. Tibial translation after anterior cruciate ligament rupture. J Bone Joint Surg Br 1994;96:745.

33. Dejour H, Neyret P, Boileau P, Donell ST. Anterior cruciate reconstruction combined with valgus tibial osteotomy. Clin Orthop 1994;299:220–228.

34. Moroni A, Pezzuto V, Pompili M, Zinghi G. Proximal osteotomy of the tibia for the treatment of genu recurvatum in adults. J Bone Joint Surg Am 1992;74:577–586.

35. Coventry MB. Upper tibial osteotomy for osteoarthritis. J Bone Joint Surg Am 1985;67:1140.

36. Insall JN, Joseph DM, Msika C. High tibial osteotomy for varus gonarthrosis. A long-term follow-up study. J Bone Joint Surg Am 1984;66:1040–1048.

37. Yasuda K, Majima T, Tsuchida T, Kaneda K. A ten- to 15-year follow-up observation of high tibial osteotomy in medial compartment osteoarthrosis. Clin Orthop 1992;186–195.

38. Billings A, Scott DF, Camargo MP, Hofmann AA. High tibial osteotomy with a calibrated osteotomy guide, rigid internal fixation, and early motion. Long-term follow-up. J Bone Joint Surg Am 2000;82:70–79.

39. Harding ML. A fresh appraisal of tibial osteotomy for osteoarthritis of the knee. Clin Orthop 1976;114:234.

40. Aglietti P, Manchetti PP. Distal femoral varus osteotomy in the valgus osteoarthritic knee. Am J Knee Surg 2000;13:89–95.

41. Cole BJ, Harner CD. Degenerative arthritis of the knee in active patients: evaluation and management. J Am Acad Orthop Surg 1999;7:389–402.

15

Realignment of the Patellofemoral Joint

Giles R. Scuderi

BACKGROUND

Patellar instability has been implicated as a cause of recurrent knee pain and disability. Initial treatment should focus on a supervised physiotherapy program. Surgical treatment is reserved for patients sustaining severe and unremitting symptoms that have not responded to at least 3 to 6 months of therapy. Surgical treatment is also indicated for an acute patellar dislocation with disruption of the medial patellar retinaculum or associated with an osteochondral fracture. Several surgical procedures are available to correct patellar instability and are directed toward correcting the underlying pathology. In correcting lateral patellar instability, the surgical procedures release the tight and contracted lateral retinaculum, transfer the vastus medialis, or reorient the tibial tubercle. Surgical procedures include lateral retinacular release, proximal realignment, distal realignment, and combined procedures. Because no single procedure corrects all cases of patellar instability, variables such as the patient's age and level of activity, the condition of the articular cartilage, and etiology of the instability must be considered in selecting the ideal operation (Table 15.1).

LATERAL RETINACULAR RELEASE

Merchant and Mercer first described the lateral retinacular release in 1974 for patients with patellofemoral pain and lateral patellar tilt, or subluxation.[1] The indications and contraindications are listed in Table 15.2. Acceptable results can be expected in patients who have a tight lateral retinaculum, limited medial patella glide, and no evidence of severe patellar malalignment or ligament laxity. Poor prognostic factors include (1) increased quadriceps angle; (2) generalized ligament hyperlaxity; (3) patellar hypermobility; (4) excessive genu varum, valgum, or recurvatum; (5) increased femoral anteversion; (6) increased internal tibial torsion; and (7) abnormal foot pronation.[2]

Surgical Technique

ARTHROSCOPIC LATERAL RELEASE

A diagnostic arthroscopy is performed through the standard anteromedial and anterolateral portal. Following a diagnostic evaluation and concomitant intraarticular surgery, attention is directed to performing the lateral retinacular release. The knee is placed in full extension, with the arthroscope in the anteromedial portal and the instrumentation in the anterolateral portal. While directly visualizing the lateral retinaculum, an arthroscopic knife or electrocautery is used to cut the lateral retinaculum approximately 5 to 10 mm from the lateral border of the patella. The release extends from the inferior fibers of the vastus lateralis to the joint line. As the retinaculum is released, the subcutaneous fat will be seen. Care should be taken to avoid cutting into the subcutaneous fat because of its close proximity to the overlying skin. When the lateral release is complete, the lateral border of the patella should be able to be passively lifted approximately 60° to 90° degrees. If a pneumatic tourniquet is used, it should be deflated at this point and hemostasis should be obtained with an electrocautery. Inevitably, branches of the superior and inferior lateral geniculate vessels are cut and should be cauterized.

Postoperatively, the knee is placed in a soft compressive dressing and the patient is allowed weight bearing as tolerated. The patients are started on a supervised rehabilitation program within 48 h of surgery. Emphasis is placed on range of motion and quadriceps strengthening. Patients are allowed to return to sports and recreational activities once their strength is 90% of the opposite uninvolved leg.

OPEN LATERAL RELEASE

Following an arthroscopic evaluation of the knee, the leg is positioned in full extension. A 2-cm longitudinal skin incision is made along the lateral border of the patella. Subcutaneous dissection proximally and distally permits visualization of the lateral retinaculum. The lateral retinaculum is then divided longitudinally about 1 cm from the lateral border of the patella. The lateral release should extend from the lower fibers of the vastus lateralis to the lateral bor-

TABLE 15.1   Patellar instability and suggested surgical procedure.

Diagnosis	Surgical procedure
Lateral patellar compression syndrome	Lateral retinacular release
Patellar subluxation	Lateral retinacular release
	Proximal realignment
	Distal realignment
Acute patellar dislocation	Repair medial retinaculum and lateral retinacular release
	Proximal realignment
Recurrent patellar dislocation	Proximal realignment
	Distal realignment
	Combined proximal and distal realignment
Malalignment with severe chondromalacia	Tibial tubercle elevation
	Tubercle anteromedialization

TABLE 15.3   Complications of lateral retinacular release.

Hemarthrosis
Arthofibrosis
Medial patellar subluxation
Reflex sympathetic dystrophy

der of the patella tendon. If possible, the synovium may be preserved; however, if it is divided, this is of no clinical significance. Following the release, if a pneumatic tourniquet is used, it should be released to obtain hemostasis. Inevitably, branches of the superior and inferior lateral geniculate vessels are cut and should be cauterized. The subcutaneous layer and skin are closed in a routine fashion and a soft compression dressing. Postoperatively, the patient is allowed full weight bearing as tolerated and physiotherapy is started within 48 hours as described above.

Results

Comparison of the results of arthroscopic lateral release is difficult because various techniques, follow-up examinations, and selection criteria are used.[3] Most studies show 70% success.[4–6] Aglietti et al. reviewed the various techniques and results and noted a large range of satisfactory results, from 14% to 99%. Reported results of lateral release in patients with patellofemoral arthritis are also variable.[7] Jackson et al.[8] reviewed the results in patients with unremitting patellofemoral pain in the presence of malalignment and reported 75% good and excellent results at 4 years, but the results deteriorated over time to 56% at 6 years. Dzioba[5] has documented that the predictors of a successful lateral retinacular release include pain with knee flexion against resistance, a positive apprehension sign with lateral deviation, a tight lateral retinaculum with limited patella glide, a positive Merchant view, and evidence of lateral patella overhang. Although the procedure may be simple to perform, it is not without complication (Table 15.3).

TABLE 15.2   Lateral retinacular release.

Indications
  Lateral patellar compression syndrome
  Lateral patellar subluxation
Contraindications
  Patellofemoral pain without lateral tilt
  Normal tracking patella
  Hypermobile patella

PROXIMAL PATELLAR REALIGNMENT

Although lateral retinacular release is an appealing procedure, it does not restore normal orientation to a malaligned extensor mechanism. This procedure releases the tight lateral retinaculum and reinforces the pull of the vastus medialis. The indications for proximal patellar realignment include recurrent patellar subluxation and recurrent patellar dislocation. Insall et al.[9,10] originally described the proximal "tube" realignment that was later modified to the proximal patellar realignment with advancement of the vastus medialis and imbrication of the medial capsule with a lateral retinacular release.

Surgical Technique

A straight midline skin incision over the patella permits exposure of the extensor mechanism. A medial parapatellar arthrotomy is performed along the medial border of the quadriceps tendon over the patella and along the medial border of the patellar tendon. A lateral retinacular release is then performed approximately 1 cm from the lateral border of the patella. The synovium can be preserved unless it is fibrotic and acts as a restricting band. The lateral release should extend from the inferior fibers of the vastus lateralis to the joint line. The lateral superior geniculate artery is often sacrificed during the release and should be cauterized to avoid a hemarthrosis.

Advancement of the vastus medialis and medial retinaculum is accomplished by overlapping the medial flap on the patella and quadriceps tendon. This advancement is provisionally set at 10 to 15mm from the original position, and patellar tracking is checked (Figure 15.1). With the tourniquet released, the patella should track entirely within the femoral sulcus with no medial or lateral tilt through a full range of motion. If the patella continues to maltrack or tilt, then further lateral advancement of the vastus medialis and the medial retinaculum should be performed. Care should be taken not to overtighten the medial retinaculum or rotate the patella at the time of closure. A hemovac drain is placed in the joint, and the closure can be performed with number 0 absorbable or nonabsorbable interrupted sutures. The subcutaneous layer and skin are then closed in a routine fashion and a soft compressive dressing is applied.

Postoperatively, continuous passive motion (CPM) is begun in the recovery room and the patient is started on a structured rehabilitation program that focuses on range of motion and muscle strengthening. The patient is allowed to resume sports and recreational activities when the quadriceps strength is 90% of the opposite knee, as tested by a kinematic dynometer.

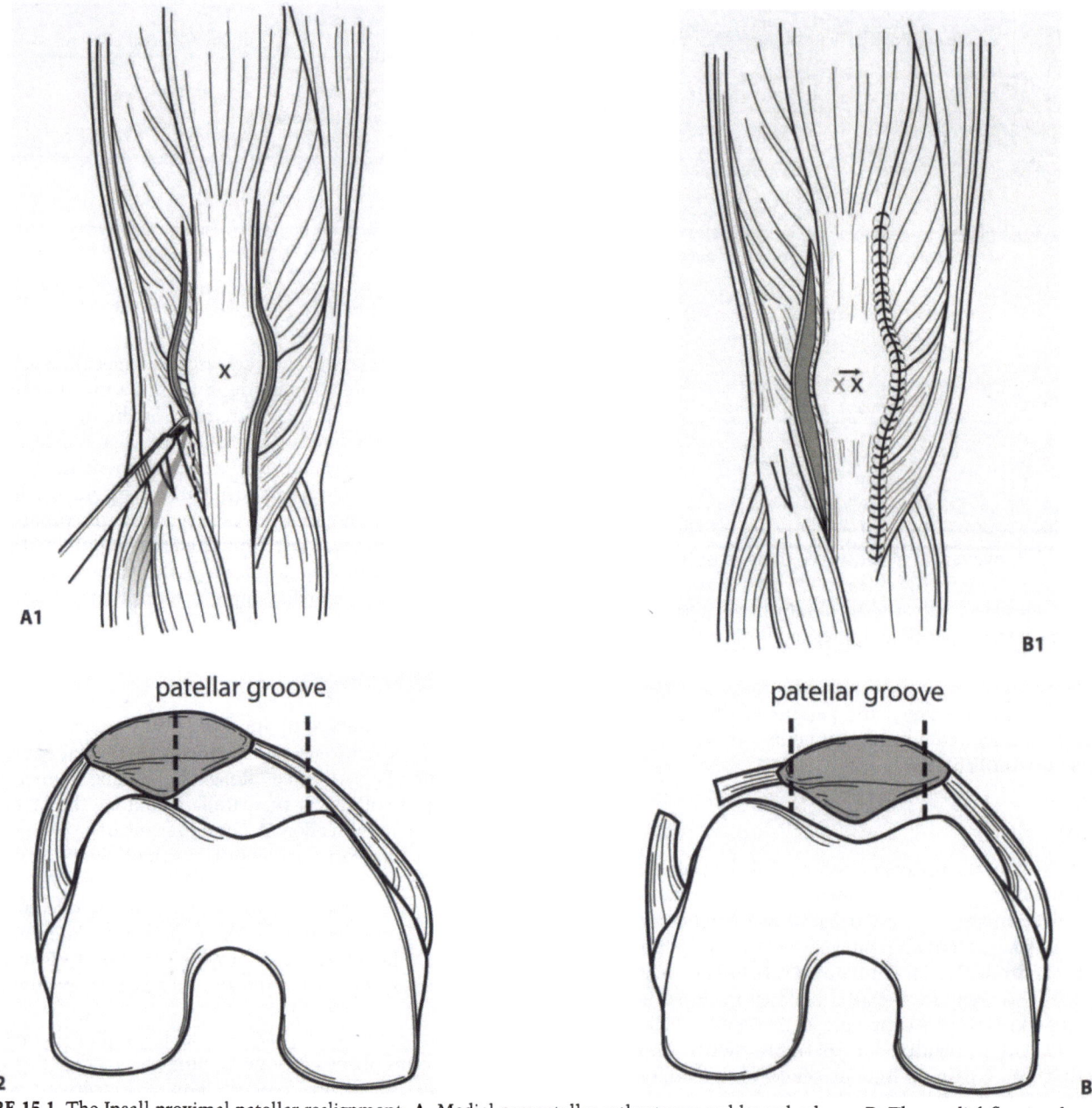

FIGURE 15.1 The Insall proximal patellar realignment. **A.** Medial parapatellar arthrotomy and lateral release. **B.** The medial flap is advanced laterally and secured in position.

Results

In one of the initial reviews of the proximal patella realignment, Insall et al.[10] reported on 75 cases with a 91% incidence of good and excellent results at follow-up of 2 to 10 years. The results suggested that clinical improvement correlated with the correction of the patellar axial alignment, although there was no correlation with the degree of chondromalacia. In a review of 60 knees, Scuderi et al.[11] reported 81% good and excellent results with both patellar subluxation and dislocation, and the successful results were sustained for as long as 9 years. Abraham et al.[12] reported similar satisfactory to excellent results in 11 of 12 knees (92%) for recurrent dislocation, but when performed for chondromalacia the results deteriorate with time, with only 55% satisfactory results at 5 to 11 years.

Although redislocation is a common complication of patellar realignment, Scuderi et al. reported a 1.2% rate of redislocation with a proximal realignment, which is superior to redislocation rates, noted to be as high as 25% with other procedures.[11,13]

DISTAL REALIGNMENT

Distal realignment procedures transfer the tibial tubercle and patellar tendon medially, reducing the quadriceps angle. The procedure is indicated for recurrent patellar subluxation or dislocation. Distal realignment procedures are contraindicated in the skeletally immature patient with open epiphyseal plates and those patients with a normal quadriceps or tubercle sulcus angle. Transferring the tibial tubercle in a skeletally immature patient can cause premature closure of the proximal tibial epiphyseal growth plate, resulting in a genu varum or genu recurvatum deformity; it may also result in contracture of the patellar tendon and patella infera.[13] Our current distal realignment procedure is the Fulkerson tubercle osteotomy or anteromedialization procedure.[14]

Surgical Procedure: Fulkerson Osteotomy

This distal tubercle osteotomy is performed though a straight anterior skin incision from the midlateral patella to the distal aspect of the tibial tubercle. Under direct visualization a lateral retinacular release is performed, the patella everted, and the condition of the patellar articular surface assessed. The degree and pattern of damage to the patellar articular surface determine the degree of anteromedialization. The tubercle osteotomy is 5 to 8 cm long with the distal aspect tapering to 2 to 3 mm. The slope of the osteotomy dictates the amount of anteriorization. If no anteriorization is necessary, then the slope of the osteotomy is eliminated. Upon completing the osteotomy, the tibial tubercle is hinged distally and pushed medially up the tibial slope. Holding the tibial tubercle in the transposed position, the patella tracking is assessed and, if appropriate, the position is secured with two bicortical screws (Figure 15.2). Anteriorization of 12 to 15 mm is possible without supplemental bone graft. The wound is then closed in layers over a suction drain.

Following surgery, the knee is placed in a soft compressive dressing and CPM is started in the recovery room. The patient is allowed partial weight bearing with crutches for 6 weeks or until the osteotomy is healed.

TABLE 15.4 Complications with distal realignment procedures.
Fracture
Loss of fixation
Wound healing problems
Infection
Compartment syndrome
Avascular necrosis

Results

Fulkerson et al. have reported consistent long term results in patients carefully selected for anteromedialization; 93% of patients with patellofemoral pain and degenerative arthritis demonstrated excellent or good results. A 2-year study of 26 patients reported 89% good or excellent results, and 75% of patients with severe patellar arthritis had good results.[15] In a group of 11 patients observed for more than 5 years, 90% had stable results without evidence of deterioration.[16] Complications are attributable to error in surgical technique (Table 15.4).

PROXIMAL AND DISTAL REALIGNMENT

At times a proximal or distal realignment alone is not sufficient to correct patellar instability. Therefore, a combined procedure such as the Elmslie–Trillat procedure is indicated. The indications include (1) recurrent patellar subluxation or dislocation; (2) patellofemoral pain with malalignment of the extensor mechanism; (3) acute dislocation in the skeletally mature patient with malalignment of the extensor mecha-

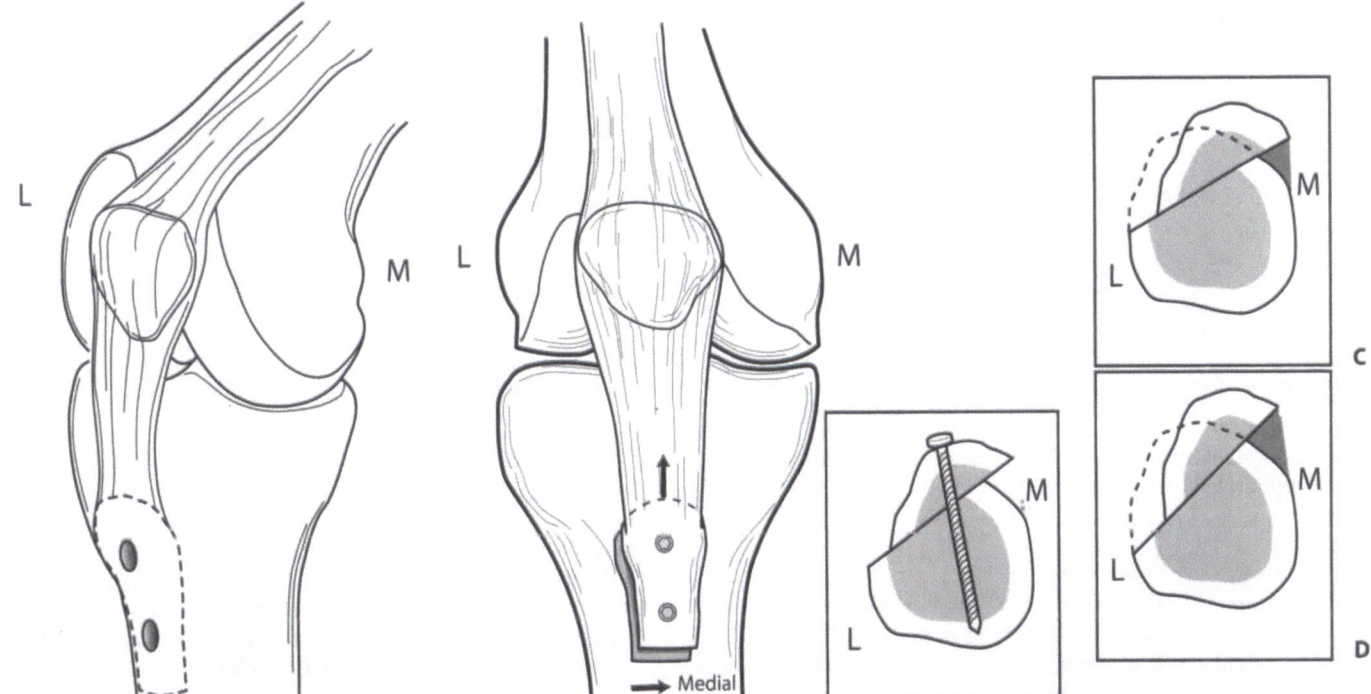

FIGURE 15.2 The Fulkerson distal realignment. **A, B.** Anteromedialization is obtained by an oblique osteotomy of the tibial tubercle. **C, D.** The slope of the osteotomy determines the degree of anteriorization.

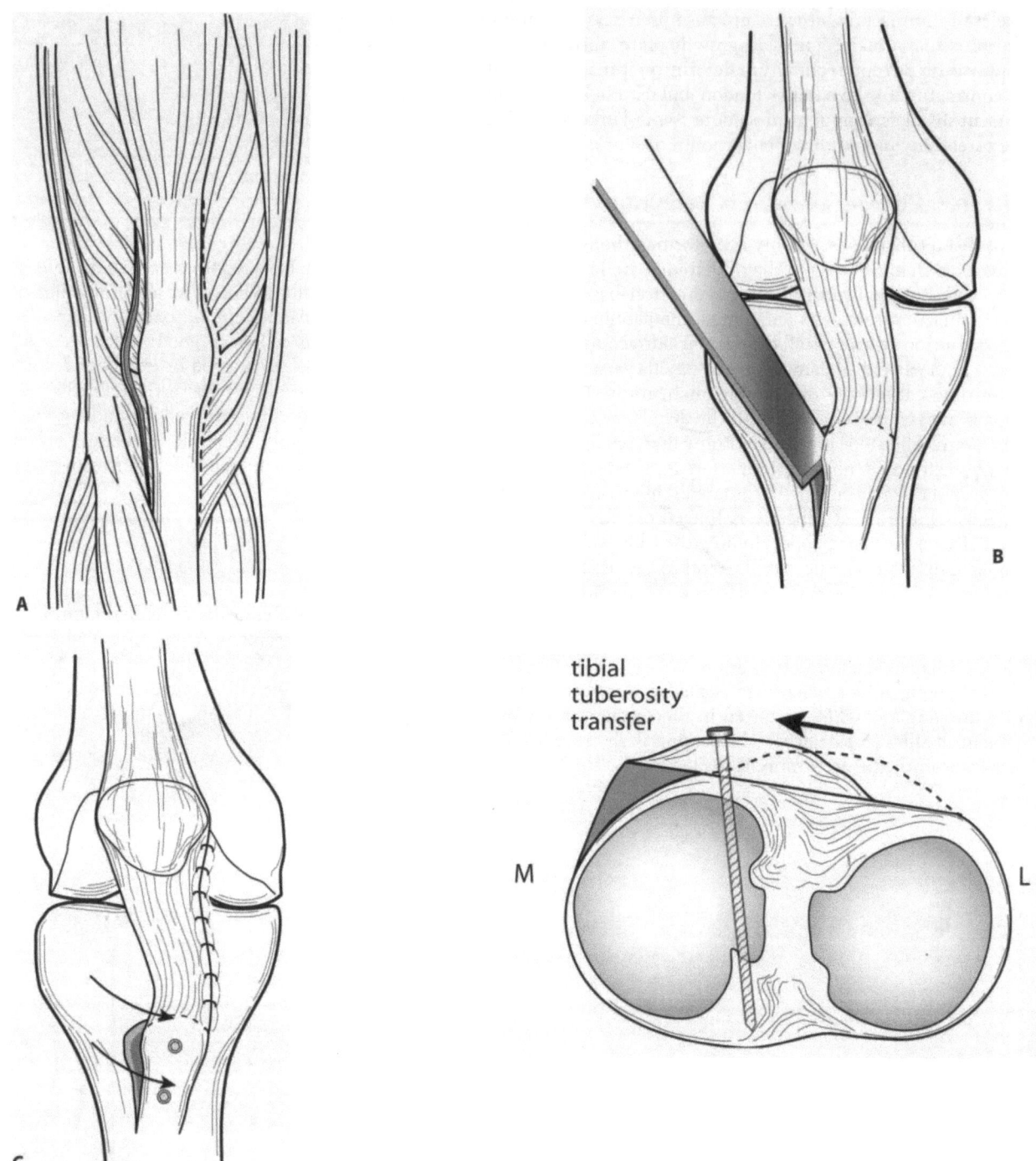

FIGURE 15.3 The Elmslie–Trillat procedure. **A.** Planned medial arthrotomy and lateral release. **B.** The tibial tubercle is osteotomized and transferred medially. **C.** The tibial tubercle is secured with two bicortical screws. **D.** Axial view of the medialized tubercle.

nism; and (4) failed prior proximal realignment with an abnormal tubercle sulcus angle.[13,17–19]

Surgical Technique: Elmslie–Trillat Procedure

The Elmslie–Trillat procedure realigns the patella medially with a tibial tubercle transfer, proximal realignment, and lateral retinacular release. An anterior midline skin incision exposes the extensor mechanism. Following a lateral retinacular release, a 4- to 6-cm osteotomy of the tibial tubercle is performed maintaining the distal attachment. The osteotomy is cut flat without any slope so that the transfer can be directed medially without any elevation of the tibial tubercle. To hinge the distal attachment, the plane of the osteotomy should thin out to 2 to 3 mm distally. The tibial tubercle is then rotated medially around its distal attachment and fixed to the anteromedial tibia with a screw. If this distal transfer is not sufficient to centralize the patella, then a proximal realignment is performed with lateral advancement of the vastus medialis and the medial retinaculum, similar to the foregoing description. In this new position, the patella should track in the femoral sulcus without tilt through a full range of motion (Figure 15.3). The wound is then closed in layers over a suction drain.

Following surgery, the knee is placed in a soft compressive dressing and CPM is started in the recovery room. The patient is allowed partial weight bearing with crutches for 6 weeks or until the osteotomy is healed.

Results

In a 2-year minimum follow-up study of 114 knees, DeBurge and Chambat[20] reported that 81% of the patients were satisfied and the redislocation rate was 1.7%. However, 19% of the patients were experiencing pain, which was attributed to the development of lateral patellofemoral degenerative arthritis. Radiographic evaluation on the Merchant view showed that 70% were well positioned, 11% were undercorrected with a residual lateral position, and 19% were overcorrected with medial subluxation. Cerullo et al. also reported that patients treated for patellar dislocation had a higher incidence of satisfactory results when compared to the subluxation group.

ACUTE PATELLA DISLOCATION

In the presence of an acute patellar dislocation, the medial retinaculum and the insertion of the vastus medialis may be torn and avulsed from the medial border of the patella, or the medial patellofemoral ligament may tear from its femoral origin on the adductor tubercle. In performing an open repair, a straight midline skin incision provides the best exposure for inspection of the extensor mechanism. Following a thorough inspection of the joint to remove any loose bony or chondral fragments, the medial retinaculum and vastus medialis are repaired to the medial border of the patella and quadriceps tendon with number 0 nonabsorbable sutures. A lateral retinacular release should also be performed to balance the extensor mechanism. Tensioning of the repair and closure of the defect is critical. The repair is placed in enough tension to balance the patella in the femoral sulcus through a full range of motion without tilt (Figure 15.4). Following wound closure

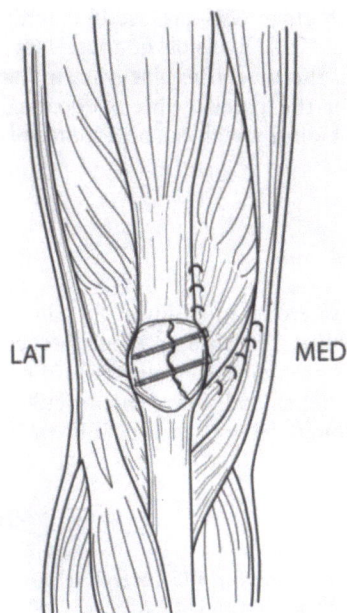

FIGURE 15.5 The large bone fragment is reattached to the patella and fixed with two bicortical screws.

over a suction drain, a light compressive dressing is applied. CPM and cryotherapy are initiated in the recovery room. The rehabilitation program is similar to the proximal realignment procedure that was described previously.

The need for anatomic repair of the medial patellofemoral ligament following an acute patella dislocation has been reported.[22] The vastus medialis obliquus muscle origin is repaired to the adductor magnus tendon using interrupted nonabsorbable sutures. The torn medial patellofemoral ligament is repaired to its stump on the adductor tubercle and adjacent fascia with nonabsorbable sutures. The patellar tracking is then assessed and the wound is closed in layers. Postoperatively, the knee is immobilized about 2 weeks until the patient has regained sufficient quadriceps function. The patient then begins active and passive range-of-motion exercises, as well as a strengthening program, and can return to sports when muscle strength is comparable to the contralateral side.

There are certain intraoperative situations that may require some modification in this technique. If a small osteochondral fragment from the medial border of the patella or odd facet has avulsed with the medial retinaculum, it should be excised and the medial retinaculum reattached to the medial border of the patella. This repair can be achieved by creating a small bone trough along the medial margin of the patella at the site of the avulsion and placing drill holes in the anterior cortex of the patella. Multiple number 0 nonabsorbable sutures are placed in the medial retinaculum and passed through the drill holes in the patella. As the sutures are tied, the medial retinaculum is secured to the patella. An alternative is to place multiple soft tissue anchors at the base of the bony trough and then secure the medial retinaculum to the patella.[13]

Another intraoperative problem is a large osteochondral fracture, which tends to include the medial and odd facet of the patella. Similar to a longitudinal fracture of the patella, it requires secure anatomic fixation. Once the open reduction is

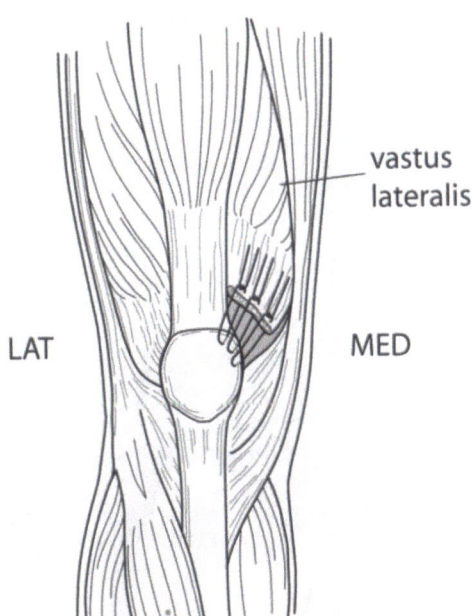

vastus lateralis

LAT   MED

FIGURE 15.4 The medial retinaculum is reattached to the patella.

performed, the fragments are secured with two bicortical screws (Figure 15.5). Excision of these large fragments and imbrication of the medial retinaculum may result in medial maltracking of the patella with overloading of the medial patellofemoral joint, which can be a source of continued post-operative pain.[13]

SUMMARY

There are numerous procedures for the management of patellar instability. Because no single procedure corrects all patellofemoral problems, a careful assessment of the etiology of the problem, the condition of the articular surface, and the level of patient activity should influence the course of treatment.

References

1. Merchant AC, Mercer RL. Lateral release of the patella: a preliminary report. Clin Orthop 1974;103:40–45.
2. Gecha SR, Torg JS. Clinical prognostications for the efficacy of retinacular release surgery to treat patellofemoral pain. Clin Orthop 1990;253:203–208.
3. Cushner FD, Scott WN. Arthroscopy of the patellofemoral joint. In: Scuderi, GR (ed) The Patella. New York: Springer-Verlag; 1995:201–221.
4. Aglietti P, Pisaneschi A, Buzzi R, et al. Arthroscopic lateral release for patellar pain or instability. Arthroscopy 1989;5:176–183.
5. Dzioba RB. Diagnostic arthroscopy and longitudinal open lateral release: a four year follow-up study to determine predictors of surgical outcome. Am J Sports Med 1990;18:343–348.
6. Henry JH, Goletz TH, Williamson B. Lateral retinacular release in patellar subluxation. Indications, results and comparison to open patellofemoral reconstruction. Am J Sports Med 1986;14:121–129.
7. Bullek DD, Kelly MA. Management of patellofemoral arthritis. In: Scuderi, GR (ed) The Patella. New York: Springer-Verlag; 1995:291–308.
8. Jackson RW, Kunkel SS, Taylor GJ. Lateral retinacular release for patellofemoral pain in the older patient. Arthroscopy 1991;7:283–286.
9. Insall J, Bullough PG, Burstein AH. Proximal "tube" realignment of the patella for chondromalacia patellae. Clin Orthop 1979;244:63–69.
10. Insall JN, Aglietti P, Tria AJ. Patellar pain and incongruence. II. Clinical application. Clin Orthop 1983;176:225–232.
11. Scuderi G, Cuomo F, Scott WN. Lateral release and proximal realignment for patellar subluxation and dislocation. J Bone Joint Surg 1988;70A:856–861.
12. Abraham E, Washington E, Huang TL. Insall proximal realignment for disorders of the patella. Clin Orthop 1989;248:61–65.
13. Scuderi GR. Surgical Management of Patellar Instability. In Scuderi, GR (ed) The Patella. New York: Springer-Verlag; 1995:223–245.
14. Post WR, Fulkerson JP. Distal realignment of the patellofemoral joint: Indications, effects, results and recommendations. Orthop Clin North Am 1992;23:631–643.
15. Fulkerson JP. Anteromedialization of the tibial tuberosity for patellofemoral malalignment. Clin Orthop 1983;177:176–181.
16. Fulkerson JP, Becker GJ, Meaney JA, et al. Anteromedial tibial tubercle transfer without bone graft. Am J Sports Med 1990;18:490–497.
17. Cox JS. Evaluation of the Roux–Elmslie–Trillat procedure for knee extensor alignment. Am J Sports Med 1982;10:303–310.
18. Cox JS. An evaluation of the Elmslie–Trillat procedure for management of patellar dislocations and subluxation. A preliminary report. Am J Sports Med 1976;4:72–77.
19. Trillat A, DeJour H, Couette A. Diagnostic et traitement des sublux-recidivates de la rotule. Rev Chir Orthop Reparatrice Appar Mot 1979;50:185–191.
20. Deburge A, Chambat P. La transposition de la tuberosite tibiale anterieure. Rev Chir Orthop Reparatrice Appar Mot 1980;66:218.
21. Cerullo G, Puddu G, Conteduca F, et al. Evaluation of the results of extensor mechanism reconstruction. Am J Sports Med 1988;16:93–98.
22. Ahmad CS, Stein BES, Matuz D, Henry JH. Immediate surgical repair of the medial patellar stabilizers for acute patellar dislocation. A review of eight cases. Am J Sports Medicine 2000;28:804–810.

16

Emerging Technologies in Cartilage Repair

Daniel A. Grande

BACKGROUND

The long-held axiom in orthopaedic science as put forth by Hunter in 1743, that cartilage once injured is incapable of healing, has been essentially refuted by the technique of autologous chondrocyte transplantation. This conceptual change in the way orthopaedic surgeons approach the problem of cartilage repair has spawned a myriad of new and innovative treatment modalities. This chapter focuses on the new techniques and directions researchers are exploring in their efforts to perfect restoration of a functional articular surface.

CELL SEEDED APPROACHES TO CARTILAGE REPAIR

The original work published by our group described the use of autologous culture-expanded chondrocytes[1] as the principal method of cell-based cartilage repair, which is currently practiced today and marketed by Genzyme Biosurgery (Cambridge, MA, USA). This technique was later repeated in human patients with similar successful results.[2] Thus, the concept of using cells as the basis for effecting cartilage repair is well founded in the biologic principle that they are the machines effectively synthesizing the extracellular matrix and able to maintain the integrity of the matrix. It is therefore not surprising that a number of groups have concentrated their efforts on incorporating cells as part of their strategies. Of particular note are the attempts to reconstitute cartilage tissue without any scaffold material at all. These approaches utilize the cellular synthetic machinery alone to engineer a new cartilage tissue. Specialized media and different perfusion methods are incorporated to culture cartilage tissue that can be then implanted into cartilage defects without the use of any biomaterial scaffolds.[3,4]

Methods for actually obtaining good in situ fixation as well as incorporation with host tissue remain to be determined. The key disadvantage of actually "manufacturing" a piece of cartilage tissue is that it is not much different from a piece of donor allograft cartilage. Integration of cell-based tissue constructs with the host recipient remains a difficult challenge in this area of research. The most intriguing and innovative aspect regarding the work by Adkisson et al.[3] is that it was counterintuitive to that traditionally performed in tissue-engineered approaches to cartilage. Instead of feeding these cell cultures with complete medium containing all the required nutrients, they weaned these cultures to a serum-free and nutrient-starved type of media, which resulted in a superior cartilage tissue with a high collagen and aggrecan content, especially when compared with cells grown under conditions containing typical serum and nutrient levels.

A number of different and innovative approaches have utilized not only differentiated chondrocytes as cells for repair but also cells from a variety of different cell compartments and levels of chondrogenic differentiation. The most widely used cell type other then chondrocytes are marrow-derived mesenchymal stem cells (MSCs), originally described by Caplan.[5] Various stem cells with mesenchymal potential from other tissue compartments, such as skeletal muscle,[6] adipose tissue,[7] periosteum,[8] perichondrium,[9] and most recently the synovial membrane, have also recently been identified.[10]

The primary advantage of using undifferentiated stem cells over chondrocytes is that one does not need to harvest good-quality articular cartilage and thus destroy more articular cartilage at the risk of repairing another damaged site. Furthermore, in theory these stem cells are taken from tissue that is able to easily replenish the cell number without ill effect. Under ideal conditions, these stem cells will differentiate into cartilage under the proper local cuing. In some instances, differentiation may require special media supplements to "push" a cell down a chondrocyte lineage or an idealized geometric orientation or surface treatment.[11,12]

TISSUE ENGINEERING AND SCAFFOLD APPROACHES

Scaffold design as related to cartilage growth and differentiation has been the focus of a number of reports. In addition to the widely utilized polyanhydrides such as polyglycolic acid (PGA) and polylactic acid (PLA), a number of new materials are being developed. Chondroinduction of mouse mesenchymal stem cells was demonstrated using a highly porous polyvinyl formal (PVF) resin.[13] Scaffolds fabricated from chitosan hold potential promise and have recently been shown to have no significant immunologic respons in spite of their invertebrate origins.[14] There is also a trend toward hybrid types of scaffolds such as coating various materials with biologic components to render them more biocompatible or potentially chondroinductive. For instance, porous scaffolds made from a biodegradable copolymer of trimethylene carbonate and glycolide were coated with fibronectin,[15] which resulted in better ingrowth of cells into the porous scaffolds.

In a similar fashion, hyaluronic acid has been used in conjunction with collagen sponges. Chondrocytes cultured with a concentration as low as 2% (w/w) expressed a fourfold increase in collagen type II mRNA expression.[16] Studies have also demonstrated the feasibility of improved methods of incorporating hyaluronic acid within type II collagen sponges by direct cross-linking.[17] Hyaluronic acid scaffolds have been used as vehicles for delivery of important chondroinductive proteins[18] such as bone morphogenic protein 2 (BMP-2).

Scaffolds that are viscoelastic in nature, as compared to classic solid materials of which we usually think for cartilage tissue engineering, also have potential clinical applications. Development of a photopolymerizing hydrogel system can provide an efficient method to encapsulate chondrocytes and localize them within a defect in a clinically relevant manner.[19] This technology would have broad applications for growth factor and drug delivery as well as local cell delivery. Viscous or liquid types of scaffolds such as alginate can even be molded into highly complex shapes for use in certain anatomic regions.[20] Changing the ratios of components can add new and stronger material properties to the hydrogels.[21] Novel hydrogels made from oligopolyethylene—glycol fumarate can be custom made to have a range of material properties depending on the application desired.[22] Hydrogel properties can also influence extracellular matrix (ECM) production by photoencapsulated chondrocytes using different equilibrium swelling ratios.[23] Fibrin has been well explored as a method for holding various cells and molecules in situ.[24] Steps to actually deliver the cells as injectable cell-fibrin composites have also met with success.[25,26]

In addition to the plethora of new materials and composites used for tissue engineering scaffolds, new concepts and techniques to manufacture these scaffolds are being actively investigated. Li et al.[27] have fabricated a novel electrospun nanofibrous structure made from polylactic-co-glycolic acid (PLGA) fibers ranging from 500 to 800 nm in diameter that features morphologic similarity to the ECM of natural tissues with a wide range of pore-size distribution. Scaffold pore size is a key parameter in the success of various scaffolds, either allowing proper cell infiltration throughout the matrix or inhibiting migration to cause cell clumping at the scaffold surfaces and cell free spaces within the interior. When implanted into cartilage defects, such scaffolds typically result in fibrous tissue repair (unpublished data). Limited studies have attempted to define an optimum pore size for the application of cartilage repair[28] and more work is needed. Many investigators agree on a range of 100 to 200 μm.

Bioreactor systems for culturing cartilage tissue constructs can grow a greater quantity of cartilage tissue in a shorter time than is possible with static culture. Additionally, the cartilage construct contains significantly higher levels of aggrecan and collagen than those constructs grown under static tissue culture conditions.[29] Medium perfusion has been shown to stimulate more rapid deposition of matrix components.[30] Although the material and chemical properties of bioreactor-grown cartilage constructs appear to be superior to statically cultured cartilage constructs, there are drawbacks to this approach in the application of articular resurfacing. The well-developed cartilage does not readily incorporate with host (native) articular cartilage. Similarly, cartilage with a high degree of aggrecan resists vascular invasion and remodeling in the region of the subchondral bone. Bioreactor-grown cartilage may find its most useful niche in the field of plastic surgery.

GROWTH FACTORS, GENE THERAPY, TISSUE ENGINEERING AND COMBINATION THERAPY

Recent work by our laboratory and others has further elaborated on the theme of combining methods of gene therapy with tissue engineering. We have recently demonstrated transduction of periosteal cells with the gene for bone morphogenetic protein 7 (BMP-7), when seeded onto PGA scaffolds, can be effectively used to repair defects in articular cartilage[31] (Figure 16.1). In continuation of that work[32] a method was developed whereby a bilayer approach using insulin-like growth factor I (IGF-I)-transduced cells within scaffolds were placed to address cartilage repair at the surface (cartilage layer) and cells transduced by BMP-7 seeded in scaffolds were placed in the subchondral bone region. This method resulted in rapid bone repair in the subchondral region coupled with rapid hyaline cartilage repair in the articular surface layer. Recent work in our laboratory has incorporated the gene for the sonic hedgehog articulated periosteal cell line. We have observed complete restoration of cartilage defects using this gene, with hyaline cartilage of impressive quality. However, there would appear to be a persistence of the cartilage tissue in areas normally remodeled into subchondral bone. These results suggest that introduction of potent developmental genes can lead to untoward results in attempts at perfecting a natural development process.

Other laboratories have shown adenoviral transfer of chondrocytes with the gene for transforming growth factor beta (TGF-β).[33] This potent growth factor has tremendous therapeutic potential for cartilage repair and was shown to increase proteoglycan and collagen production in a dose-dependent manner. Its role in cartilage repair using this method is still not known. A natural extension of the attempt to promote rapid high-quality cartilage repair is the local introduction of growth factors known to be anabolic for chondrocytes or chondroinductive in some manner. The methods primarily investigated to date have been the direct pharmacologic approach whereby the growth factor is delivered directly or by time release in some type of polymer, natural or synthetic, into the local defect environment. IGF-I has received significant interest because of its known anabolic properties on the matrix synthetic apparatus of articular chondrocytes.[24] IGF-I also shows constitutive levels of expression that increases in regions of cartilage immediately adja-

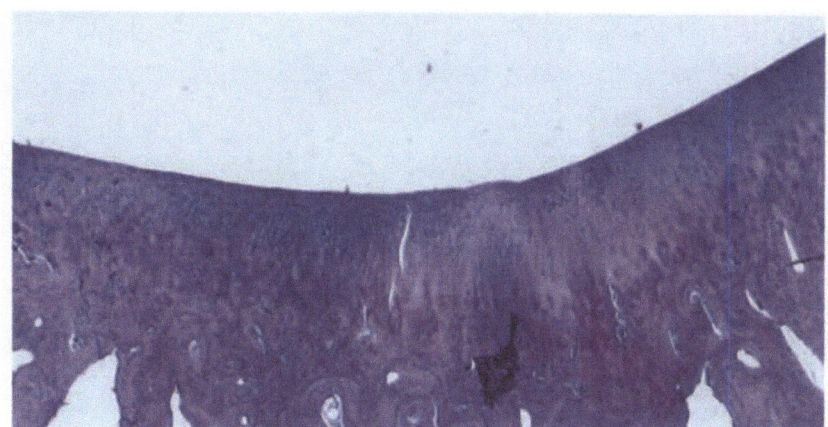

FIGURE 16.1 Histological view of cartilage surface repaired using a cell seed PGA scaffold containing cells transduced with the BMP-7 gene. (×100 orig. mag. H&E stain.)

cent to defects following cartilage injury,[34] leading to speculation of its importance in cartilage wound repair. This molecule has also been demonstrated to promote mesenchymal stem cells toward cartilage differentiation under different in vitro conditions.[35] A promising new growth factor is the growth and differentiation factor 5 (GDF-5), which acts early in development[36] and may be useful in directing early chondrogenesis either alone or in combination with gene therapy. It should also be appreciated that growth factors may have a differential effect on tissue-engineered cartilage, that may not be true in the native situation.[37]

One of the most promising new molecules with significant clinical implications in cartilage repair is the novel synthetic thrombin peptide 508 or TP-508. It is a simple 28-amino-acid fragment of the thrombin molecule with mitogenic effects on stem cells without any of the fibrinogenic activities of the complete molecule. Work done in our laboratory with the rabbit, as well as in others, has shown that when delivered within poly-L-lactic acid (PLLA) microspheres at total dosages between 10 and 50 μg within a 3 mm cartilage defect, rapid repair of cartilage defects can be achieved[38] (Figure 16.2). The de novo cartilage is hyaline-like in its appearance and the cartilage surfaces are completely restored. Current investigations are underway to provide efficient and reproducible in vivo delivery. The importance of this molecule is that, compared with all the various complicated technologies discussed in this chapter, the application of a single simple peptide was able to obtain a result equal to or better than any of these more costly approaches. The lesser cost of management of cartilage lesions with an effective off-the-shelf device would revolutionize orthopaedic surgery.

Coupled with the aforementioned emerging approaches designed to simplify and lower the cost of treatment of orthopaedic lesions is the general emphasis recently placed upon methods that do not incorporate cells at all but are driven solely by the use of specialized biomaterial scaffolds. An implantable scaffold that by nature of its geometry or material properties could be used as an effective "off the shelf" repair device is a hotly researched area for both commercial and academic groups. One key question that remains unresolved as it relates to clinical orthopaedics is exactly what is an acceptable clinical endpoint or result. For instance, academic scientists constantly strive to repair cartilage that is

completely hyaline in its biochemical and biomechanical properties, a highly ambitious goal given the nature of the clinical problem.

However, the clinical scientist who routinely treats these lesions is faced with the daunting task of what to do at the moment he is within the joint addressing a significant cartilage lesion. The available methods such as microfracture, abrasion and other techniques that involve bringing vascular access to the joint space eventually result in clinical sequelae in which the patient appears to function clinically with less pain. Thus, the concept of placing into the defect a material or scaffold that ideally is off the shelf and readily available and which can serve to augment the known reparative response that will occur, is becoming an acceptable alternative to the more expensive and complex techniques covered in this chapter. One of the more promising biomaterial scaffold materials, which has already been granted U.S. Food and Drug Administration (FDA) approval for shoulder repair, is porcine-derived small intestine submucosa (SIS). Work by Cook and coworkers[39] has shown tremendous utility for this natural biomaterial in repair of the meniscus. A different configuration of the material may be used in a similar fashion for articular cartilage. Work by Grande et al.[40] (Figure 16.3) and Slivka et al.,[41] and Athanasiou et al.[42] has actively developed PLGA composite materials designed to allow cell infiltration and migration from the host tissue. Other groups have investigated the use of hyaluronic acid as an implantable scaffold.[43] This method essentially takes advantage of what we term the extrinsic repair response and attempts to organize it into a reliable repair tissue. Although it may not have all the composition of hyaline cartilage, it can function as a bearing surface for a period of perhaps 5 to 10 years and thus it merits strong consideration in clinically delaying the need for total joint replacement.

SUMMARY AND CONCLUSIONS

From this overview, it is apparent that a significant research as well as economic effort is focused on addressing the clinical problem of cartilage repair. It is apparent cell-based therapies such as autologous chondrocyte transplantation are currently the leading, and thus driving, technologies for clinical use. However, recent events such as the recent FDA

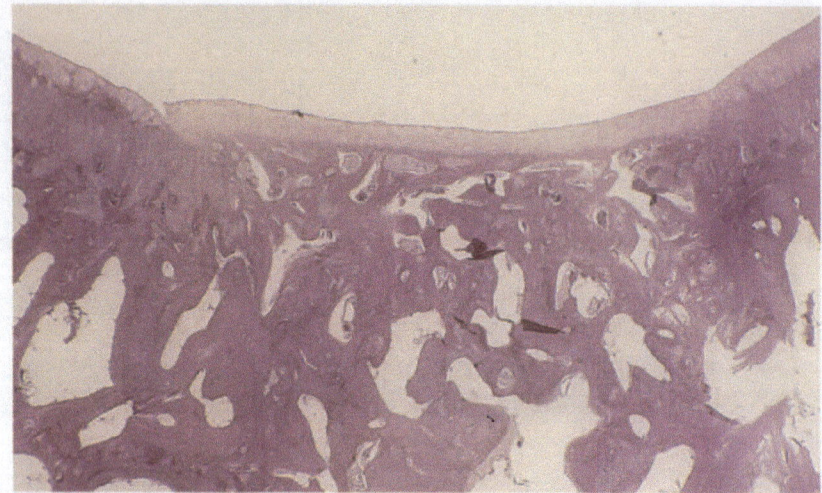

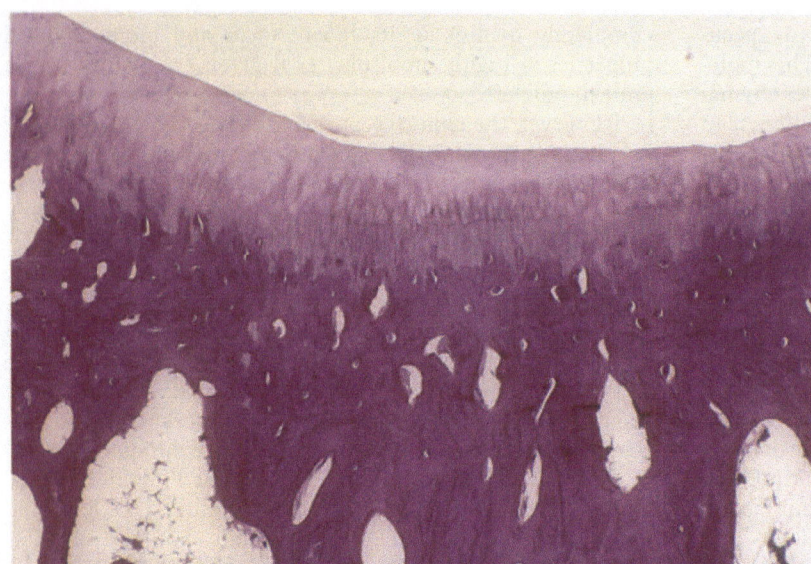

FIGURE 16.2 A. Histological results of cartilage defect in a rabbit knee not treated (empty control). **B.** Defect similar to A treated with 10 ug of TP-508. Both are at 8 weeks postoperative. (×40 orig. mag. H&E stain.)

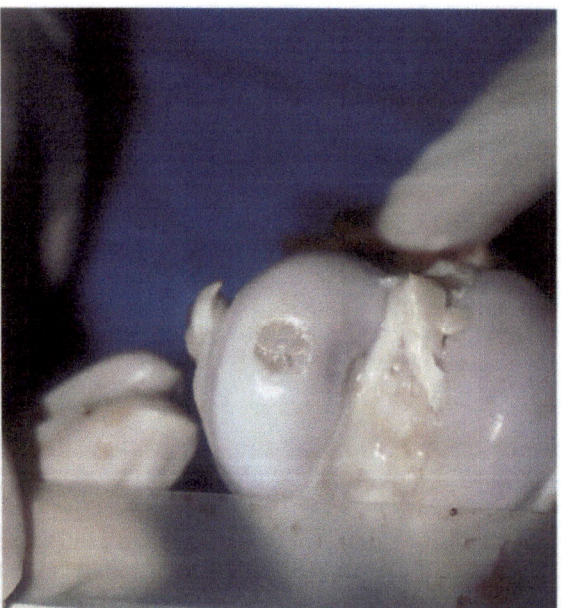
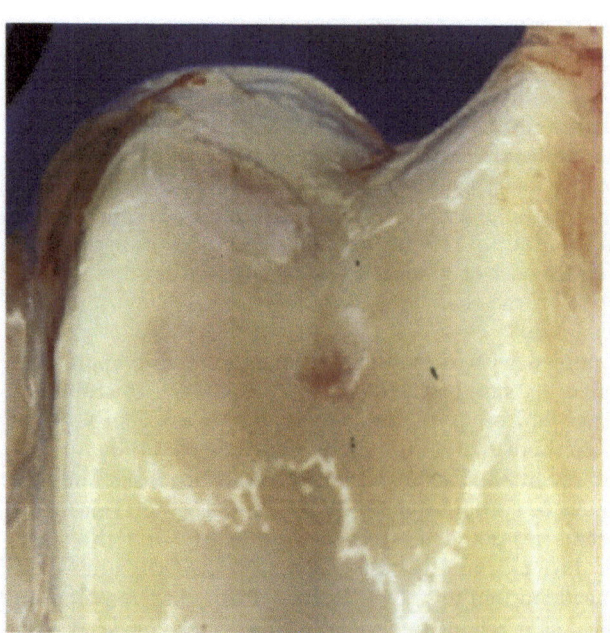

FIGURE 16.3 Macroscopic views of two goat knee joints treated with scaffolds made of PLGA without any cell seeding prior to implantation. This was developed to be used at time of surgery. **A** is a view of the MFC at 3 weeks. **B** is at 6 weeks.

approval of BMP-2 for spine fusion points the way to technologies that will be growth factor and device driven and, thus, "off the shelf" type technologies. Factors such as TP-508 coupled with some of the novel bioabsorbable scaffold materials are most likely the next generation of treatment options in the orthopaedist's armamentarium.

GLOSSARY

PGA: Polyglycolic acid is often used as a matrix or scaffold material for culturing cells in a three-dimensional environment. Its relative degradative half-life is approximately 2 weeks.

PLA: Poly-L-lactic acid is used as a scaffold for tissue engineering similarly to PGA. Its degradation time is much longer, on the order of 6 months to 1 year.

BMP-7: Bone morphogenetic protein-7 has been linked to a variety of regulatory processes and also supports ectopic cartilage and bone formation. It also plays a role in differentiation, development, and physiologic tissue development.

BMP-2: Bone morphogenetic protein-2 is important in osteogenic differentiation and may stimulate adipogenesis as well as osteogenesis. It also plays a role in differentiation, development, and physiologic tissue development.

IGF-1: Insulin-like growth factor-1 is important as an anabolic regulator of cartilage metabolism and may play a role in bone reformation.

Transduction: The transfer of genetic material from one organism to another.

Scaffold: A three-dimensional biomaterial growing environment or matrix.

Bioreactor: A closed culture system for growing tissue-engineered constructs.

TGF-β: Transforming growth factor beta-1 stimulates bone metabolism and may be a factor in bone fracture repair as well as cartilage formation.

GDF-5: Growth and differentiation factor-5 is involved in the growth and development of cartilage.

References

1. Grande D, Pitman M, Peterson L, Menche D, Klein M. The repair of experimentally produced defects in rabbit articular cartilage by autologous chondrocyte transplantation. J Orthop Res 1989;7:208–214.
2. Brittberg M, Lindahl A, Nilsson A, et al. Treatment of deep cartilage defects in the knee with autologous chondrocyte transplantation. N Engl J Med 1994;331:889.
3. Adkisson DH IV, Gillsi MP, Davis EC, Maloney W, Hruska K. In vitro generation of scaffold independent neocartilage. Clin Orthop 2001;39(suppl):1S.
4. Boyle J, Luan B, Cruz TF, Kandel RA. Characterization of proteoglycan accumulation during formation of cartilaginous tissue in vitro osteoarthritis. Cartilage 1995;3:117–125.
5. Caplan AI. Mesenchymal stem cells. J Orthop Res 1991;9:641–650.
6. Grande DA, Southerland SS, Manji R, Schwartz RE, Lucas PA. Repair of articular cartilage defects using mesenchymal stem cells. Tissue Eng 1995;1(4):345–353.
7. Erickson G, Franklin D, Gimble J, Guilak F. Adipose tissue-derived stromal cells display a chrondrogenic phenotype in culture. Trans Orthop Res Soc 2001;198.
8. O'Driscoll S, Marx R, Beaton D, Miura Y, Gallay S, Fitzsimmons J. Validation of a simple histological-histochemical cartilage scoring system. Tissue Eng 2001;7:313.
9. Coutts R, Woo S, Amiel D, von Shroeder HP, Kwan M. Rib perichondrial autografts in full thickness articular cartilage defects in rabbits. Clin Orthop Res 1992;275:263–273.
10. DeBari C, Dell'Accio F, Tylzanowski P, Luyten F. Multipotent mesenchymal stem cells from adult human synovial membrane. Arthritis Rheum 2001;44:8.
11. Papadaki M, Mahmood T, Gupta P, et al. The different behaviors of skeletal muscle cells and chondrocytes on PEGT/PBT block copolymers are related to the surface properties of the substrate. J Biomed Mater Res 2001;54:47.
12. Martin I, Shastri V, Padera R, et al. Selective differentiation of mammalian bone marrow stromal cells cultured on three dimensional polymer foams. J Biomed Mater Res 2001;55:229.
13. Aung T, Miyoshi H, Tun T, Ohshima N. Chondroinduction of mouse mesenchymal stem cells in three-dimensional highly porous matrix scaffolds. J Biomed Mater Res 2002;61:75.
14. VandeVord P, Matthew H, DeSilva S, Mayton L, Wu B, Wooley P. Evaluation of the biocompatibility of a chitosan scaffold in mice. J Biomed Mater Res 2001;59:585.
15. Bhati R, Mukherjee D, McCarthy K, Rogers S, Smith S, Shalaby S. The growth of chondrocytes into a fibronectin-coated biodegradable scaffold. J Biomed Mater Res 2001;56:74.
16. Alleman F, Mizuno S, Eid K, Yates KE, Zaleske D, Glowacki J. Effects of hyaluronan on engineered articular cartilage extracellular gene expression in 3-dimensional collagen scaffolds. J Biomed Mater Res 2001;55:13–19.
17. Taguchi T, Ikoma T, Tanaka J. An improved method to prepare hyaluronic acid and type II collagen composite matrices. J Biomed Mater Res 2002;61:330.
18. Kim H, Valentini R. Retention and activity of BMP-2 in hyaluronic acid based scaffolds in vitro. J Biomed Mater Res 2002;59:573.
19. Elisseeff J, Mcintosh W, Anseth K, Riley S, Langer R. Photoencapsulation of chondrocytes in poly(ethylene oxide)-based semi-interpenetrating networks. J Biomed Mater Res 2000;51:164.
20. Chang S, Rowler J, Tobias G, et al. Injection molding of chondrocyte/alginate constructs in the shape of facial implants. J Biomed Mater Res 2001;55:503.
21. Wong M, Siegrist M, Wang X, Hunziker E. Development of mechanically stable alginate/chondrocyte constructs: effects of guluronic acid content and matrix synthesis. J Orthop Res 2001;19:493.
22. Temenoff K, Athanasiou K, LeBaron R, Mikos A. Effect of poly(ethylene glycol) molecular weight on tensile swelling properties of oligo(poly(ethylene glycol)fumarate) hydrogens for cartilage tissue engineering. J Biomed Mater Res 2002;59:429.
23. Bryant S, Anseth K. Hydrogel properties influence ECM production of chondrocytes photoencapsulated in poly(ethylene glycol) hydrogels. J Biomed Mater Res 2002;59:63.
24. Nixon A, Saxer R, Brower-Toland B. Exogenous insulin-like growth factor-I stimulates an autoinductive IGF-I autocrine/paracrine response in chondrocytes. J Orthop Res 2001;19:26.
25. Passaretti D, Silverman R, Huang W, et al. Cultured chondrocytes produce injectable tissue-engineered cartilage in hydrogel polymer. Tissue Eng 2001;7:805.

26. Perka C, Arnold U, Spitzer R, Lindenhayn K. The use of fibrin beads for tissue engineering and subsequential transplantation. Tissue Eng 2001;7:359.

27. Li W-J, Laurencin C, Caterson E, Tuan R, Ko F. Electrospun nanofibrous structure: a novel scaffold for tissue engineering. J Biomed Mater Res 2002;60:613.

28. Bhardwaj T, Pilliar R, Grynpas M, Kandel R. Effect of material geometry on cartilaginous tissue formation in vitro. J Biomed Mater Res 2001;57:190.

29. Vunjak-Novakovic G, Martin I, Obradovic B, et al. Bioreactor cultivation conditions modulate the composite and mechanical properties of tissue-engineered cartilage. J Orthop Res 1999; 17:130–138

30. Mizuno S, Allemann F, Glowacki J. Effects of medium perfusion on matrix production by bovine chondrocytes in three dimensional collagen sponges. J Biomed Mater Res 2001;56:368.

31. Mason J, Breitbart AS, Barcia M, Porti D, Pergolizzi R, Grande DA. Cartilage and bone regeneration using gene-enhanced tissue engineering. Clin Orthop Res 2000;379(suppl):S171–S178.

32. Grande DA, Tomin A, Mason JM, Wollowick AL, Garone E, Lane J. A dual gene therapy approach to osteochondral defect repair using a bilayer implant containing BMP-7 and IGF-1 transduced periosteal cells. Trans Orthop Res Soc 2001.

33. Shuler F, Georgescu H, Niyibizi C, et al. Increased matrix synthesis following adenoviral transfer of a transforming growth factor β1 gene into articular chondrocytes. J Orthop Res 2000;18:585.

34. Fortier L, Balkman C, Sandell L, Ratcliffe A, Nixon A. Insulin-like growth factor-I gene expression patterns during spontaneous repair of acute articular cartilage injury. J Orthop Res 2001;19:720.

35. Worster A, Brower-Toland B, Fortier L, Bent S, Williams J, Nixon A. Chondrocytic differentiation of mesenchymal stem cells sequentially exposed to transforming growth factor-β1 in monolayer and insulin-like growth factor-I in a three dimensional matrix. J Orthop Res 2001;19:738.

36. Mikic B, Schalet B, Clark R, Gaschen V, Hunziker E. GDF-5 deficiency in mice alters the ultrastructure, mechanical properties and composition of the achilles tendon. J Orthop Res 2001; 19:365.

37. Blunk TM, Sieminski A, Gooch K, et al. Differential effects of growth factors on tissue-engineered cartilage. Tissue Eng 2002;8:73.

38. Grande D, Karnaugh RD, Ryaby JT, et al. In vivo evaluation of the synthetic thrombin peptide, TP508, in articular cartilage repair. Trans Orthop Res Soc 2002;447.

39. Cook J, Tomlinson J, Arnoczky S, Fox D, Cook C, Kreeger J. Kinetic study of the replacement of porcine small intestinal submucosa rafts and the regeneration of meniscal-like tissue in large avascular meniscal defects in dogs. Tissue Eng 2001;7:321.

40. Grande DA, Halberstadt C, Schwartz R, Lingben Z, Linton J, Naughton G. Evaluation of matrix scaffolds for tissue engineering of articular cartilage grafts. J Biomed Mater Res 1997; 34(2):211–220.

41. Slivka MA, Leathebury NC, Kieswetter K, Niederauer GG. Porous, resorbable, fiber-reinforced scaffold tailored for articular cartilage repair. Tissue Eng 2001;7:6.

42. Athanasiou K, Schmitz JP, Agrawal CM. The effects of porosity on in vitro degradation of polyactic acid-polyglycolic acid implants used in repair of articular cartilage. Tissue Eng 1995;4:299.

43. Solchaga L, Dennis J, Goldberg V, Caplan A. Hyaluronic acid-based polymers as cell carriers for tissue-engineered repair of bone and cartilage. J Orthop Res 1999;17:205–213

17

Unicondylar Arthroplasty

R. Michael Meneghini and Mitchell B. Sheinkop

BACKGROUND

Isolated unicompartmental arthritis of the knee is often a therapeutic challenge. Preservation of the unaffected compartments was thought to be essential by Duncan McKeever, who performed the first unicompartmental knee arthroplasty in 1952.[1] In 1973, Marmor reported his initial experience with the unicompartmental replacement, composed of a stainless steel femoral component and a polyethylene tibial component.[2] Since then, the unicompartmental knee arthroplasty has been controversial, primarily because a few early studies reported discouraging results.[3,4] In 1976, Insall and Walker reported 30% poor results in unicompartmental replacement; however, more than half the patients in the study had undergone a concomitant patellectomy.[3] In a 2-year follow-up study on the Marmor modular knee replacement in 1978, Lasker reported a 22% revision rate. Thin polyethylene inserts and overcorrection of angular deformity contributed to the high rate of failure in this series.[4]

High tibial osteotomy and unicompartmental knee arthroplasty have been debated as the most appropriate treatment for the younger, active patient with isolated unicompartmental disease of the knee. Broughton et al. reported superior results and fewer complications in unicompartmental arthroplasty when compared to high tibial osteotomy.[5] The two groups were reevaluated at 12- to 17-year follow-up, with a much higher revision rate in the osteotomy group.[6] Scott and Santore reported their initial results of unicondylar arthroplasty and noted improved pain relief and fewer postoperative complications when compared to high tibial osteotomy.[7] Furthermore, conversion of a high tibial osteotomy to a total knee arthroplasty is associated with increased postoperative morbidity such as infection and patellar tendon rupture when compared to conversion of a unicondylar replacement to a total knee arthroplasty.[8]

Despite improved outcomes and few postoperative complications, many surgeons are reluctant to perform a unicompartmental knee arthroplasty in young patients with an active lifestyle. Engh and McAuley reported a subset of unicompartmental knee arthroplasties in patients between 40 and 60 years of age.[9] After accounting for failures resulting from excessively thin polyethylene, they reported an acceptable 86% survivorship rate at 7 years.[9] Unicompartmental arthroplasty appears to be an acceptable option in young, active patients over age 45 when a polyethylene of adequate thickness is utilized.

In the properly selected patient, unicompartmental knee replacement has advantages over total knee arthroplasty. Preservation of the cruciate ligaments and patellofemoral articulation in unicompartmental arthroplasty allows maintenance of a normal gait and quadriceps mechanism with a closer return to preoperative knee flexion when compared to total knee arthroplasty.[10,11] Furthermore, patients who received a unicondylar and a total knee arthroplasty during the same hospitalization report a subjectively better knee with increased range of motion in the knee with the unicompartmental arthroplasty.[12] Unicompartmental knee arthroplasty is also associated with shorter hospital stays, fewer serious complications, improved ambulatory function, and less cost than total knee arthroplasty.[13,14]

An additional advantage of unicompartmental knee arthroplasty is preservation of native bone stock. Reports of revision surgery for unicompartmental knee arthroplasty demonstrate that the simplicity and complications compare favorably with those for total knee arthroplasty.[15,16] Levine et al. corroborated these results following failed unicompartmental knee arthroplasty and reported early results comparable to primary total knee arthroplasty.[17] Preservation of bone stock, maintenance of near-normal knee kinematics and ease of revision makes unicompartmental arthroplasty an attractive option for patients with isolated medial or lateral compartment degenerative disease.

INDICATIONS

Proper patient selection is critical to the successful outcome of unicondylar knee arthroplasty. The indication for a unicompartmental knee replacement is osteoarthritis or osteonecrosis, isolated to the medial or lateral compartment without any evidence of patellofemoral disease. Furthermore, the uninvolved and patellofemoral compartments should exhibit no more than grade 2 chondromalacia[18] inspection at

TABLE 17.1   Indications and contraindications for unicompartmental arthroplasty.

Indications	Contraindications
Isolated medial or lateral compartment arthrosis	Inflammatory arthropathy
Grade 2 or less chondromalacia of opposite and patellofemoral compartments	Grade 3 or more chondromalacia of opposite or patellofemoral compartments
Weight less than 91 kg (200 lb)	Weight greater than 91 kg (200 lb)
Age greater than 60 years	Age less than 40 years or heavy laborer
Knee flexion greater than 90°	Knee flexion limited to less than 90°
Knee flexion contracture less than 10°	Knee flexion contracture 10° or greater
Varus angular deformity less than 10°	Severe varus or valgus angular deformity
Valgus angular deformity less than 15°	Absent anterior cruciate ligament
Intact anterior cruciate ligament	Ligamentous instability or subluxation

the time of index unicompartmental arthroplasty. Kozinn and Scott have documented strict selection criteria for unicompartmental knee arthroplasty.[19] The ideal candidate should be at least 60 years of age and not perform heavy labor. Additionally, the senior author believes the patient should weigh less than 82 kg (180 lbs). The patient should have at least 90° of knee flexion preoperatively and a flexion contracture of 10° or less. The preoperative angular deformity of the knee is an important consideration, and the patient should demonstrate less than 10° of varus or less than 15° of valgus. These strict selection criteria serve as a guideline, as a patient who satisfies all but one or two of these criteria may remain a reasonable candidate for unicompartmental knee arthroplasty.

As mentioned, intraoperative evidence of greater than grade 2 chondromalacia in the opposite compartment or the patellofemoral articulation is a contraindication for unicondylar arthroplasty. Furthermore, any patient with an inflammatory arthropathy is precluded from unicondylar replacement and should have a total knee arthroplasty.[4] Patients with previous patellectomy[3] or high tibial osteotomy[20] typically have poor results as well. Finally, patients without an intact anterior cruciate ligament (ACL) should not have a unicondylar arthroplasty, because early failure is more likely to occur.[21] Selection criteria and contraindications are summarized in Table 17.1.

TECHNIQUE

The authors initially utilized a longitudinal midline incision and parapatellar arthrotomy to perform the unicompartmental knee arthroplasty. At our institution, currently a minimally invasive surgical approach is used with an 8- to 10-cm incision placed directly over the medial or lateral femoral condyle to allow access to the affected compartment. The technique described here details the procedure for a medial unicompartmental knee replacement; however, a lateral unicompartmental knee replacement is performed via a similar incision of the same length lateral to the patella and patellar tendon. Furthermore, femoral intramedullary and tibial extramedullary instrumentation allows the proper placement of the components and is recommended by the authors as described in this technique.

Under general or regional anesthesia, the patient is placed in the supine position with a pneumatic tourniquet on the proximal thigh. The lower extremity is prepped in standard

fashion, the foot and ankle are placed in a foot holder, and the tourniquet is inflated after exsanguination of the lower extremity. The hip is flexed to 70° to 90° and the knee flexed to approximately 100° to 120°.

An anteromedial longitudinal skin incision is made beginning at the superior pole of the patella, extending distally 8 to 10 cm along the medial edge of the patella and patellar tendon (Figure 17.1). The medial joint capsule is incised starting at the superior medial edge of the patella and extending distally to approximately 2 cm below the joint line, just medial to the patellar tendon and tibial tubercle. The vastus medialis oblique muscle may be incised 1 to 2 cm in line with its fibers to facilitate proximal exposure, if necessary. Once the capsular incision is made, it is critical that exposed synovium,

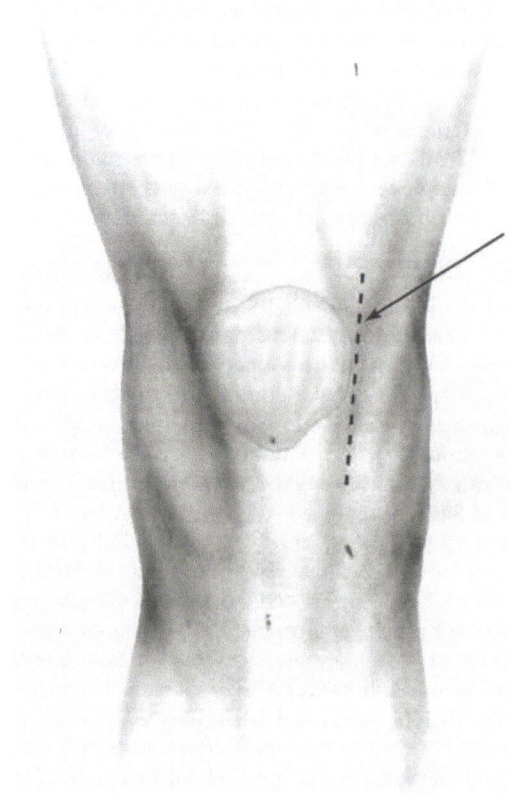

FIGURE 17.1 Anteromedial skin incision (*arrow*), extending along the medial edge of the patella and patellar tendon, approximately 8–10 cm in length.

medial fat pad, and meniscal remnant are excised to facilitate visualization of the entire medial compartment. In addition, release a portion of the deep medial collateral ligament along the tibial articular surface, but avoid excessive soft tissue release that may overcorrect the varus deformity. Carefully debride any intercondylar or patellar osteophytes that may impinge on the tibial spines or femoral component, respectively. Finally, inspect the lateral compartment and patellofemoral articular surfaces to ensure isolated medial compartment disease before implanting the unicompartmental components. If grade 3 chondromalacia is found in either location, the unicondylar replacement should be aborted and a total knee arthroplasty performed.

Flex the knee to approximately 30° without everting the patella and slide the patella laterally. Establish access into the distal femur with an intramedullary drill with a starting point 1 cm anterior to the insertion of the ACL in the intercondylar notch (Figure 17.2). With the knee flexed at 30°, place the intramedullary femoral resection guide into the distal femur (Figure 17.3A) and impact the guide while flexing the knee to approximately 120° until the guide lies flush with the femoral condyle articular surface (Figure 17.3B). The distal femur

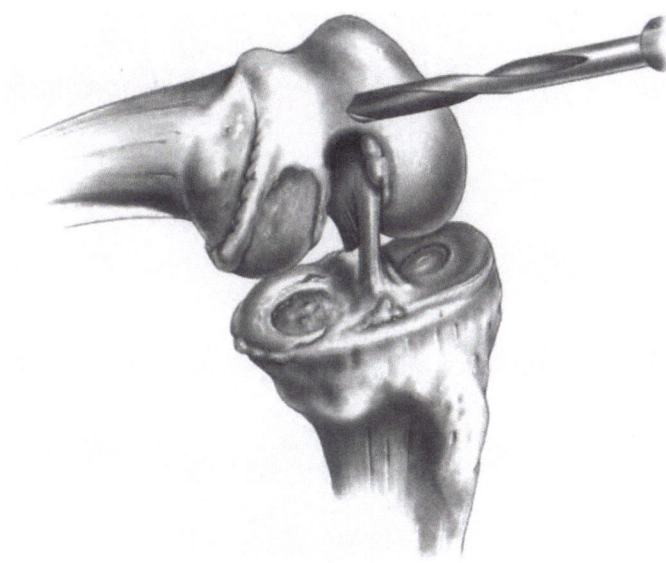

FIGURE 17.2 Intramedullary drill starting point, 1 cm anterior to the anterior cruciate ligament insertion in the intercondylar notch of the femur.

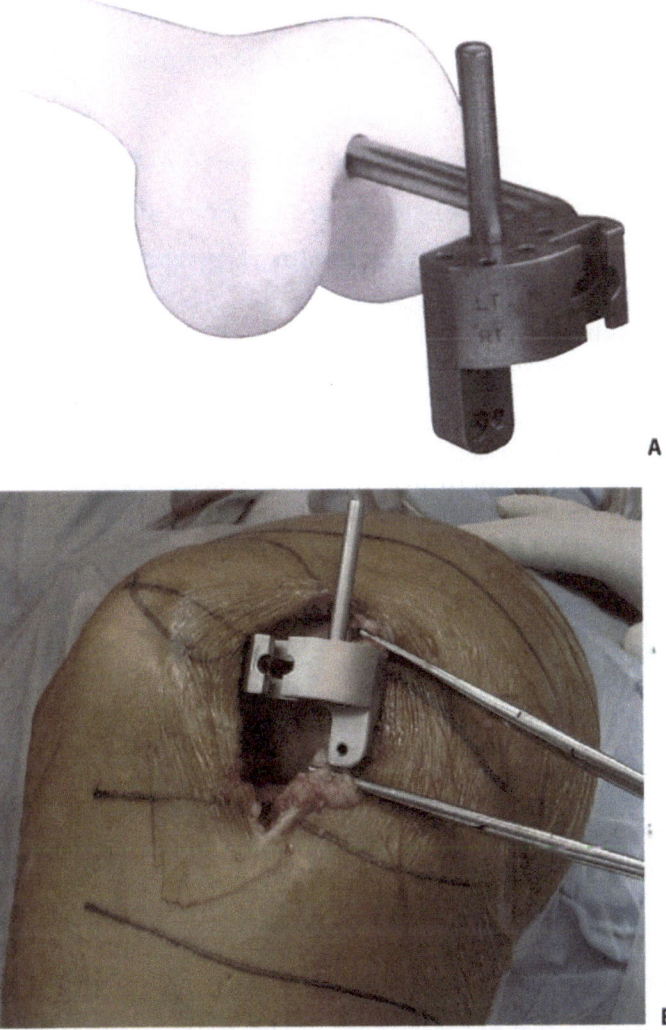

FIGURE 17.3 A. Illustration of intramedullary femoral resection guide insertion. **B.** Intraoperative position of the intramedullary guide, impacted flush against the femoral condyle articular surface.

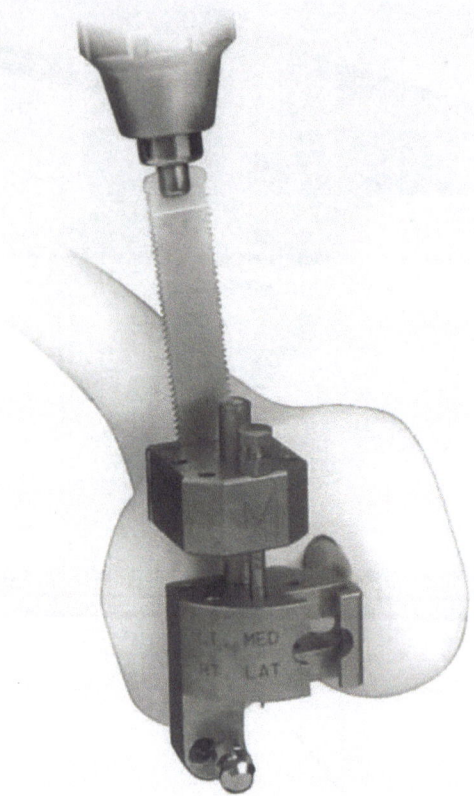

FIGURE 17.4 Resection of the distal femoral articular surface is accomplished through a cutting guide, positioned at approximately 5°–7° with respect to the anatomic axis of the femur.

nent. The trial femoral and tibial components are then inserted, along with a trial polyethylene articulating surface, and the knee is taken through a full range of motion. The surgeon should pay particular attention to ensure that there is no impingement of the patella on the anterior surface of the femoral component. Furthermore, the tibial and femoral components should align perfectly in the coronal plane. Finally, 2 mm of laxity should be present between the components with slight manual valgus stress to prevent excessive biomechanical loads in the medial compartment.

The trial components are removed, the bone surfaces are irrigated with pulsatile lavage, and the final femoral and

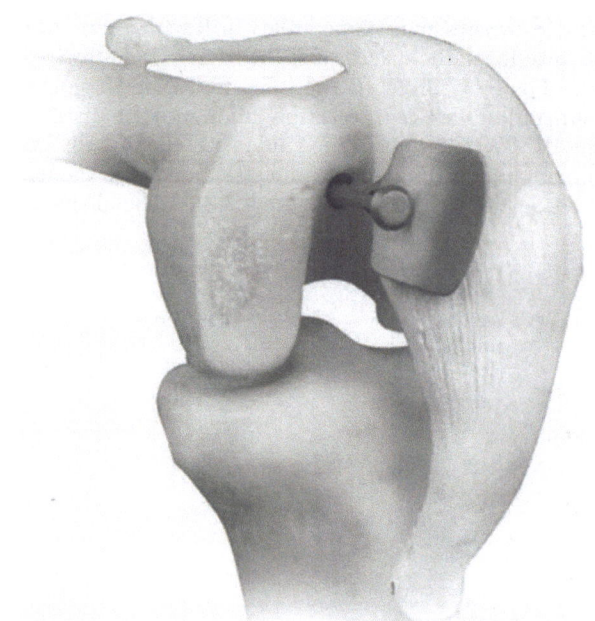

articular surface is resected with an oscillating saw through an alignment guide (Figure 17.4) set at the appropriate valgus angle with respect to the femoral anatomic axis. The angulation of the articular surface with respect to the anatomic axis of the femur is determined from preoperative mechanical axis radiographs and typically measures 5° to 7° of valgus. Insert an intramedullary patellar retractor (Figure 17.5) and attach the distal femoral finishing guide (Figure 17.6), using the oscillating saw to make the remaining posterior condyle and chamfer cuts. The surgeon may encounter difficulty in positioning the femoral finishing guide in the proper amount of flexion. If this occurs, the tibial articular surface resection may be performed before the final femoral cuts, as described next; this allows positioning of the femoral finishing guide in the proper degree of flexion, preventing untoward impingement of the patella on the final femoral component.

Extramedullary instrumentation is utilized to ensure correct positioning of the tibial component, perpendicular to the anatomic axis of the tibia in the coronal plane. The extramedullary alignment guide is positioned so that a depth resection gauge placed on the tibial cutting platform (Figure 17.7) provides an appropriate tibial surface resection to allow insertion of a polyethylene articular insert of at least 8 mm. The sagittal cut is made just medial to the medial tibial spine (Figure 17.8), taking care not to damage the ACL. Once the tibial articular surface is resected, the posterior capsule is visualized (Figure 17.9A) and any posterior osteophytes or meniscal remnants should be removed. Use a tibial sizer (Figure 17.9B) to choose the appropriate-size tibial compo-

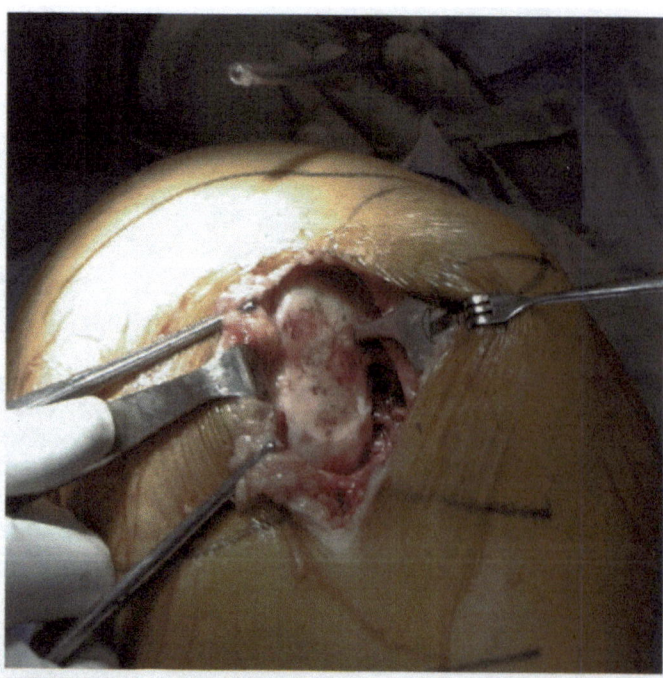

B

FIGURE 17.5 A. Illustration of intramedullary patellar retractor. B. Intraoperative photograph demonstrates the excellent visualization obtained with the patellar retractor in position.

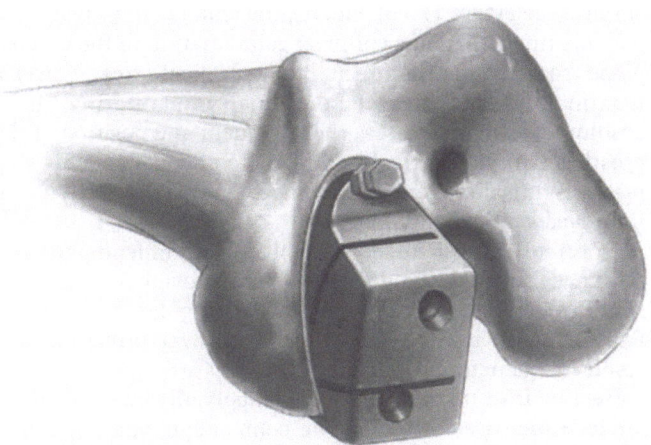

FIGURE 17.6 Illustration of the distal femoral finishing guide used to make the final cuts to accommodate the femoral component.

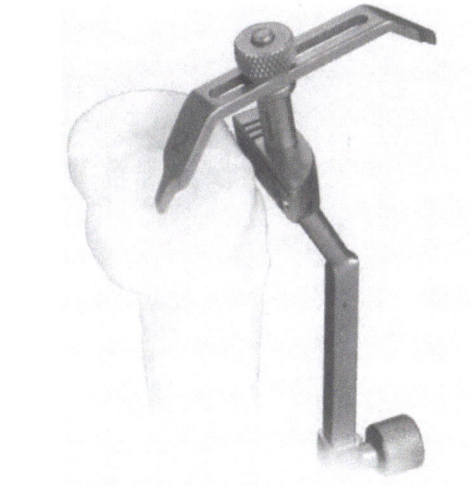

A

tibial components are cemented into place. The cement is allowed to cure with the trial polyethylene spacer in place and the knee in full extension. All extraneous cement is removed from the knee, and the final tibial polyethylene articular surface is inserted. The final position of the components are confirmed (Figure 17.10), the tourniquet is deflated, and hemostasis is obtained. The capsular incision is closed over a small drain, the skin incision is closed, and a bulky dressing is applied.

SURGICAL PEARLS AND PITFALLS

The success of unicompartmental knee arthroplasty is highly dependent on proper patient selection. However, proper surgical technique is essential in establishing a unicompartmental replacement with proper component position, minimizing the biomechanical stresses on the components and remaining articular cartilage. Patella impingement on the femoral component may occur if the component is improperly positioned and is strongly correlated with subsequent patellofemoral pain and need for revision.[22] In a recent study, patellar impingement was associated with placement of the femoral component in an anterior position relative to the trochleocondylar junction and occurred more frequently in lateral unicondylar arthroplasty.[22] The surgeon should ensure the anterior edge of the femoral component is flush with the articular surface of the trochlear groove, especially with regard to unicondylar arthroplasty of the lateral compartment. Anterior placement may occur if excessive bone is resected from the posterior femoral condyle, placing the femoral component in extension relative to the femoral axis.[22]

Careful attention should be directed to placing the tibial component in the correct alignment. Proper position of the tibial component is attained with adequate intraoperative exposure as well as proper use of an extramedullary alignment guide. The tibial component should be properly placed in the mediolateral position to prevent overhang of the component relative to the underlying tibial plateau. Excessive overhang will result in ligamentous tethering as well as aseptic loosening with subsequent early failure of the prosthesis.

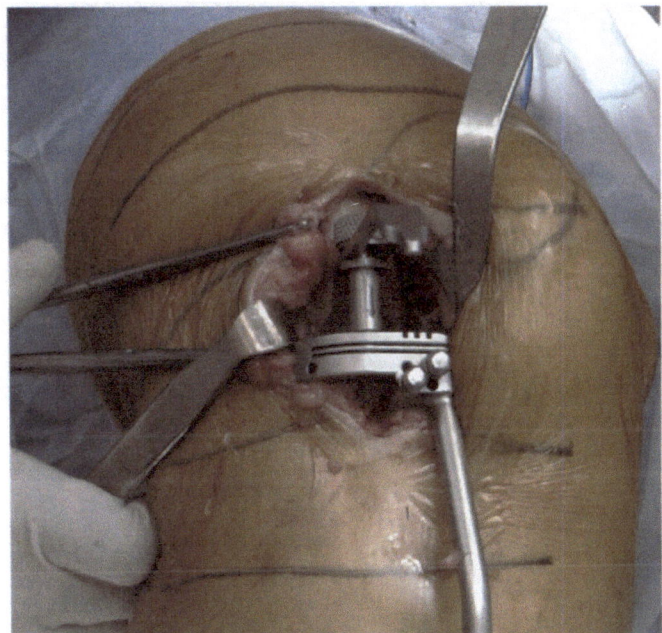

B

FIGURE 17.7 A. Illustration of depth resection guide on the tibial resection platform of the extramedullary alignment guide. **B.** Corresponding operative picture shows the depth resection guide attached to the tibial resection platform of the extramedullary alignment guide.

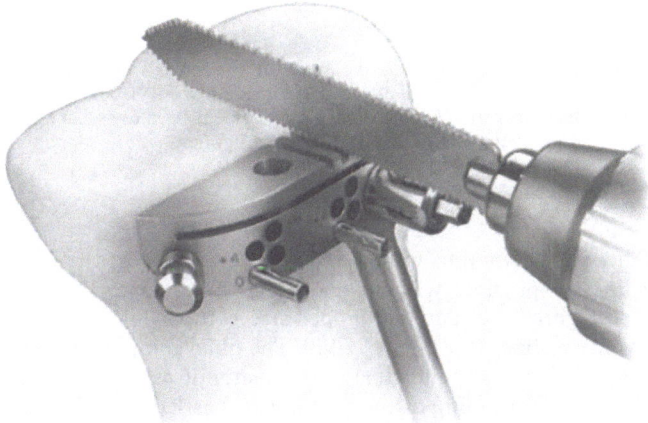

FIGURE 17.8 Illustration of the tibial surface sagittal cut made just medial to the medial tibial spine.

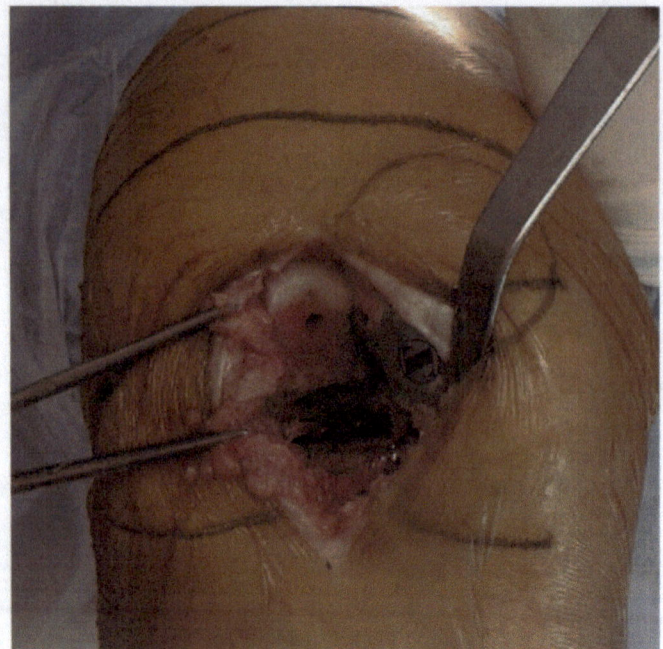

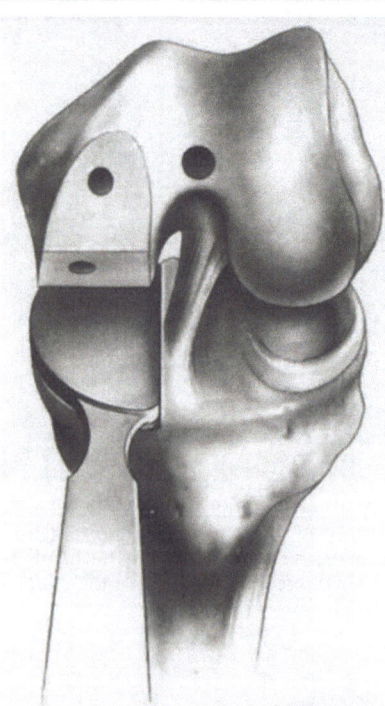

surface (see Figure 17.7B). Finally, the femoral and tibial components must align in a collinear configuration in the coronal plane, so as to distribute the biomechanical stresses over a maximal surface area. Before final implantation, it is absolutely critical to assess the alignment and position of the prosthesis intraoperatively with trial components. This step prevents misalignment or impingement and will result in improved surgical outcomes.

Currently, most surgeons involved with unicompartmental knee arthroplasty do not advocate overcorrecting the slight preoperative varus or valgus angular deformity.[24] Extensive soft tissue releases to obtain overcorrection may result in ligamentous instability, whereas attempting to overcorrect by inserting too large a tibial polyethylene will likely produce increased stress on the components and polyethylene, resulting in early failure of the prosthesis. Furthermore, overcorrection of a medial unicondylar replacement into valgus alignment will place excessive loads and stress in the lateral compartment, leading to subsequent early degeneration. Conversely, some authors have recently correlated an increased rate of failure and revision of unicompartmental knee replacements with undercorrection of the angular deformity[23]; however, the undercorrection was also correlated with a thin polyethylene insert causing high failure rates due to excessive wear. Additionally, thin polyethylene inserts (less than 8 mm) have been associated with increased polyethylene wear and subsequent early failure.[15] We recommend using a polyethylene thickness of at least 8 mm, while avoiding overcorrection of the angular deformity with soft tissue releases or excessive bone resection.

One of the advantages of the unicompartmental knee arthroplasty is preservation of native bone stock because of the minimal bone resection required for implantation of the components. Although the surgeon must resect enough tibial bone to insert a polyethylene of sufficient thickness, careful attention must be paid to prevent excessive tibial plateau resection. Subsequent tibial surface and metaphyseal bone loss will make an eventual revision procedure more difficult, likely necessitating wedge or bulk graft augmentation. The surgical pitfalls in unicompartmental knee arthroplasty and the subsequent complications are summarized in Table 17.2.

FIGURE 17.9 A. Intraoperative view of the medial compartment after resection of the tibial articular surface, allowing visualization of the posterior capsule. **B.** The tibial sizing guide is used to assess alignment and prevent overhang of the final component.

The tibial component should be placed as close to the tibial spines as possible without damaging the cruciate ligament (see Figure 17.8) and the proper size component chosen to avoid overhang (see Figure 17.9B). The tibial component must also be placed perpendicular to the anatomic axis of the tibia, as varus positioning of the component has led to early loosening and subsequent failure.[23] This placement is accomplished by correctly aligning the extramedullary guide with the anatomic axis of the tibia when resecting the articular

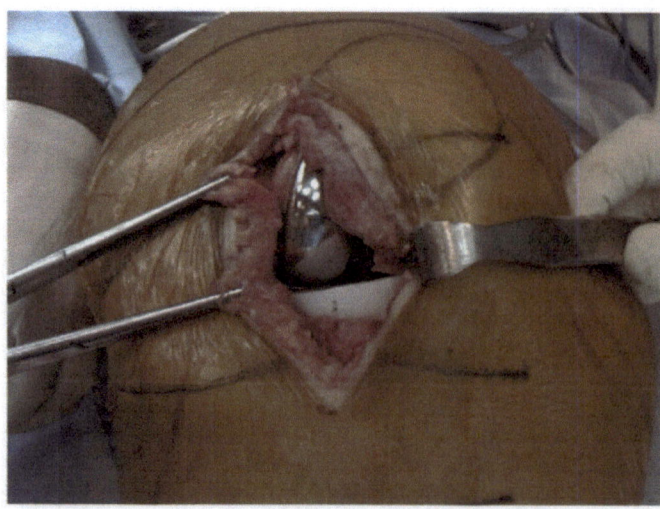

FIGURE 17.10 Intraoperative view of the final unicompartmental components cemented in place.

TABLE 17.2 Surgical pitfalls in unicompartmental knee arthroplasty.	
Surgical pitfall	*Complication*
Improper patient selection	Early failure
Polyethylene less than 8 mm	Excessive polyethylene wear, early failure
Femoral component placed anteriorly	Patellar impingement, patellofemoral pain, failure
Femoral component placed in extension	Patellar impingement, patellofemoral pain, failure
Tibial component placed with plateau overhang	Aseptic loosening, early failure
Tibial component placed in relative varus alignment	Aseptic loosening, early failure
Overcorrection of preoperative angular deformity	Aseptic loosening, progressive arthosis, early failure
Excessive tibial/femoral bone resection	Difficult and complicated revision surgery

REHABILITATION

The postoperative care and rehabilitation of a patient with a unicompartmental knee arthroplasty is similar to that of a total knee arthroplasty. All patients should receive preoperative and postoperative prophylactic antibiotics, as well as postoperative deep venous thrombosis prophylaxis with pharmacologic anticoagulation in the form of coumadin or low molecular weight heparin. The intraarticular drain and bulky dressing are removed the morning of postoperative day 1. Physical therapy is initiated on postoperative day 1 with gait training with assisted weight bearing in the form of a crutch or walker.

Physical therapy should emphasize both quadriceps strengthening and knee motion. Quadriceps strengthening may be initiated on postoperative day 1 and consists of quad sets and assisted straight-leg raises. The patient should be encouraged to attain quadriceps strength, especially when the minimally invasive surgical approach, which minimizes trauma to the quadriceps mechanism, has been used. Range-of-motion exercises are initiated on postoperative day 1, emphasizing full terminal knee extension as well as maximal passive and active knee flexion. Appropriate goals by postoperative day 3 are achievement of passive knee flexion from full extension to greater than 90° of flexion, with active motion from minus 10° of full extension to 90° of knee flexion. Patients should continue outpatient physical therapy five times weekly for the first 3 weeks, then three times weekly for the next 3 weeks. A study of unicompartmental knee replacement with a minimally invasive approach demonstrated that attainment of straight-leg raise, knee flexion to 70°, and functional independence including stair climbing occurred three times faster than in total knee arthroplasty.[25]

COMPLICATIONS

Unicompartmental knee replacement is a technically challenging and demanding surgery, because the precise placement of the components in the proper position is critical to the success of the procedure. Appropriately, a learning curve exists for the unfamiliar surgeon. An outcome study of unicompartmental knee arthroplasties from the Swedish Knee Arthroplasty Register demonstrated a positive association between the number of procedures performed annually by a particular surgeon and the rate of revision.[26] Furthermore, as the minimally invasive surgical approach continues to become more widespread, appropriate instrumentation is necessary to ensure proper component positioning in a reliable and reproducible fashion.

Failure of unicompartmental knee arthroplasty is most commonly caused by aseptic loosening of the components or progressive degenerative disease of the remaining articular cartilage.[15-17,22,27] Aseptic loosening of the tibial component is frequently associated with polyethylene inserts less than 8 mm in thickness, resulting in accelerated wear and subsequent failure of the prosthesis.[15] Patients typically complain of startup pain relieved with further ambulation and exhibit progressive radiolucency at the cement–bone interface of the involved component. The most recent long-term studies of unicompartmental knee arthroplasty report aseptic loosening rates of 0% to 9%.[28-33] This potential will be diminished by maintaining a polyethylene thickness of at least 8 mm. The recent long-term follow-up of unicompartmental arthroplasties performed at our institution did not demonstrate any aseptic loosening at an average 12-year follow-up.[34] All polyethylene components used in this series of patients were 8 mm thick or greater.

Progressive arthritis of the unresurfaced compartment is another leading cause for failure of the unicompartmental knee replacement.[16-17] A recent series of 35 revision arthroplasties for failed unicompartmental replacements reported 5 (14%) were secondary to progression of opposite compartment arthrosis. However, the recent long-term outcome studies report rates of arthritis progression leading to failure of unicondylar arthroplasty between 0% and 5%.[28-33] Progressive degeneration of the remaining articular cartilage is minimized by proper patient selection, ensuring that minimal chondromalacia exists at the time of unicompartmental knee arthroplasty, and by strict adherence to the principles outlined earlier in this chapter.

Patellofemoral complications in unicompartmental arthroplasty predominantly consist of progression of osteoarthritis and impingement of the patella on the femoral component. A recent investigation of patellofemoral complications following unicompartmental knee arthroplasty reported impingement of the patella on the femoral component resulted in significant patellofemoral pain.[22] Radiographic evidence of impingement occurred in 28% of the unicompartmental arthroplasties in the study and was associated with anterior placement of the femoral component; however, only one knee required surgical intervention. The study further reported 29% of knees demonstrated radiographic evidence of patellofemoral osteoarthritis at an average 14-year follow-up, none of which required revision.[22]

Finally, most investigators familiar with revision surgery for failed unicondylar knee arthroplasty maintain conversion to total knee arthroplasty is relatively straightforward and is not associated with an increased rate of complications.[15,17,27] A study of 73 revision arthroplasties for failed unicondylar replacement due to aseptic loosening and progression of

TABLE 17.3   Long-term results of unicompartmental knee arthroplasty.

Author	Publication year	Number of knees	Mean age (years)	Mean follow-up (years)	Percent revised	10-year survivorship[a] (%)
Marmor[34]	1988	60	65	11	15	70
Scott[28]	1991	100	71	8–12	13	85
Heck[29]	1993	294	68	6	5	91
Cartier[30]	1996	60	65	12	4	93
Murray[21]	1998	143	71	7	3	98
Squire[31]	1999	136	71	18	10	—[b]
Svard[32]	2001	124	70	12	5	95
Berger[c]	2003	62	68	12	3	98

[a] Survivorship based on revision for any reason.
[b] Ten-year survivorship not reported; 15-year survivorship is 90%.
[c] Presented at the 70th Annual Meeting of the American Academy of Orthopaedic Surgeons, New Orleans, LA, February 2003.

arthritis demonstrated 79% good to excellent results at an average of 56 months.[27]

RESULTS

Although unicompartmental knee arthroplasty has been controversial since its introduction in the 1970s, reported outcomes have been steadily improving. Marmor[35] reported 70% of his initial 60 unicondylar arthroplasties had a satisfactory result at 10-year follow-up. There was a substantial 15% revision rate, predominantly from aseptic loosening secondary to thin, 4-mm polyethylene tibial components. In 1991, Scott et al.[28] reported 85% 10-year survivorship using the unicondylar prosthesis. Thirteen knees in this series of 100 unicompartmental arthroplasties required revision, with 9 of the 13 secondary to aseptic loosening. The authors concluded this relatively high revision rate was a result of poor selection criteria,[28] as many of those patients revised would not meet the selection criteria outlined in this chapter.

With improvements in selection criteria, surgical technique, and component design, improved outcomes of unicompartmental knee arthroplasty were reported in the 1990s. In 1993, Heck et al.[29] published a multicenter study involving 294 unicompartmental knee arthroplasties and reported a 10-year survivorship of 91% with an improved revision rate of only 5%. A study of 60 unicondylar knee arthroplasties published in 1996 reported a 10-year survivorship of 93% and a revision rate of 4%.[30]

Insight into the outcomes of patients who have a unicompartmental knee arthroplasty into the second decade was provided in a study by Squire et al.[31] The study reported a 15-year minimum follow-up of 140 cemented unicompartmental knee arthroplasties with a 15-year survivorship of 90%. A revision rate of 10% was reported at an average 18-year follow-up, comparable to that of total knee arthroplasty. The long-term problems were progression of degenerative disease and tibial component wear and subsidence.[31]

Reports of congruent, mobile-bearing unicompartmental knee arthroplasty have recently emerged and demonstrate encouraging long-term outcomes.[21,33] In 1998, Murray et al. reported the results of 143 Oxford medial unicompartmental arthroplasties with an average 7-year follow-up.[21] The study reported a 10-year survivorship of 98% with a minimal 3.5% revision rate. None of the failures requiring revision were

caused by aseptic loosening.[21] An independent study of 124 mobile-bearing unicompartmental knee arthroplasties published in 2001 confirmed these long-term results. The study reported a 10-year cumulative survivorship of 95% with a 5% rate of revision.[32] However, both studies involving mobile-bearing unicompartmental arthroplasties documented revisions resulting from to dislocation of the mobile polyethylene bearing.[21,32]

The long-term results of unicompartmental knee arthroplasty at our institution have been recently reviewed and are extremely encouraging. Berger et al.[33] reported our initial clinical experience at an average 7-year follow-up, documenting 98% good or excellent results. These 62 consecutive unicompartmental arthroplasties currently have an average 12-year follow-up, with a 10-year survivorship equal to 98%. There have been only 2 revisions for opposite compartment degeneration, at 7 and 10 years, respectively (Table 17.3). The authors attribute the successful outcomes to strict selection criteria, proper surgical technique, and a well-designed prosthesis (Figure 17.11).

FUTURE DIRECTIONS

With improved long-term outcome studies, unicompartmental knee arthroplasty has become less controversial and is currently considered an excellent surgical option in patients with isolated unicompartmental disease. Improvements in component materials, such as highly cross-linked polyethylene, may allow improved results in younger patients previously considered inappropriate candidates for unicondylar arthroplasty.

The surgeons at our institution currently utilize a minimally invasive surgical approach, as opposed to the previous patella-everting arthrotomy. As reported by other authors,[25] we are experiencing shorter hospital stays (typically 1–2 postoperative days) and accelerated rehabilitation with the newer minimally invasive approach, without compromising component position. Further long-term studies of the new minimally invasive approach are in progress to confirm our belief that results will be equal or superior to those obtained with the traditional surgical exposure. In the meantime, unicompartmental knee arthroplasty remains an excellent surgical option for the properly selected patient with isolated unicompartmental articular disease of the knee.

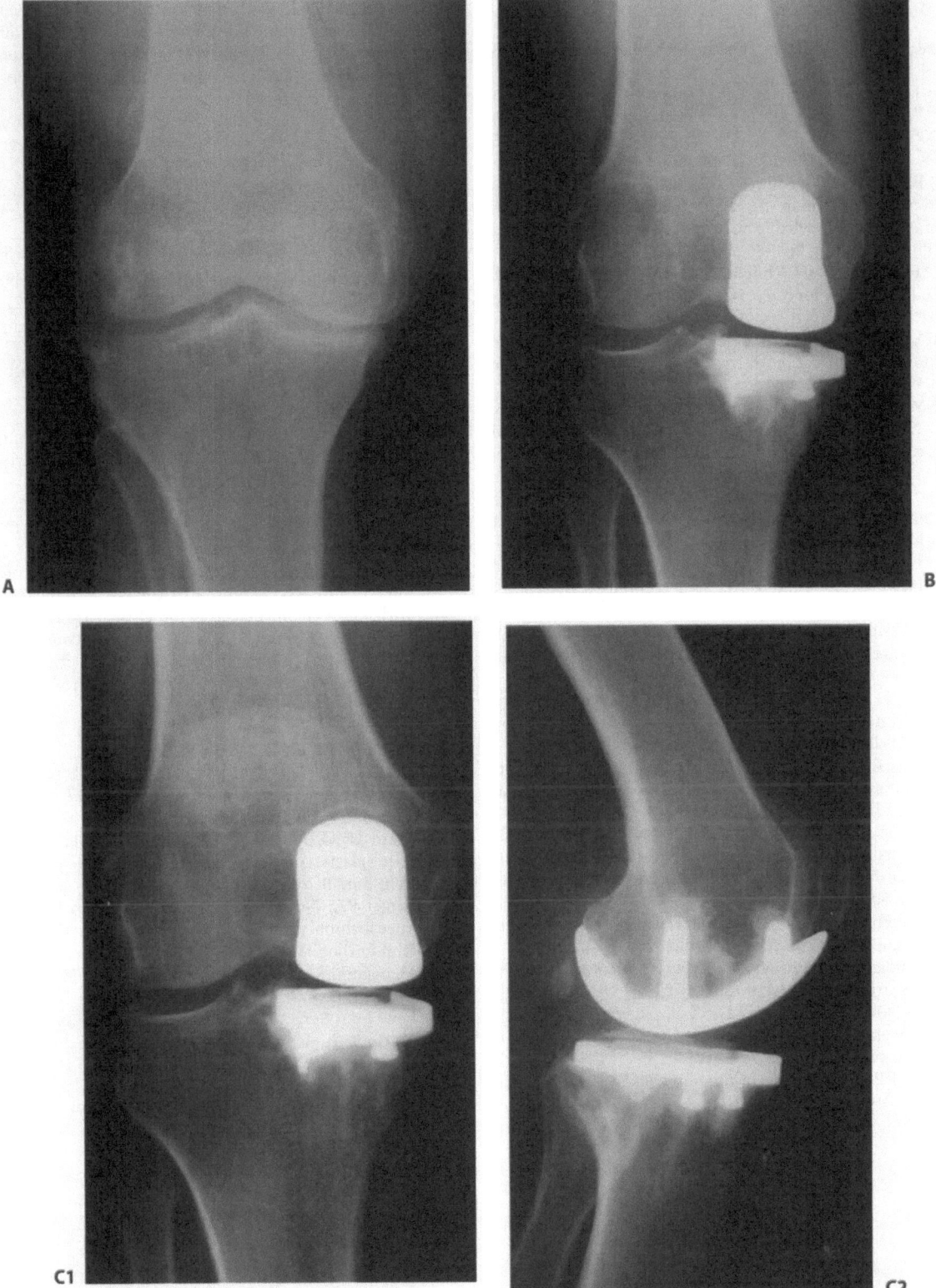

FIGURE 17.11 A. Preoperative, anteroposterior (AP) radiograph of a patient with isolated medial compartment degenerative joint disease of the knee. **B.** Six-week postoperative AP radiograph of the medial unicompartmental knee arthroplasty with components in appropri-ate alignment. **C.** AP (*left*) and lateral (*right*) radiographs of the uni-compartmental knee arthroplasty 10 years after the index procedure with no evidence of component loosening.

References

1. McKeever, D. Tibial plateau prosthesis. Clin Orthop 1960;18: 86–95.
2. Marmor L. The modular knee. Clin Orthop 1973;94:242–248.
3. Insall J, Walker P. Unicondylar knee replacement. Clin Orthop 1976;120:83–85.
4. Laskin R. Unicompartmental tibiofemoral resurfacing arthroplasty. J Bone Joint Surg Am 1978;60:82–185.
5. Broughton NS, Newman JH, Baily RA. Unicompartmental replacement and high tibial osteotomy for osteoarthritis of the knee. J Bone Joint Surg Br 1986;68:447–452.
6. Weale AE, Newman JH. Unicompartmental arthroplasty and high tibial osteotomy for osteoarthrosis of the knee. Clin Orthop 1994;302:134–137.
7. Scott RD, Santore RF. Unicondylar unicompartmental replacement for osteoarthritis of the knee. J Bone Joint Surg Am 1981;63:536–544.
8. Jackson M, Sarongi PP, Newman JH. Revision total knee arthroplasty: Comparison of outcome following primary proximal tibial osteotomy or unicompartmental arthroplasty. J Arthroplasty 1994;9:539–542.
9. Engh GA, McAuley JP.: Unicondylar arthroplasty: an option for high-demand patients with gonarthrosis. Instr Course Lect 1999;48:143–148.
10. Andriacchi TP, Galante J, Fermier RW. The influence of total knee replacement on walking and stair climbing. J Bone Joint Surg Am 1982;64:1328–1335.
11. Chassin EP, Mikosz RP, Andriacchi TP, et al. Functional analysis of cemented medial unicompartmental knee arthroplasty. J Arthroplasty 1996;11:553–559.
12. Laurencin CT, Zelicof SB, Scott RD, et al. Unicompartmental versus total knee arthroplasty in the same patient. Clin Orthop 1991;273:151–156.
13. Rougraff BT, Heck DA, Gibson AE. A comparison of tricompartmental and unicompartmental arthroplasty for the treatment of gonarthrosis. Clin Orthop 1991;273:157–164.
14. Robertsson O, Borgquist L, Knutson K, et al. Use of unicompartmental instead of tricompartmental prostheses for unicompartmental arthrosis in the knee is a cost-effective alternative. Acta Orthop Scand 1999;70:170–175.
15. McAuley JP, Engh GA, Ammeen DJ. Revision of failed unicompartmental knee arthroplasty. Clin Orthop 2001;392:279–282.
16. Bohm I, Landsiedl F. Revision surgery after failed unicompartmental knee arthroplasty. J Arthroplasty 2000;15:982–989.
17. Levine WN, Ozuna RM, Scott RD, et al. Conversion of failed modern unicompartmental arthroplasty to total knee arthroplasty. J Arthroplasty 1996;11:797–801.
18. Outerbridge RE. The aetiology of chondromalacia patelae. J Bone Joint Surg Br 1961;43:752–757.
19. Kozinn S, Scott R. Current concepts review: unicondylar knee arthroplasty. J Bone Joint Surg Am 1989;71:145–150.
20. Rees JL, Price AJ, Lynskey TG, et al. Medial unicompartmental arthroplasty after failed high tibial osteotomy. J Bone Joint Surg Br 2001;83:1034–1036.
21. Murray DW, Goodfellow JW, O'Connor JJ. The Oxford medial unicompartmental arthroplasty. A ten-year survival study. J Bone Joint Surg Br 1998;80:983–989.
22. Hernigou P, Deschamps G. Patellar impingement following unicompartmental arthroplasty. J Bone Joint Surg Am 2002;84: 1132–1137.
23. Ridgeway SR, McAuley JP, Ammeen DJ, et al. The effect of alignment of the knee on the outcome of unicompartmental knee replacement. J Bone Joint Surg Br 2002;84:351–355.
24. Laskin RS. Unicompartmental knee replacement: some unanswered questions. Clin Orthop 2001;392:267–271.
25. Price A, Webb J, Topf H, et al. Oxford unicompartmental knee replacement with a minimally invasive technique. J Bone Joint Surge Br 2000;Suppl I:24.
26. Robertsson O, Knutson K, Lewold S, et al. The routine of surgical management reduces failure after unicompartmental knee arthroplasty. J Bone Joint Surg Br 2001;83:45–49.
27. Chakrabarty G, Newman JH, Ackroyd CE. Revision of unicompartmental arthroplasty of the knee. Clinical and technical considerations. J Arthroplasty 1998;13:191–196.
28. Scott RD, Cobb AG, McQueary FG, et al. Unicompartmental knee arthroplasty. Eight- to twelve-year follow-up evaluation with survivorship analysis. Clin Orthop 1991;271:96–100.
29. Heck DA, Marmor L, Gibson A. Unicompartmental knee arthroplasty: a multicenter investigation with long term follow up evaluation. Clin Orthop 1993;286:154–159.
30. Cartier P, Sanouiller JL, Grelsamer RP. Unicompartmental knee arthroplasty surgery. Ten-year minimum follow-up period. J Arthroplasty 1996;11:782–788.
31. Squire MW, Callaghan JJ, Goetz DD, et al. Unicompartmental knee arthroplasty. A minimum fifteen year followup study. Clin Orthop 1999;367:61–72.
32. Svard UCG, Price AJ. Oxford medial unicompartmental knee arthroplasty. A survival analysis of an independent series. J Bone Joint Surg Br 2001;83:191–194.
33. Berger RA, Nedeff DD, Barden RM, et al. Unicompartmental knee arthroplasty. Clinical experience at 6- to 10-year followup. Clin Orthop 1999;367:50–60.
34. Meneghini RM, Berger RA, Jacobs JJ, et al. Modern unicompartmental knee arthroplasty at a minimum 10-year follow-up. J Bone Joint Surg 2004 (accepted for publication).
35. Marmor L. Unicompartmental knee arthroplasty. Ten- to thirteen-year follow-up study. Clin Orthop 1988;226:14–20.

PART III

Case Studies

Brian J. Cole and
Michael G. Dennis

EDITORS

Introduction to Case Studies

The illustrated case studies in Part III were prepared to help solidify the decision-making required for patients who are diagnosed with chondral disease of the knee. The cases are organized by level of complexity, taking into consideration substantial comorbidities such as tibiofemoral and patellofemoral malalignment, ligament disruption, and meniscal deficiency. The cases are presented in increasing level of difficulty based upon the defect- and patient-specific factors considered in the final treatment recommendation. Similar to the way a downhill ski run is graded for its level of difficulty, the cases are rated using green circles (easiest decision-making), blue squares (intermediate decision-making), black diamonds (advanced decision-making), and double black diamonds (expert decision-making). Within each cate-gory, the cases are organized by increasing complexity as well. Based upon the reader's practice experience, some may feel more comfortable with the decisions made in one category versus another. We believe, however, that this is the best way to convey the implicit level of complexity, thereby allowing the reader to better understand how these cases fall within the treatment algorithm. When off-label usage of tech-nology was implemented, it is clearly indicated within the body of the case. While mastering the techniques and per-forming a thorough evaluation of all patient- and defect-specific factors is a prerequisite to sound judgment, the bullet points at the end of each cases that emphasize the final ratio-nale for the treatment chosen will be of particular interest and value to the reader.

PATHOLOGY
Osteochondritis dissecans of the medial femoral condyle with documented long-term natural history

TREATMENT
Nonoperative treatment

SUBMITTED BY
Brian J. Cole, MD, MBA, Rush Cartilage Restoration Center, Rush University Medical Center, Chicago, Illinois, USA

CHIEF COMPLAINT AND HISTORY OF PRESENT ILLNESS

The patient is currently a 39-year-old male orthopedic surgeon who was diagnosed with symptomatic osteochondritis dissecans of his medial femoral condyle of his left knee at the age of 14. At that time, he complained of weight-bearing pain and discomfort on the medial aspect of his left knee with activity-related swelling. When initially diagnosed as having osteochondritis dissecans, he was treated with 8 weeks of nonweight bearing with crutches and asked to refrain from sports or impact activities thereafter. He remained asymptomatic, but was followed up regularly for radiographic evaluation to assess for evidence of instability.

PHYSICAL EXAMINATION

He ambulates with a nonantalgic gait and stands in symmetric physiologic varus. He has no effusion and full range of motion. He has no tenderness over his medial femoral condyle. His entire knee examination is normal.

RADIOGRAPHIC EVALUATION

A series of radiographs obtained from the age of 14 to the present demonstrate persistence of the osteochondritis dissecans lesion with no progression or evidence of instability. Radiographs demonstrate a lesion of osteochondritis dissecans of the medial femoral condyle of his left knee (Figures C1.1 through C1.3).

FOLLOW-UP

The patient remains completely asymptomatic and active in several high-level sports including skiing and running. Serial radiographs demonstrate persistence of the lesion.

DECISION-MAKING FACTORS

1. Diagnosed early at a time when growth plates remained open.
2. Initial attempt at nonoperative treatment with protected weight bearing was successful in rendering him asymptomatic.
3. Despite persistence of the lesion demonstrated on plain radiographs and magnetic resonance imaging (MRI), he remains asymptomatic and highly active.
4. An identified target lesion that can be reliably followed clinically and radiographically for evidence of progression or instability.

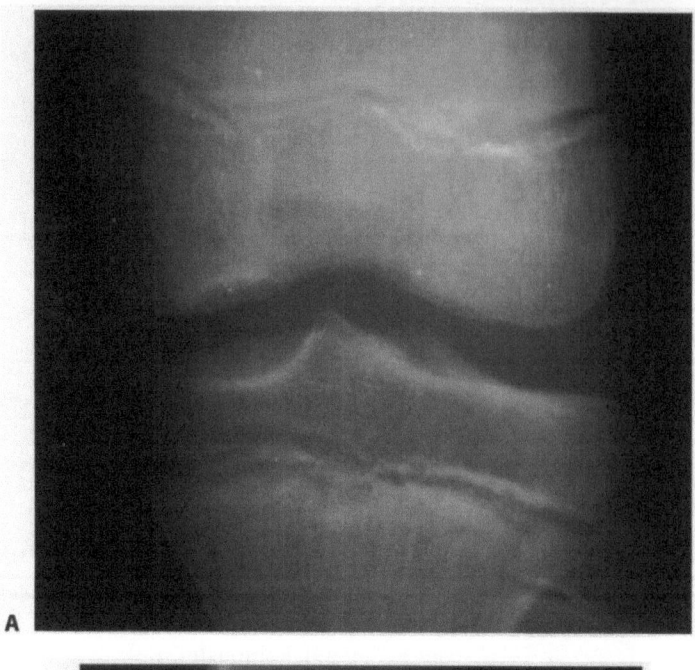

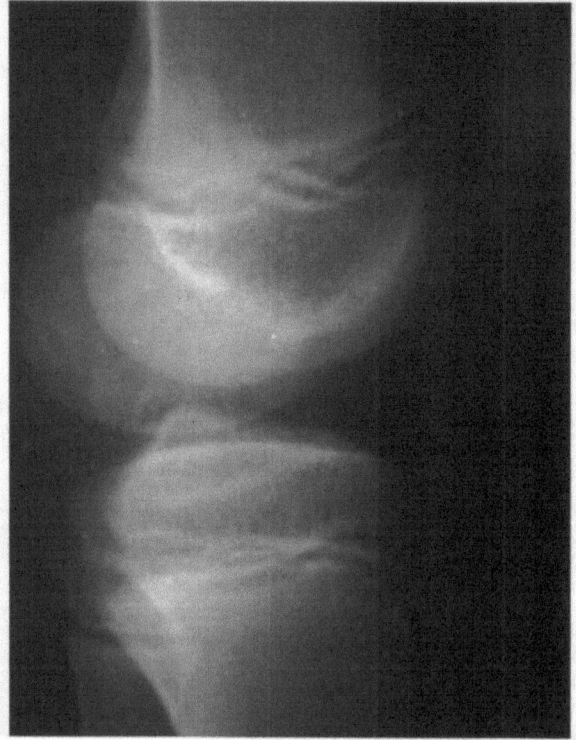

FIGURE C1.1 Initial radiographs of a 14-year-old male with symptomatic osteochondritis dissecans of the left knee. Anteroposterior (**A**) and lateral (**B**) radiographs demonstrate an in situ lesion of osteochondritis dissecans of the medial femoral condyle.

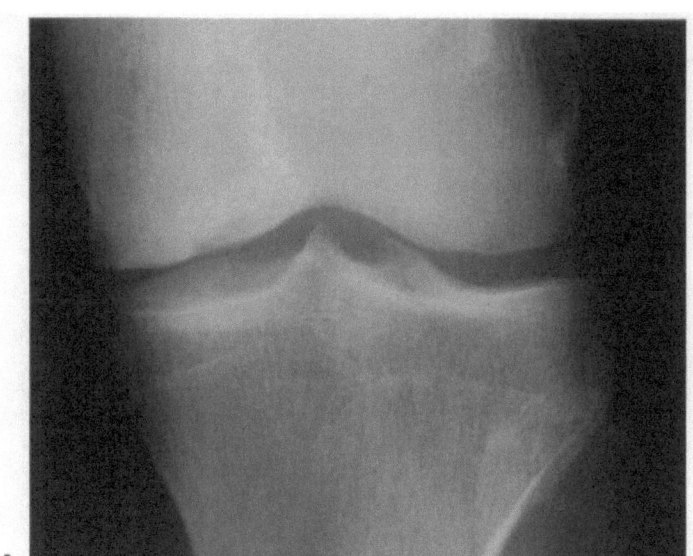

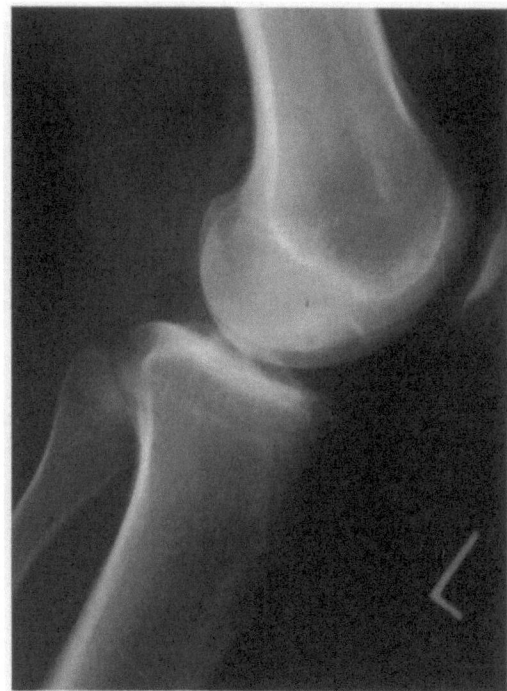

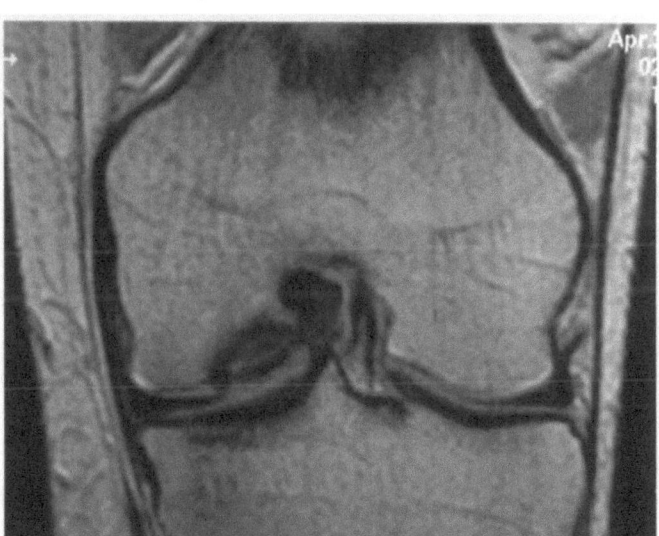

FIGURE C1.2 Radiographs obtained 24 years later. Anteroposterior (**A**) and lateral (**B**) radiographs demonstrate no evidence of fragmentation or collapse. (**C**) Coronal MRI demonstrates no fragmentation or evidence of significant instability.

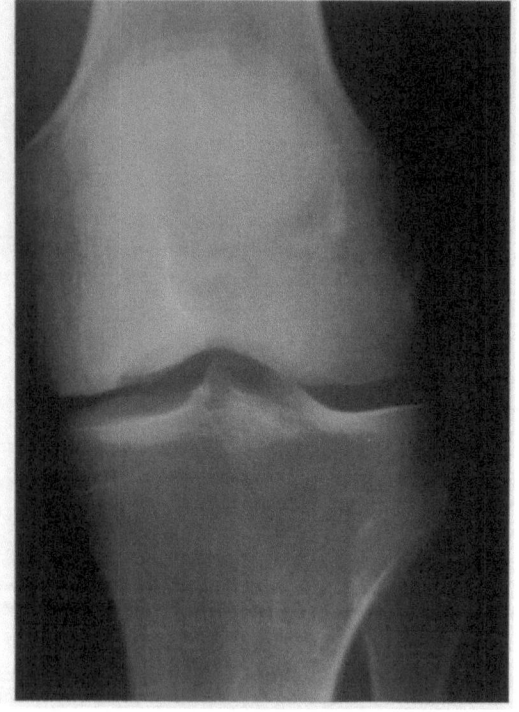

A

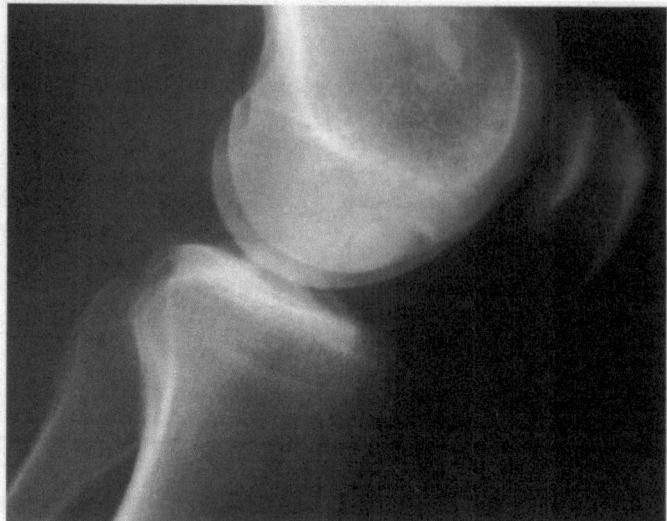

B

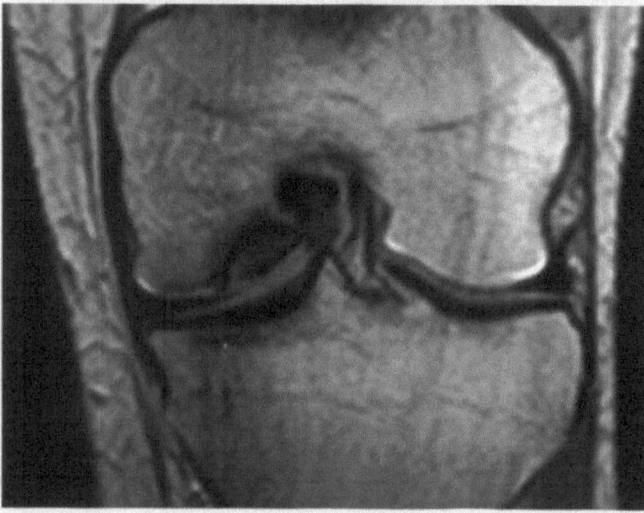

C

FIGURE C1.3 Radiographs obtained 29 years later. Anteroposterior (**A**) and lateral (**B**) radiographs demonstrate no evidence of fragmentation or collapse. (**C**) Coronal MRI demonstrates no fragmentation or evidence of significant instability. No significant interval change is seen compared to Figure C1.2.

2

PATHOLOGY
Avascular necrosis

PROCEDURE
Total knee replacement

SUBMITTED BY
Tom Minas, MD, and Tim Bryant, RN, Cartilage Repair Center, Brigham and Women's Hospital, Boston, Massachusetts, USA

CHIEF COMPLAINT AND HISTORY OF PRESENT ILLNESS

The patient is a 55-year-old man with a long-standing history of ulcerative colitis. His acute episodes have been treated with high-dose steroids. Recently, he has developed severe right knee weight-bearing discomfort. He also has pain at rest and at night. The joint pain is confined to his right knee only. He denies generalized malaise, fever, or erythema of the knee joint. Antiinflammatory medications and corticosteroid injections have not helped. He is unable to walk without the use of a cane.

PHYSICAL EXAMINATION

Height, 5 ft, 11 in.; weight, 185 lb. Clinical examination demonstrates a severe antalgic gait without the use of a cane. He has a large joint effusion that limits his range of motion to 95 degrees of flexion. He has a 30-degree fixed flexion deformity. Tricompartmental crepitus is present with generalized tenderness. Ligament examination is unremarkable.

RADIOGRAPHIC EVALUATION

Plain radiographs demonstrate diffuse patchy osteopenia of the distal femur, patella, and proximal tibia with well-maintained joint spaces and some early flattening to the medial femoral condyle consistent with multifocal avascular necrosis (Figure C2.1). A magnetic resonance imaging (MRI) scan demonstrates diffuse distal femoral avascular necrosis (not shown), with an osteochondral fragment of the medial femoral condyle

SURGICAL INTERVENTION

A cruciate-retaining total knee arthroplasty was performed (Figure C2.2). Aggressive physical therapy was required to restore full extension that was obtained at the time of surgery. A Dyasplint™ was utilized to assist in regaining extension and for stretching of the hamstrings and joint capsule.

FOLLOW-UP

Three months postoperatively, the patient regained 0 to 110 degrees of flexion. He walks with no gait disturbance and is

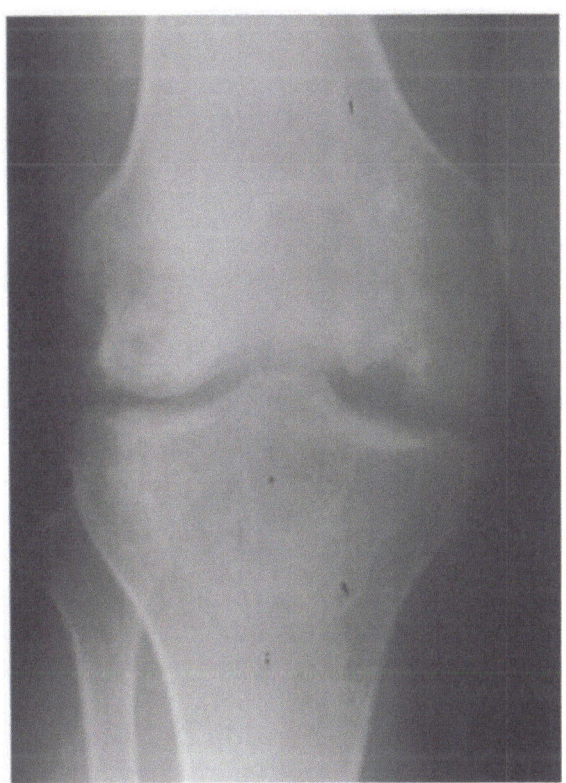

FIGURE C2.1 Standing anteroposterior radiograph demonstrates normal tibiofemoral joint space, osteochondral defect of medial femoral condyle, early peripheral lateral osteophytes, and patchy sclerosis and lucency of the distal femur compatible with avascular necrosis.

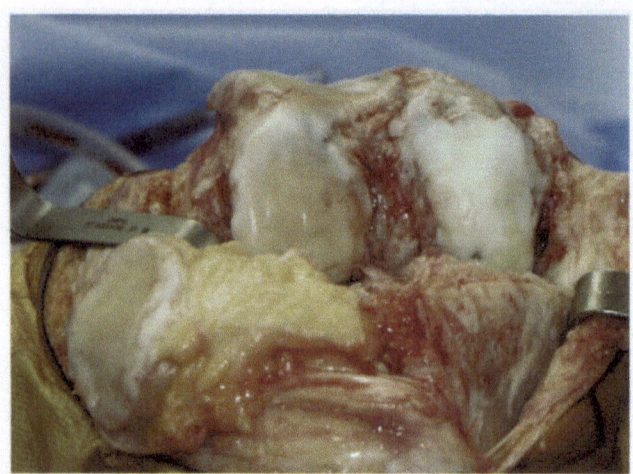
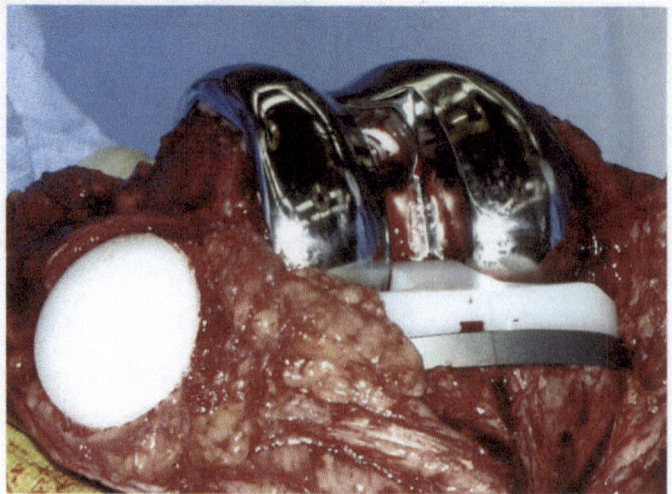

FIGURE C2.2 **(A)** Clinical photograph at the time of arthrotomy reveals discolored articular cartilage that is easily peeled off the distal femur. **(B)** Intraoperative appearance of total knee prosthesis.

painfree. Two years postoperatively his result remains excellent.

DECISION-MAKING FACTORS

1. Low-demand, 55-year-old male with severely symptomatic multifocal avascular necrosis.

2. Ongoing use of oral steroids.

3. Global nature of avascular necrosis and ongoing steroid insult contraindicates the implementation of cartilage restoration.

CHIEF COMPLAINT AND HISTORY OF PRESENT ILLNESS

The patient is a 14-year-old girl with a 1-year history of weight-bearing pain and discomfort on the medial aspect of her right knee with activity-related swelling and mechanical symptoms. When initially diagnosed as having osteochondritis dissecans, she was treated with 8 weeks of nonweight bearing with crutches and asked to refrain from sports or impact activities thereafter. Despite these efforts, she remained symptomatic and was referred for definitive treatment.

PHYSICAL EXAMINATION

Height, 5 ft, 3 in.; weight, 115 lb. She ambulates with a slightly antalgic gait and stands in symmetric physiologic valgus. Her right knee has a moderate-sized effusion. Her range of motion is 0 to 130 degrees. She is tender to palpation over the medial femoral condyle. Meniscal findings are absent. Her patellofemoral joint demonstrates normal tracking with no evidence of crepitus or apprehension. Her ligament examination is within normal limits.

Radiographs demonstrate an unstable lesion of osteochondritis dissecans of the medial femoral condyle of her right knee (Figure C3.1).

SURGICAL INTERVENTION

Because of persistent symptoms, she was indicated for arthroscopic reduction and internal fixation using a headless titanium screw. At arthroscopy, a lesion approximately 20 mm by 20 mm was found to be in situ, but unstable, with two palpably loose fragments. The fragments were elevated from the bed while leaving it hinged on an intact portion of the articular cartilage, and the base was debrided and microfractured. The fragments were repaired with two titanium headless screws (Acutrak, Mansfield, MA, USA) (Figure C3.2). Postoperatively, the patient was made nonweight bearing for approximately 8 weeks and utilized a continuous passive motion machine. At 8 weeks, she returned for hardware removal whereby the defect was believed to be stable and fully healed (Figures C3.3, C3.4). She was permitted to return to all activities at 4 months following her hardware removal.

FOLLOW-UP

At the patient's 6-month follow-up visit, she had no symptoms and had returned to all activities. Radiographs demonstrate a healed osteochondritis dissecans lesion of the medial femoral condyle (Figure C3.5).

DECISION-MAKING FACTORS

1. Young patient with symptomatic lesion of osteochondritis dissecans.
2. Persistent symptoms despite initial treatment with nonoperative protocol.
3. In situ, but unstable, lesion without significant fragmentation and clinically viable osteochondral fragment large enough to be repaired with screws.
4. Despite need for hardware removal, compression fixation used to maximize chances for healing.

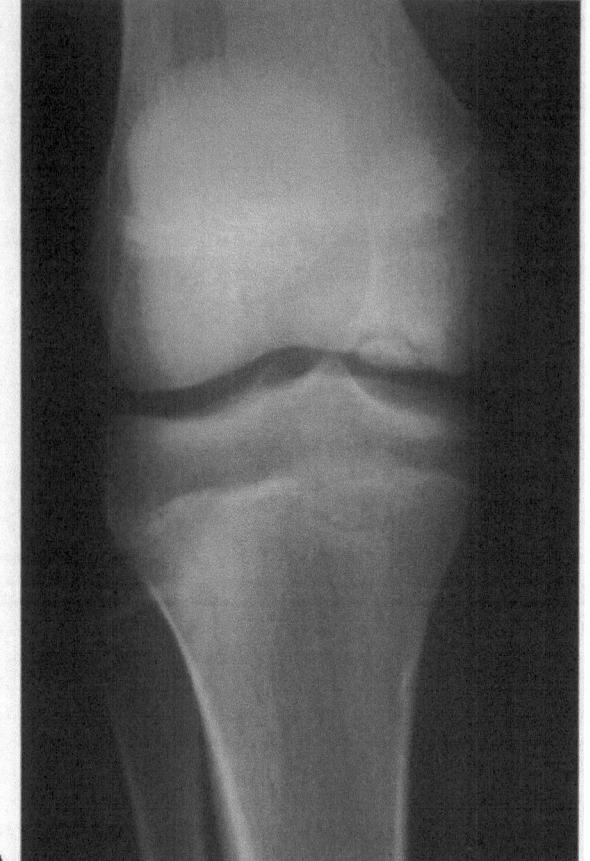

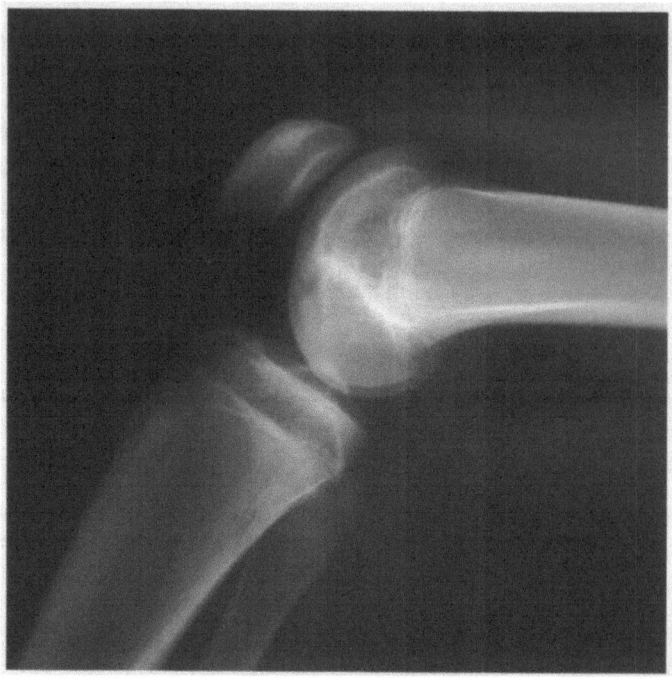

A   B

FIGURE C3.1 Anteroposterior (A) and lateral (B) radiographs demonstrate in situ lesion of osteochondritis dissecans of the medial femoral condyle in the right knee of a skeletally immature adolescent. Note the fragmentation best seen on the lateral radiograph.

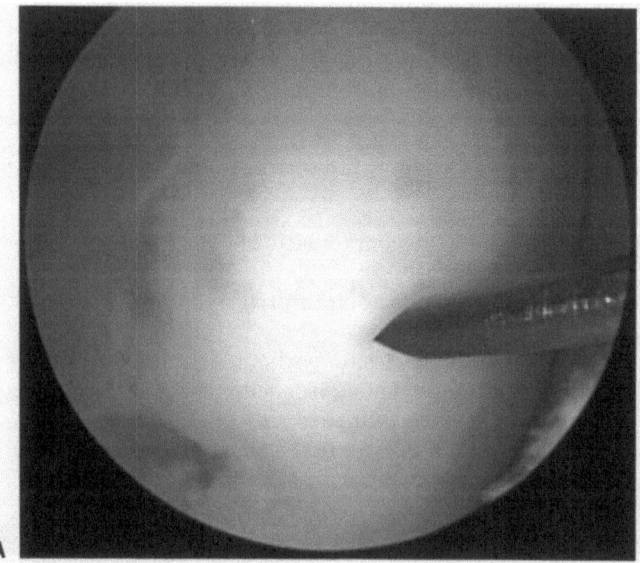

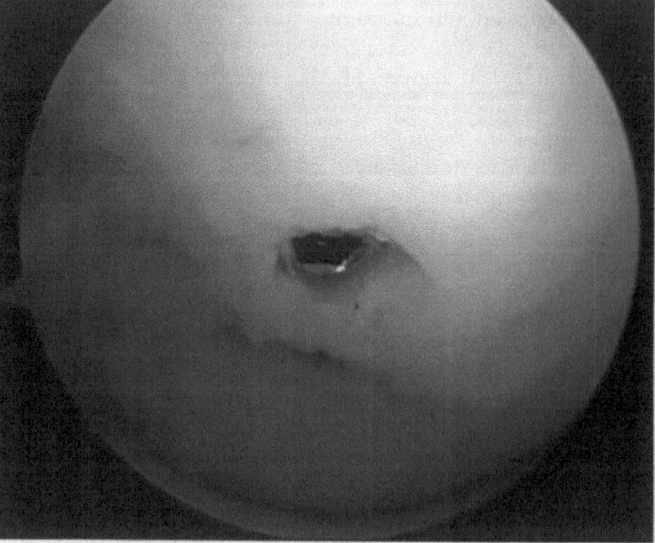

A   B

FIGURE C3.2 (A) An unstable lesion of osteochondritis dissecans seen arthroscopically along the medial femoral condyle. (B) The lesion bed has been prepared with debridement and microfracture followed by arthroscopic fixation using headless titanium screws for compression.

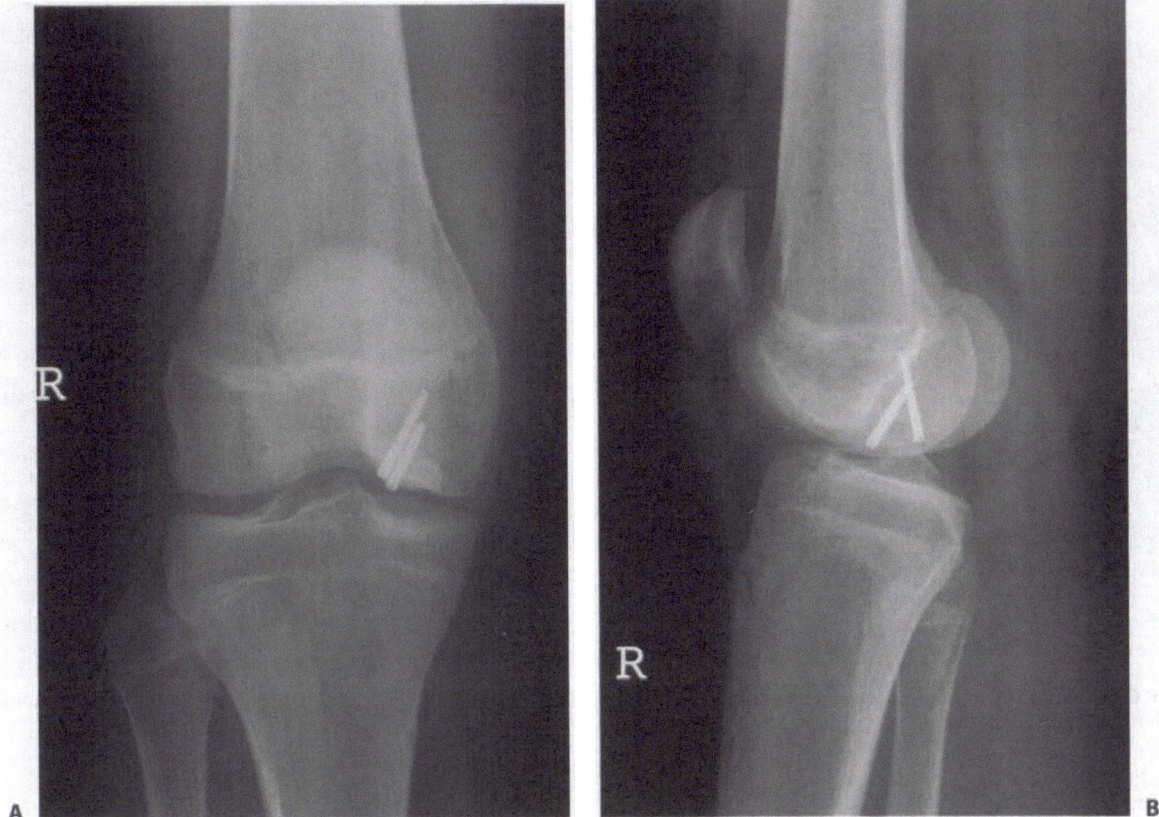

FIGURE C3.3 Anteroposterior (**A**) and lateral (**B**) radiographs obtained 8 weeks postoperatively demonstrate excellent healing of the fragment with no evidence of displacement.

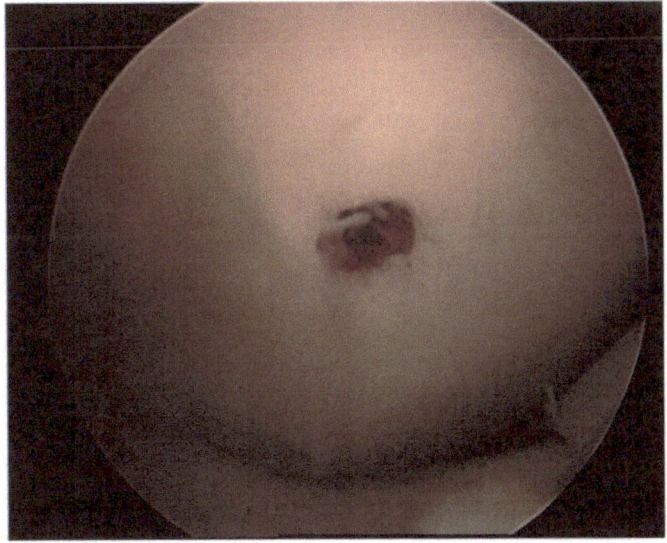

FIGURE C3.4 Eight-week arthroscopic view immediately following screw removal demonstrates clinical evidence of union of the osteochondral fragment.

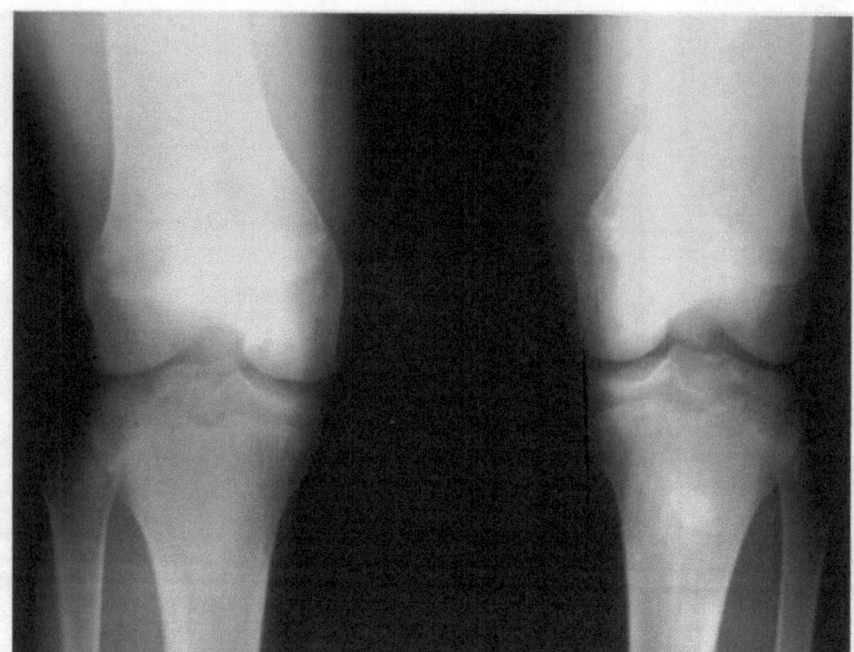
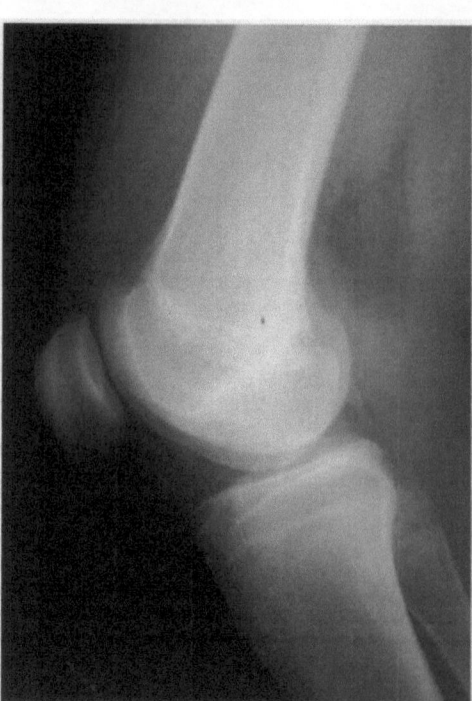

A

B

FIGURE C3.5 Six-month postoperative anteroposterior (**A**) and lateral (**B**) radiographs demonstrate integration of the fragment with no evidence of further fragmentation.

PATHOLOGY
Unstable in situ osteochondritis dissecans of the medial femoral condyle

TREATMENT
Arthroscopic fixation of osteochondral fragment followed by loose body removal

SUBMITTED BY
Brian J. Cole, MD, MBA, Rush Cartilage Restoration Center, Rush University Medical Center, Chicago, Illinois, USA

CHIEF COMPLAINT AND HISTORY OF PRESENT ILLNESS

The patient is an active 35-year-old woman who had no previous history of knee problems until the insidious onset of medial-sided right knee pain, swelling, and weight-bearing discomfort that began 6 months before presentation. She denied any trauma and was actively participating in snow skiing, running, and aerobics before the onset of these symptoms. She does not ever recall knee symptoms as a child or adolescent. She was referred for treatment of an unstable lesion of osteochondritis dissecans (OCD).

PHYSICAL EXAMINATION

Height, 5 ft, 5 in.; weight, 135 lb. She ambulates with a non-antalgic gate. She stands in symmetric physiologic valgus. Her right knee has a moderate-sized effusion. Her range of motion is 0 to 130 degrees. She is tender to palpation over the medial femoral condyle and has crepitus along the medial side of her knee with range of motion. Meniscal findings are absent. Her ligament examination is within normal limits.

RADIOGRAPHIC EVALUATION

Preoperative radiographs demonstrate a fragmented lesion of OCD along the medial femoral condyle in the right knee (Figure C4.1).

SURGICAL INTERVENTION

Because of the nature of her symptoms and the radiographic findings, she was indicated for an initial attempt at arthroscopic reduction and fixation of the OCD lesion. At the time of arthroscopy, an unstable lesion measuring approximately 2 cm by 3 cm by 1 cm (depth) was found in situ. A single major fragment was appreciated with a smaller minor fragment. This entire lesion was elevated from its bed, and the base was debrided and microfractured to promote healing. The major fragment was reduced and repaired with a single headless titanium screw (Acutrak, Mansfield, MA). The minor fragment was too small for screw fixation, and a single bioabsorbable pin was used (Orthosorb Pin; Johnson and Johnson, Canton, MA) (Figure C4.2). Postoperatively, the patient was made nonweight bearing for approximately 8 weeks and utilized continuous passive motion at 6 h/day. Thereafter, she was allowed to gradually return to higher-level activities.

FOLLOW-UP

The patient did exceptionally well until she presented again 1 year later with complaints of mechanical locking. However, the weight-bearing pain along the medial aspect of her knee was completely eliminated. Postoperative radiographs taken at 1 year demonstrated a loose body within the suprapatellar pouch, seen best on the lateral radiograph (Figure C4.3). She was indicated for arthroscopy for removal of the loose body. The defect was inspected and found to be entirely intact with no identifiable source for the loose body, although it was suspected that the minor fragment had displaced and its bed had filled with fibrocartilage (Figure C4.4). The headless screw was deep within the subchondral bone and completely overgrown with fibrocartilage and was, therefore, not removed. The patient returned to all activities, and radiographs taken at 2 years postoperatively demonstrated no evidence of further fragmentation with osseous integration of the major fragment (Figure C4.5).

DECISION-MAKING FACTORS

1. In situ defect with a viable plate of subchondral bone attached to the defect.
2. The ability to achieve anatomic fixation within the defect bed and a strong desire to avoid future treatment required for cartilage restoration should the fragment otherwise be removed.
3. Compression fixation used despite potential need for hardware removal to maximize chances for healing.

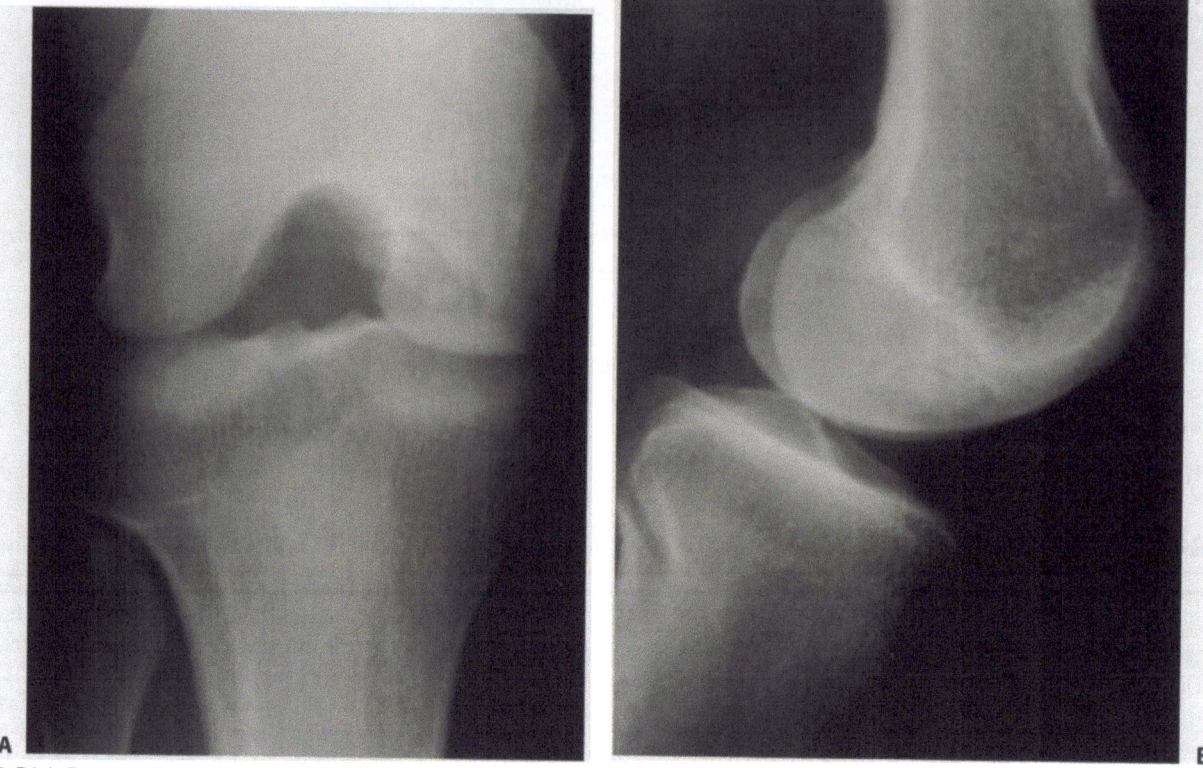

FIGURE C4.1 Preoperative anteroposterior (**A**) and lateral (**B**) radiographs demonstrate a fragmented lesion of osteochondritis dissecans (OCD) along the medial femoral condyle of the right knee.

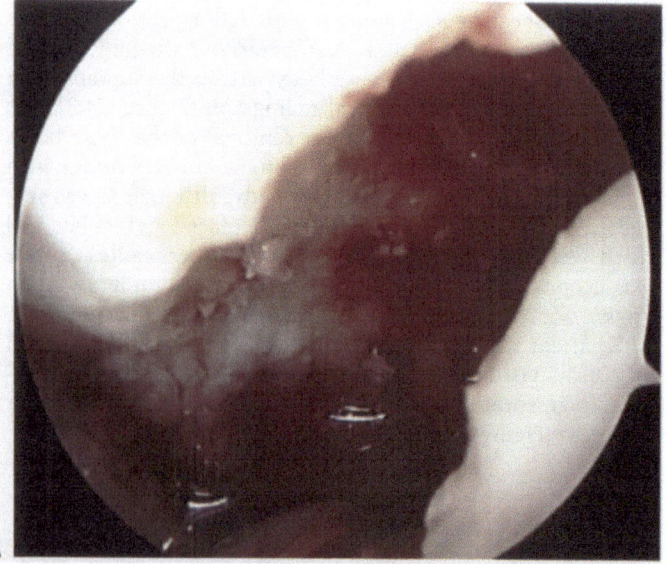 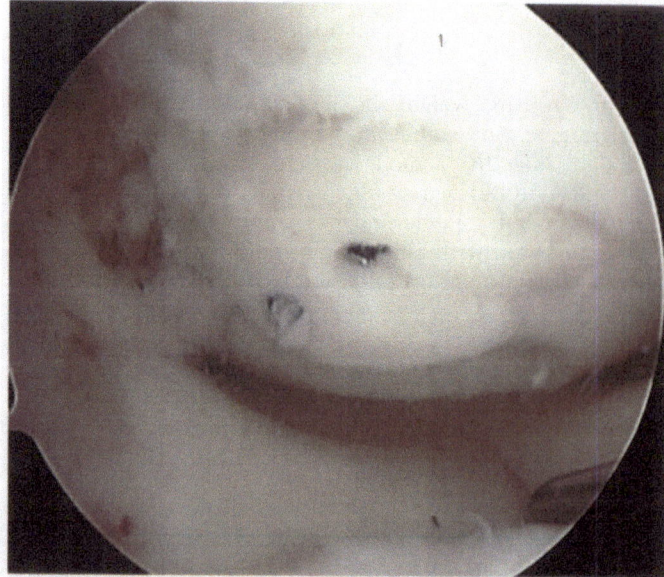

FIGURE C4.2 (A) An unstable lesion of OCD is seen arthroscopically along the medial femoral condyle with the lesion hinged open on intact articular cartilage. The base is debrided and microfractured to promote healing. **(B)** Arthroscopic fixation achieved with a headless titanium screw (Acutrak, Mansfield, MA) and a single bioabsorbable pin (Orthosorb Pin, Johnson and Johnson, Canton, MA).

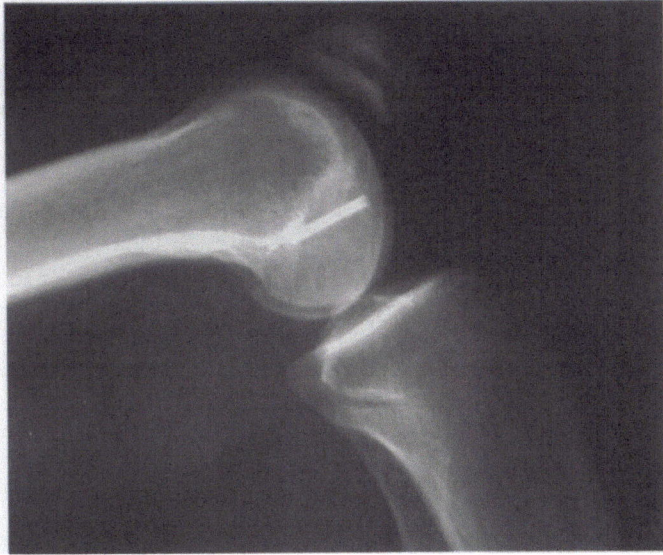

FIGURE C4.3 Lateral radiographs obtained at 1 year demonstrate a loose body within the suprapatellar pouch. Otherwise, the main fragment appears intact with the hardware still in place.

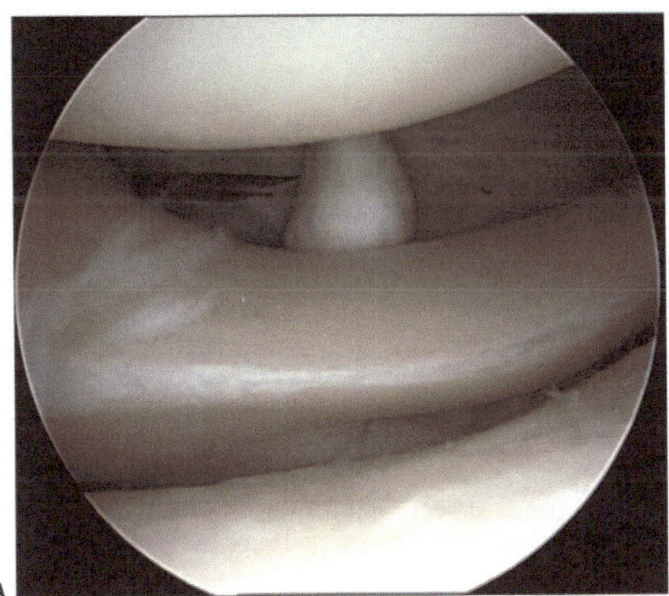

A

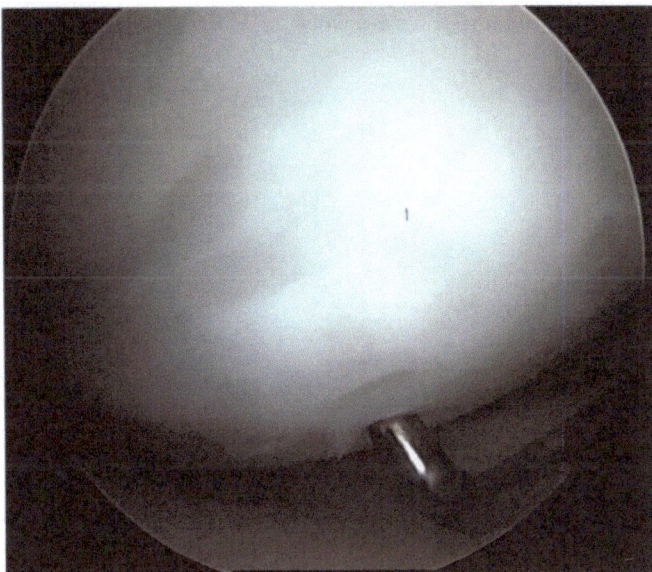

B

FIGURE C4.4 (A) Arthroscopic view of the loose body within the posterior aspect of the lateral compartment near the popliteal tendon. **(B)** Arthroscopic view of the defect without any obvious source of the loose body. The defect is stable to palpation and the areas are covered with fibrocartilage.

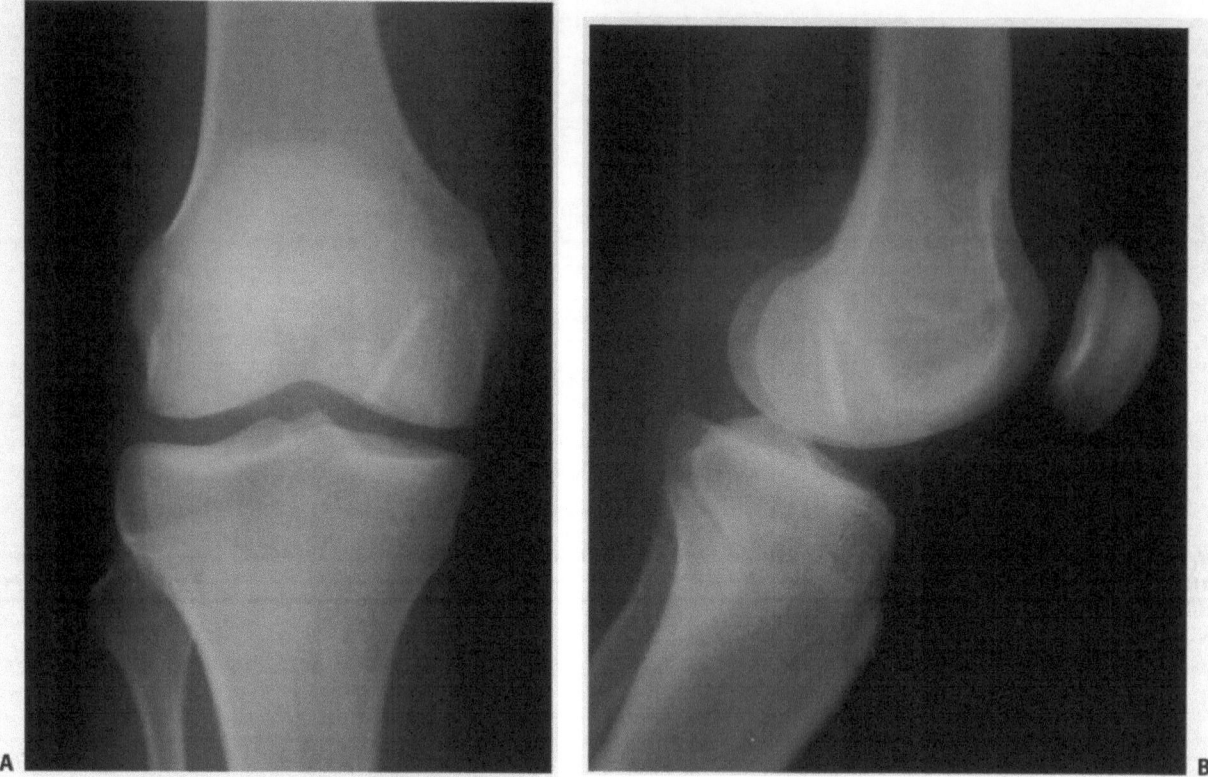

FIGURE C4.5 Two-year postoperative anteroposterior (**A**) and lateral (**B**) radiographs demonstrate osseous integration of the main fragment and no evidence of further fragmentation.

5

PATHOLOGY
Concomitant medial meniscus tear and focal chondral defect of the medial femoral condyle

TREATMENT
Medial meniscectomy and microfracture medial femoral condyle

SUBMITTED BY
Brian J. Cole, MD, MBA, Rush Cartilage Restoration Center, Rush University Medical Center, Chicago, Illinois, USA

CHIEF COMPLAINT AND HISTORY OF PRESENT ILLNESS

This 40-year-old woman had no preexisting knee problems until a twisting event occurred while attempting to squat. She noted the sudden onset of right knee pain and locking along the medial aspect of her knee. Her pain did not remit despite the passage of approximately 12 weeks time, and she continued to complain of locking. Because of her clinical symptoms, she was indicated for arthroscopy with a presumed diagnosis of medial meniscus tear.

PHYSICAL EXAMINATION

Height, 5 ft, 4 in.; weight, 130 lb. She ambulated with a slight antalgic gait. She stood in slight symmetric physiologic valgus. Her right knee has a small effusion. She is tender to palpation over the medial joint line. She has a positive flexion McMurray's test. Her range of motion is 0 to 120 degrees, with pain upon further attempt at flexion. Ligamentous testing is within normal limits.

RADIOGRAPHIC EVALUATION

Plain radiographs were within normal limits. No magnetic resonance image (MRI) was obtained.

SURGICAL INTERVENTION

At the time of the arthroscopy, she was noted to have a posterior horn medial meniscus tear with an irreparable parrot-beak configuration. The patient underwent a partial arthroscopic meniscectomy with debridement to a stable rim (Figure C5.1). Additionally, an incidental grade IV chondral lesion of the medial femoral condyle measuring approximately 15 mm by 15 mm was noted, which was questionably contributing to her symptoms. In part because the lesion was present in the ipsilateral symptomatic compartment, a formal microfracture technique was performed (Figure C5.2). Postoperatively, the patient was made nonweight bearing for 6 weeks and placed on continuous passive motion. Thereafter, she gradually progressed to activities as tolerated.

FOLLOW-UP

At 2 years of follow-up, she has continued to do well with the absence of any activity-related effusions, swelling, or ongoing discomfort.

DECISION-MAKING FACTORS

1. Simple irreparable meniscus tear that should predictably respond favorably to meniscectomy.
2. An incidental chondral lesion of the medial femoral condyle that could or might be a cause of persistent symptoms if left untreated.
3. A chondral lesion of relatively small size (i.e., less than 2–3 cm^2) in an otherwise low activity level and low physical demand patient.
4. Anticipated willingness of the patient to comply with the early-phase rehabilitation requirements to optimize the results following a marrow-stimulating technique.

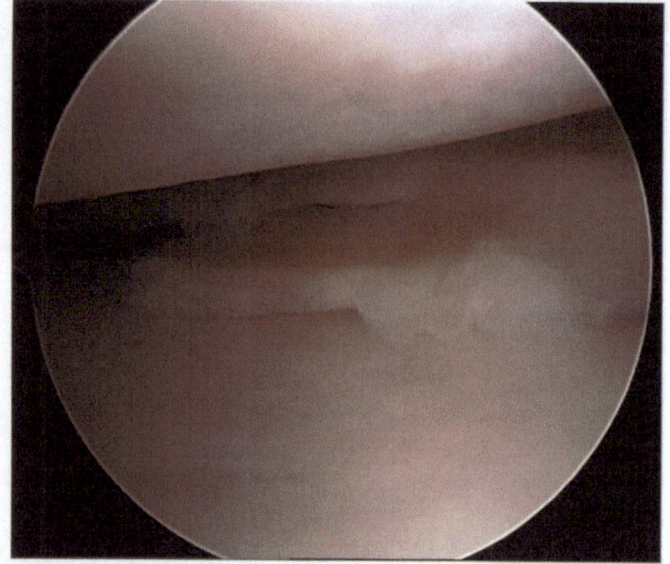 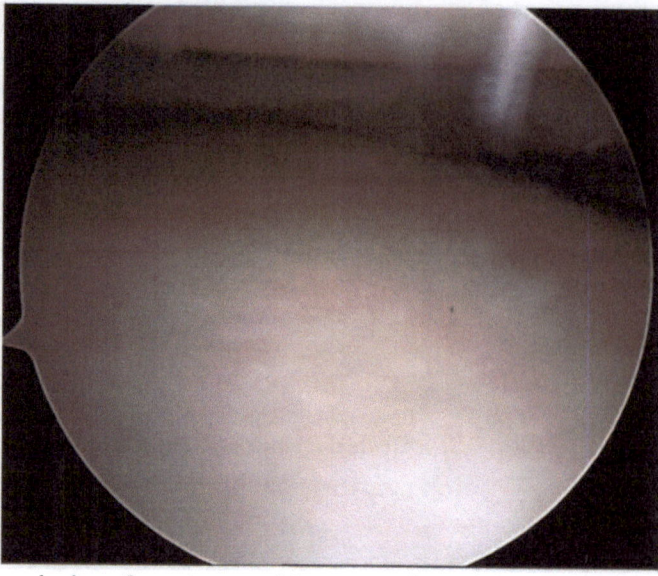

A   B

FIGURE C5.1 Arthroscopic photographs demonstrating an irreparable, parrot-beak configuration tear of the posterior horn of the medial meniscus before (**A**) and after (**B**) partial meniscectomy back to a stable rim.

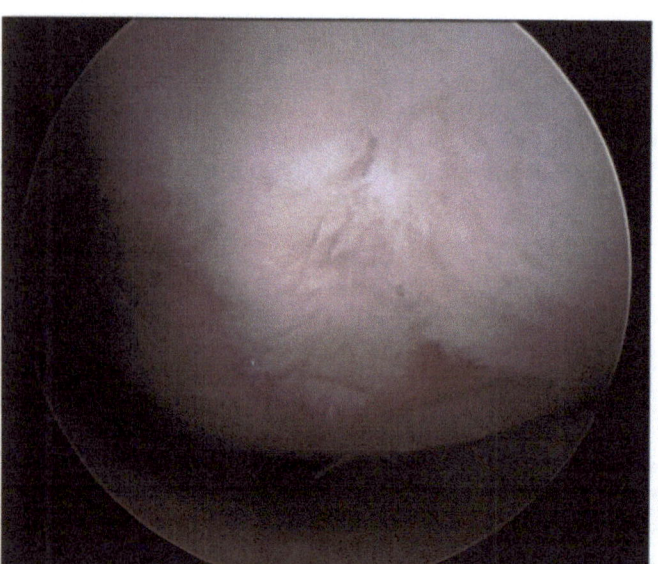 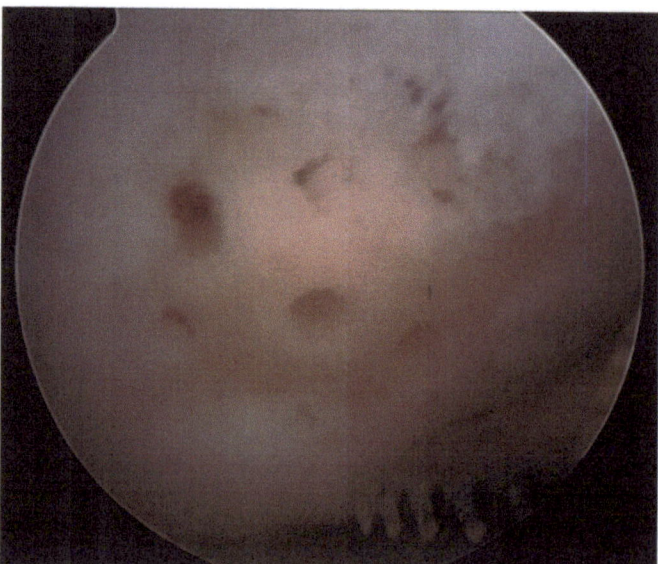

A   B

FIGURE C5.2 Photographs of grade III/IV chondral lesion of the medial femoral condyle measuring approximately 15 mm by 15 mm before (**A**) and after (**B**) formal microfracture technique was performed.

6

PATHOLOGY
Isolated focal chondral defect of the medial femoral condyle

TREATMENT
Microfracture

SUBMITTED BY
Tom Minas, MD and Tim Bryant, RN, Cartilage Repair Center, Brigham and Women's Hospital, Boston, Massachusetts, USA

CHIEF COMPLAINT AND HISTORY OF PRESENT ILLNESS

The patient is a 48-year-old woman who sustained an injury to the medial femoral condyle of her right knee. This lesion was treated with arthroscopic debridement alone for a grade II, partial-thickness chondral defect. This intervention alleviated her catching symptoms; however, her medial-sided weight-bearing pain persisted. She had significant limitations of her activities of daily living. She was not a particularly athletic or active individual, but desired pain relief with activities of daily living.

PHYSICAL EXAMINATION

Height, 5 ft, 3 in.; weight, 125 lb. Clinical examination demonstrated a slim woman with neutrally aligned lower extremities. She had no gait disturbance. Her range of motion was full and symmetric. There was no effusion. She had tenderness over the weight-bearing portion of her medial femoral condyle. Her ligament and meniscal examinations were normal.

RADIOGRAPHIC EVALUATION

Plain films were unremarkable and were without evidence of joint space narrowing or degenerative changes.

SURGICAL INTERVENTION

At arthroscopy, a small 10 mm by 10 mm grade III lesion of the medial femoral condyle was identified. A formal microfracture technique was performed, including removal and curettage of damaged repair tissue and cartilage back to stable intact normal articular cartilage; this involved removal of the tidemark. A sharp microfracture awl was used peripherally around the defect and then centrally at intervals of 3 to 5 mm without connecting or destabilizing the subchondral plate (Figure C6.1). Postoperatively, the patient was made protected weight bearing for 6 weeks and used continuous passive motion.

FOLLOW-UP

The patient was full weight bearing by 3 months and returned to sporting activities by 6 months. She is presently 1 year after her surgery and is pain-free (Figure C6.2).

DECISION-MAKING FACTORS

1. Low-demand patient with small focal chondral defect which represented a relatively large area of the entire width of the medial femoral condyle.
2. Failure of previous arthroscopic debridement.
3. Osteochondral autograft was not chosen due to concerns for donor site morbidity given relatively small size of the trochlea.
4. Willingness to remain compliant with postoperative rehabilitation required to achieve successful result following microfracture.
5. Patient understanding that excessive activity levels, despite fibrocartilage fill, may lead to recurrent symptoms and further treatment attempts.

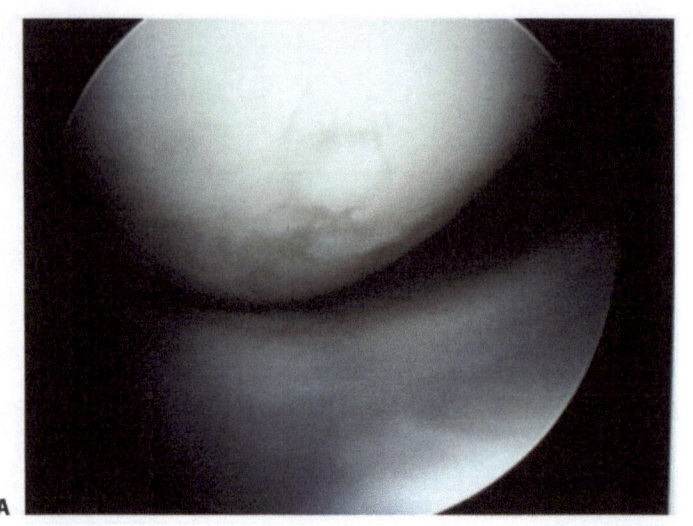

A

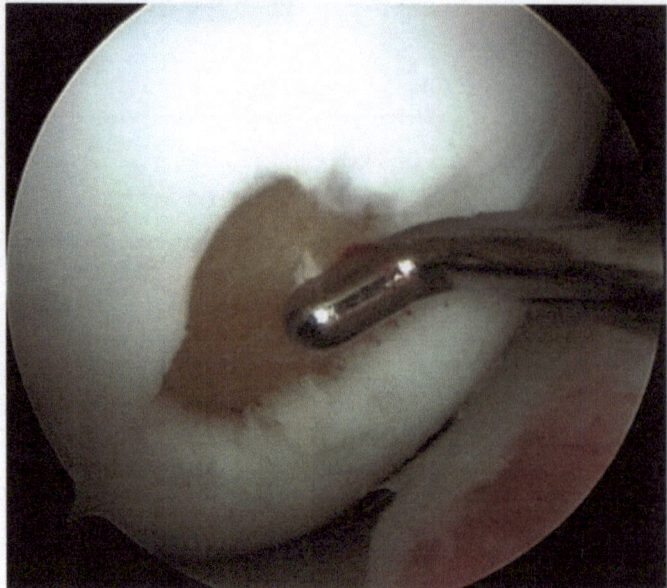

B

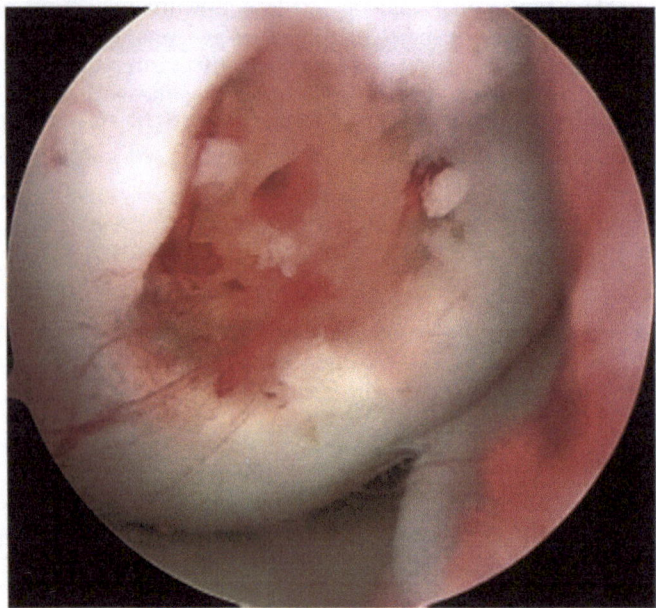

C

FIGURE C6.1 Arthroscopic photographs identifying (**A**) 10 mm by 10 mm defect treated with (**B**) defect preparation and (**C**) microfracture technique.

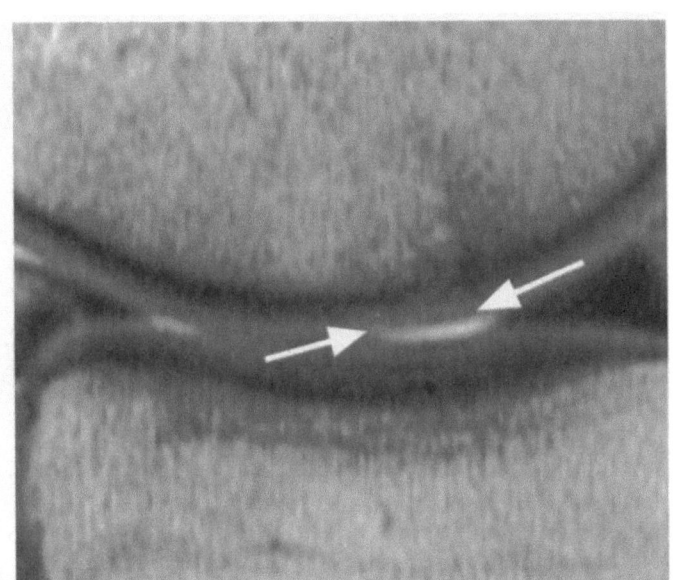
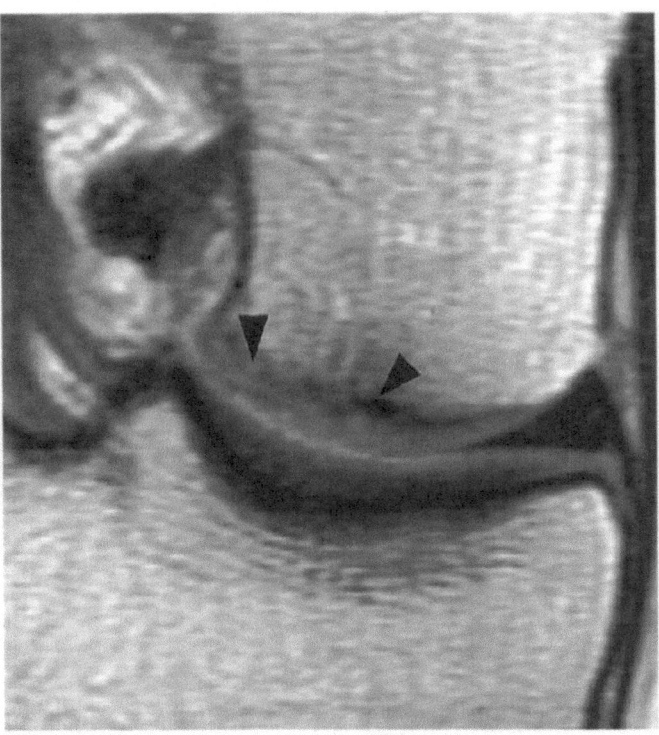

A
B

FIGURE C6.2 One-year postoperative magnetic resonance imaging (MRI) demonstrates on sagittal (**A**) and coronal (**B**) images that repair tissue is filling the defect area, where former microfracture was performed (*arrows*).

PATHOLOGY
Symptomatic focal chondral defect of lateral femoral condyle

TREATMENT
Microfracture of lateral femoral condyle with biopsy for possible future autologous chondrocyte implantation

SUBMITTED BY
Brian J. Cole, MD, MBA, Rush Cartilage Restoration Center, Rush University Medical Center, Chicago, Illinois, USA

CHIEF COMPLAINT AND HISTORY OF PRESENT ILLNESS

This patient is a 39-year-old, very active architect who had a hyperextension injury to his left knee while playing basketball. He had immediate onset of swelling and weight-bearing pain along the lateral aspect of his left knee. He failed to respond to conservative care. Because of his persistent symptoms that remained unresponsive to relative rest, a magnetic resonance image (MRI) was obtained; based upon this information, he was indicated for arthroscopy.

PHYSICAL EXAMINATION

Height, 5 ft, 10 in.; weight, 180 lb. The patient ambulates with a slightly antalgic gait. He stands in symmetric neutral alignment. His left knee has a moderate-sized effusion. His range of motion is from 0 to 130 degrees. He is tender to palpation over the lateral femoral condyle. Meniscal findings are absent. Patellofemoral joint demonstrates good tracking with no evidence of crepitus. His ligamentous examination is within normal limits.

RADIOGRAPHIC EVALUATION

Plain radiographs were evaluated and found to be within normal limits (Figure C7.1). MRI showed subchondral edema and violation of the chondral surface of the lateral femoral condyle (Figure C7.2).

SURGICAL INTERVENTION

At the time of arthroscopy, a full-thickness 10 mm by 16 mm chondral injury of the lateral femoral condyle within the weight-bearing zone in extension was identified (Figure C7.3). A formal microfracture procedure was performed (Figure

C7.4). Because of the patient's relatively active lifestyle, the location of the lesion, and the possibility for fibrocartilage breakdown in the future, a concomitant biopsy of 200 to 300 mg cartilaginous tissue was obtained from the intercondylar notch (Figure C7.5). [The author of this case (B.J.C.) currently does not routinely biopsy a patient unless there is an explicit intention to treat a defect with autologous chondrocyte implantation in the near future.] Postoperatively, the patient was made nonweight bearing for approximately 6 weeks. He was placed on continuous passive motion, which he performed for 6 weeks at 6 h/day.

FOLLOW-UP

The patient continues to do well nearly 2 years after his microfracture and has returned to all sports without any symptoms of weight-bearing pain, activity-related swelling, or discomfort. There is no intention in the near future to perform any further management of his defect unless he were to become symptomatic again.

DECISION-MAKING FACTORS

1. Relatively young active male with acute onset of symptoms related to a symptomatic femoral condyle chondral lesion.
2. Microfracture indicated as a first-time treatment for a relatively small chondral defect. Alternative treatment could also include primary osteochondral autograft transplantation.
3. Potential for failure of a marrow-stimulating technique in an otherwise active male, leading to the concomitant biopsy during this procedure.
4. Ability and willingness to be compliant with the postoperative rehabilitation required of a microfracture technique.

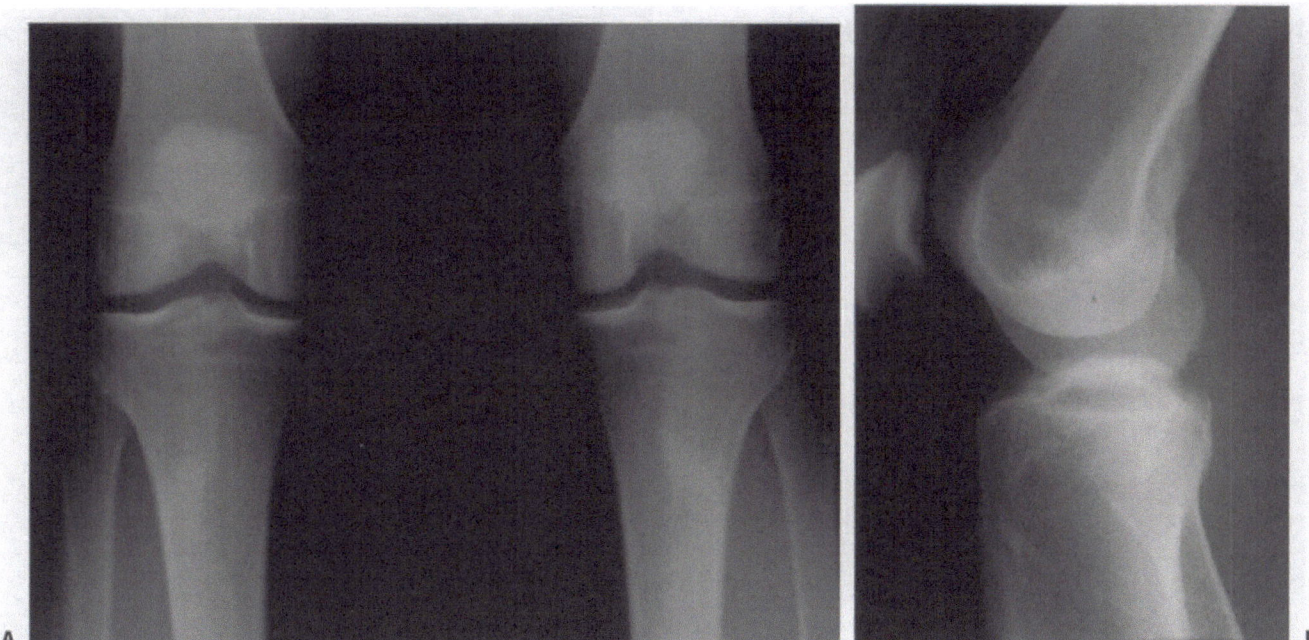

FIGURE C7.1 Forty-five-degree flexion weight-bearing posteroanterior (**A**) and lateral (**B**) radiographs demonstrate no abnormalities.

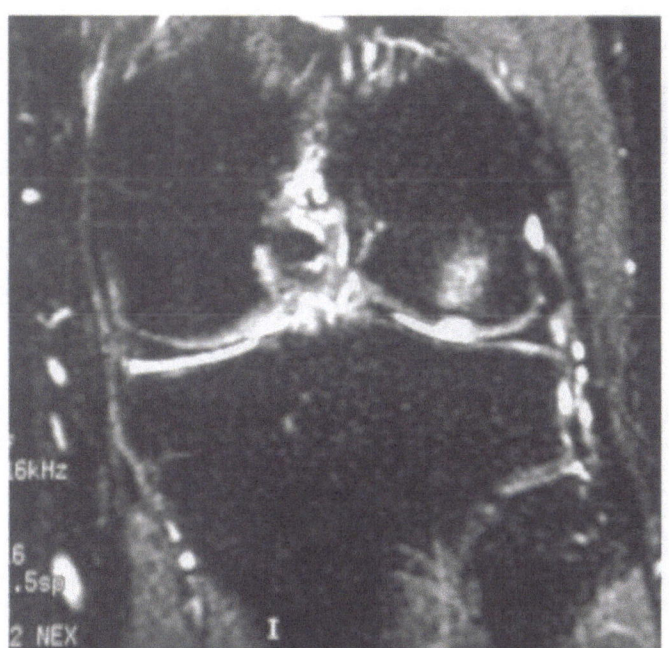

FIGURE C7.2 Coronal MRI demonstrates subchondral edema as well as violation of the chondral surface of the lateral femoral condyle.

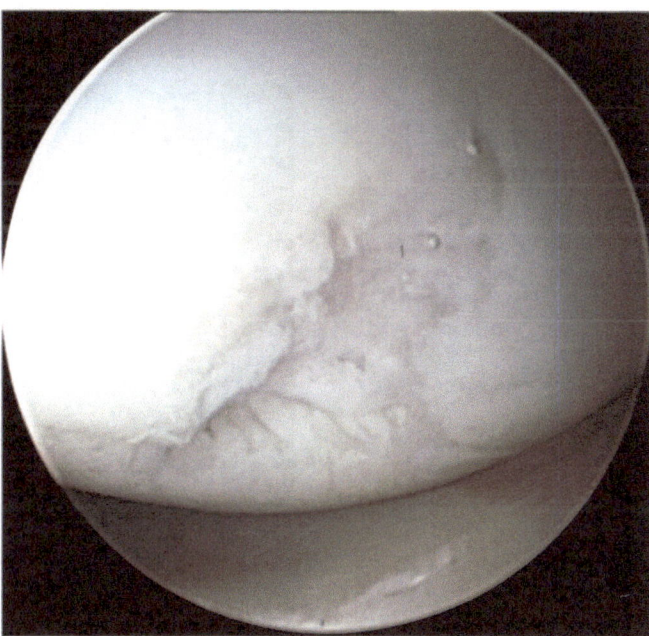

FIGURE C7.3 Arthroscopic photograph reveals a 10 mm by 16 mm full-thickness chondral dect of the lateral femoral condyle within the weight-bearing zone.

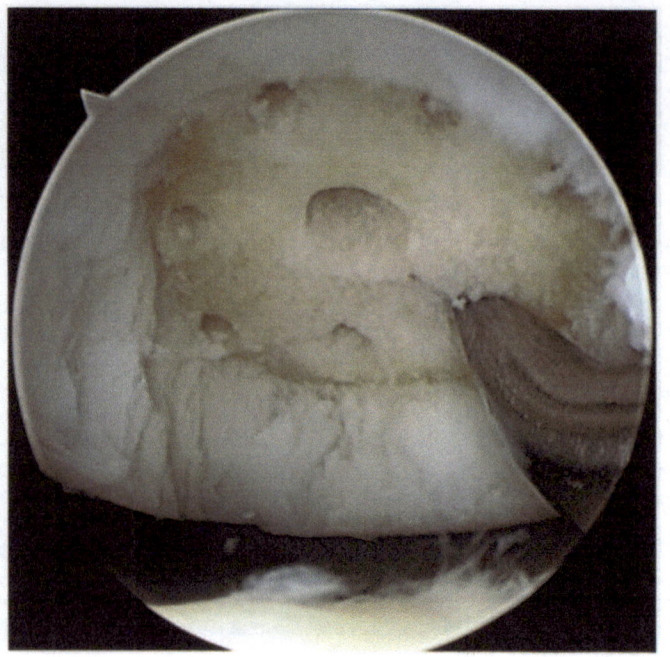
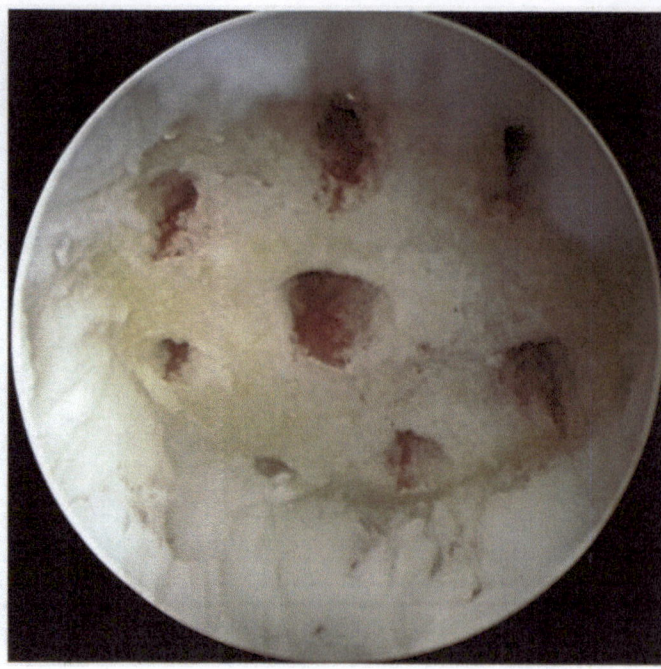

A

FIGURE C7.4 Arthroscopic views of the microfracture technique being performed. **(A)** Bloody return is shown from the holes penetrating the subchondral bone **(B)**.

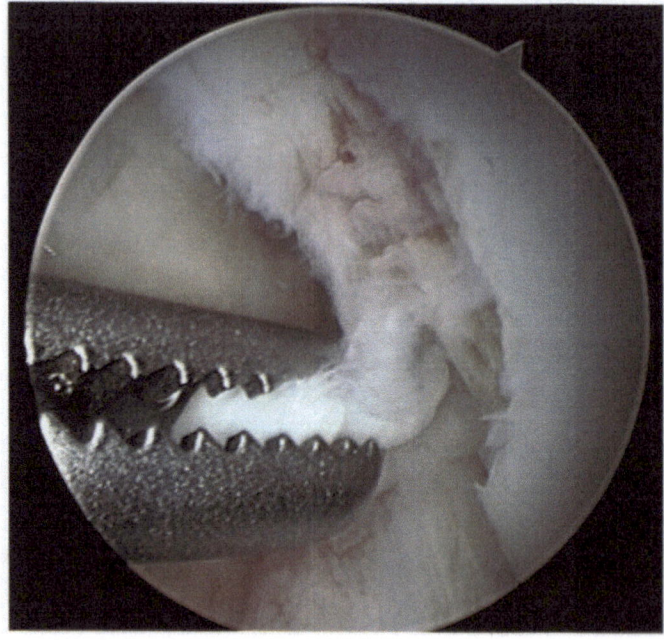

FIGURE C7.5 Arthroscopic view of biopsy of 200 to 300 mg cartilaginous tissue obtained from the intercondylar notch for potential future autologous chondrocyte implantation should the need arise.

8

PATHOLOGY
Isolated small grade IV medial femoral condyle chondral lesion

TREATMENT
Primary osteochondral autograft transplantation

SUBMITTED BY
Brian J. Cole, MD, MBA, Rush Cartilage Restoration Center, Rush University Medical Center, Chicago, Illinois, USA

CHIEF COMPLAINT AND HISTORY OF PRESENT ILLNESS

This patient is a 31-year-old man who sustained a single, giving-way episode of his left knee, after a misstep approximately 4 months before evaluation. Since his initial injury, he has had several hyperextension-type giving-way episodes. He complains of activity-related swelling and medial knee pain with weight bearing. He is unable to participate in any impact-type activities.

PHYSICAL EXAMINATION

Height, 6 ft, 2 in.; weight, 188 lb. He ambulates with a non-antalgic gait. He stands in neutral alignment. His left knee has a moderate effusion. His range of motion is 0 to 130 degrees. He is tender to palpation over the medial femoral condyle. Meniscal findings are absent. His ligament examination is within normal limits.

RADIOGRAPHIC EVALUATION

Plain radiographs and magnetic resonance imaging (MRI) are within normal limits.

SURGICAL INTERVENTION

Because of his persistent symptoms, he was indicated for a diagnostic arthroscopy and evaluation for possible chondral injury. At the time of arthroscopy, he was noted to have a 10 mm by 10 mm grade IV lesion along the weight-bearing portion of his medial femoral condyle (Figure C8.1). It was elected to proceed with primary osteochondral autograft transplantation (Figure C8.2). Postoperatively, the patient was made partial weight bearing for approximately 4 to 6 weeks and placed on continuous passive motion for 6 weeks at approximately 6 h/day. Thereafter, he progressed to activities as tolerated.

FOLLOW-UP

At his 2-year follow-up, the patient complains of no pain. He has full range of motion and enjoys all sports without any symptoms such as swelling, locking, or weight-bearing discomfort.

DECISION-MAKING FACTORS

1. Defect less than $2\,cm^2$ in the weight-bearing zone of the femoral condyle.

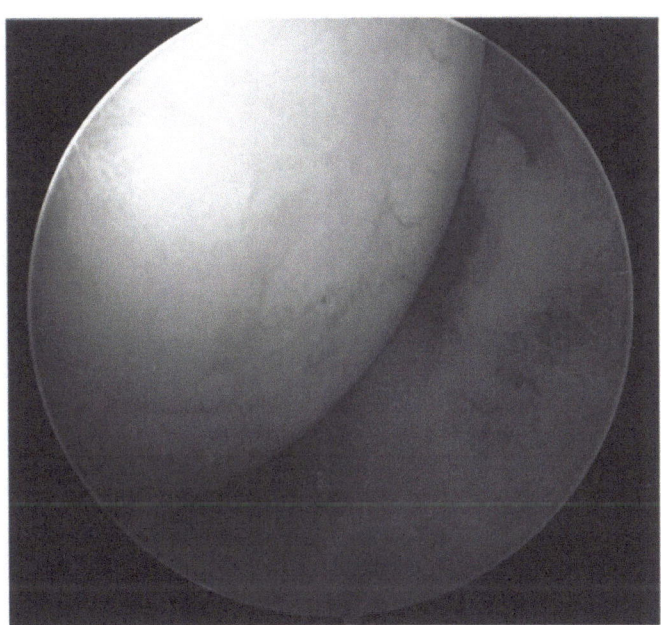

FIGURE C8.1 Arthroscopic photograph of the 10 mm by 10 mm lesion along the weight-bearing portion of his medial femoral condyle.

2. Isolated pathology in a young, active male with expectations and activity levels likely to exceed any benefit that microfracture might provide.

3. First-line treatment aimed at cartilage restoration because his activity level and the defect characteristics warranted this relatively higher level of treatment.

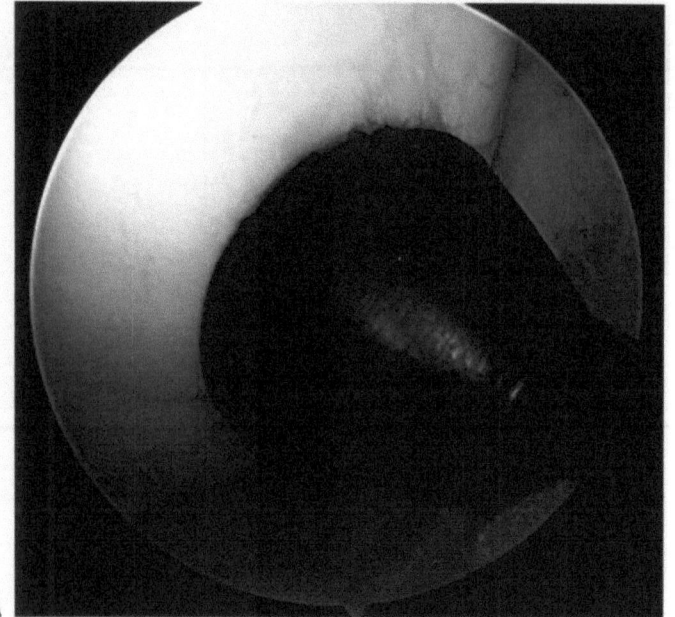

A

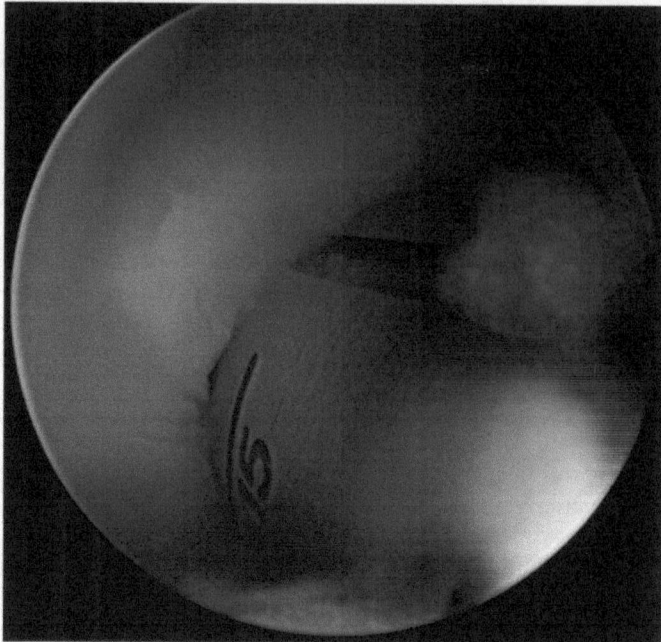

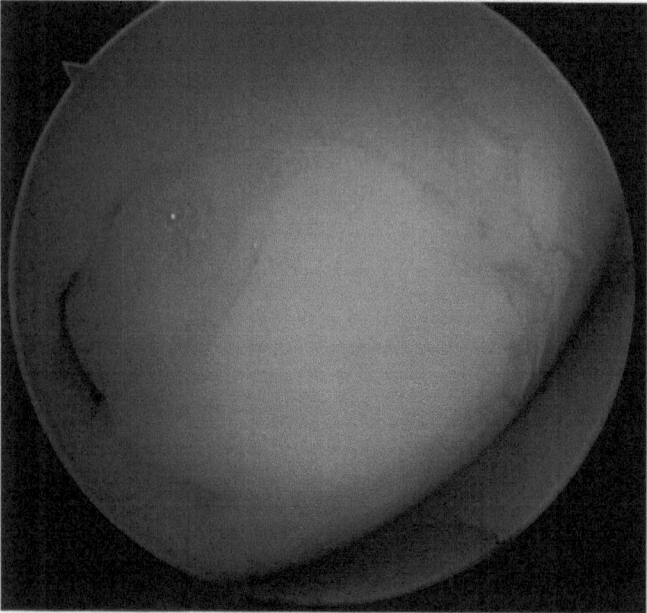

C

FIGURE C8.2 The defect was (A) sized and (B) subsequently extracted using a 10-mm coring reamer. (C) Autograft plug obtained from region of lateral sulcus terminalis is impacted into place.

9

PATHOLOGY
Isolated medial compartment osteoarthritis

TREATMENT
Unicompartmental knee replacement

SUBMITTED BY
Tom Minas, MD, and Tim Bryant, RN, Cartilage Repair Center, Brigham and Women's Hospital, Boston, Massachusetts, USA

CHIEF COMPLAINT AND HISTORY OF PRESENT ILLNESS

The patient is a 60-year-old man with severe left knee medial joint line pain with weight bearing. He has difficulty walking even short distances. He also has difficulty with stairs. He has severe limitations with activities of daily living, and wishes to have pain relief with these activities as well as with nonimpact recreational sports. He has failed attempts at treatment with corticosteroid injections, unloader bracing, antiinflammatories, and physical therapy.

PHYSICAL EXAMINATION

Height, 5 ft, 11 in.; weight, 185 lb. The patient is a slender 60-year-old man who appears physiologically younger than his chronologic age. He has mild symmetric varus alignment of both lower extremities. He walks with an antalgic gait on the left side only. His range of motion is 0 to 125 degrees of flexion. He has medial joint line tenderness and medial tibiofemoral crepitus. There is no effusion and no patellofemoral or lateral compartment crepitus or tenderness. There are palpable medial osteophytes, and his alignment corrects almost to neutral with a valgus-producing force. There is a good medial endpoint. His ligament examination is within normal limits.

RADIOGRAPHIC EVALUATION

Plain radiographs demonstrate complete loss of the medial joint space, and a healthy lateral and patellofemoral joint compartment without evidence of tibiofemoral subluxation (Figure C9.1).

SURGICAL INTERVENTION

Because of his age, low-demand activities, and need to return to work in a short period of time, it was decided to pursue surgical reconstruction by medial unicompartmental arthroplasty (Figure C9.2). Postoperatively, the patient was advanced to weight bearing and range of motion as tolerated. He progressed to activities as tolerated by 16 weeks (Figure C9.2).

FOLLOW-UP

Within a few weeks postoperatively his pain was completely resolved allowing early return to work. He returned to golf within 3 months and to recreational skiing within 9 months after reconstruction (Figure C9.3). His range of motion was comparable to his preoperative condition.

DECISION-MAKING FACTORS

1. An otherwise healthy, 60-year-old male with end-stage bipolar medial compartment osteoarthritis and slight varus alignment.
2. Goals: to return to low-demand activities and work within a few weeks of surgery.
3. No evidence of significant patellofemoral or lateral tibiofemoral symptoms by history, radiographs, or physical examination.

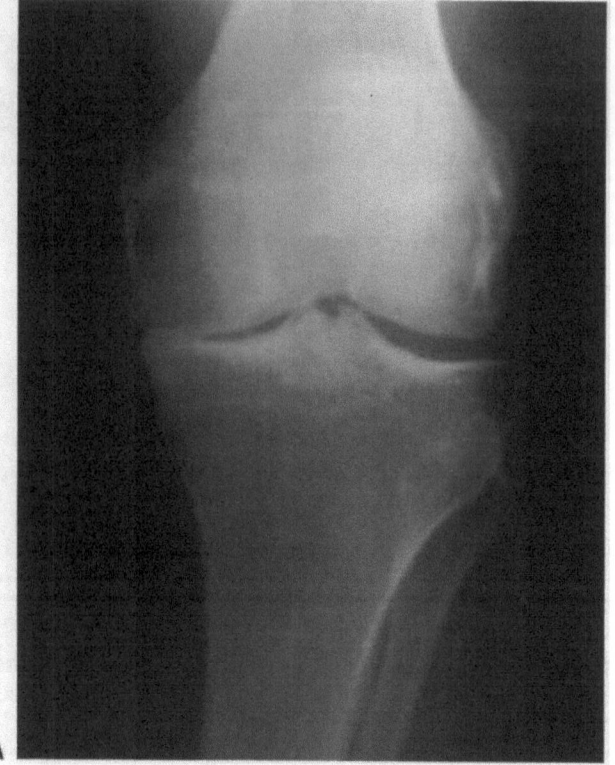

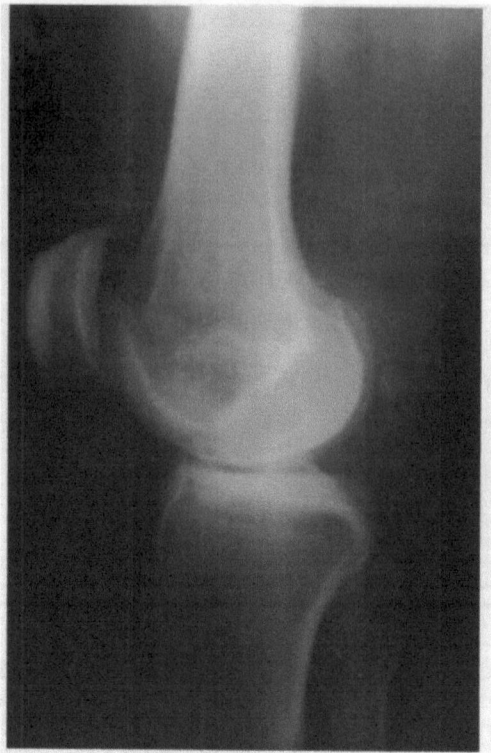

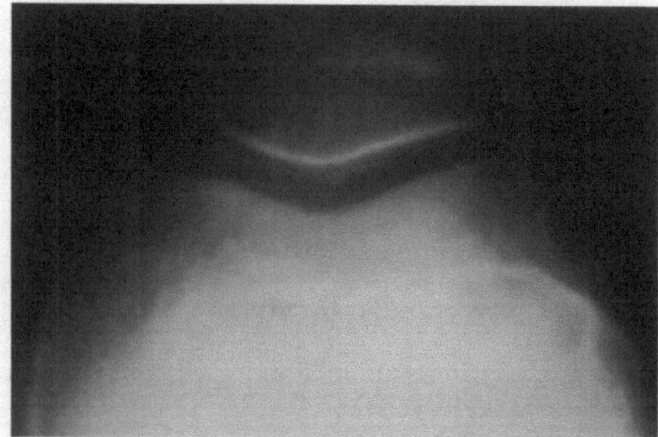

FIGURE C9.1 Preoperative (A) standing anteroposterior, (B) lateral, and (C) skyline radiographs demonstrate nearly complete loss of medial joint space with healthy lateral and patellofemoral compartments without evidence of tibiofemoral subluxation.

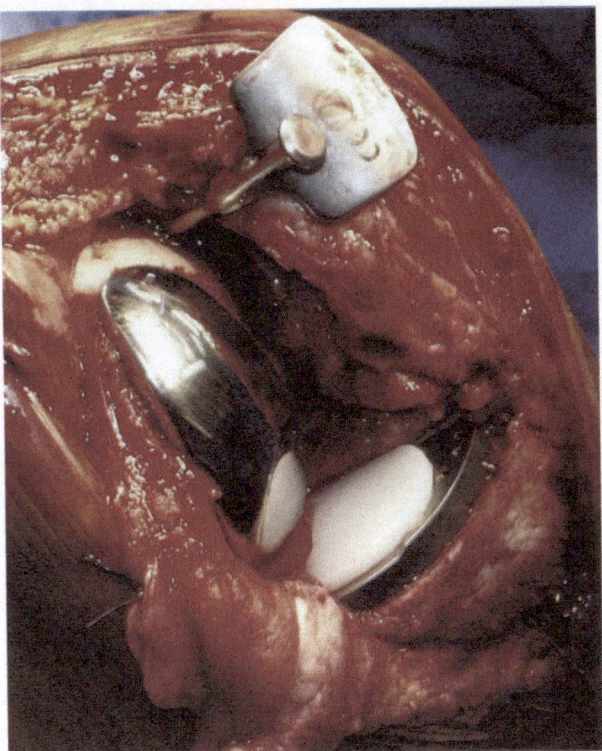

FIGURE C9.2 Intraoperative photograph of implanted tibiofemoral unicompartmental prosthesis through a minimally invasive incision without a quadriceps split.

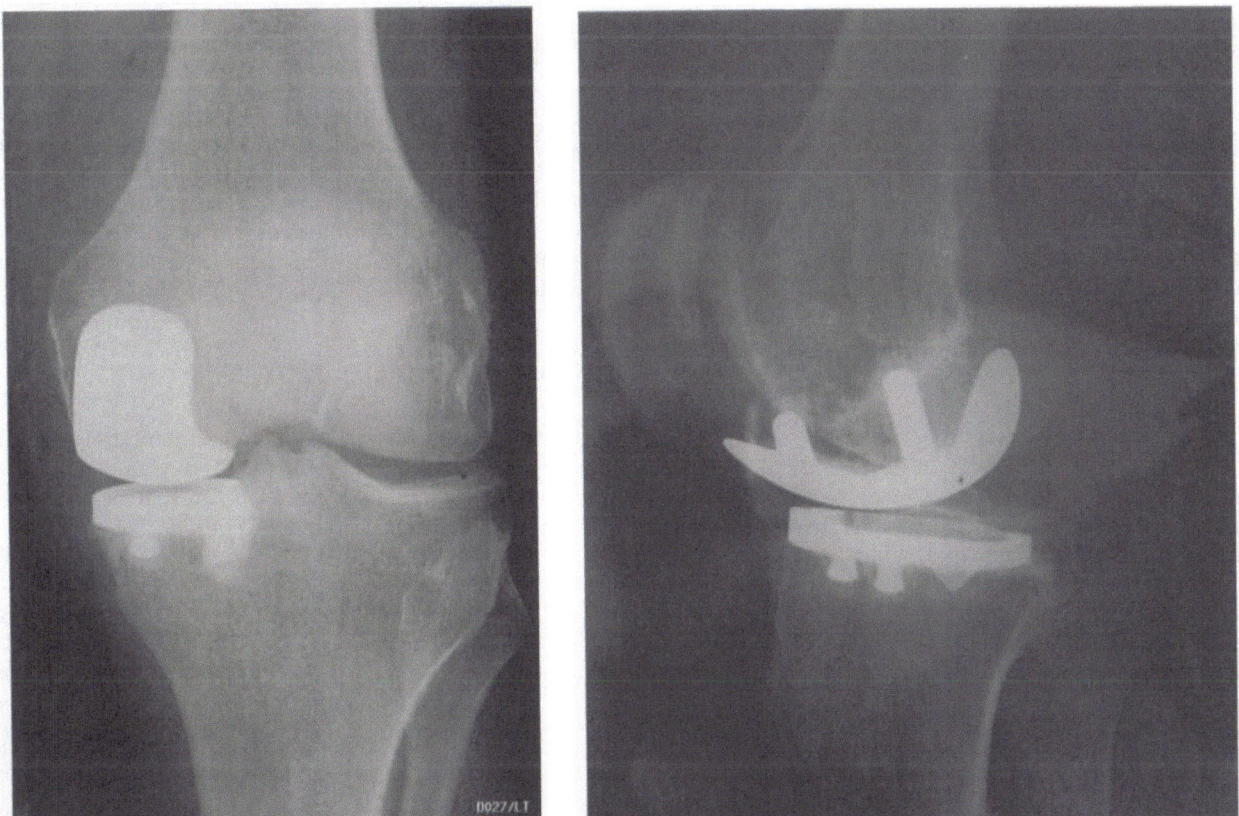

FIGURE C9.3 Postoperative anteroposterior (**A**) and lateral (**B**) radiographs of well-functioning medial unicompartmental prosthesis.

10

PATHOLOGY
Unicompartmental bipolar disease

TREATMENT
Unispacer

SUBMITTED BY
Jack Farr, MD, Cartilage Restoration Center of Indiana, OrthoIndy, Indianapolis, Indiana, USA.

CHIEF COMPLAINT AND HISTORY OF PRESENT ILLNESS

This male patient is a 44-year-old, large-machine mechanic with progressive, left greater than right, medial-sided knee pain. The quality is sharp with twisting and turning activities and at other times deep, dull aching. The severity is intense and the timing is per weight-bearing activity, although he does have some aching at rest. The patient has unsuccessfully worn an unloader knee brace for the past 2 years. He reports a history of an open meniscectomy and arthroscopy of his right knee performed more than 20 years previously. He smokes 1 to 2 packs per day and has for the past 20 years.

PHYSICAL EXAMINATION

Height, 5 ft, 9 in.; weight, 150 lb; BMI (body mass index), 22.5. The patient ambulates with an antalgic gait. He stands in slight symmetric varus. Bilateral range of motion is from 5 to 130 degrees of flexion. He has a mild effusion on the right knee and moderate effusion on the left knee. He has bilateral focal medial joint line tenderness. There is no increased ligamentous laxity.

RADIOGRAPHIC EVALUATION

Anteroposterior and lateral radiographs demonstrate medial compartment joint space narrowing (Figure C10.1). The Merchant view shows a central patella with maintenance of joint space. The posteroanterior standing notch view shows significant joint space loss in the right medial compartment and moderate narrowing in the left medial compartment. The long-leg alignment view shows 4 to 5 degrees varus on the right and 3 to 4 degrees varus on the left.

SURGICAL INTERVENTION

The arthroscopy revealed minimal chondrosis except medially where both the femoral condyle and tibial plateau had extensive grade III and early IV chondrosis. The meniscus was relatively absent. The anterior cruciate ligament was intact. Following arthroscopic preparation of the joint surfaces, a unispacer was inserted through a miniarthrotomy (Figure C10.2). Postoperatively, the patient was immediately allowed weight bearing and range of motion as tolerated. Advance to unrestricted activities was permitted after 3 months.

FOLLOW-UP

At 3 months, radiographs demonstrate good placement of the unispacer (Figure C10.3). The patient has returned to work and, at 6 months, he is now limited by his nonoperative knee. He still has some minor complaints of residual discomfort along the medial side of his right knee, albeit less than he had preoperatively.

DECISION-MAKING FACTORS

1. Relatively advanced unicompartmental bipolar disease of the medial compartment in a young patient who is unwilling to take time off work to allow the healing required of a high tibial osteotomy.
2. A heavy smoker with a relative contraindication to osteotomy.
3. Considered to be relatively young for unicompartmental knee replacement.
4. Unispacer should allow successful revision, if necessary, to unicompartmental or total knee arthroplasty, without compromising the result of those procedures.

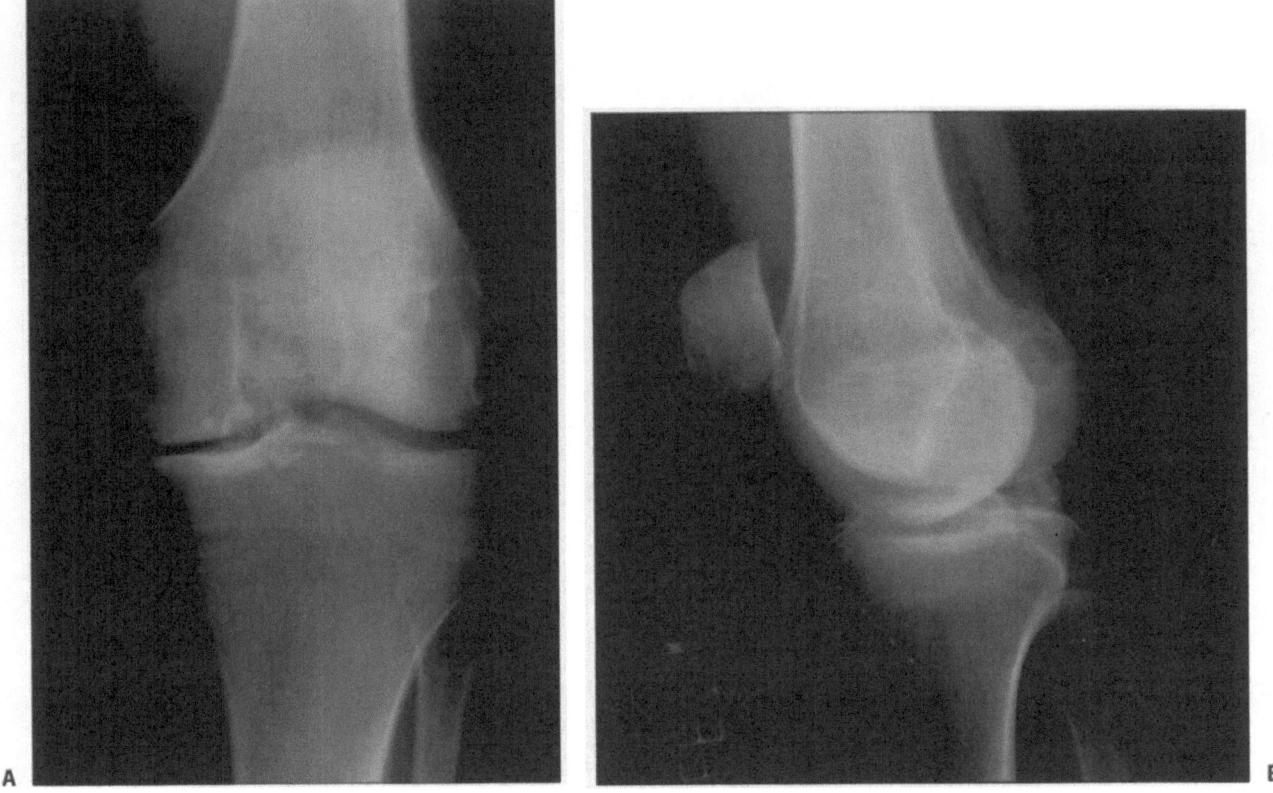

FIGURE 10.1 Preoperative anteroposterior (**A**) and lateral (**B**) radiographs show narrowing of medial joint space with slight varus deformity.

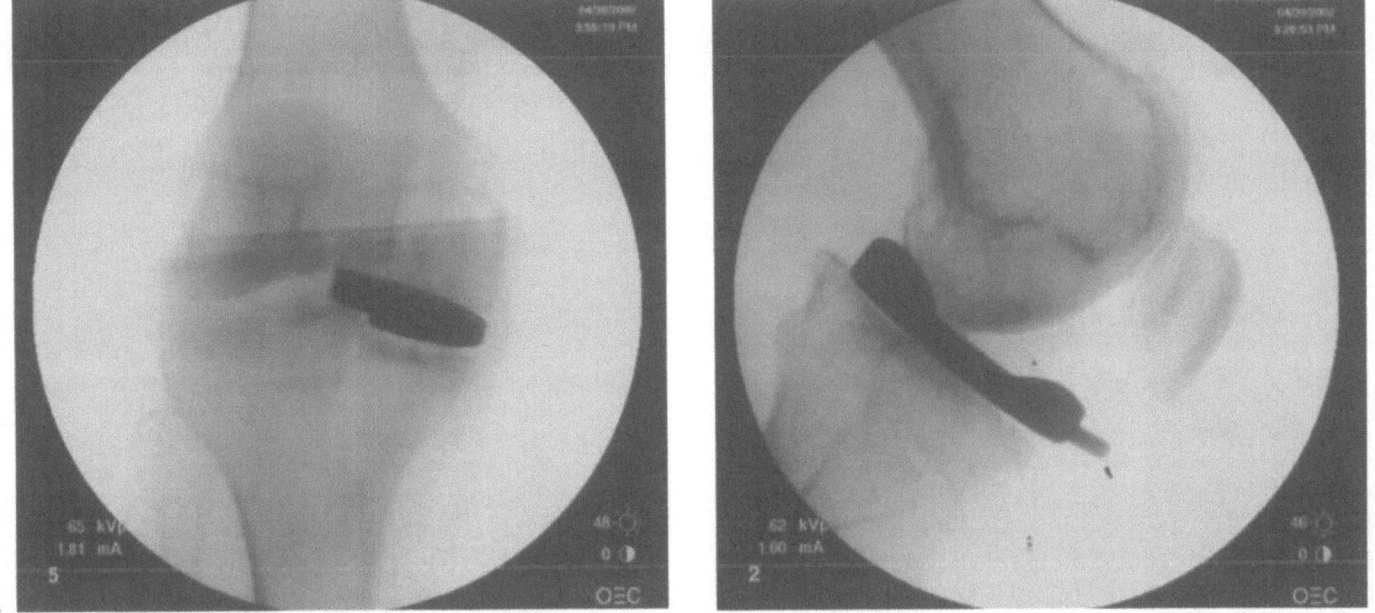

FIGURE 10.2 Intraoperative anteroposterior (**A**) and lateral (**B**) radiographs show proper placement of the unispacer.

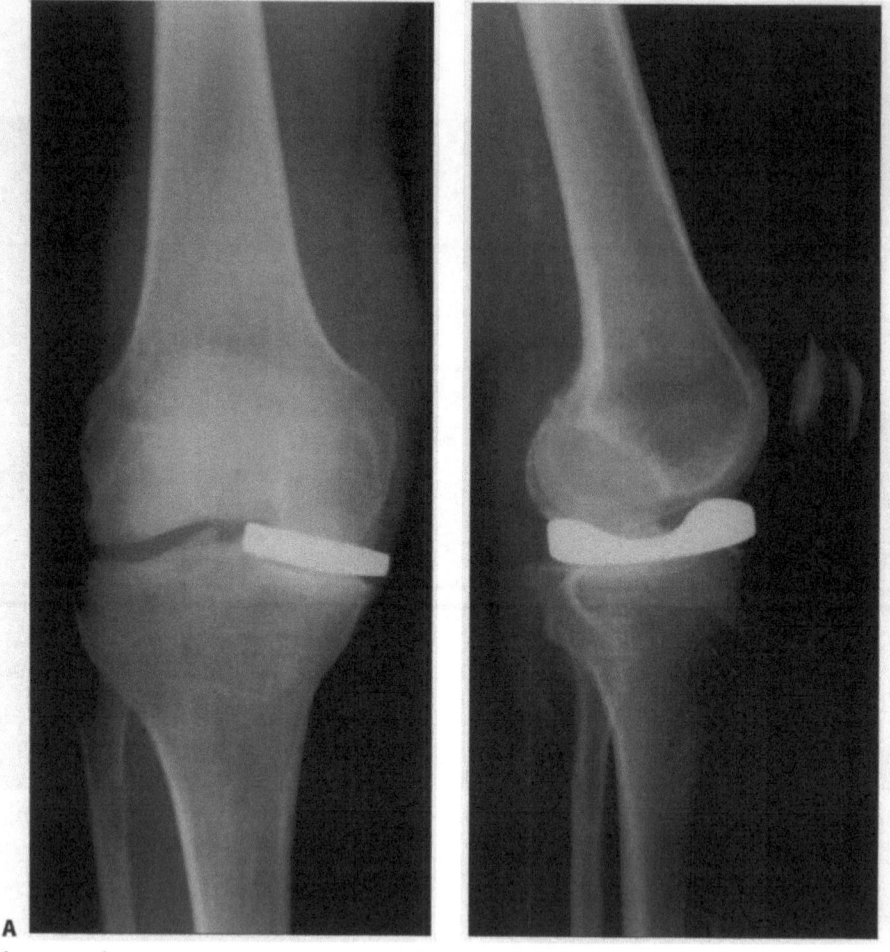

FIGURE 10.3 Three-month postoperative anteroposterior (**A**) and lateral (**B**) radiographs of unispacer in satisfactory position.

11

PATHOLOGY
Medial femoral condyle focal chondral defect

TREATMENT
Osteochondral autograft transplant

SUBMITTED BY
Brian J. Cole, MD, MBA, Rush Cartilage Restoration Center, Rush University Medical Center, Chicago, Illinois, USA

CHIEF COMPLAINT AND HISTORY OF PRESENT ILLNESS

This patient is a 42-year-old woman who had an acute twisting event and developed the onset of medial-sided right knee pain. She continued to complain of persistent right knee medial-sided weight-bearing pain and discomfort in addition to activity-related swelling. Her symptoms were not alleviated by a trial of antiinflammatory medication as well as a course of physical therapy.

PHYSICAL EXAMINATION

Height, 5 ft, 4 in.; weight, 155 lb. She has an antalgic gait. Her right knee has a moderate effusion. Her range of motion is 0 to 130 degrees. She is tender to palpation over the medial joint line and femoral condyle. Meniscal findings are equivocal, with pain reported with a varus axial load and rotation, but no palpable click. Her ligament examination is within normal limits.

RADIOGRAPHIC EVALUATION

Plain radiographs were unremarkable (Figure C11.1). A magnetic resonance image (MRI) was obtained and found to be within normal limits.

SURGICAL INTERVENTION

Initially, it was believed that she had a medial meniscus tear and was therefore indicated for arthroscopy. At arthroscopy, she was diagnosed as having an isolated grade III to IV chondral defect measuring 12 mm by 12 mm in the weight-bearing zone of the medial femoral condyle. As this was the only pathology identified, it was treated with an isolated microfracture technique (Figure C11.2). Postoperatively, the patient was made nonweight bearing for approximately 6 weeks and was placed on continuous passive motion for a similar period of time. She did well for approximately the first 8 months. As her activity level increased, however, she developed activity-related effusions and persistent medial-sided symptoms.

Because of persistent symptoms, she was indicated for osteochondral autograft transplantation of the medial femoral condyle. At the time of surgery, there was significant fibrocartilage fill of the medial femoral condyle, which was replaced with a 10-mm osteochondral autograft harvested from the lateral aspect of the trochlea (Figure C11.3).

FOLLOW-UP

At 18 months postoperatively, the patient remains painfree and has resumed all her activities. Follow-up radiographs demonstrate excellent incorporation of the osteochondral autograft with no joint space narrowing, cystic change, or joint incongruity (Figure C11.4).

DECISION-MAKING FACTORS

1. Index microfracture in a symptomatic patient indicated for isolated lesion less than $2\,cm^2$ as a first-line treatment.
2. Failure of primary microfracture as index treatment in a young intermediate-demand patient with a relatively small isolated defect.
3. Ability to replace fibrocartilage fill with a single osteochondral autograft plug.

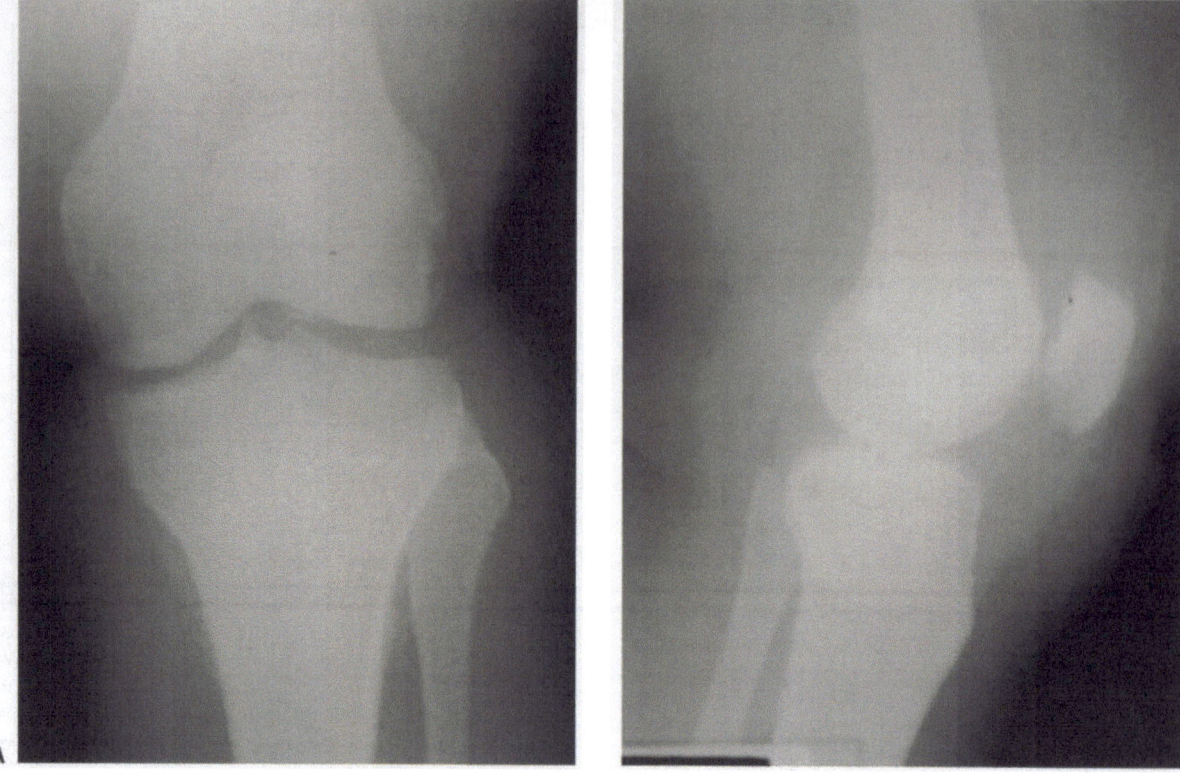

FIGURE C11.1 Anteroposterior (**A**) and lateral (**B**) radiographs of patient with a symptomatic medial femoral condyle chondral lesion diagnosed at arthroscopy, but with no evidence of defect demonstrated by plain radiographs or MRI.

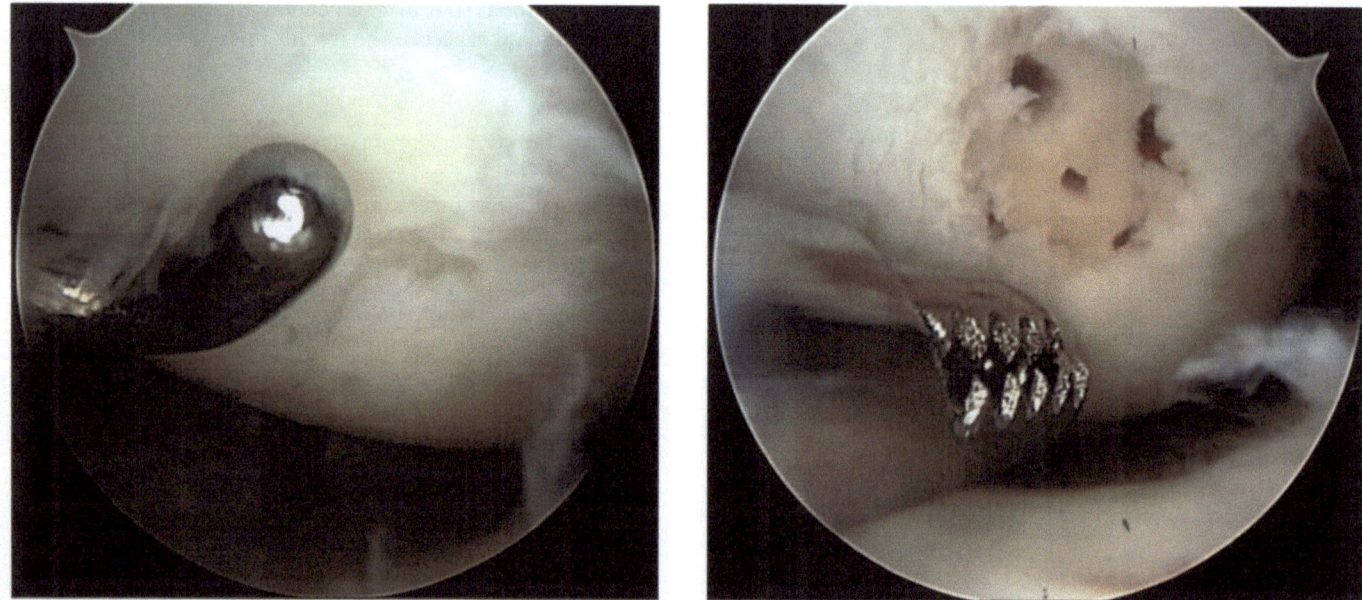

FIGURE C11.2 (**A**) Arthroscopic photograph of a grade III to grade IV lesion of the weight-bearing zone of the medial femoral condyle with delamination. (**B**) Microfracture technique used to treat this lesion.

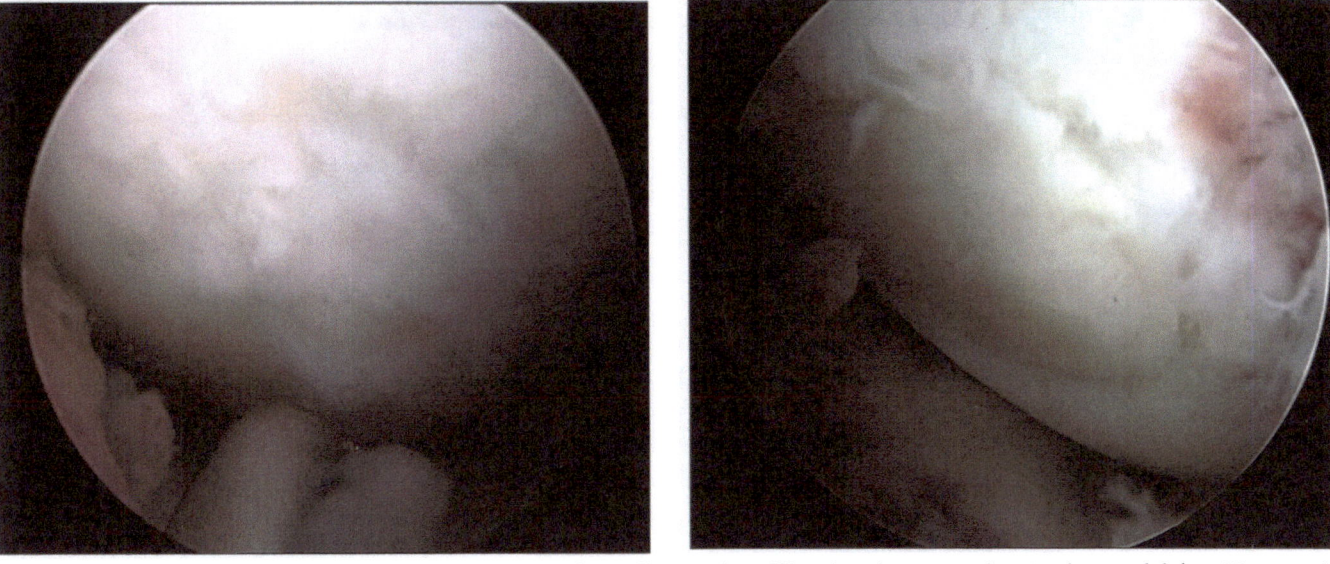

FIGURE C11.3 At second-look arthroscopy (**A**), there is significant fibrocartilage fill within the previously microfractured defect. However, it is soft to palpation and the patient remains symptomatic. (**B**) Ten-millimeter osteochondral autograft plug impacted into place.

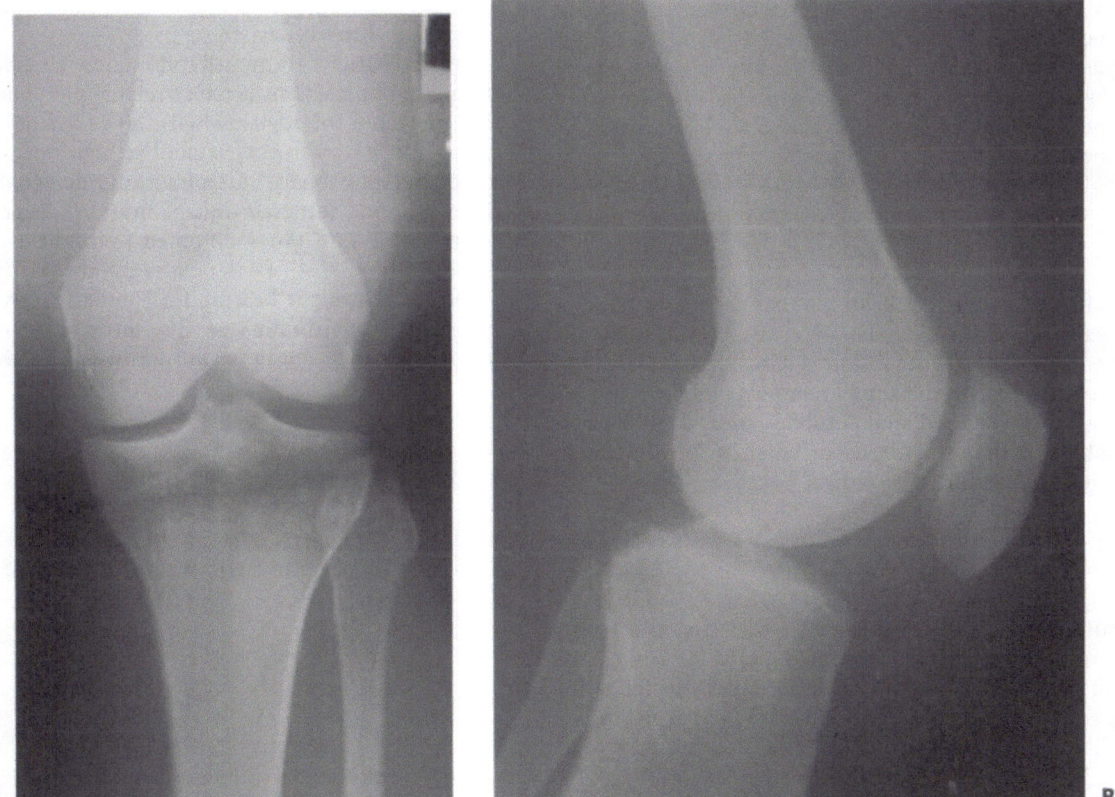

FIGURE C11.4 Anteroposterior (**A**) and lateral (**B**) radiographs, at 1-year follow-up demonstrate excellent incorporation of the osteochondral autograft without evidence of joint space narrowing, cystic change, or joint incongruity.

12

PATHOLOGY
Lateral femoral condyle focal chondral defect

TREATMENT
Osteochondral autograft transplant

SUBMITTED BY
Brian J. Cole, MD, MBA, Rush Cartilage Restoration Center, Rush University Medical Center, Chicago, Illinois, USA

CHIEF COMPLAINT AND HISTORY OF PRESENT ILLNESS

This patient is a 34-year-old emergency room nurse who sustained a work-related injury following a twisting event. She heard a pop and had the immediate onset of swelling and lateral-sided right knee pain. Subsequently, she reported a catching sensation but denied any episodes of giving-way. Her symptoms have not improved with a trial of antiinflammatory medication.

PHYSICAL EXAMINATION

Height, 5 ft, 4 in.; weight, 135 lb. She has a slightly antalgic gait with neutral alignment. Her right knee has a moderate-sized effusion. Her range of motion is 0 to 130 degrees. She is tender to palpation over the lateral femoral condyle. Meniscal findings are equivocal. Patellofemoral joint demonstrates good tracking with no evidence of crepitus. Her ligament examination is within normal limits.

RADIOGRAPHIC EVALUATION

Posteroanterior 45-degree flexion weight-bearing and lateral views were within normal limits (Figure C12.1). A magnetic resonance (MRI) was obtained that was significant for a suggestion of a type II signal within the lateral meniscus but was otherwise considered normal.

SURGICAL INTERVENTION

Because of failure to respond to conservative treatment, she was indicated for arthroscopic evaluation and treatment. At the time of arthroscopy, she was noted to have an isolated chondral lesion of the lateral femoral condyle measuring approximately 12 mm by 12 mm. This lesion was treated with a formal microfracture technique (Figure C12.2). Following the microfracture, the patient was placed nonweight bearing for approximately 4 to 6 weeks and used continuous passive motion for 4 to 6 h/day.

At the patient's 6-month follow-up visit, she continued to complain of persistent activity-related pain and swelling and was indicated for revision with an osteochondral autograft transplant. At arthroscopy, she had significant fibrocartilage fill of her previously microfractured defect (Figure C12.3). Osteochondral autograft transplantation was performed using 9-mm and 7-mm plugs obtained from the lateral trochlear ridge (Figure C12.4). Postoperatively, the patient was placed on protected weight bearing for approximately 4 to 6 weeks and utilized continuous passive motion. At 6 months, she was permitted to engage in activities as tolerated.

FOLLOW-UP

At nearly 1 year postoperatively, the patient has full range of motion, no swelling, and minimal complaints of activity-related pain.

DECISION-MAKING FACTORS

1. Index microfracture in a symptomatic patient indicated for isolated lesion less than 2 cm^2 as a first-line treatment.
2. Failure of primary microfracture as index treatment in a young intermediate-demand patient with a relatively small isolated defect.
3. Ability to replace fibrocartilage fill with two or fewer osteochondral autograft plugs.

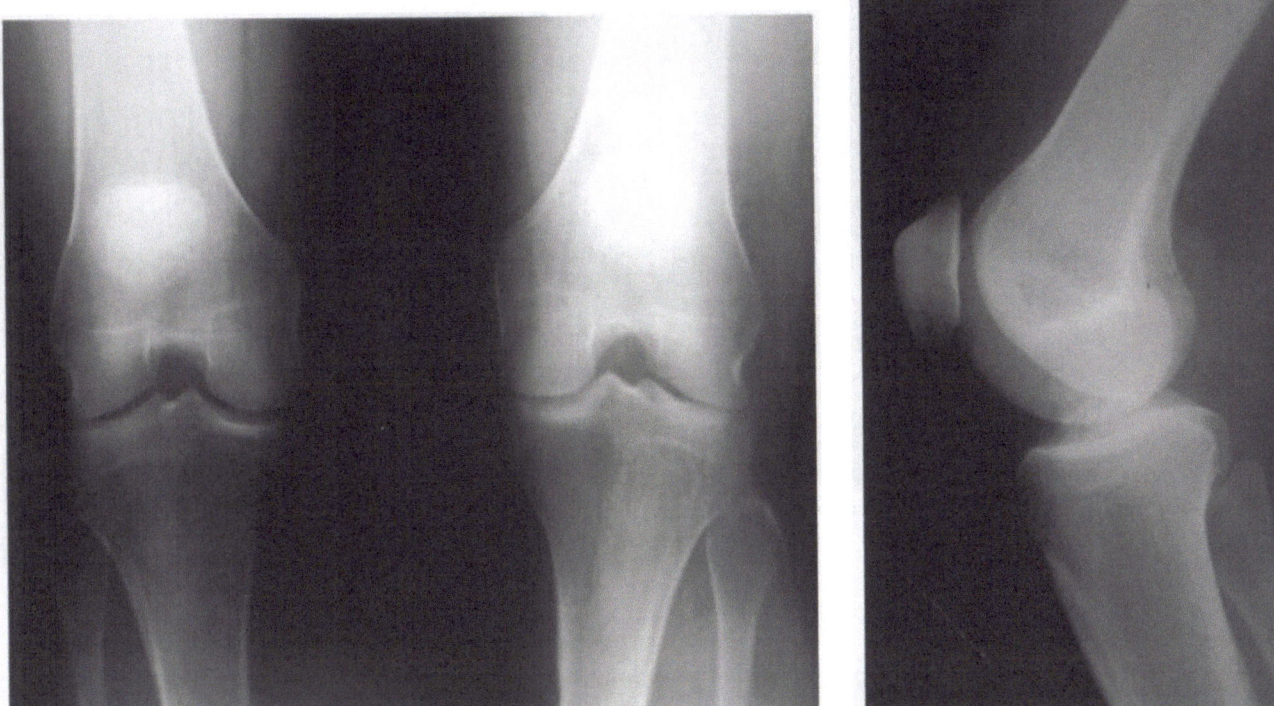

FIGURE C12.1 Forty-five-degree flexion posteroanterior weight-bearing (**A**) and lateral (**B**) radiographs without abnormalities.

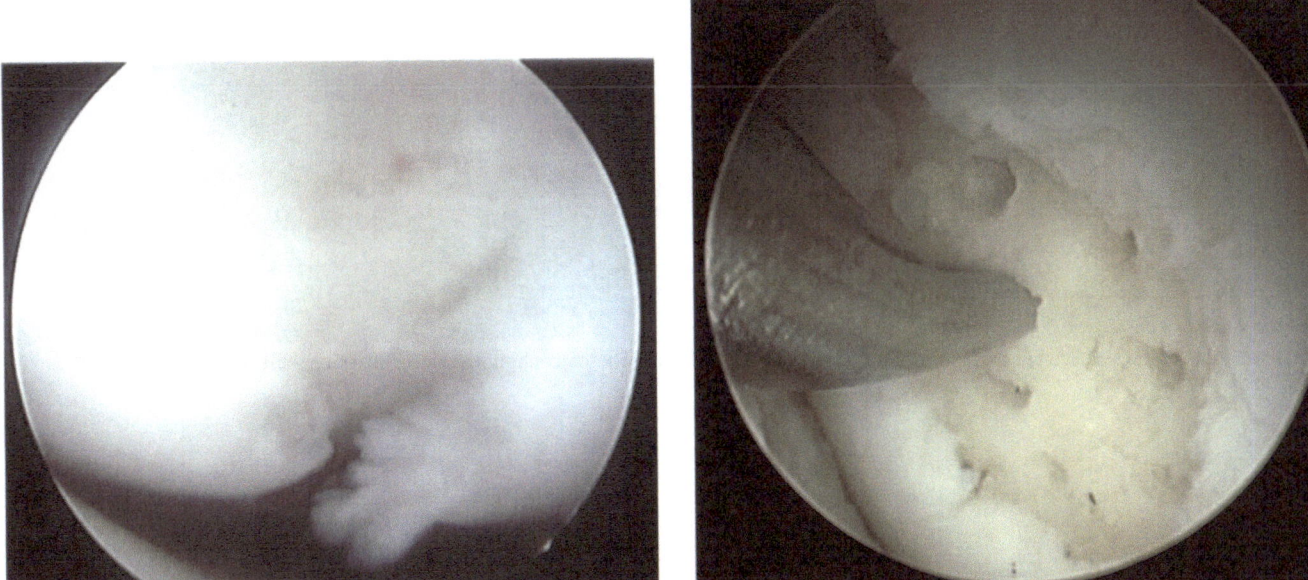

FIGURE C12.2 Index microfracture treatment of isolated 12 mm by 12 mm defect of the lateral femoral condyle. Arthroscopic view of the lesion (**A**) before microfracture and (**B**) after microfracture technique performed with creation of vertical walls surrounding the defect.

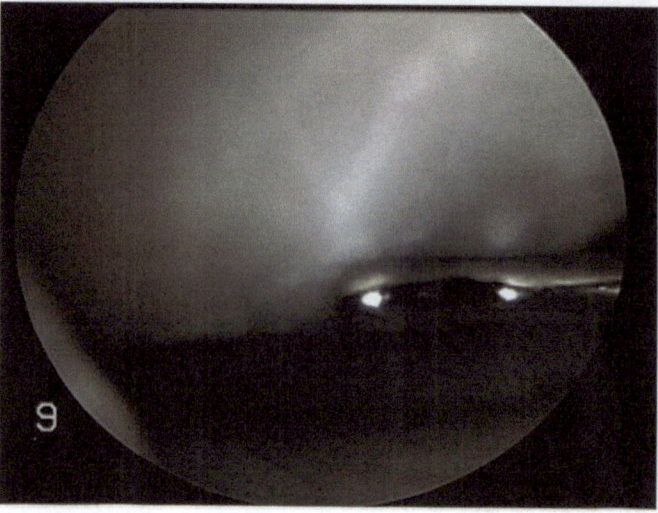

FIGURE C12.3 Arthroscopic view obtained 8 months after microfracture in which the defect was found to be filled with soft fibrocartilaginous tissue.

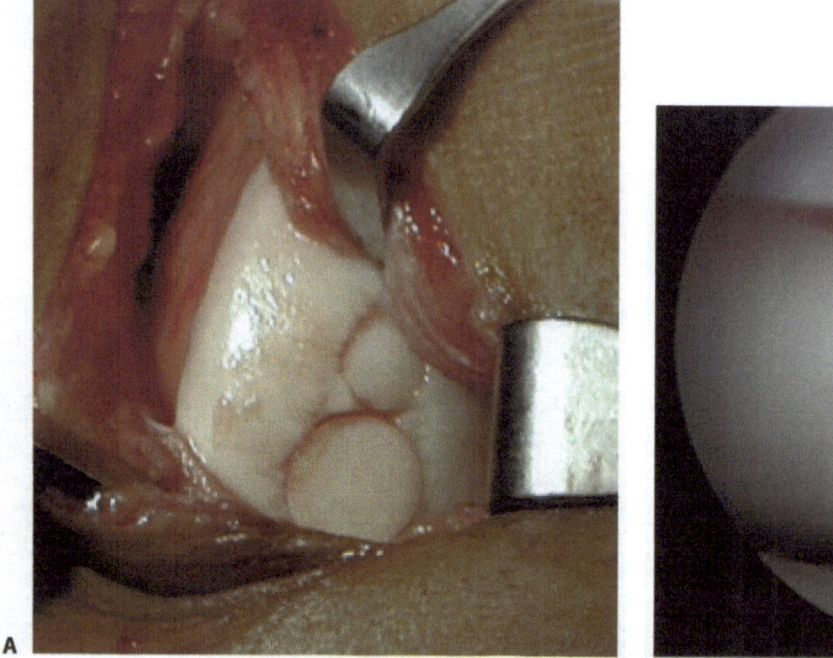

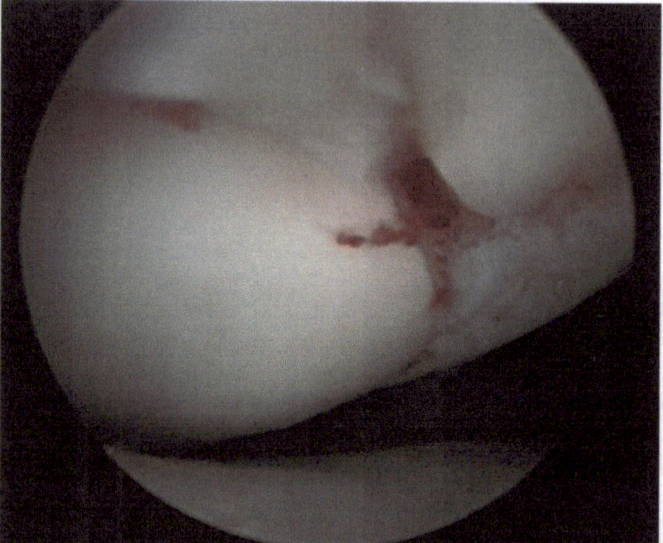

A   B

FIGURE C12.4 Intraoperative photograph (**A**) and arthroscopic view (**B**) of the osteochondral autograft transplant plugs, measuring 9 mm and 7 mm, respectively.

13

PATHOLOGY
Focal chondral defect of the medial femoral condyle and patella

TREATMENT
Osteochondral autograft of the medial femoral condyle and microfracture of the patella

SUBMITTED BY
Brian J. Cole, MD, MBA, Rush Cartilage Restoration Center, Rush University Medical Center, Chicago, Illinois, USA

CHIEF COMPLAINT AND HISTORY OF PRESENT ILLNESS

The patient is a 44-year-old woman with a chief complaint of anterior knee pain and pain with weight bearing along the medial aspect of her right knee. Additionally, she has recurrent mechanical symptoms, swelling, difficulty doing her work, and inability to participate in her hobby as a sport barrel jumper. Two years prior, she had an arthroscopic chondral debridement, and was diagnosed with a full-thickness chondral defect of her medial femoral condyle documented to be the "size of a dime" and a similarly sized, nearly full thickness lesion of her patella. She did not respond favorably to this arthroscopy and remained symptomatic. Before being indicated for repeat surgical intervention, she demonstrated a failure to respond to a rigorous patellofemoral rehabilitation program.

PHYSICAL EXAMINATION

Height, 5 ft, 4 in.; weight, 130 lb. The patient walks with a nonantalgic gait, and her alignment is symmetric in slight physiologic valgus. She has a small effusion. Her range of motion is 0 to 130 degrees. She is tender to palpation over the medial femoral condyle in flexion. She has palpable patellofemoral crepitus at 45 degrees of knee flexion with no patellar apprehension. Meniscal findings are absent, and her ligament examination is within normal limits. She has no quadriceps atrophy and has a Q angle of less than 8 degrees.

RADIOGRAPHIC EVALUATION

Plain radiographs were within normal limits. Magnetic resonance studies demonstrated both chondral lesions with subchondral edema behind the medial femoral condyle lesion.

SURGICAL INTERVENTION

Because of her persistent symptoms and failure to respond to previous debridement, she was indicated for a repeat right knee arthroscopy. An 8 mm by 8 mm, nearly grade IV chondral defect located centrally within the patella and an 8 mm by 8 mm, grade IV chondral defect of the weight-bearing zone of the medial femoral condyle were identified. The patellar lesion was treated with a formal microfracture technique (Figure C13.1). The medial femoral condyle lesion was treated with an osteochondral autograft transplant (Figure C13.2).

FOLLOW-UP

In an effort to clear her for competitive barrel jumping and because she had mild anterior knee pain, the patient was indicated for second-look arthroscopy 6 months following her treatment. The patella demonstrated excellent fill with relatively soft fibrocartilaginous tissue, and the osteochondral plug demonstrated excellent integration with no evidence of degeneration (Figure C13.3). At 1 year, she reported only minimal activity-related symptoms, and at 2 years she was successfully competing at barrel jumping with no radiographic abnormalities (Figure C13.4).

DECISION-MAKING FACTORS

1. Physically demanding patient in her fifth decade with chondral lesions that failed to respond to initial arthroscopic debridement and physical therapy.
2. Small patellar lesion amenable to microfracture with few other viable or appropriate solutions. Other options considered could include anteromedialization osteotomy, depending on the severity of her symptoms.
3. Small lesion of the medial femoral condyle easily treated with a second-line treatment using a single-plug osteochondral autograft.

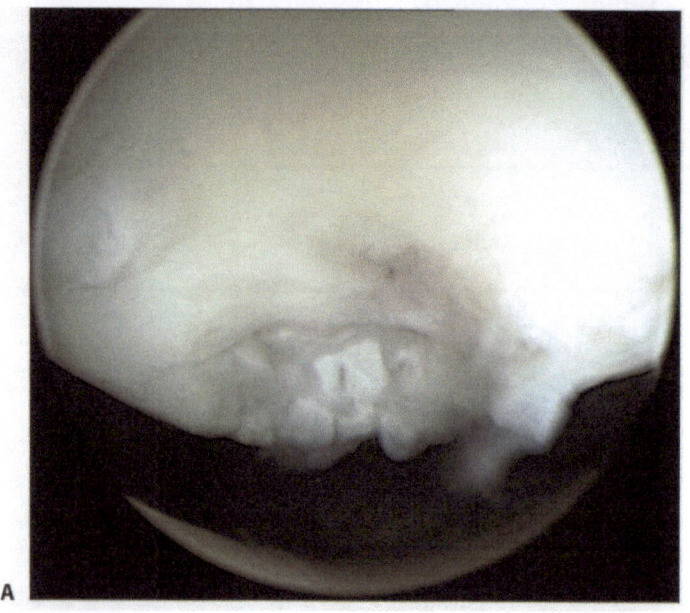

A

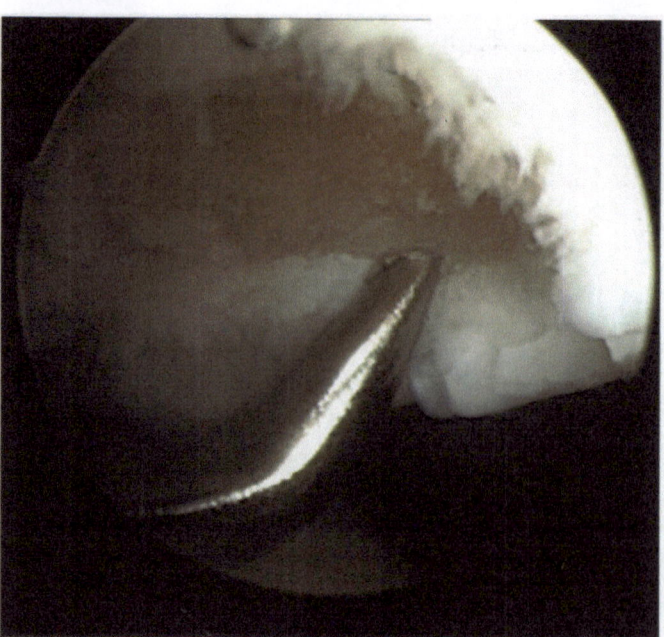

B

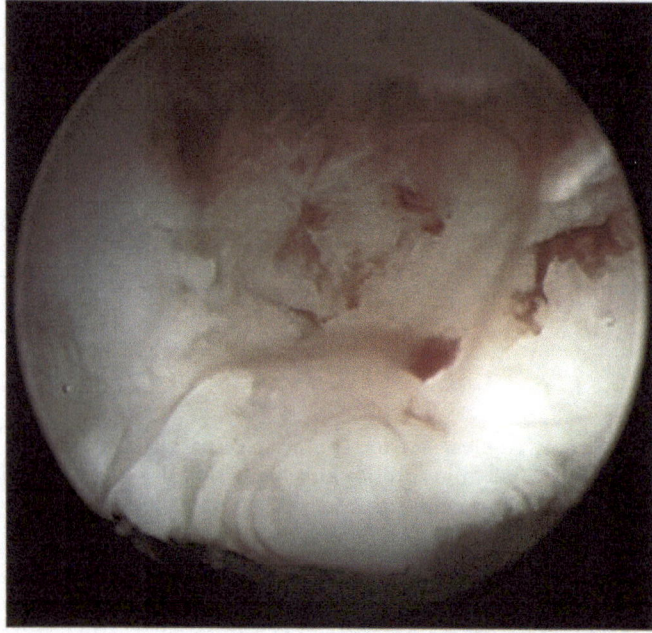

C

FIGURE C13.1 Arthroscopic pictures demonstrate treatment of patellar defect. (**A**) Central, nearly grade IV patellar defect measuring 8 mm by 8 mm. (**B**) Microfracture technique of the patella with debridement through the calcified layer and penetration with a microfracture awl. (**C**) Subchondral bone demonstrates bleeding through the microfracture holes.

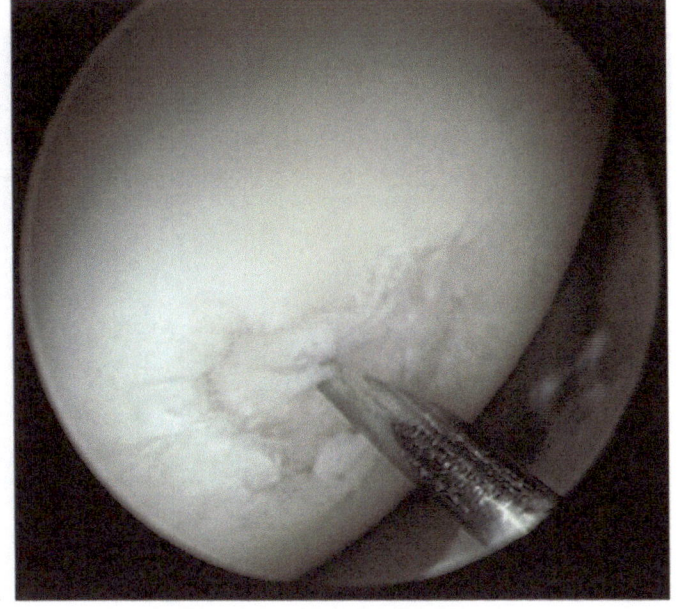

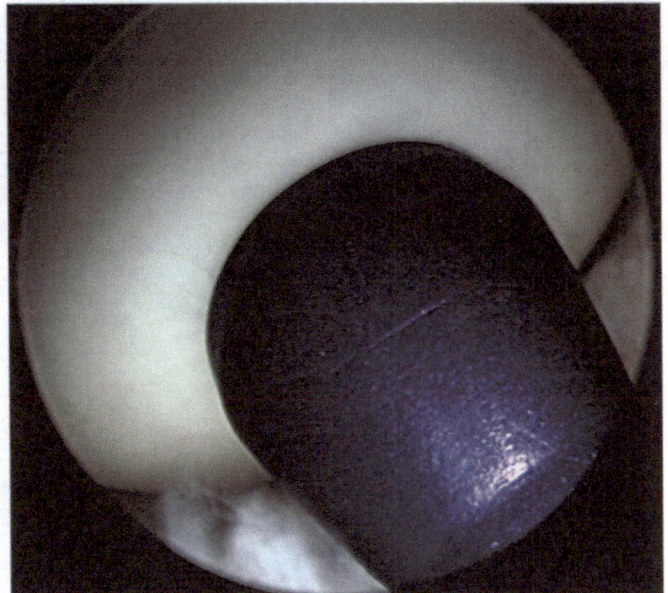

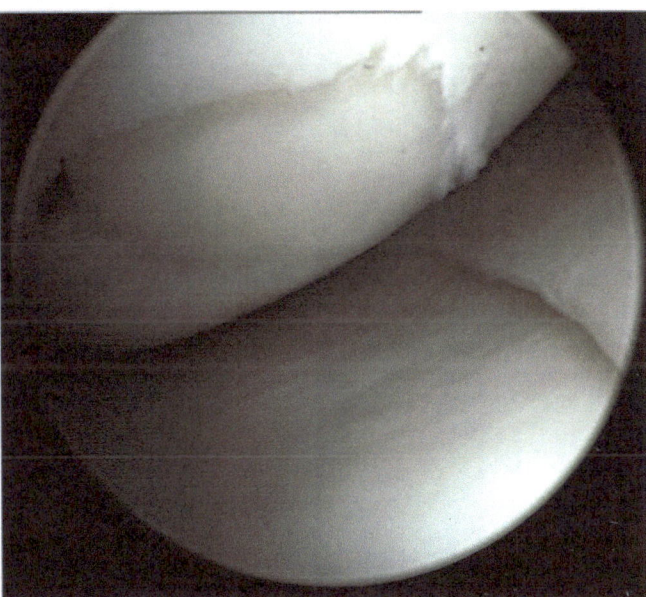

FIGURE C13.2 Arthroscopic pictures demonstrate treatment of the medial femoral condyle. (**A**) Medial femoral condyle defect of the weight-bearing zone (**B**) being measured at approximately 8 mm by 8 mm. (**C**) The osteochondral plug in place.

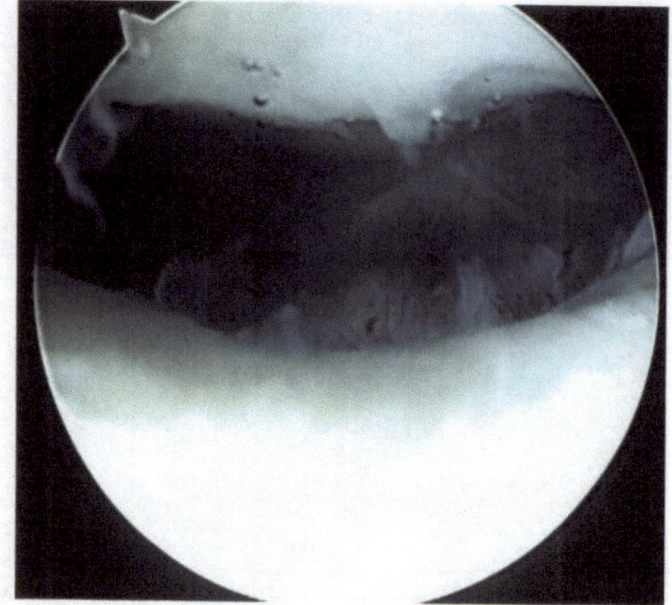
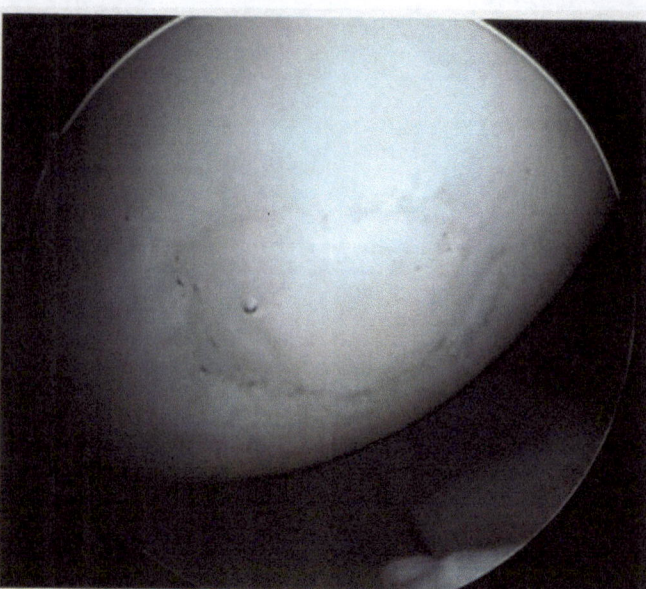

FIGURE C13.3 Six-month second-look arthroscopy of the patella (**A**) demonstrates soft fibrocartilage within the defect and the medial femoral condyle (**B**), with a well-healed and integrated osteochondral autograft plug without signs of degeneration.

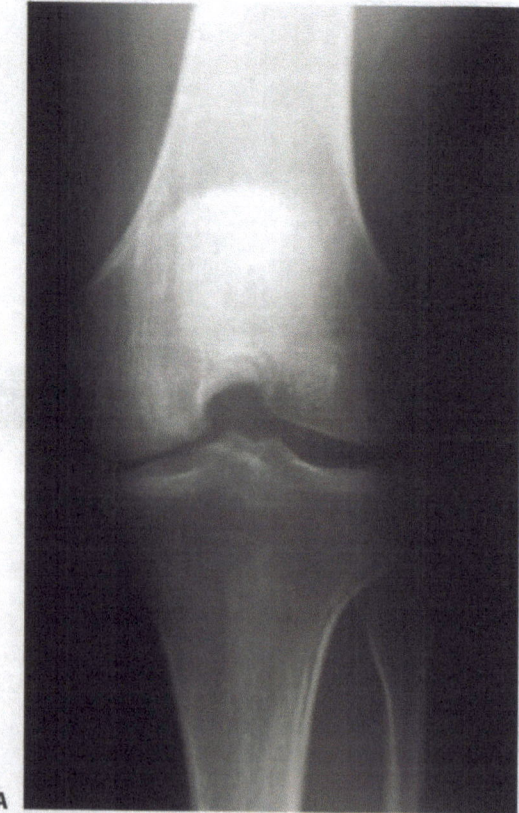
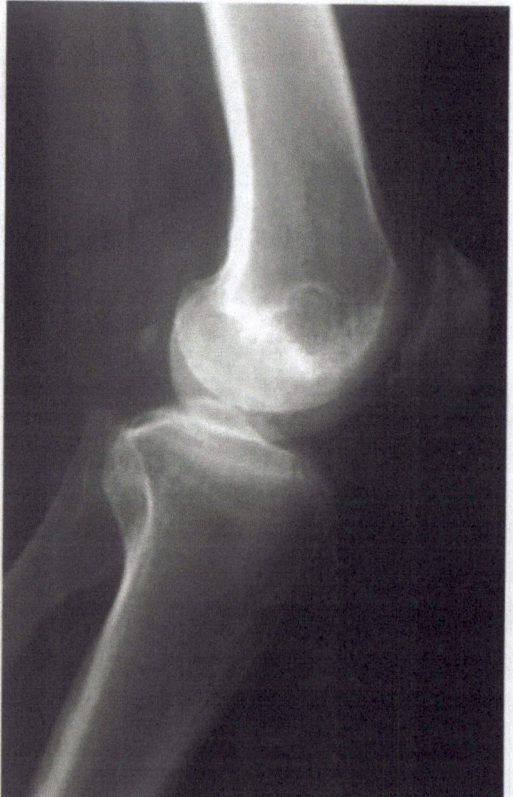

FIGURE C13.4 Two-year anteroposterior (**A**) and lateral (**B**) radiographs demonstrate virtually no evidence of the osteochondral plug and the absence of subchondral sclerosis or joint space narrowing.

14

PATHOLOGY
Lateral femoral condyle osteochondritis dissecans

TREATMENT
Fresh osteochondral allograft transplantation

SUBMITTED BY
Brian J. Cole, MD, MBA, Rush Cartilage Restoration Center, Rush University Medical Center, Chicago, Illinois, USA

CHIEF COMPLAINT AND HISTORY OF PRESENT ILLNESS

This patient is a 19-year-old male college student whose chief complaint is that of activity-related lateral-sided left knee pain, with associated swelling, stiffness, locking, and a sense of giving-way. His symptom onset began suddenly 2 years previously while playing soccer. His symptoms are made worse with weight bearing, running, impact activities, and prolonged standing. He desires to participate in collegiate-level sports.

He was initially treated 1 year previously with arthroscopy and removal of a necrotic 2.5 cm by 2.5 cm osteochondral fragment consistent with chronic osteochondritis dissecans of the lateral femoral condyle (Figure C14.1). He failed to improve following loose body removal and was referred for definitive treatment.

PHYSICAL EXAMINATION

Height, 6 ft, 2 in.; weight, 185 lb. He has a normal gait. Alignment reveals slight symmetric physiologic varus of approximately 2 degrees. He has a mild effusion with tenderness along the lateral femoral condyle. His range of motion is from 0 to 130 degrees. There is no evidence of any meniscal findings. He has slight patellofemoral and lateral compartment crepitus with range of motion. He has no evidence of quadriceps atrophy. He has a normal patellofemoral joint and a normal ligament examination.

RADIOGRAPHIC EVALUATION

Forty-five-degree posteroanterior flexion weight-bearing and lateral radiographs demonstrate osteochondritis dissecans of the lateral femoral condyle of the left knee with a large cavitary defect involving more than 5 to 8 mm of subchondral bone at the base of the defect (Figure C14.2).

SURGICAL INTERVENTION

Because of the size, location, and depth of the lesion, the patient was indicated for fresh osteochondral allograft transplantation (Figure C14.3). Postoperatively, he was made nonweight bearing for approximately 8 weeks and used continuous passive motion for 6 weeks for 6 to 8 h/day. At 6 months, he was permitted to engage in high-impact activities.

FOLLOW-UP

Two years following his allograft transplant, he complains of no pain, swelling, or catching. He has returned to all activities. He has radiographic evidence of graft incorporation and preservation of joint space (Figure C14.4).

DECISION-MAKING FACTORS

1. A young high-demand patient with osteochondritis dissecans of the weight-bearing zone of the lateral femoral condyle.
2. Failure of previous treatment involving fragment removal with persistent symptoms.
3. A large (6.25 cm²) and deep lesion (greater than 6 to 8 mm of subchondral bone involvement) of the lateral femoral condyle considered otherwise difficult if not contraindicated to manage with osteochondral autograft or autologous chondrocyte implantation.
4. Rehabilitation tolerance and willingness to be compliant with initial nonweight-bearing status.

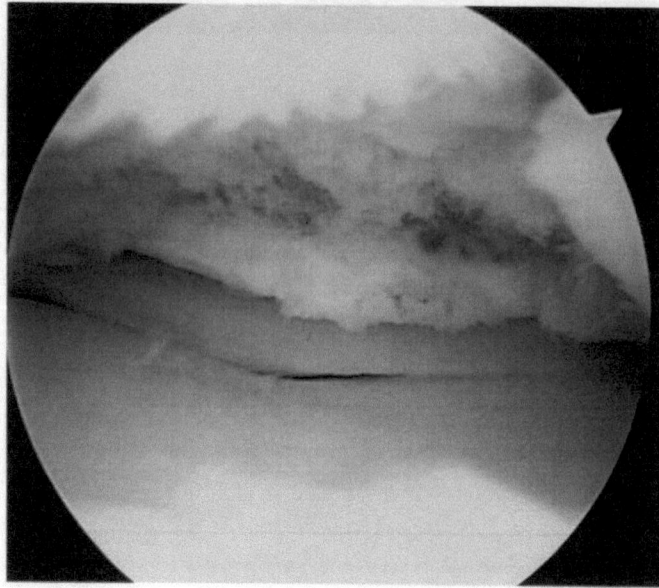

FIGURE C14.1 Arthroscopic photograph of the defect obtained at the time of fragment removal demonstrates exposed subchondral bone with normal meniscus and normal lateral tibial plateau.

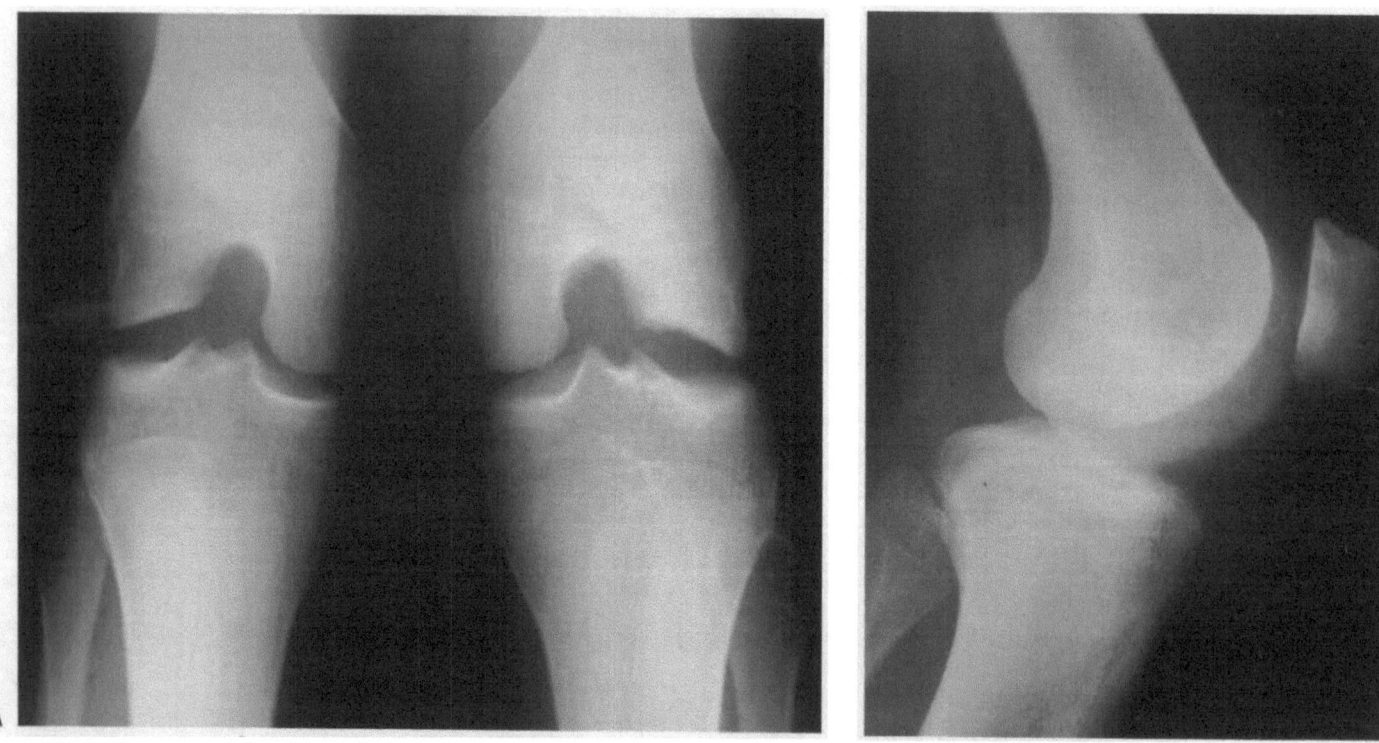

FIGURE C14.2 Forty-five-degree flexion posteroanterior weight-bearing (**A**) and lateral (**B**) radiographs demonstrate osteochondritis dissecans of the lateral femoral condyle of the left knee with a large cavitary defect.

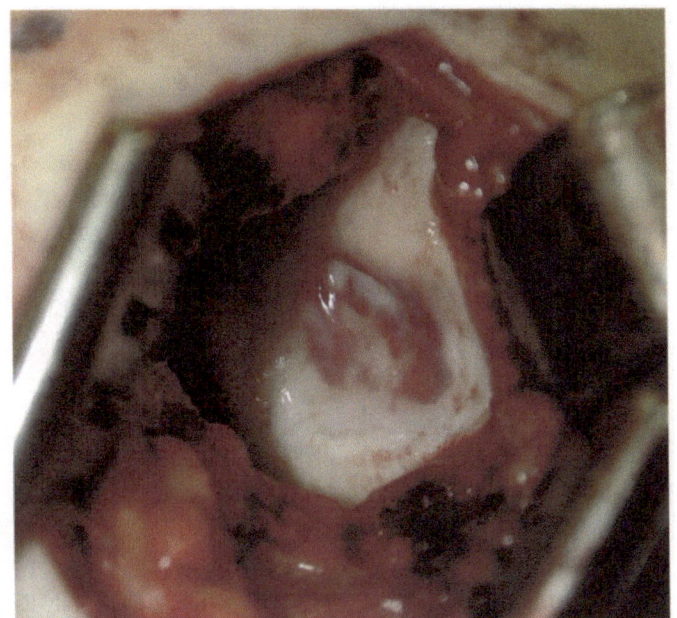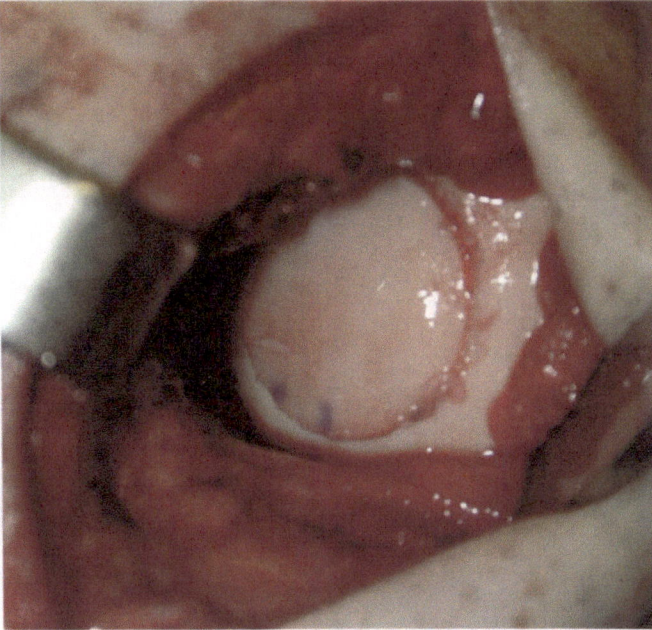

FIGURE C14.3 Twelve months following fragment removal, intraoperative photographs demonstrate fibrocartilage covering the subchondral bone (**A**). (**B**) Fresh osteochondral allograft, measuring 25 mm by 25 mm, is press-fit within the lateral femoral condyle.

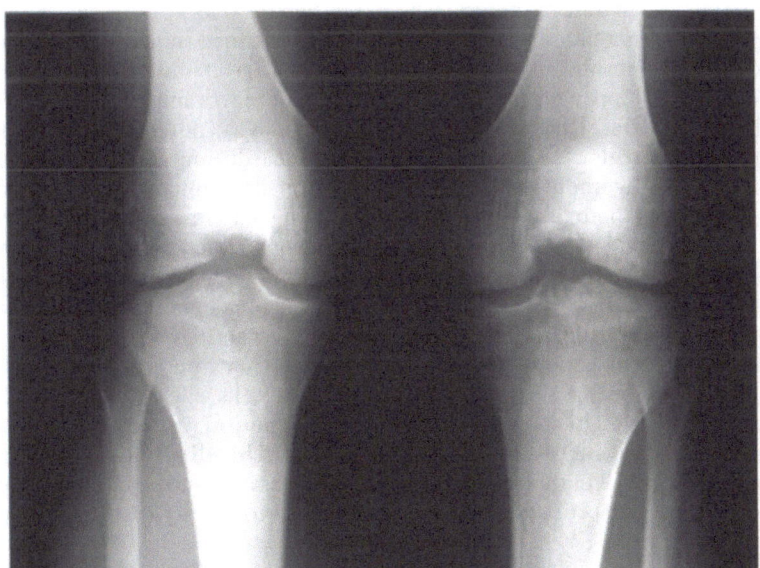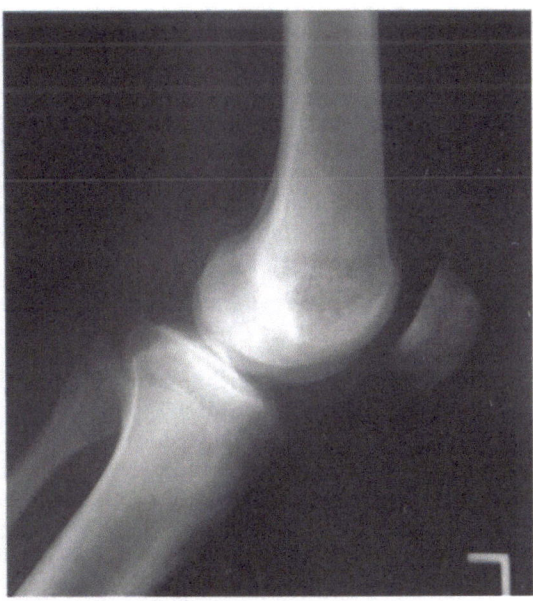

FIGURE C14.4 Two-year postoperative 45-degree flexion posteroanterior weight-bearing (**A**) and nonweight-bearing (**B**) flexion lateral radiographs demonstrate excellent incorporation of the lateral femoral condyle osteochondral allograft.

15

PATHOLOGY
Focal chondral defect of the lateral femoral condyle

TREATMENT
Autologous chondrocyte implantation of the lateral femoral condyle

SUBMITTED BY
Brian J. Cole, MD, MBA, Rush Cartilage Restoration Center, Rush University Medical Center, Chicago, Illinois, USA

CHIEF COMPLAINT AND HISTORY OF PRESENT ILLNESS

The patient is a 27-year-old woman with a long-standing history of right knee patellar instability. As a child, before she was skeletally mature, she underwent two lateral releases that failed to resolve her instability. Subsequently, when she had reached skeletal maturity, she underwent an anteromedialization of her tibial tubercle. Although her patellar instability was successfully treated, she developed locking and mechanical symptoms requiring arthroscopic removal of several loose bodies approximately 2 years before presentation for cartilage treatment. At the time of the arthroscopy, she was noted to have an approximately 3 cm by 3 cm grade IV lesion in the lateral femoral condyle. She experienced some relief from the removal of the loose bodies; however, she still reports significant lateral-sided knee pain, swelling, and giving-way. Repeated attempts at formal physical therapy failed to alleviate her symptoms.

PHYSICAL EXAMINATION

Height, 5 ft, 3 in.; weight, 125 lb. She has a nonantalgic gait. She stands in slight symmetric physiologic valgus. She has a large lateral incision extending down inferiorly from her anteromedialization procedure and previous lateral releases. She has a trace effusion with mild patellofemoral crepitus. Her range of motion is from 0 to 135 degrees. She has a positive J sign with active extension. She has mild patellar apprehension with lateral glide testing in 30 degrees of flexion. She has significant tenderness over the lateral femoral condyle. Her medial and lateral joint lines are not tender. Her ligament exam is within normal limits.

RADIOGRAPHIC EVALUATION

Plain radiographs of the right knee (Figure C15.1) reveal hardware fixation from the previous anteromedialization procedure in place as well as an incongruity on the lateral femoral condyle of her left knee. Magnetic resonance imaging (MRI) examination reveals a chondral defect of the lateral femoral condyle with a full-thickness lesion extending into the subchondral bone with subchondral edema present.

SURGICAL INTERVENTION

The patient underwent arthroscopy in which a lateral femoral condyle defect with soft fibrocartilaginous tissue measuring 20 mm by 25 mm was noted (Figure C15.2). The defect was noted to be contained with a well-defined transition zone and normal surrounding articular cartilage. An articular cartilage biopsy for future autologous chondrocyte implantation (ACI) was harvested from the intercondylar notch, in the same region as a notchplasty performed during anterior cruciate ligament (ACL) reconstruction is typically performed. Approximately 2 months later, the patient underwent ACI to the lateral femoral condyle lesion, which was noted to be 32 mm by 18 mm in dimension following debridement (Figure C15.3). Postoperatively, she was made heel-touch weight bearing for approximately 8 weeks and continued to use a continuous passive motion (CPM) machine for 6 to 8 h/day for that same period of time. At 8 weeks, she was advanced to weight bearing and range of motion as tolerated. She advanced through the traditional rehabilitation protocol for ACI of the femoral condyle. She was asked to refrain from any impact or ballistic activities for 12 to 18 months.

FOLLOW-UP

The patient is now 18 months status post ACI. She states that she is totally painfree; however, she is still unable to fully perform high-impact activities due to muscular deconditioning. Her knee physical examination is entirely within normal limits. Radiographs obtained at 12 months demonstrate slight improvement in the contour of the lateral femoral condyle.

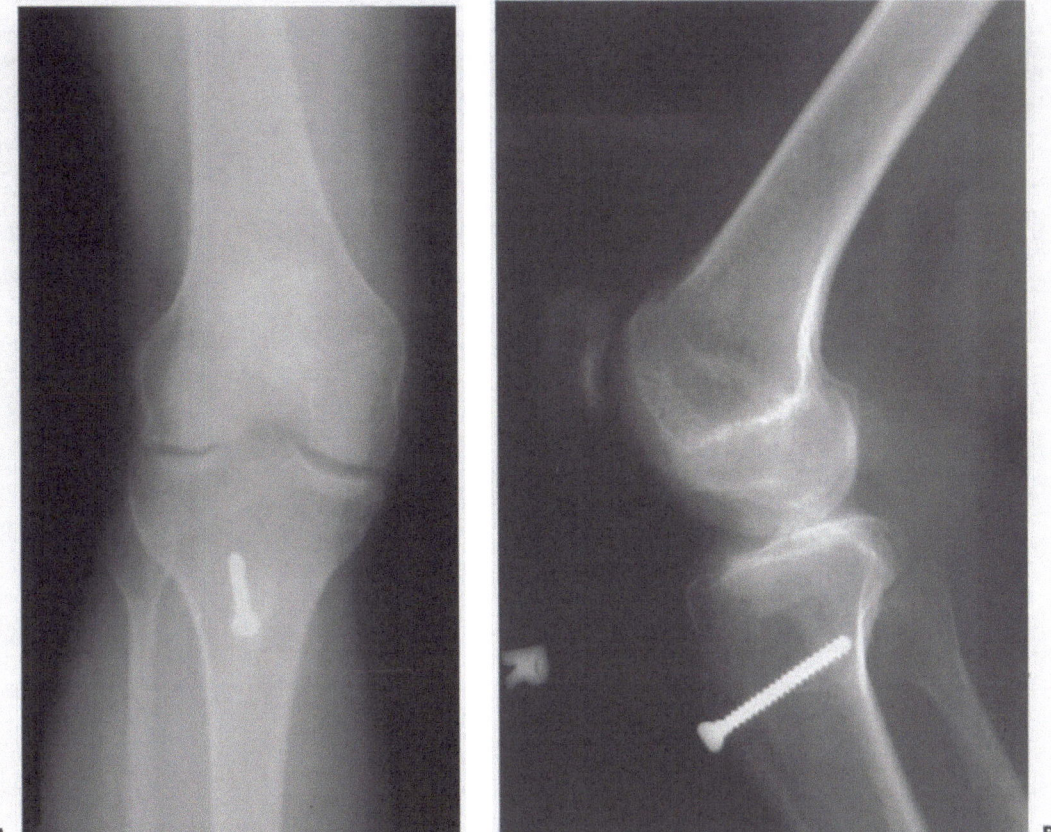

FIGURE C15.1 Preoperative anteroposterior (AP) **(A)** and lateral **(B)** radiographs of the right knee demonstrate fixation hardware from prior osteotomy procedure as well as flattening and irregularity of the lateral femoral condyle.

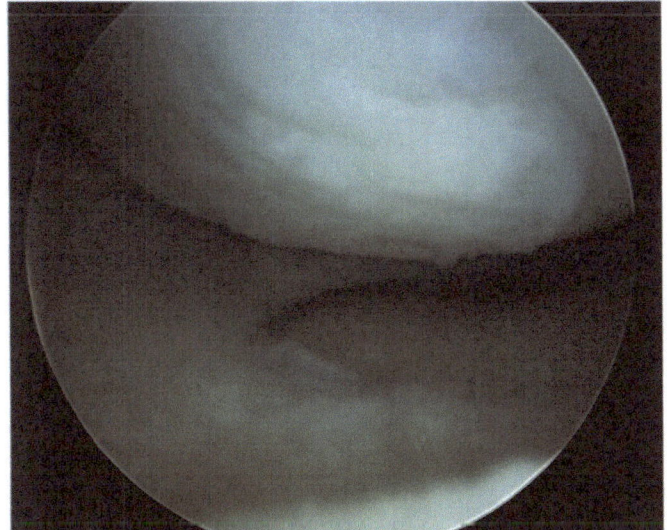

FIGURE C15.2 Arthroscopic photograph of the lateral femoral condyle of the right knee demonstrates large chondral defect filled with fibrocartilaginous tissue.

DECISION-MAKING FACTORS

1. Persistent symptoms despite several failed surgical attempts at patellar stabilization and loose body removal.
2. Young, high-demand patient with a large superficial chondral lesion amenable to chondrocyte transplantation or fresh osteochondral allograft. Lesion size precludes optimal result with microfracture or osteochondral autograft transplantation.
3. Patient preference for her own tissue and surgeon preference for ACI given the relatively young age of this patient and the desire to avoid the creation of a subchondral defect otherwise required for fresh osteochondral allograft transplantation.
4. Ability and willingness to be compliant with the postoperative course.

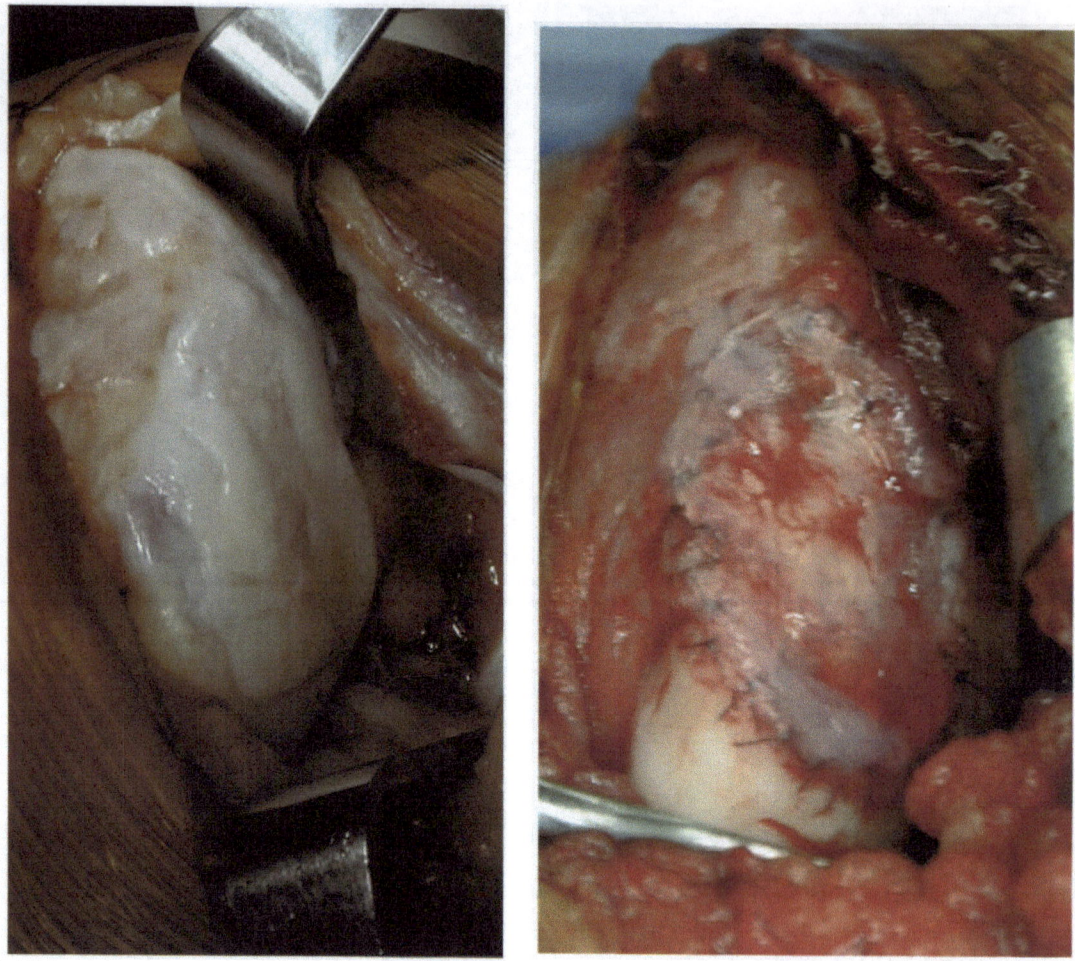

FIGURE C15.3 **(A)** Intraoperative photograph demonstrates large lateral femoral condyle lesion with full-thickness cartilage loss noted, with the central area filled with fibrocartilaginous tissue. **(B)** Lateral femoral condyle lesion with periosteal patch sewn in place, sealed by fibrin glue.

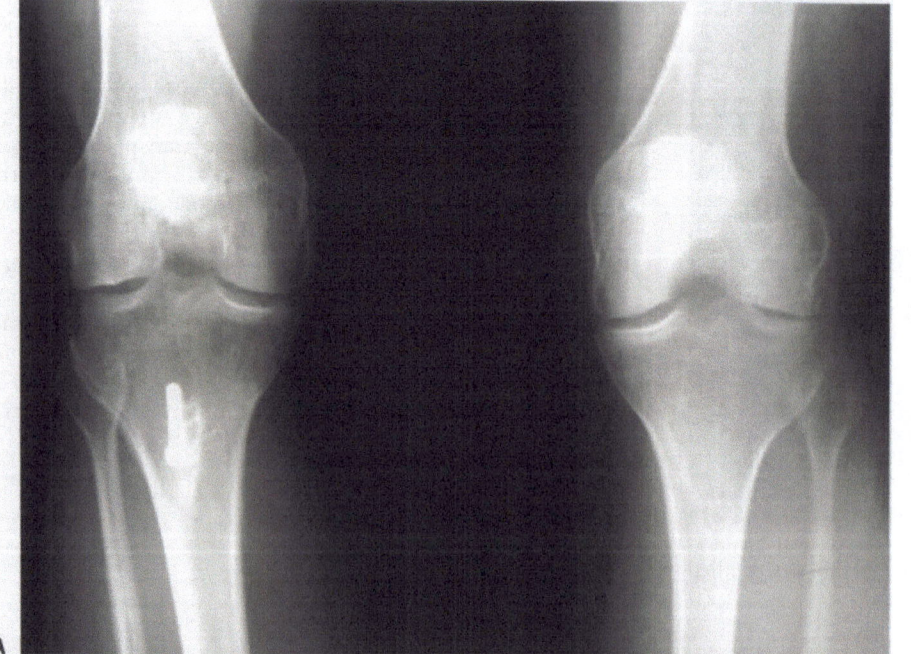
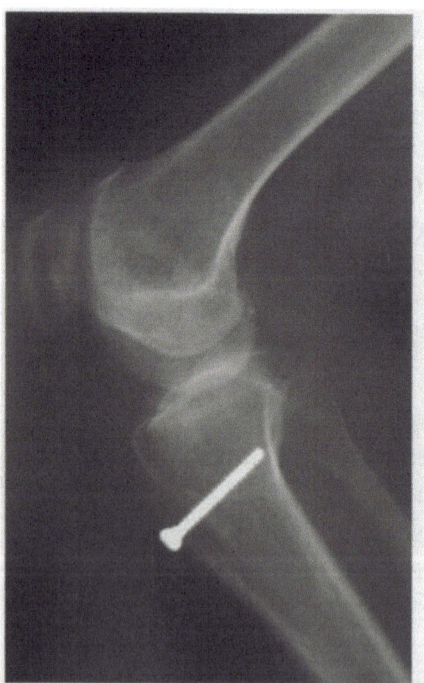

FIGURE C15.4 Twelve-month postoperative 45-degree posteroanterior flexion weight-bearing radiograph **(A)** and lateral radiograph **(B)** demonstrate slight improvement in the contour of the left lateral femoral condyle. No change in joint space is observed compared to preoperative radiographs.

CHIEF COMPLAINT AND HISTORY OF PRESENT ILLNESS

The patient is a 35-year-old woman who sustained a traumatic injury to her right knee while playing intramural softball 6 months before presenting for treatment. She complained of persistent medial joint line pain and activity-related swelling and effusions. She denied any giving-way or mechanical symptoms. Physical therapy failed to relieve her symptoms.

PHYSICAL EXAMINATION

Height, 5 ft, 3 in.; weight, 120 lb. The patient ambulates with a nonantalgic gait. Her alignment is in slight symmetric valgus. She has full range of motion. A trace effusion is present with tenderness over the medial femoral condyle and medial joint line. Meniscal findings are present only on the medial side. Her ligament examination is normal.

RADIOGRAPHIC EVALUATION

Preoperative radiographs were within normal limits (Figure C16.1).

SURGICAL INTERVENTION

Due to her persistent symptoms, she was indicated for arthroscopy. At the time of arthroscopy, she was diagnosed as having a posterior horn medial meniscus tear involving approximately 20% of the medial meniscus as well as a grade IV focal chondral defect of the medial femoral condyle in the weight-bearing zone measuring approximately 25 mm by 20 mm (Figure C16.2). This lesion was simply debrided, and a concomitant articular cartilage biopsy was taken from the intercondylar notch. The patient did well initially with resolution of her medial joint line pain but complained of persistent weight-bearing discomfort. She continued to have activity-related effusions and complaints of discomfort with changes in barometric pressure. Because of her ongoing symptoms, the nature of her focal chondral defect, and the relatively small amount of previous medial meniscectomy, it was believed that the persistent symptoms were caused by the focal chondral defect. Thus, the patient underwent autologous chondrocyte implantation (ACI) (Figure C16.3).

Postoperatively, she was made nonweight bearing for approximately 4 weeks and subsequently advanced to full weight bearing. Additionally, during that time she used continuous passive motion for approximately 6 h/day. She advanced through the remainder of the rehabilitation protocol over the ensuing 12 months and was asked to refrain from impact activities for at least 12 months.

FOLLOW-UP

She followed a fairly typical postoperative course but developed mechanical-type symptoms around the eighth postoperative month following autologous chondrocyte implantation. Further efforts at rehabilitation failed, and the patient was indicated for a repeat arthroscopy 1 year postoperatively under the pretext that she may have periosteal patch detachment or hypertrophy. At the time of arthroscopy, the defect was well filled with soft, hyaline-like-appearing tissue with an unstable flap along the medial edge of the repair site (Figure C16.4). Indentation testing was performed that demonstrated that the implant was slightly softer than the normal native surrounding articular cartilage but still had a high degree of inherent stiffness (Figure C16.5). The region of periosteal delamination was debrided, and a 2-mm core biopsy was obtained for histologic evaluation (Figure C16.6). The histologic evaluation demonstrated a well-integrated graft at the junction of the subchondral bone and variable amounts of proteoglycan production visibly decreasing from the subchondral bone junction toward the graft surface. Following this debridement, the patient went on to do well with no complaints of residual mechanical symptoms, minimal activity-related effusions, and has returned to intramural sports.

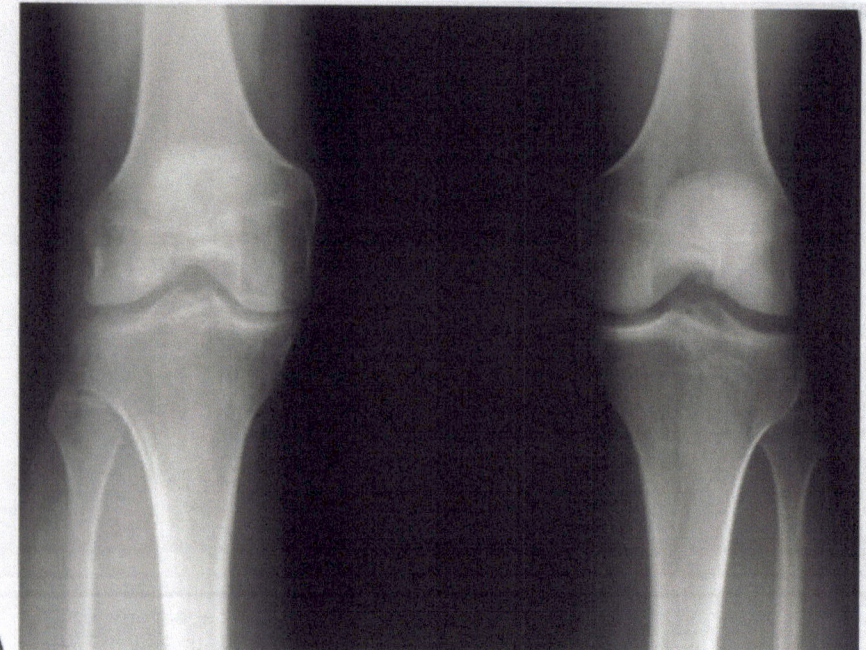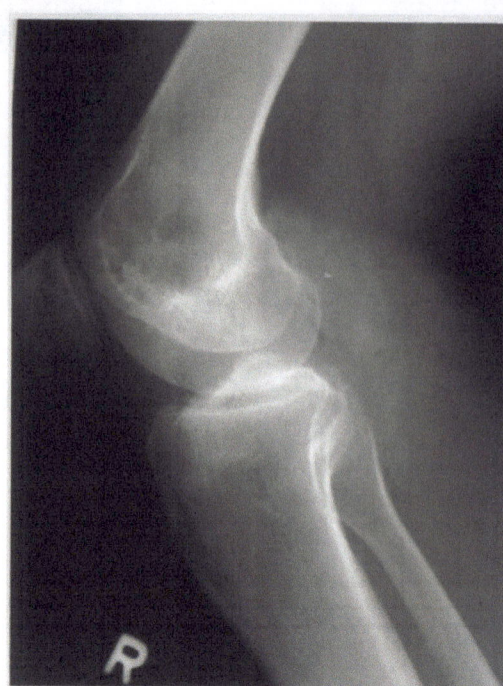

A

FIGURE C16.1 Posteroanterior 45-degree flexion weight-bearing (**A**) and lateral (**B**) radiographs obtained before index arthroscopy were essentially within normal limits save for some possible mild medial joint space narrowing.

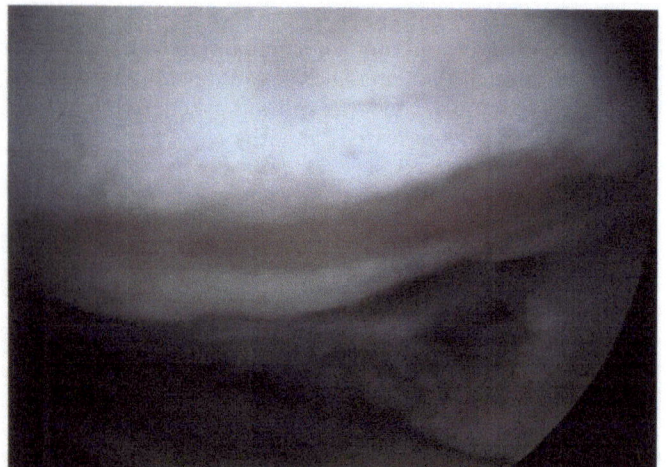

FIGURE C16.2 Arthroscopic photograph of a grade IV medial femoral condyle focal chondral defect obtained at the time of chondral debridement and partial medial meniscectomy.

DECISION-MAKING FACTORS

1. Recurrent symptoms despite previous partial medial meniscectomy in a setting where the focal chondral defect was believed to initially represent an incidental finding requiring only simple debridement.
2. Persistent symptoms of pain and swelling in the exact location of the defect.
3. Normal alignment and ligament status with a defect measuring approximately 5 cm². As opposed to fresh osteochondral allograft transplantation, ACI performed in this relatively young patient will not compromise any future treatment options should they become necessary, that is, no violation of subchondral bone with ACI.

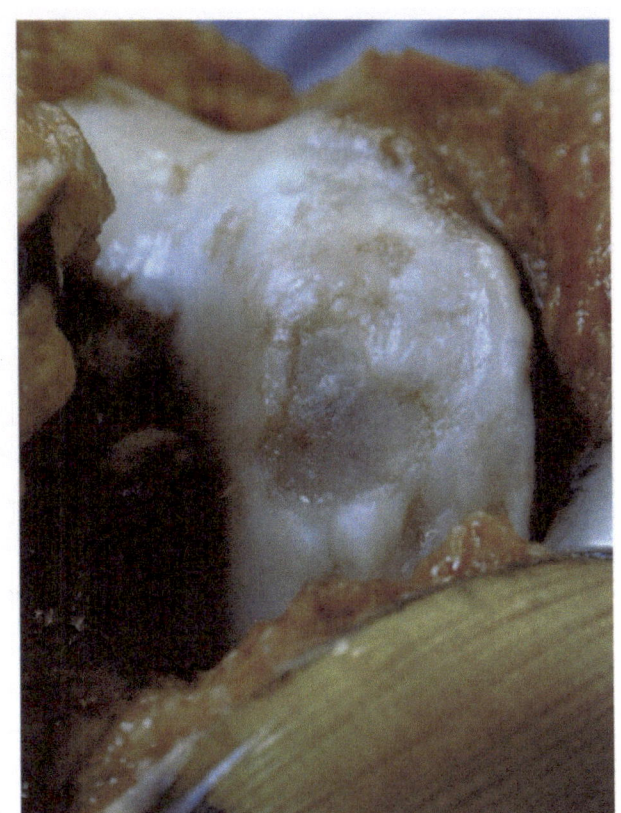

A

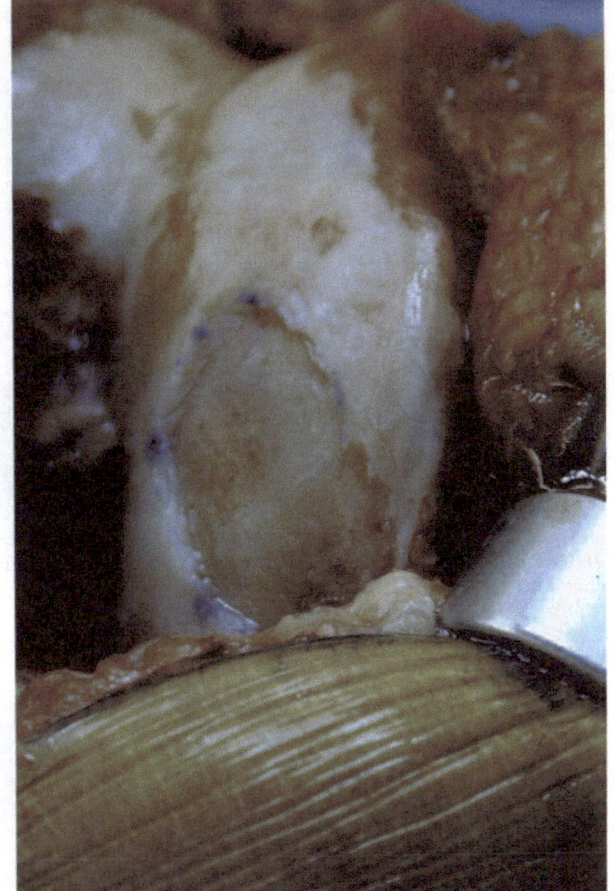

B

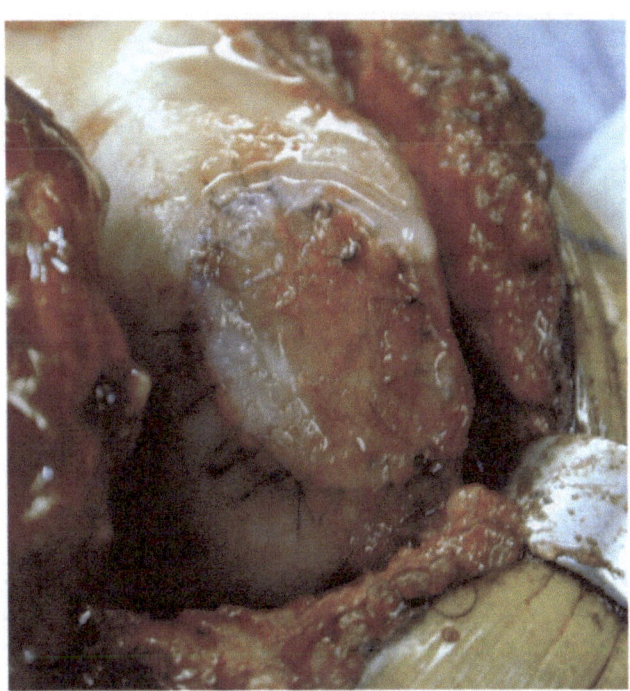

C

FIGURE C16.3 Clinical photographs at the time of autologous chondrocyte implantation demonstrate (**A**) the defect in the medial femoral condyle predebridement; (**B**) the defect postdebridement with vertical walls and no violation of the subchondral bone or calcified layer; and (**C**) the defect prepared with the periosteal patch sewn into place and fibrin glue applied.

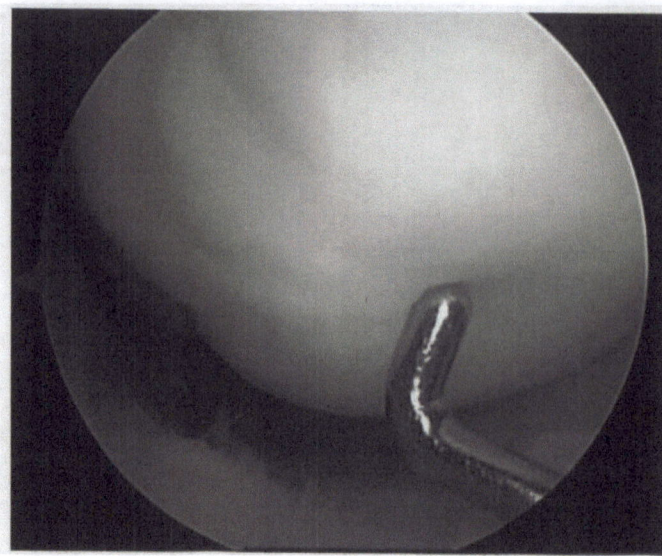

FIGURE C16.4 Second-look arthroscopy at 12 months demonstrates the defect filled and well integrated with hyaline-like tissue that is somewhat softer than the surrounding adjacent cartilage.

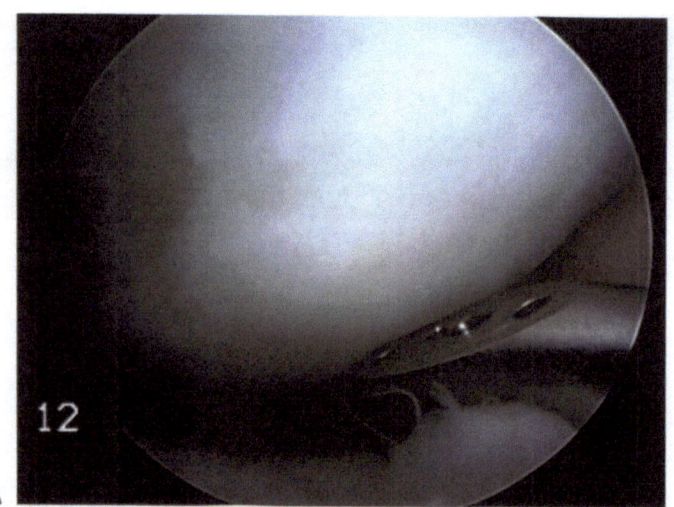

A

Native Articular Cartilage Stiffness vs ACI Implant at 1 Year

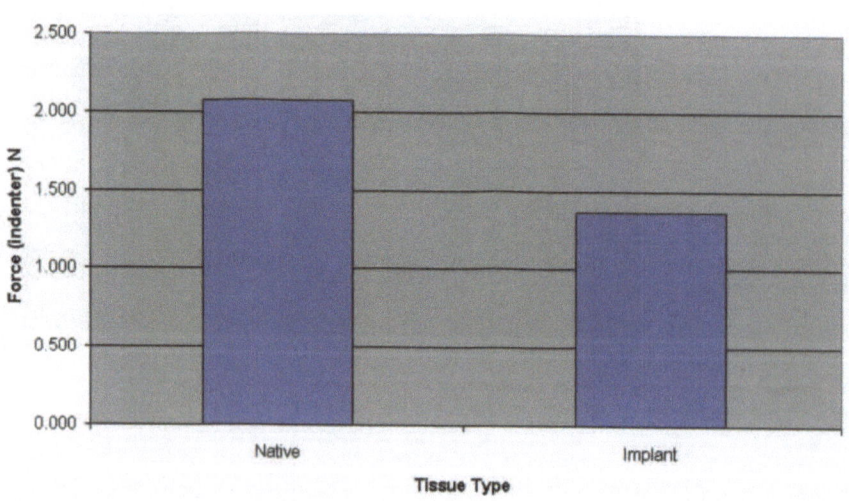

B

FIGURE C16.5 (A) Indentation testing is performed with evidence of a small area of periosteal detachment on the medial aspect of the defect. (B) Bar graph demonstrates the relative differences of the native articular cartilage compared to the hyaline-like tissue.

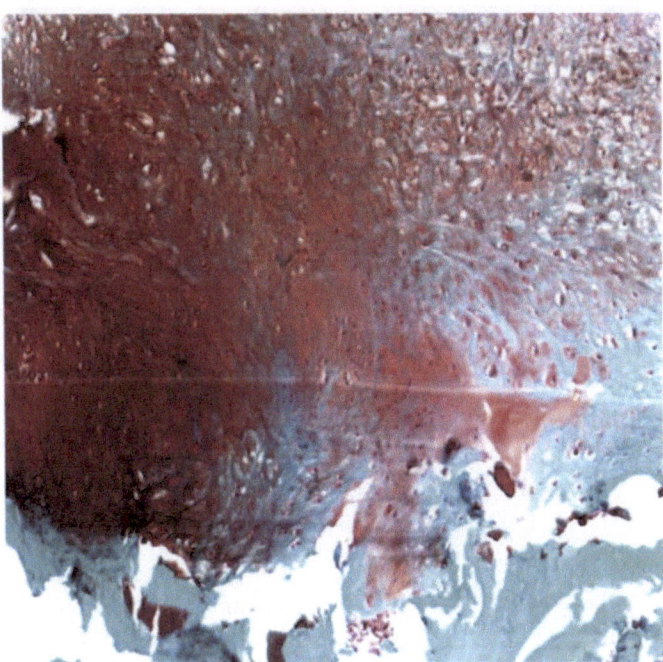

FIGURE C16.6 Safranin-O, fast green staining technique demonstrates variable degrees of proteoglycan staining within the deeper zones of the graft and integration of the hyaline-like tissue with the underlying subchondral bone. Magnification 4x original. (Courtesy of Dr. James M. Williams, PhD, Rush University.)

PATHOLOGY
Contained focal chondral defect of the medial femoral condyle

TREATMENT
Autologous chondrocyte implantation of the medial femoral condyle

SUBMITTED BY
Brian J. Cole, MD, MBA, Rush Cartilage Restoration Center, Rush University Medical Center, Chicago, Illinois, USA

CHIEF COMPLAINT AND HISTORY OF PRESENT ILLNESS

The patient is a 38-year-old man with a complaints of left knee medial-sided pain. Approximately 1 year before his initial presentation, he sustained a direct traumatic blow to the inner side of his left knee. He developed persistent weight-bearing pain and swelling. He underwent arthroscopy and was diagnosed with a grade IV medial femoral condyle focal chondral defect that was initially treated with abrasion arthroplasty at an outside institution (Figure C17.1). Postoperatively, the patient remained symptomatic with recurrent activity-related pain and effusions. He was unable to work as a waiter because of his persistent symptoms.

PHYSICAL EXAMINATION

Height, 5 ft, 10 in.; weight, 170 lb. The patient ambulates with a significant antalgic gait. His alignment is in slight symmetric varus. He has full range of motion. He has significant tenderness over his medial femoral condyle and medial joint line. Meniscal compression signs are absent. He has mild medial tibiofemoral crepitus with passive range of motion. His ligament examination is normal.

RADIOGRAPHIC EVALUATION

Plain radiographs were within normal limits.

SURGICAL INTERVENTION

At the time of arthroscopy 1 year following his abrasion arthroplasty, he demonstrated soft fibrocartilage fill of a 25 mm by 25 mm medial femoral condyle defect with a firm base and palpable subchondral bone (Figure C17.2). At that time, it was elected to perform an articular cartilage biopsy from the intercondylar notch. Approximately 8 weeks later, the patient underwent autologous chondrocyte implantation (Figure C17.3). Postoperatively, he was made nonweight bearing for approximately 6 weeks and subsequently advanced to full weight bearing. Additionally, during that time he used continuous passive motion for approximately 6 h/day. He advanced through the remainder of the rehabilitation protocol over the ensuing 12 months and had some difficulty regaining full flexion. He was asked to refrain from impact activities for at least 12 months.

FOLLOW-UP

The patient did well, and at 2 years follow-up he underwent repeat arthroscopy for a painful plica that was excised. At that time he had full range of motion with minimal tenderness over the defect, but complained of a palpable and painful catching sensation due to the plica. At the time of arthroscopic debridement, he was diagnosed as having excellent fill of the defect with hyaline-like cartilage that was palpably firm and had an excellent transition zone between it and the normal surrounding cartilage (Figure C17.4). The patient has returned to the workplace and complains of some difficulty with kneeling and squatting, with his most recent follow-up being 4 years following his index operation.

DECISION-MAKING FACTORS

1. Relatively young and active individual with a failure of a primary treatment attempt aimed at forming repair tissue within the defect.
2. Persistent symptoms of pain and swelling in the exact location of the defect.
3. A relatively contained lesion of appropriate size for autologous chondrocyte implantation offered as a second-line treatment option.
4. As opposed to fresh osteochondral allograft transplantation, ACI performed in this relatively young patient will not compromise any future treatment options should they become necessary, i.e., no violation of subchondral bone with ACI.

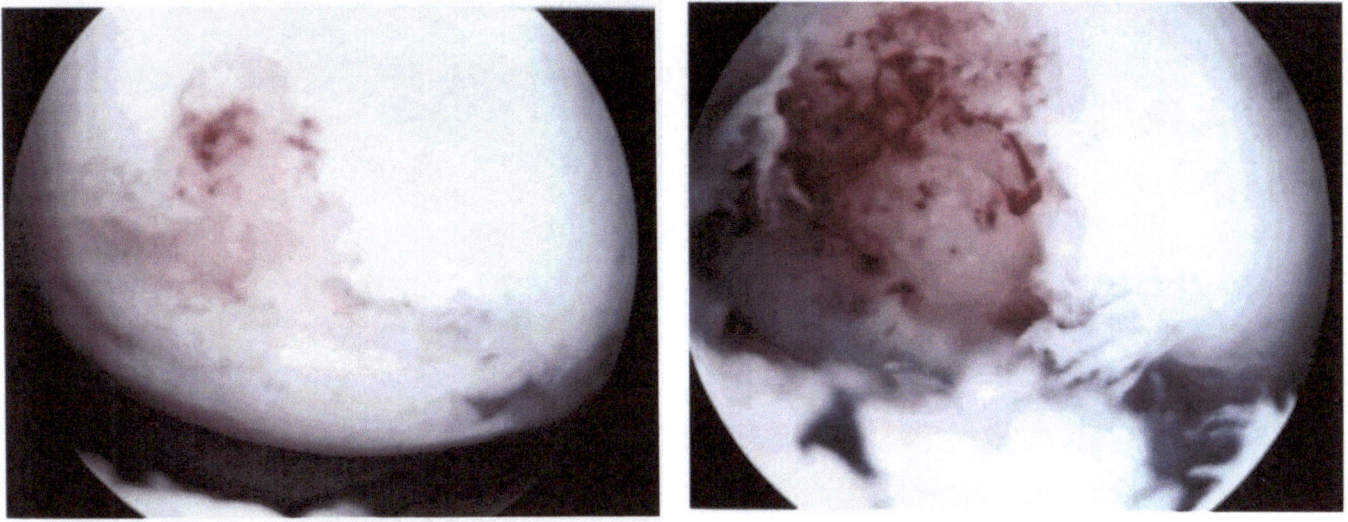

FIGURE C17.1 (**A**) Arthroscopic picture of the index defect of the medial femoral condyle. (**B**) Abrasion arthroplasty performed at the time of index surgery.

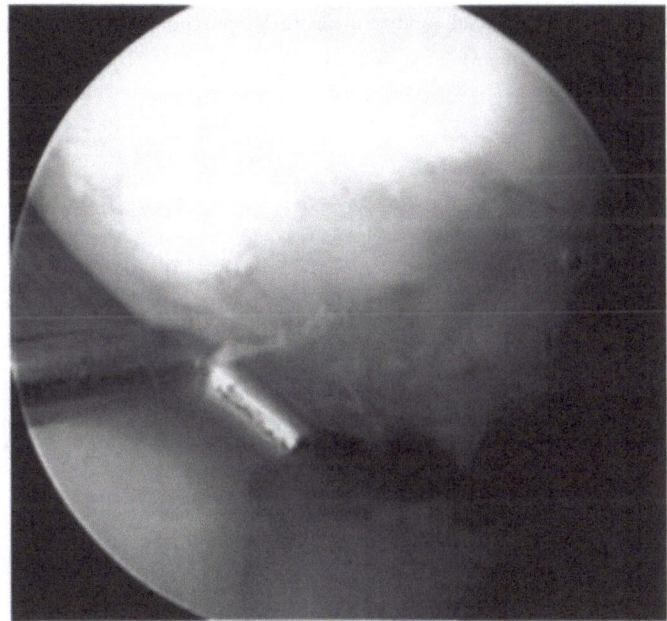

FIGURE C17.2 One-year postoperative arthroscopic picture demonstrates fibrocartilaginous fill that is soft with a firm, subchondral bed.

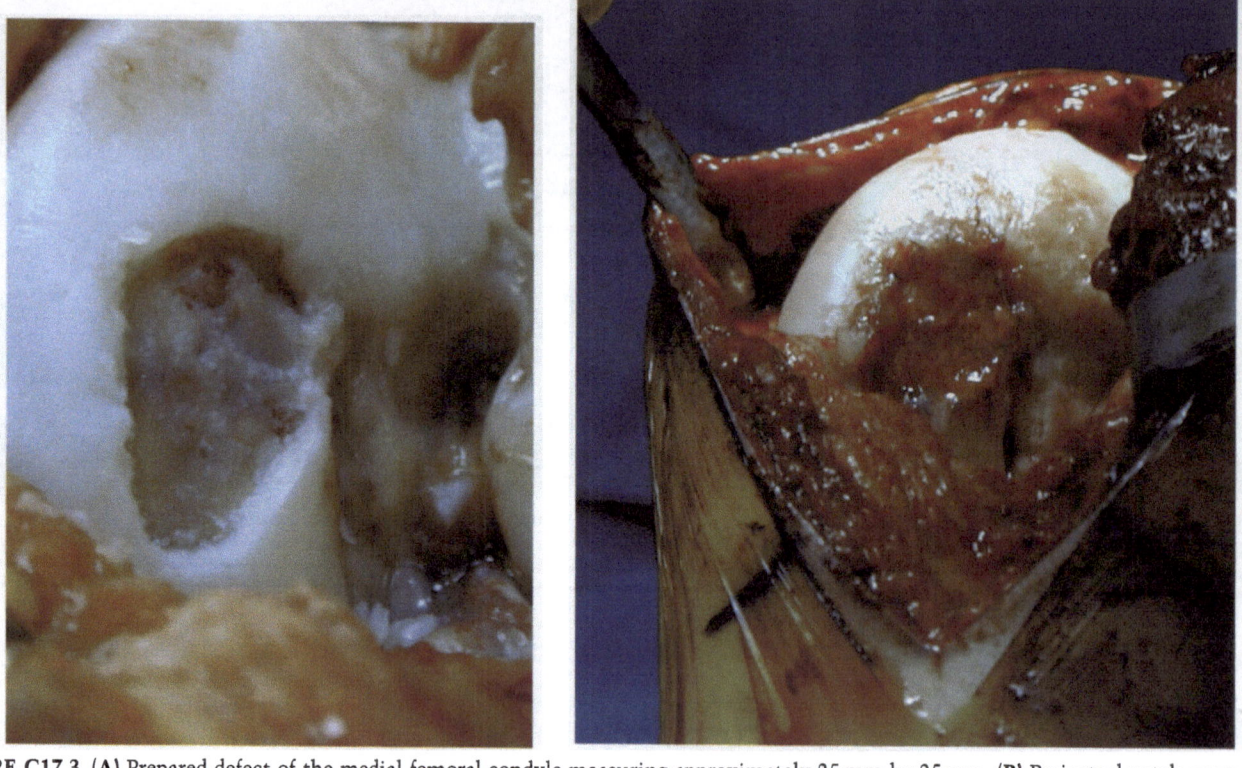

FIGURE C17.3 (A) Prepared defect of the medial femoral condyle measuring approximately 25 mm by 25 mm. **(B)** Periosteal patch sewn into place following fibrin glue placement.

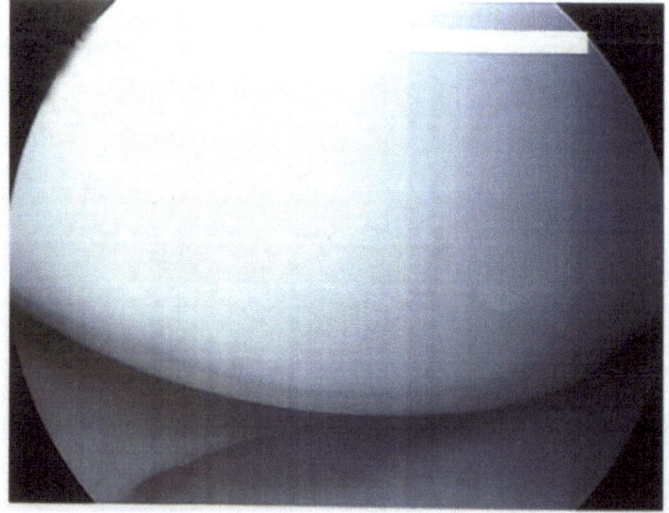

FIGURE C17.4 Second-look arthroscopy at 2 years demonstrates excellent fill with a smooth transition zone between the defect and normal surrounding articular cartilage.

18

PATHOLOGY
Osteochondritis dissecans of the medial femoral condyle

TREATMENT
Autologous chondrocyte implantation of the medial femoral condyle

SUBMITTED BY
Brian J. Cole, MD, MBA, Rush Cartilage Restoration Center, Rush University Medical Center, Chicago, Illinois, USA

CHIEF COMPLAINT AND HISTORY OF PRESENT ILLNESS

This patient is a previously active 26-year-old man with a history of left knee problems dating back to approximately 14 months before his initial evaluation for cartilage restoration. His past history includes episodes of periodic swelling and locking, which led to an arthroscopic removal of a loose body emanating from a lesion of osteochondritis dissecans of the medial femoral condyle, performed approximately 12 months before this evaluation. The patient did well initially, but developed recurrent pain and swelling with weight-bearing activities and an inability to perform any impact or pivoting sports.

PHYSICAL EXAMINATION

Height, 6 ft, 3 in.; weight, 180 lb. The patient walks with a nonantalgic gait. His standing alignment is in neutral. His left knee has a minimal effusion. His range of motion is 0 to 130 degrees. His medial femoral condyle is tender to palpation, and meniscal findings are absent. His ligament examination is within normal limits.

RADIOGRAPHIC EVALUATION

Initial radiographs demonstrate a lesion of osteochondritis dissecans in the typical zone of the medial femoral condyle of the left knee (Figure C18.1). Similarly, a magnetic resonance image (MRI) demonstrated loss of convexity of the medial femoral condyle in the region of the intercondylar notch with no evidence of a remaining fragment (Figure C18.2).

SURGICAL INTERVENTION

Because of his recurrent symptoms, the patient was indicated for arthroscopy and biopsy for autologous chondrocyte implantation (Figure C18.3). Approximately 5 weeks later, the patient underwent autologous chondrocyte implantation (ACI) (Figure C18.4). At the time of implantation, the lesion measured approximately 25 mm in length, 22 mm in width, and 6 mm in depth. Postoperatively, the patient was made nonweight bearing for approximately 4 weeks and utilized continuous passive motion for 6 weeks at 6 to 8 h/day. He advanced through the traditional rehabilitation protocol for ACI of the femoral condyle and was asked to refrain from any impact or ballistic activities for at least 12 months.

FOLLOW-UP

At his 2-year follow-up visit he complained of no residual symptoms. He was participating in several high-level activities including running marathons and performing triathlons. Radiographs at that time demonstrated restoration of the medial femoral condyle in the previous region of osteochondritis dissecans with no evidence of sclerotic change, lucency, or joint space narrowing (Figure C18.5).

DECISION-MAKING FACTORS

1. A failure of first-line treatment with persistent symptoms of activity-related weight-bearing pain in the region of the defect.
2. Young high-demand patient with symptomatic, relatively contained, shallow osteochondritis dissecans lesion considered relatively large for osteochondral autograft transplantation.
3. Patient preference for his own tissue and surgeon preference for ACI as a primary attempt at cartilage restoration to avoid creation of a deeper subchondral defect otherwise required for fresh osteochondral allograft transplantation.
4. Ability and willingness to be compliant with the postoperative course.

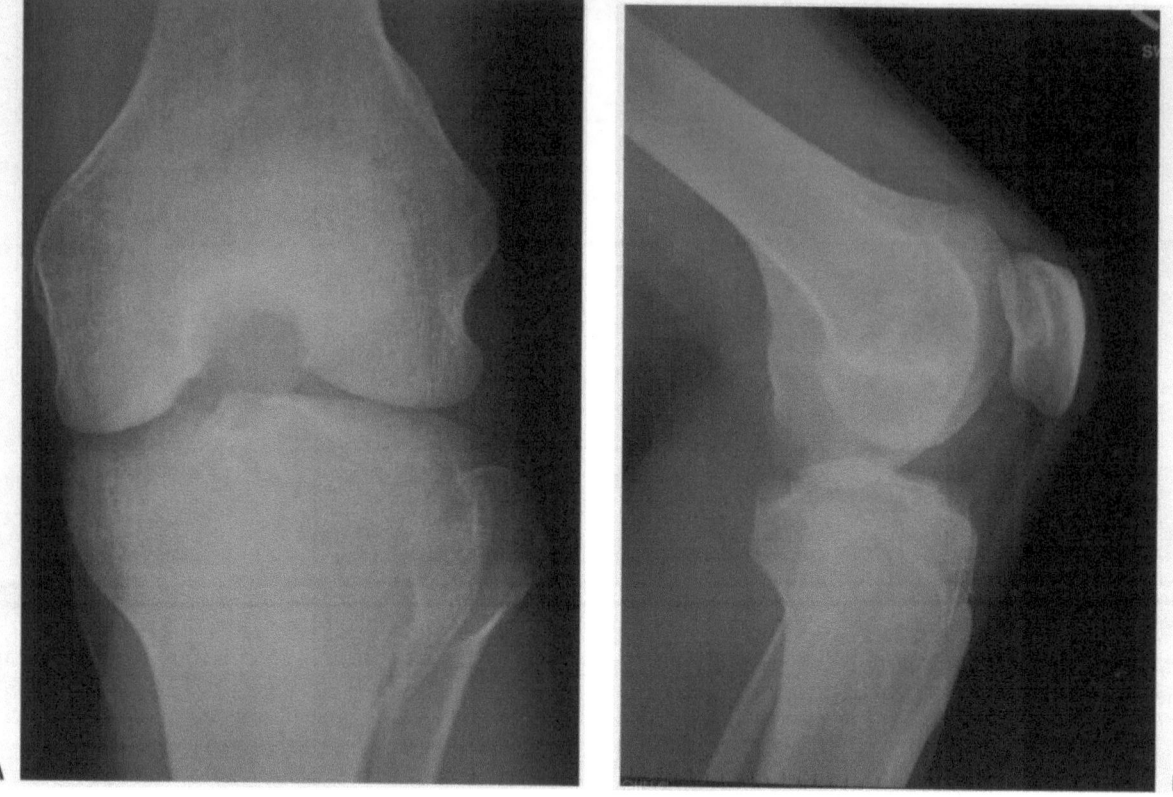

FIGURE C18.1 Preoperative posteroanterior 45-degree flexion weight-bearing (**A**) and lateral (**B**) radiographs demonstrate a lesion of osteochondritis dissecans in the typical zone of the medial femoral condyle of the left knee.

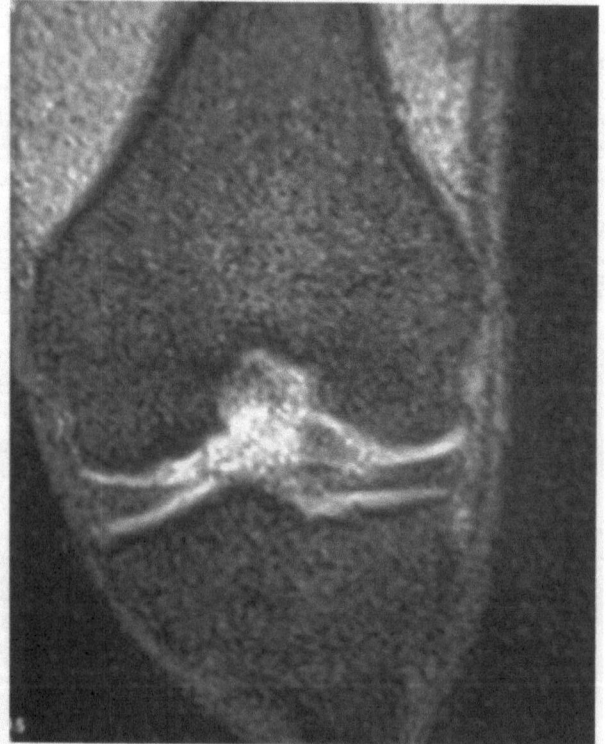

FIGURE C18.2 MRI demonstrates loss of convexity of the medial femoral condyle in the region of the intercondylar notch with no evidence of remaining fragment.

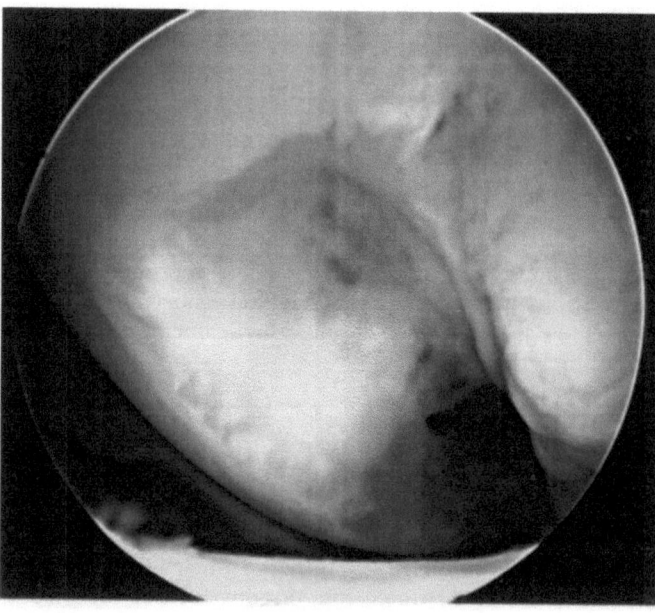

FIGURE C18.3 Arthroscopic photograph of the medial femoral condyle defect, taken at the time of biopsy.

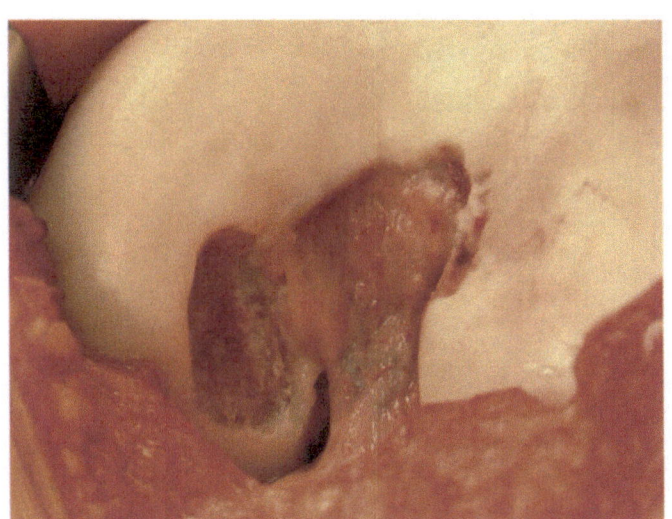
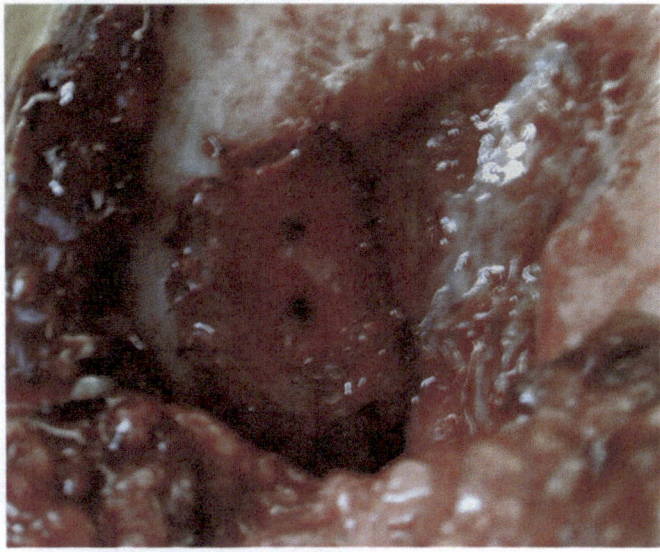

FIGURE C18.4 (A) Medial femoral condyle defect after preparation. The lesion measured approximately 25 mm in length, 22 mm in width, and 6 mm in depth. (B) After periosteal patch fixation.

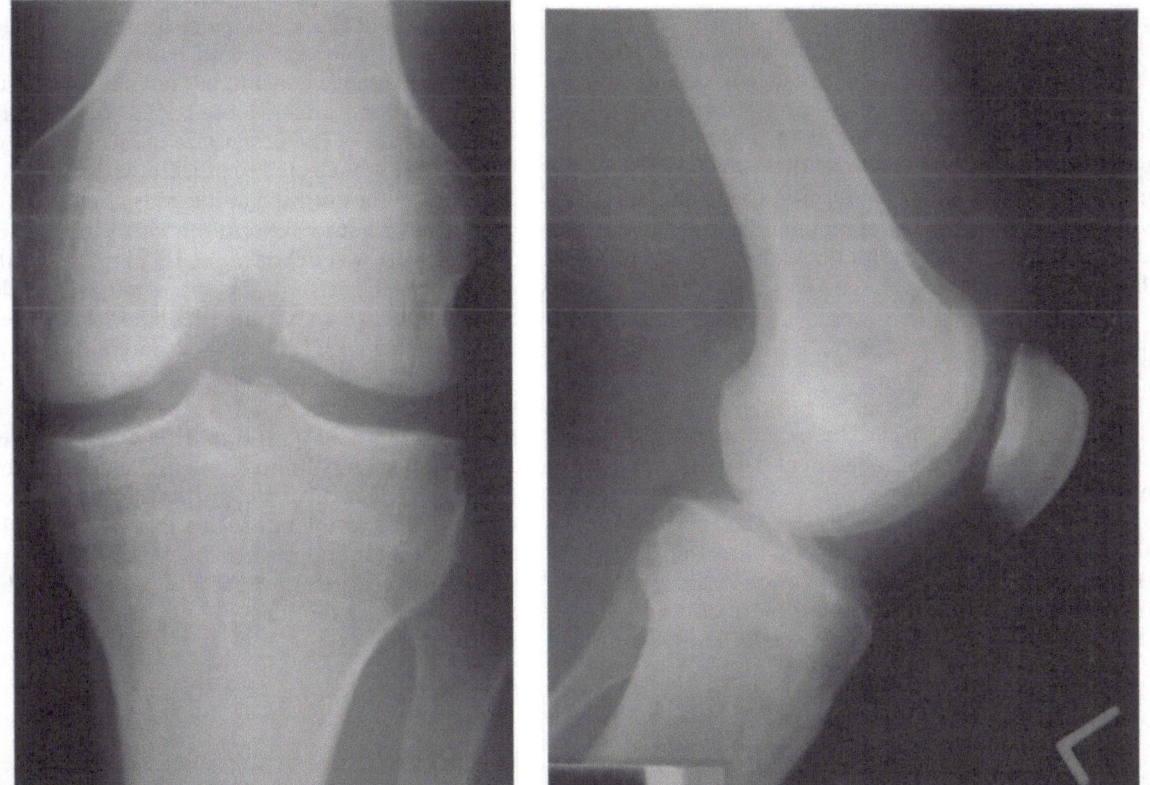

FIGURE 18.5 Two-year postoperative anteroposterior (A) and lateral (B) radiographs demonstrate restoration of the medial femoral condyle in the previous region of osteochondritis dissecans with no evidence of sclerotic change, lucency, or joint space narrowing.

CHIEF COMPLAINT AND HISTORY OF PRESENT ILLNESS

The patient is a very active 19-year-old man who reports an injury to his right knee approximately 6 months prior while jumping from a fence. He subsequently developed the onset of sudden pain and swelling of his knee. He does recall occasional clicking before that time, but it became significantly worse after this recent traumatic event. Since the time of the injury, the patient has had weight-bearing discomfort with pain along the lateral aspect of his knee. He is unable to perform high-level activities because of the pain and activity-related swelling. Additionally, he reports a catching sensation. As a result of his present symptoms, he is unable to compete in intramural college athletics as he was able to do before this injury.

PHYSICAL EXAMINATION

Height, 5 ft, 8 in.; weight, 170 lb. The patient walks with a nonantalgic gait. His standing alignment is in symmetric physiologic varus. The right knee has a moderate effusion with positive lateral joint line tenderness, no medial joint line tenderness, and no varus or valgus instability upon stress testing. His lateral femoral condyle is painful to direct palpation. His ligament examination is within normal limits. He has full range of motion and has no meniscal findings.

RADIOGRAPHIC EVALUATION

Plain radiographs of the right knee including 45-degree flexion weight-bearing posteroanterior and nonweight-bearing lateral views reveal flattening of the lateral femoral condyle consistent with chronic osteochondritis dissecans. There appears to be minimal subchondral bone loss. Magnetic resonance imaging (MRI) is also consistent with the diagnosis of osteochondritis dissecans with minimal bony involvement (Figure C19.1).

SURGICAL INTERVENTION

Based on the patient's history, age, symptoms, physical examination, and radiographic studies, he was indicated for diagnostic arthroscopy, debridement of the lateral femoral condyle lesion, and possibly microfracture depending on the size and depth of the lesion. At arthroscopy, a grade IV 28 mm by 30 mm lesion of the lateral femoral condyle was noted. The lesion extended down to but not appreciably through the subchondral bone, and no loose bodies were identified (Figure C19.2). Because of the defect size, patient activity level, and symptoms, it was elected to proceed with biopsy of the articular cartilage for eventual autologous chondrocyte implantation (ACI) and not to perform microfracture of the lesion.

The lesion was debrided, and a biopsy of 200 to 300 mg articular cartilage from the intercondylar notch was harvested. Approximately 2 months later, the patient returned and underwent ACI through a lateral-based arthrotomy (Figure C19.3). Postoperatively, the patient was made heel-touch weight bearing for 6 weeks and utilized continuous passive motion (CPM) for 6 to 8 h/day during that time. His range of motion was limited from full extension to 90 degrees of flexion. At 6 weeks, weight bearing and range of motion were advanced as tolerated. He advanced through the traditional rehabilitation protocol for ACI of the femoral condyle and was asked to refrain from any impact or ballistic activities for at least 12 months.

FOLLOW-UP

The patient is now 24 months after ACI of the lateral femoral condyle of his right knee. He has no pain and has full range of motion. He runs, bikes, and skis on a regular basis. He is actively involved with intramural sports while attending college. His radiographs show early fill and restoration of contour of the lateral femoral condyle (Figure C19.4).

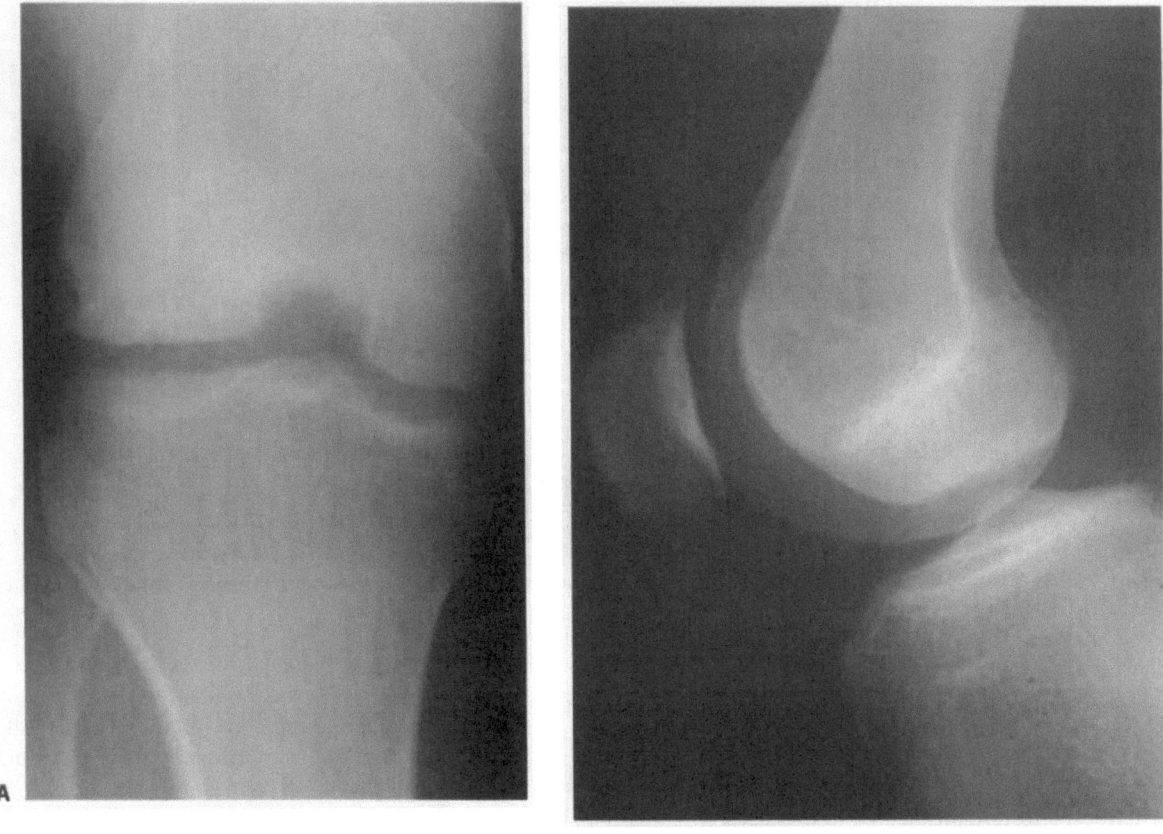

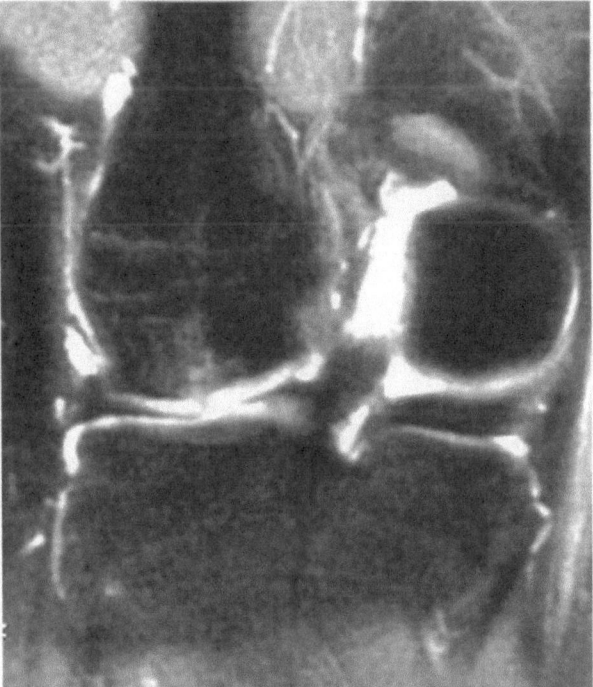

FIGURE C19.1 Preoperative (**A**) posteroanterior 45-degree flexion weight-bearing and (**B**) lateral radiographs demonstrate flattening and loss of contour of the lateral femoral condyle of the right knee with minimal loss of subchondral bone. (**C**) MRI confirms full-thickness cartilage loss of the lateral femoral condyle with minimal bony involvement.

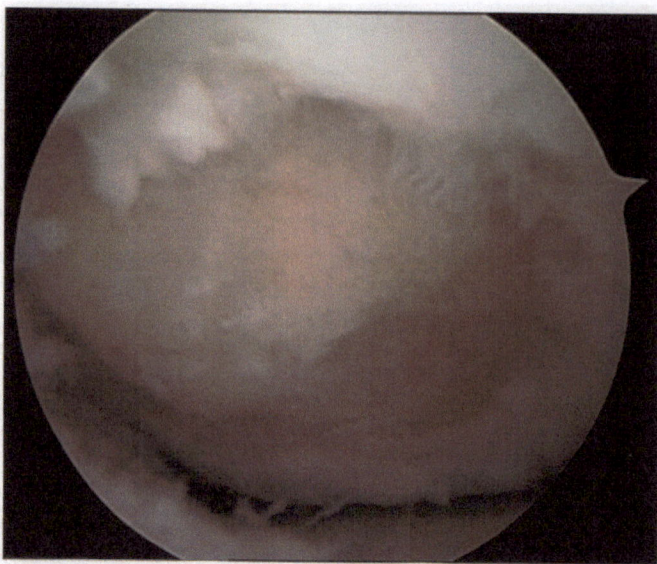

FIGURE C19.2 Arthroscopic photograph demonstrates grade IV lateral femoral condyle lesion measuring 28 mm by 30 mm, extending down to but not appreciably through the subchondral bone.

DECISION-MAKING FACTORS

1. Young, high-demand male with shallow osteochondritis dissecans lesion anticipated to be relatively unresponsive to microfracture and considered relatively large for osteochondral autograft transplantation.
2. Persistent symptoms of pain and swelling in the exact location of the defect.
3. Patient preference for his own tissue and surgeon preference for ACI as a primary cartilage restoration procedure given the relatively young age of this patient and the desire to avoid creating a subchondral defect otherwise required for fresh osteochondral allograft transplantation.
4. Ability and willingness to be compliant with the postoperative course.

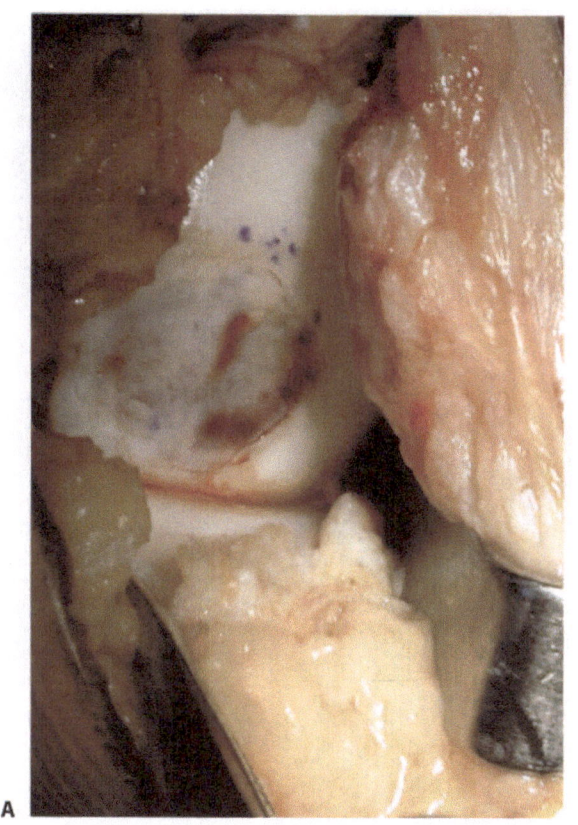

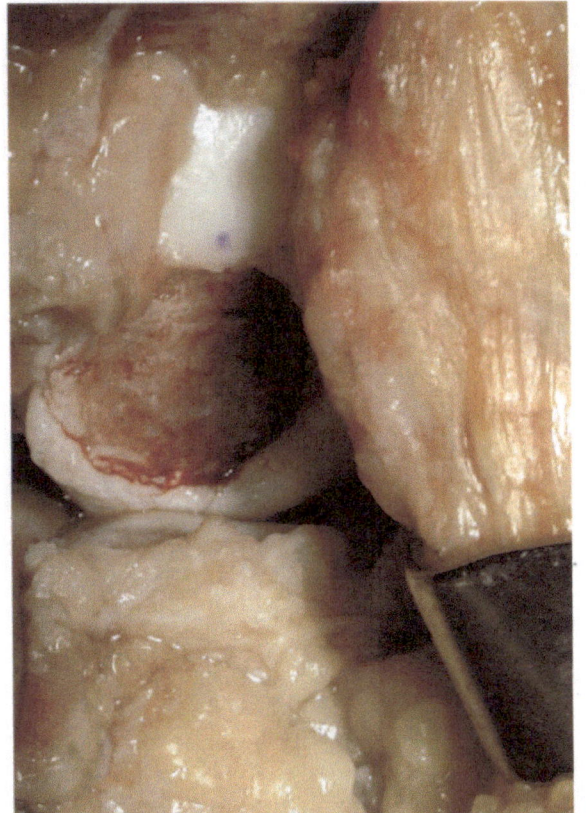

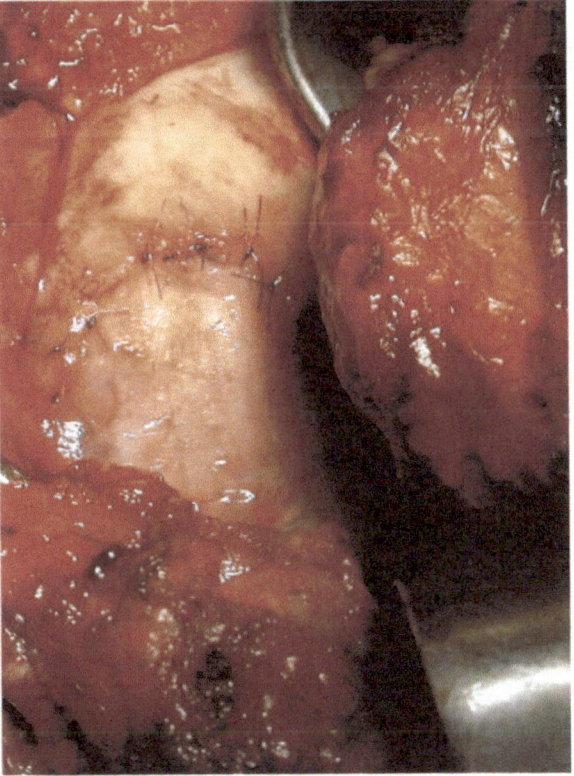

FIGURE C19.3 (**A**) Intraoperative photograph of the lateral femoral condyle lesion demonstrates full-thickness cartilage loss. (**B**) Lateral femoral condyle lesion after debridement. (**C**) Lateral femoral condyle lesion after the periosteal patch is sewn into place.

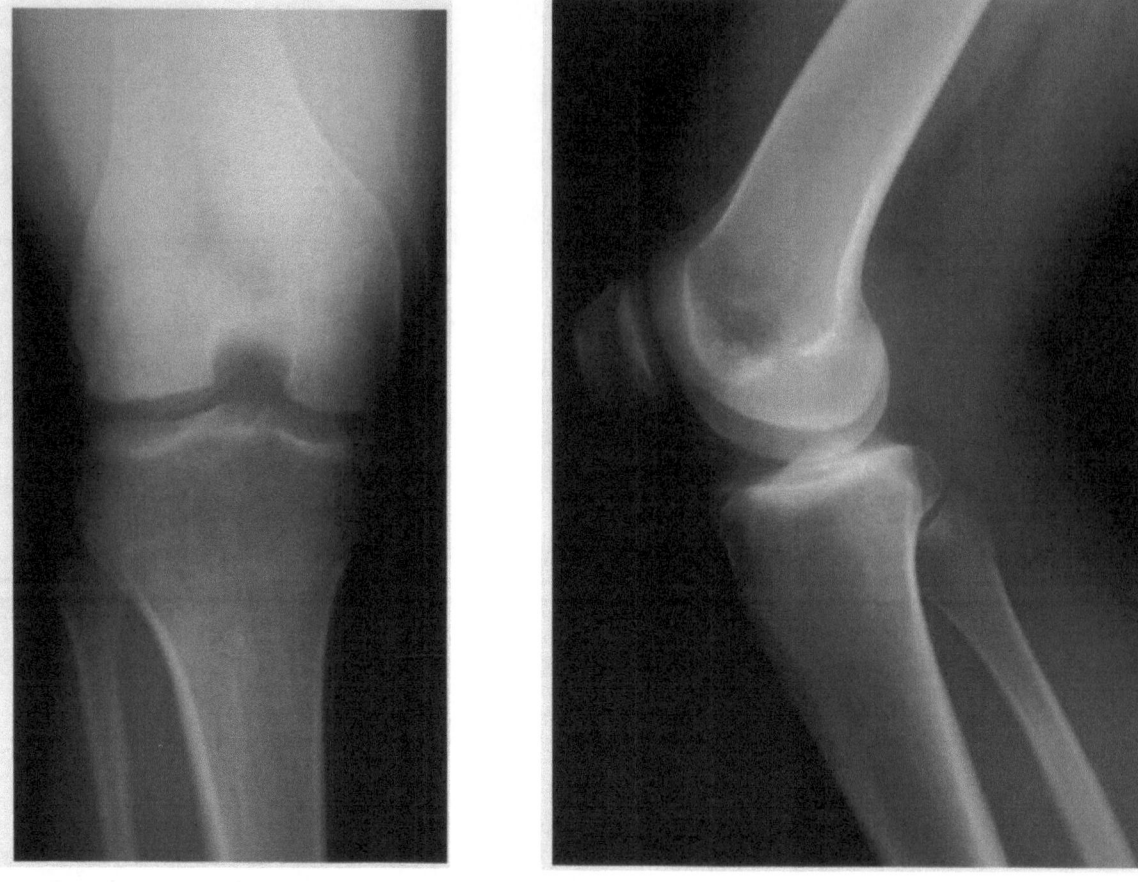

FIGURE C19.4 Postoperative anteroposterior **(A)** and lateral **(B)** radiographs at 1-year follow-up demonstrate good fill and contour of the lateral femoral condyle with no evidence of collapse.

20

PATHOLOGY
Uncontained focal chondral defect of the lateral trochlea

TREATMENT
Autologous chondrocyte implantation of the trochlea with distal realignment

SUBMITTED BY
Brian J. Cole, MD, MBA, Rush Cartilage Restoration Center, Rush University Medical Center, Chicago, Illinois, USA

CHIEF COMPLAINT AND HISTORY OF PRESENT ILLNESS

This patient is a 16-year-old girl with complaints of left knee pain and swelling of several years duration. She stated that her knee problems date back to when she was in the fourth grade at the age of 9 years. She sustained an injury that precipitated her symptoms, which have gradually worsened over the years. Two years previously, she underwent microfracture of an isolated chondral lesion of the trochlea due to her relentless symptoms of anterolateral knee pain and activity-related swelling. Initially, her symptoms were reduced. However, because of worsening complaints of swelling and pain over the ensuing 2 years, she presented for additional treatment. She indicates that although she thoroughly enjoys participating in sports, she has not been able to do so for the past few years as a result of severe knee pain. Furthermore, walking more than just a few blocks causes her knee pain and swelling, requiring her to rest and elevate her left leg. She is unable to perform stair climbing other than with a nonreciprocal gait due to severe anterolateral knee pain. Several months of aggressive patellofemoral rehabilitation failed to alleviate her symptoms.

PHYSICAL EXAMINATION

Height, 5 ft, 5 in.; weight, 122 lb. The patient ambulates with a slightly antalgic gait on the left. Her standing alignment appears to be neutral and symmetric. A moderate effusion is present in the left knee. Her range of motion is from 0 to 135 degrees. She has 1 cm of quadriceps atrophy when measured 10 cm proximal to the patella. She has a full symmetric range of motion and mild patellar apprehension. She has mild lateral joint line tenderness, no medial joint line tenderness, and her meniscal findings are grossly absent. Additionally, she has 3+ crepitus of the patellofemoral joint with active extension. Her ligament examination is within normal limits.

RADIOGRAPHIC EVALUATION

Extension weight-bearing radiographs reveal some lateral femoral condyle flattening of the left knee. Overall, her alignment is normal with no evidence of degenerative changes or joint space narrowing (Figure C20.1). Merchant views demonstrated the patella to be centered within the trochlea and no evidence of trochlear hypoplasia. Given her well-documented history and consistent symptoms, no magnetic resonance imaging (MRI) was obtained.

SURGICAL INTERVENTION

The patient underwent a left knee arthroscopy in which articular cartilage debridement was performed as well as a biopsy for autologous chondrocyte implantation (ACI). At the time of arthroscopy, a trochlear defect of approximately 30 mm by 35 mm was noted to be completely filled with soft fibrocartilage (Figure C20.2). The defect was laterally based with direct contact with the patella during the initial phases of knee flexion. Approximately 2 months later, the patient underwent ACI of her chondral lesion in addition to a distal tibial tubercle anteromedialization procedure. Due to the uncontained nature of this laterally sided trochlear lesion, two mini suture-anchors were utilized to sew the periosteal patch to the periphery (Figures C20.3, C20.4). Additionally, juxtaarticular synovial tissue was utilized to help seal the periosteal patch. Postoperatively, she was made heel-touch weight bearing for approximately 6 weeks until radiographic healing of the distal realignment was demonstrated. She utilized continuous passive motion for 6 weeks initially with partial flexion restrictions. At 8 weeks, she was advanced to weight bearing and range of motion as tolerated. She advanced through the traditional rehabilitation protocol for ACI of the trochlea. She was asked to refrain from any impact or ballistic activities for 18 months.

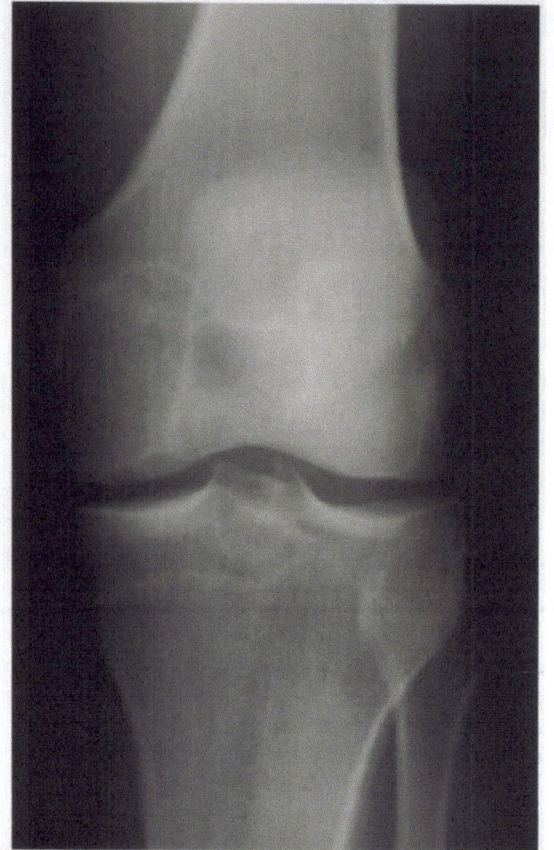

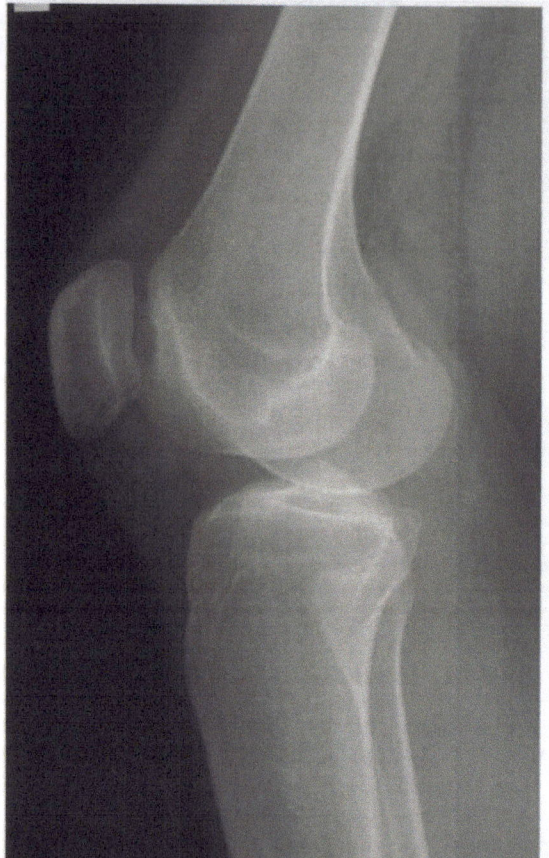

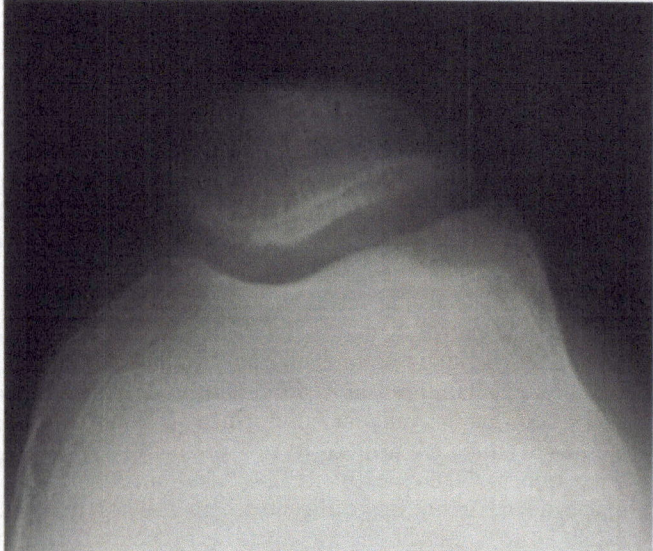

FIGURE C20.1 Anteroposterior (**A**), lateral (**B**), and merchant (**C**) radiographs of the left knee reveal mild flattening of the lateral femoral condyle without any other obvious abnormalities.

FOLLOW-UP

At her 6-month follow-up visit, she ambulated without an antalgic gait, and her knee pain and swelling had decreased substantially. At 12 months, she was walking for long distances without pain. Stair climbing was virtually painfree. She has not begun participating in gym class or sports activities as yet. However, she believes that once the protocol permits, she would be symptom free enough to allow higher-level activities.

DECISION-MAKING FACTORS

1. Previously failed microfracture technique and aggressive physical therapy program emphasizing proper patellofemoral mechanics.
2. Young, high-demand patient without viable cartilage restoration alternatives.
3. Persistent symptoms of pain and swelling in the exact location of the defect.
4. Ability and willingness to be compliant with postoperative rehabilitation.

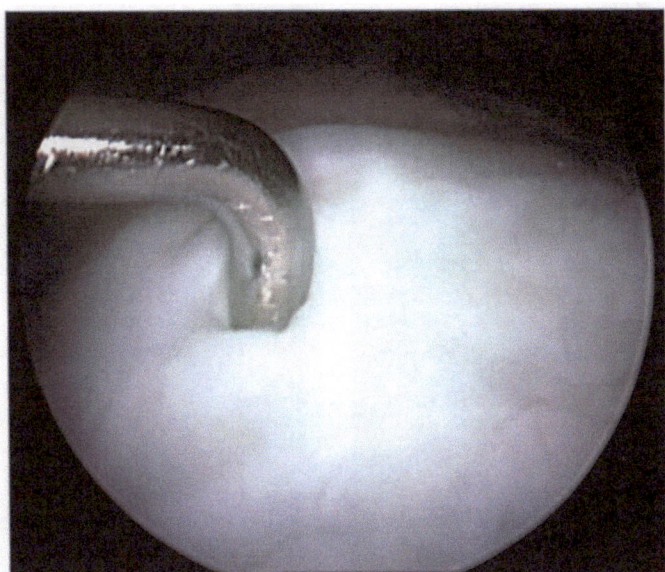

FIGURE C20.2 Arthroscopic probing of the trochlear lesion demonstrates a laterally based lesion with soft fibrocartilaginous repair tissue.

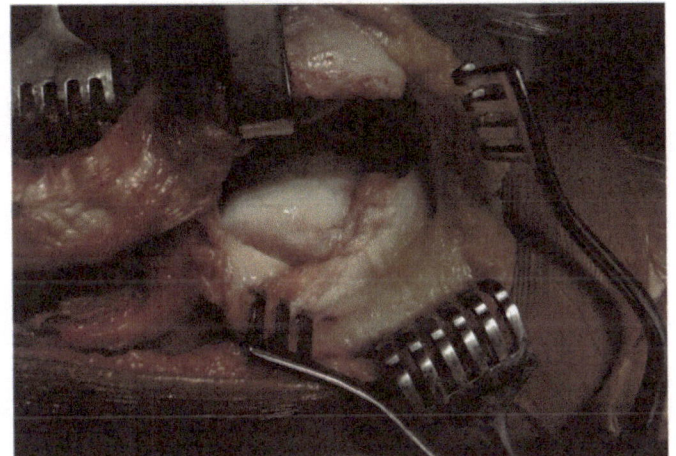

A

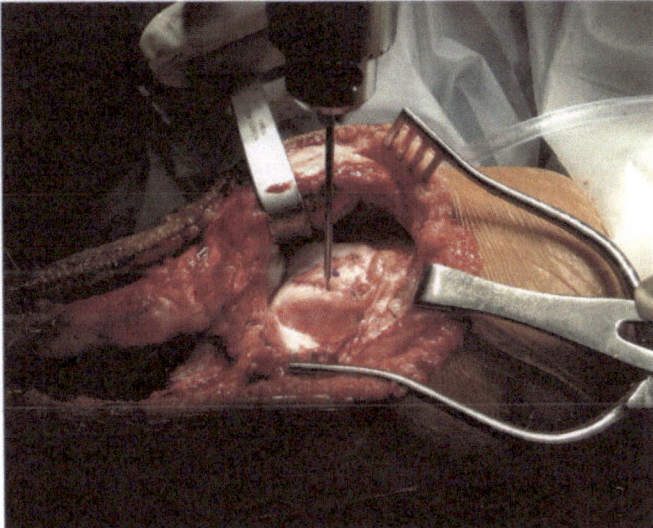

B

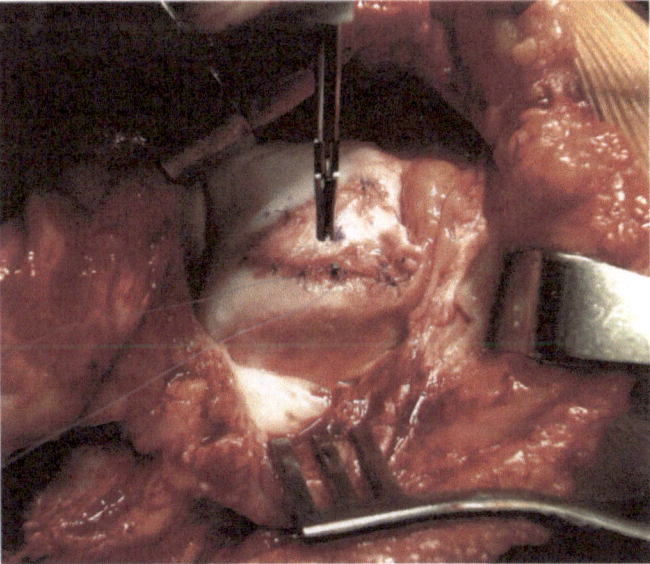

C

FIGURE C20.3 Intraoperative clinical photographs of the autologous chondrocyte implantation procedure. (**A**) Inspection of the trochlear lesion. The uncontained nature of this laterally based lesion is evident. Following initial suturing of the periosteal patch, additional fixation is provided by drilling for suture anchor placement along the lateral uncontained edge (**B**) and anchor placement before impaction (**C**).

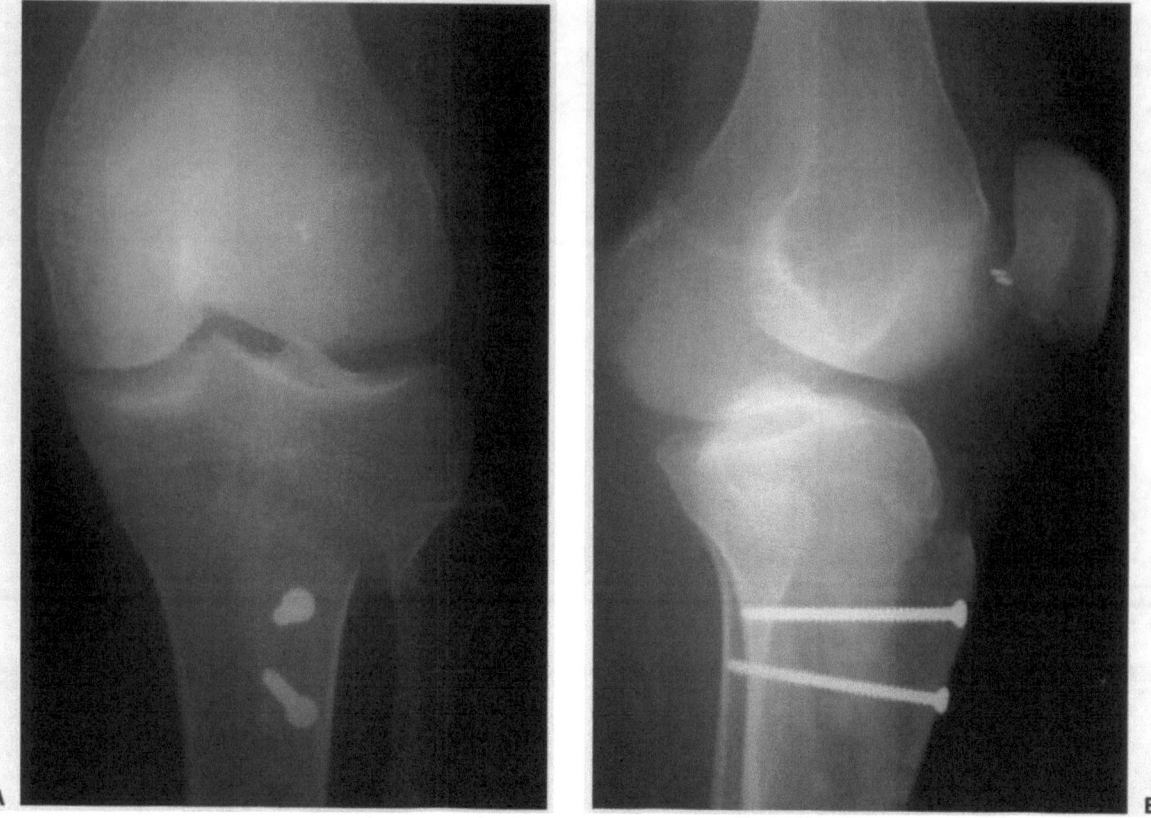

FIGURE C20.4 Postoperative anteroposterior (**A**) and lateral (**B**) radiographs of the left knee demonstrate the distal realignment procedure with hardware fixation in place. The two suture anchors utilized to secure the periosteal patch are also evident on these radiographic views.

21

PATHOLOGY
Failed prior fresh osteochondral allograft of the medial femoral condyle

TREATMENT
Revision fresh osteochondral allograft with medial opening-wedge high tibial osteotomy and iliac crest bone graft

SUBMITTED BY
Brian J. Cole, MD, MBA, Rush Cartilage Restoration Center, Rush University Medical Center, Chicago, Illinois, USA

CHIEF COMPLAINT AND HISTORY OF PRESENT ILLNESS

The patient is an 18-year-old male who has had symptoms of bilateral knee pain for 5 years before his initial evaluation. His symptom onset was sudden, occurring while playing football. Two years previously, because of ongoing symptoms of osteochondritis dissecans of both medial femoral condyles, he underwent bilateral osteochondral allograft transplantation using fresh osteochondral allografts. The right knee was treated with an opening-wedge osteotomy due to a slight varus deformity, and the left knee, because of what was believed to be a minimal varus deformity, was left untreated without an osteotomy. The patient did well with respect to the right knee and became completely asymptomatic. However, his left knee remained symptomatic, with complaints of medial knee pain on a daily basis with weight-bearing activity-related swelling, stiffness, and inability to participate in sports. He has minimal mechanical symptoms. He would like to participate in intramural and high school level sports but is unable to do so.

PHYSICAL EXAMINATION

Height, 5 ft, 10 in.; weight, 190 lb. His gait is slightly antalgic on the left. The alignment reveals a slight varus deformity on the left and normal alignment to slight valgus on the right. There is a moderate effusion in the left knee. His range of motion is 0 to 130 degrees. He is tender along the medial femoral condyle and slightly tender along the joint line. Meniscal findings, however, are grossly absent. He has 2 cm of quadriceps atrophy in the left knee when measured 10 cm proximal to the patella. His ligament examination is normal.

RADIOGRAPHIC EVALUATION

Posteroanterior flexion weight-bearing radiographs demonstrate collapse of the medial femoral condyle osteochondral allograft of the left knee. The osteochondral allograft and high tibial osteotomy previously performed on the right knee are both well healed (Figure C21.1).

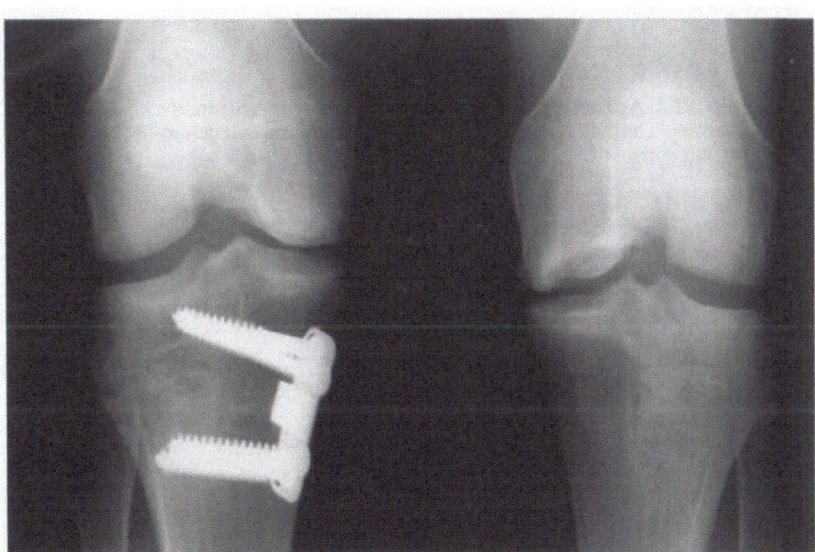

FIGURE C21.1 Flexion weight-bearing radiograph demonstrates collapse of the medial femoral condyle osteochondral allograft of the left knee and well-incorporated osteochondral allograft in the right knee with a well-healed osteotomy.

SURGICAL INTERVENTION

At the time of surgery on his left knee, there was a necrotic osteoarticular fragment and a defect measuring 30 mm by 30 mm by 8 mm in depth (Figure C21.2). The fragment was removed, and the patient underwent postoperative rehabilitation. Three months later, the patient underwent left knee osteochondral allograft reconstruction using a 30 mm by 30 mm fresh osteochondral allograft and a high tibial opening-wedge osteotomy with an 11-degree correction and iliac crest bone grafting (Figure C21.3). Postoperatively, he was made nonweight bearing for approximately 8 weeks. He utilized continuous passive motion and underwent progressive strengthening. At 8 weeks, he was advanced to weight bearing as tolerated. At 6 months, he was permitted to return to activities as tolerated.

FOLLOW-UP

At his 18-month follow-up visit, he demonstrated full range of motion, no swelling or pain, and had returned to all activities. Imaging studies reveal radiographic incorporation of his graft without collapse and a well-healed osteotomy (Figure C21.4). At the 3-year follow-up visit, he was completely asymptomatic.

DECISION-MAKING FACTORS

1. Young, active individual with symptoms related to lesion of osteochondritis dissecans.
2. Defect size greater than 3 cm^2 with subchondral bone loss beyond 6 to 8 mm.
3. Failure of primary treatment with the possibility of biomechanical and biologic failure of the osteochondral allograft.
4. Contralateral knee with similar pathology successfully treated with combined fresh osteochondral allograft and opening-wedge high tibial osteotomy.

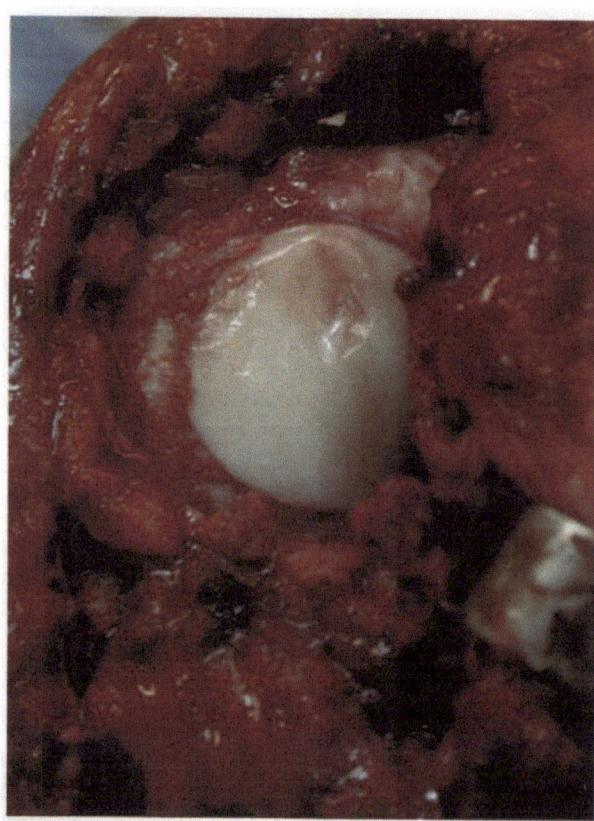

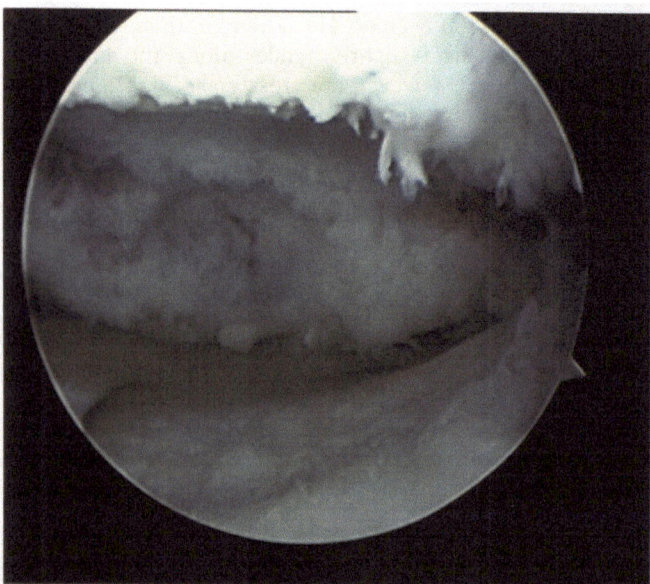

FIGURE C21.2 Arthroscopic view of the defect cavity within the medial femoral condyle following removal of the necrotic osteochondral allograft fragment.

FIGURE C21.3 Intraoperative photograph of a 30 mm by 30 mm fresh osteochondral allograft placed within the medial femoral condyle.

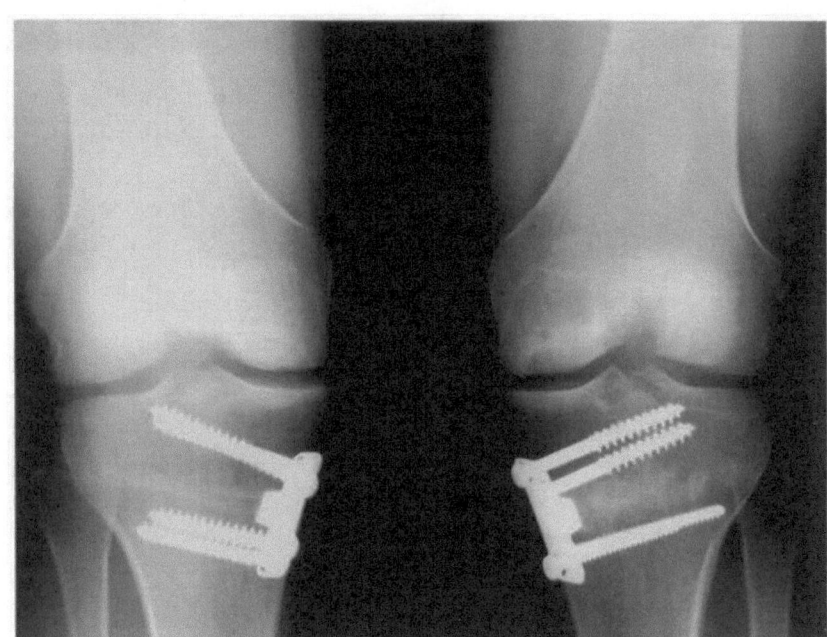

FIGURE 21.4 Eighteen-month radiograph demonstrates healing of the osteotomy and excellent incorporation of the medial femoral condyle osteochondral allograft with preservation of the medial joint space.

22

PATHOLOGY
Lateral meniscus deficiency

TREATMENT
Lateral meniscus allograft reconstruction

SUBMITTED BY
Brian J. Cole, MD, MBA, Rush Cartilage Restoration Center, Rush University Medical Center, Chicago, Illinois, USA

CHIEF COMPLAINT AND HISTORY OF PRESENT ILLNESS

This patient is an 18-year-old accomplished collegiate-level basketball player who presented following a lateral meniscectomy of her left knee performed 8 months previously, leaving her with persistent lateral joint line pain and activity-related swelling. These symptoms persisted despite having completed a rigorous postoperative physical therapy program. The symptoms occurred with routine activities and prevented her from playing basketball at a competitive level.

PHYSICAL EXAMINATION

Height, 5 ft, 9 in.; weight, 142 lb. The patient ambulates with a nonantalgic gait. She stands in slight symmetric physiologic valgus. She has a moderate effusion. There is diffuse tenderness along the lateral joint line with pain created during placement of a valgus axial load. Her range of motion was symmetric to the contralateral side. There is approximately 2 cm of quadriceps atrophy when compared to the contralateral side. She has no medial joint line tenderness and a normal ligamentous examination. There is no patellofemoral crepitus noted.

RADIOGRAPHIC EVALUATION

Plain radiographs show some flattening of the lateral femoral condyle of the left knee. There does not appear to be any bony deficit. There is no joint space narrowing, but definite irregularity is noted compared to the contralateral side.

SURGICAL INTERVENTION

Because of her persistent symptoms, she was indicated for a lateral meniscus allograft transplant. At surgery, it was noted that she had previously undergone a subtotal lateral menis-cectomy and had minimal chondral change in that compartment (Figure C22.1A). Otherwise, the knee joint was within normal limits. A lateral meniscal transplant using a keyhole technique was performed (Figure C22.1B). Postoperative rehabilitation allowed weight bearing as tolerated up to 90 degrees of flexion, which remained restricted for the first 6 weeks. Return to unrestricted activities was permitted at 6 months.

FOLLOW-UP

The patient did well initially and, although she still had mild lateral joint line pain, it was much less than what she had experienced preoperatively. At 6 months postoperative, she was able to run for conditioning, but was not yet able to participate competitively. At 9 months postoperative, she developed occasional catching without any significant pain or swelling. She had full range of motion without evidence of lateral joint line pain. However, before being fully cleared for a return to basketball, a diagnostic arthroscopy was performed to assess for meniscal healing. At second-look arthroscopy, the repair was completely intact except for a small partial tear at the junction of the posterior horn and body, which was repaired using a formal inside-out technique (Figure C22.2). Subsequent to this procedure, the patient did quite well, and is now, 2.5 years after her lateral meniscus transplant, participating in all activities without limitations. Radiographs demonstrate no change in remaining joint space compared to her preoperative views (Figure C22.3).

DECISION-MAKING FACTORS

1. Young, active, high-demand patient with ipsilateral joint line symptoms following lateral meniscectomy.
2. Intact articular cartilage.
3. Demonstrated ability and understanding to adhere to rehabilitation protocol.
4. Unresponsiveness to meniscectomy and additional nonoperative treatment.

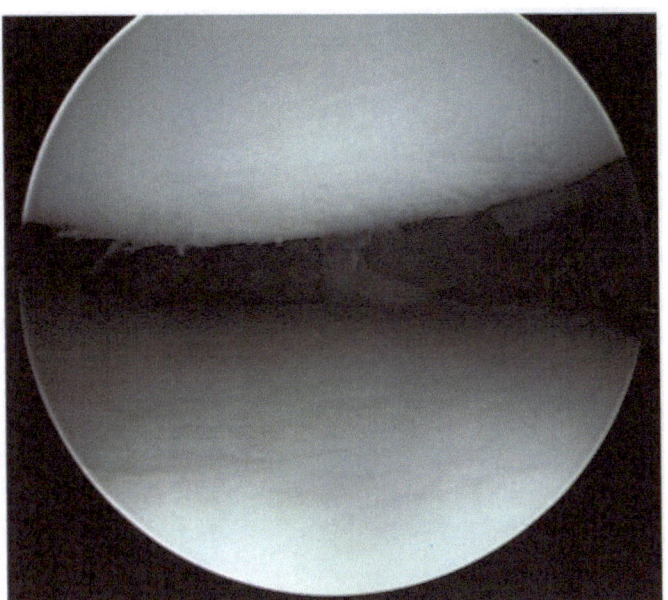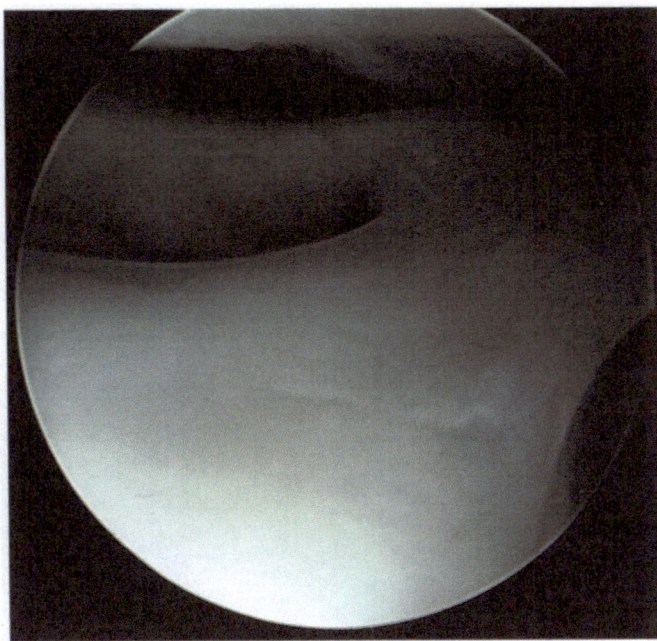

FIGURE C22.1 Arthroscopy of (**A**) the lateral compartment demonstrating prior subtotal meniscectomy and (**B**) the lateral meniscal transplant sutured into position.

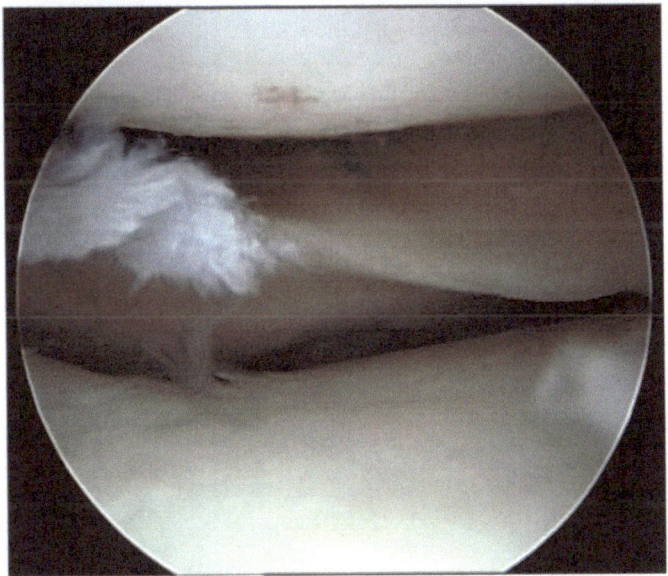

FIGURE C22.2 Arthroscopy at 9 months postoperatively shows an additional suture placed to repair a small area at the meniscal capsular junction believed to be contributing to the patient's persistent mechanical symptoms. Note the small area of degeneration at the posterior horn of the meniscus allograft.

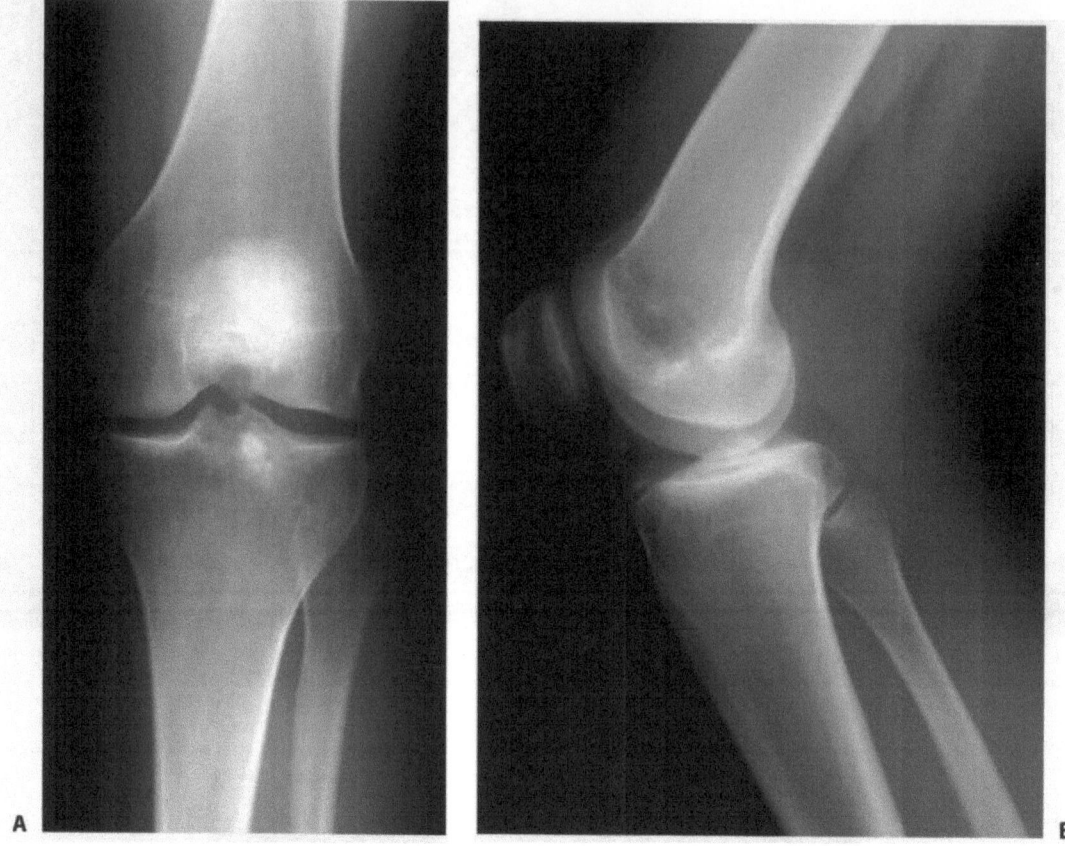

FIGURE C22.3 Two-year postoperative (**A**) anteroposterior and (**B**) lateral radiographs demonstrate maintenance of the lateral joint space with no evidence of collapse or degenerative changes.

23

PATHOLOGY
Prior medial meniscectomy and focal chondral defect medial femoral condyle

TREATMENT
Medial meniscus allograft reconstruction with osteochondral autograft transplantation

SUBMITTED BY
Brian J. Cole, MD, MBA, Rush Cartilage Restoration Center, Rush University Medical Center, Chicago, Illinois, USA

CHIEF COMPLAINT AND HISTORY OF PRESENT ILLNESS

The patient is a 40-year-old woman who had a previous medial meniscectomy of the left knee, after which she did well for approximately 5 years. She presents with moderate to severe weight-bearing pain and medial joint line discomfort. She is unable to walk more than two blocks before having to stop due to increasing discomfort. She complains of pain at night when the inner side of her knees rest against each other. Initial treatment included physical therapy and a cortisone injection that provided no relief of her symptoms.

PHYSICAL EXAMINATION

Height, 5 ft, 6 in.; weight, 130 lb. The patient walks with a slightly antalgic gait. Her left knee is in neutral alignment compared to the right knee, which is in slight physiologic valgus. The left knee has a small effusion. She has full symmetric range of motion. Her medial femoral condyle and joint line are both tender to palpation. She has full range of motion, no patellofemoral crepitus, and a normal ligament examination.

RADIOGRAPHIC EVALUATION

Preoperative radiographs demonstrate mild medial joint space narrowing with no significant flattening of the medial femoral condyle (Figure C23.1).

SURGICAL INTERVENTION

At the time of cartilage restoration surgery (Figure C23.2), she was identified as having a previous subtotal medial meniscectomy and an associated grade IV focal chondral defect along the medial femoral condyle measuring approximately 10 mm by 10 mm. She underwent allograft medial meniscus transplantation using a double bone plug technique and osteochondral autograft transplantation using a single 10-mm-diameter plug (Figure C23.3). Postoperative rehabilitation included partial weight bearing for the first 4 weeks with immediate use of continuous passive motion for 6 h/day for the first 6 weeks. Return to unrestricted activities was permitted at 6 months.

FOLLOW-UP

At the 2-year follow-up visit, she demonstrates no progression of joint space narrowing and excellent integration of the osteochondral plug (Figure C23.4). She returned to all activities with no complaints of pain or swelling.

DECISION-MAKING FACTORS

1. Active patient in her fifth decade with ipsilateral symptoms believed to be related to a prior subtotal meniscectomy and, possibly, to the associated defect of her medial femoral condyle.
2. Concomitant pathology requiring simultaneous treatment to eliminate any contraindication to either procedure being performed in isolation.
3. Absence of contraindications to meniscus transplantation including the lack of significant malalignment, the absence of bipolar disease, and a correctable grade IV lesion of the medial femoral condyle.
4. Relatively small defect (less than or equal to approximately 1 cm^2) with a single stage solution that will restore the surface with hyaline cartilage.

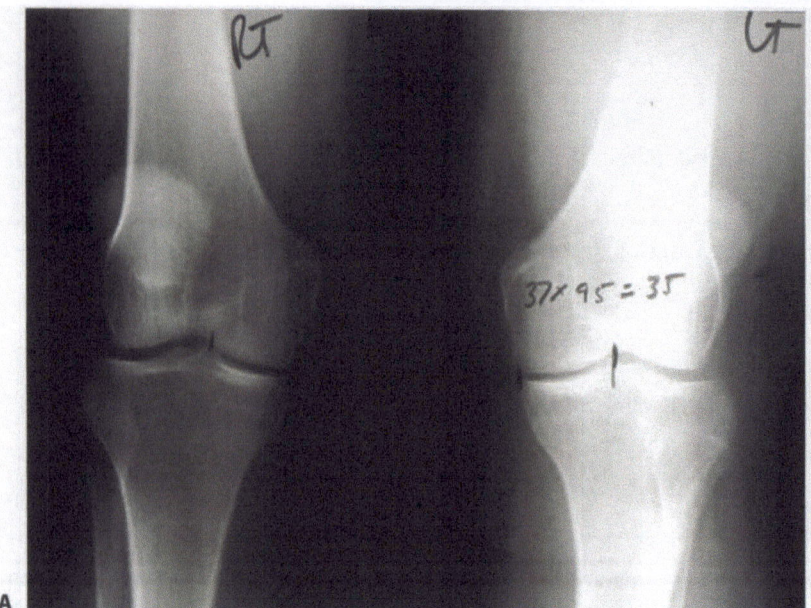
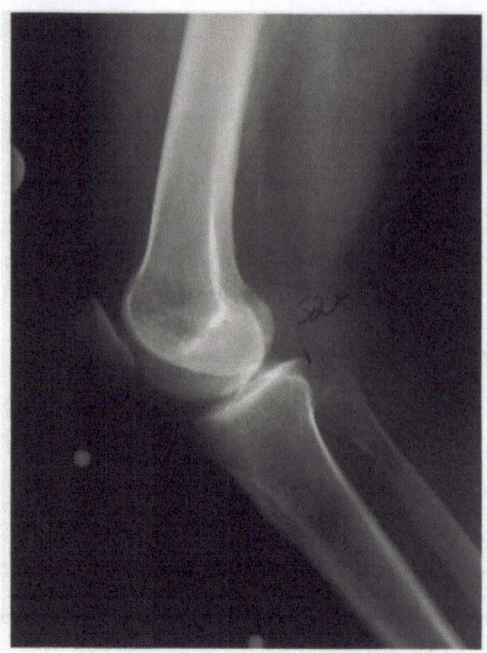

FIGURE C23.1 Extension weight-bearing anteroposterior (**A**) and lateral (**B**) radiographs demonstrate mild medial joint space narrowing without flattening of the femoral condyle or significant osteophyte formation.

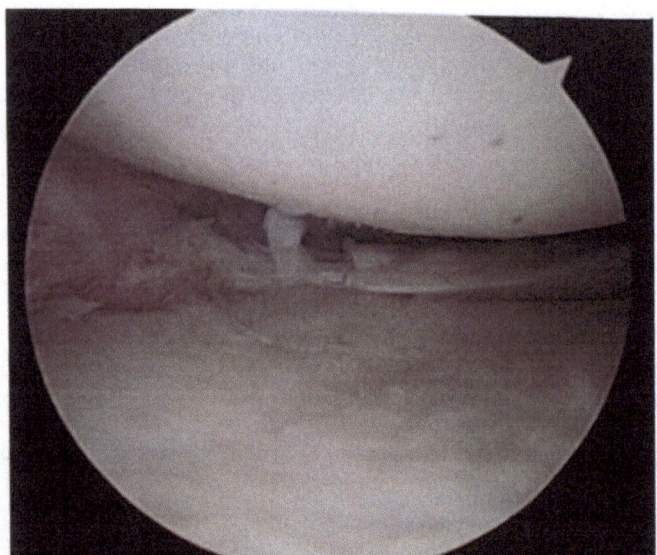
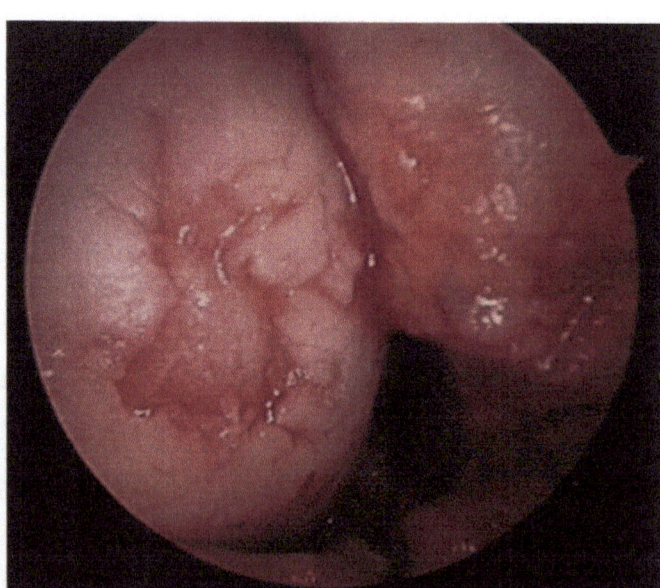

FIGURE C23.2 (A) Arthroscopic photograph obtained at the time of meniscus transplantation demonstrates prior subtotal medial meniscectomy with minimal changes in the articular surface of the tibia.

(B) Arthroscopic photograph taken through the arthrotomy shows the 10 mm by 10 mm grade IV defect of the medial femoral condyle.

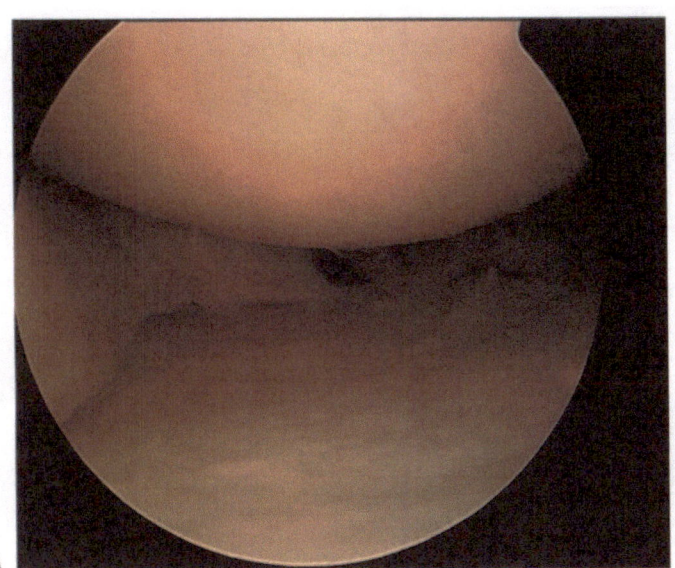
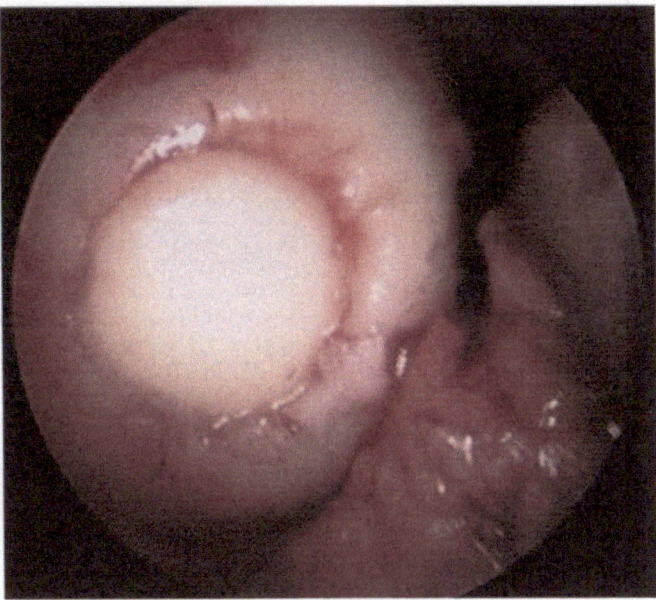

FIGURE C23.3 **(A)** Allograft medial meniscus transplant sutured in place. **(B)** The 10-mm-diameter osteochondral autograft is in place, effectively resurfacing the medial femoral condyle defect.

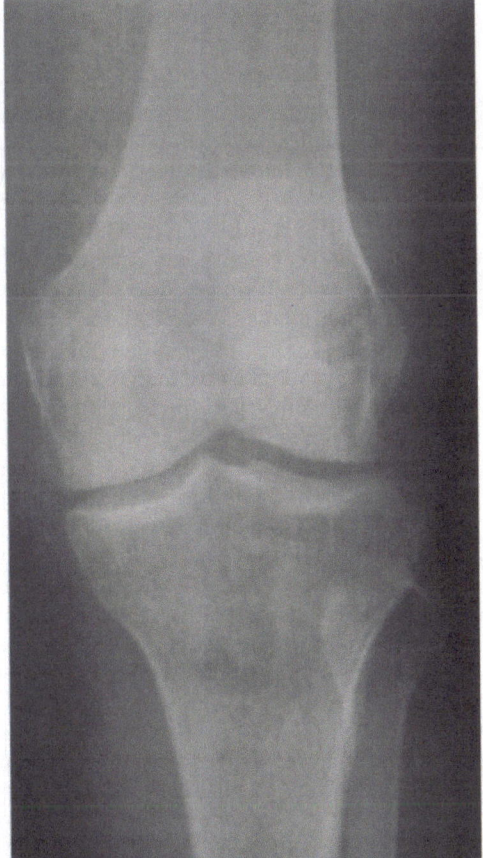
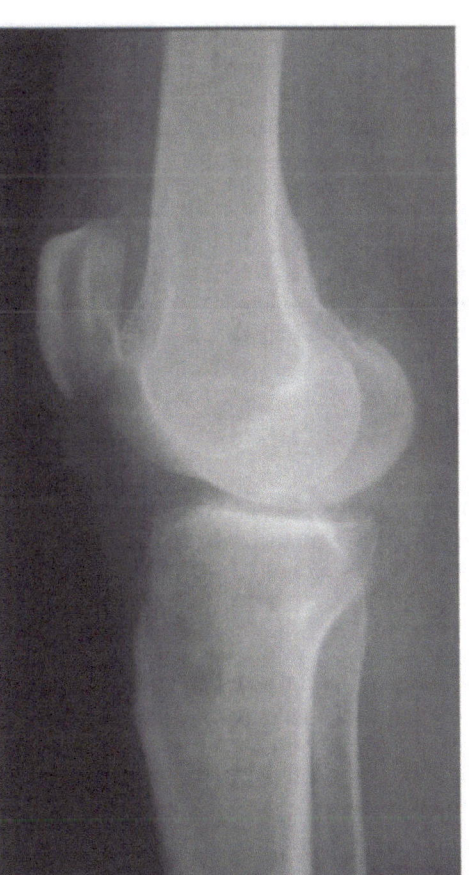

FIGURE C23.4 Two-year postoperative anteroposterior **(A)** and lateral **(B)** radiographs demonstrate preservation of joint space with no progression in degeneration and full integration of the osteochondral allograft plug with no cystic change or collapse.

24

PATHOLOGY
Failed anterior cruciate ligament reconstruction with medial meniscus deficiency

TREATMENT
Revision anterior cruciate ligament reconstruction and medial meniscus allograft reconstruction

SUBMITTED BY
Brian J. Cole, MD, MBA, Rush Cartilage Restoration Center, Rush University Medical Center, Chicago, Illinois, USA

CHIEF COMPLAINT AND HISTORY OF PRESENT ILLNESS

This 16-year-old male patient is a high school soccer player who sustained a complete tear of his anterior cruciate ligament (ACL) during a soccer game approximately 18 months before presentation. He underwent ACL reconstruction using a bone–patella tendon–bone autograft. His postoperative course was uncomplicated; he had complete relief of his pain and instability, and was able to return to playing competitive soccer. Approximately 11 months later, while playing soccer he felt a pop in his knee. He came to arthroscopic evaluation, at which time he was noted to have a large irreparable bucket-handle tear of his medial meniscus that required a subtotal meniscectomy. Although still intact, the ACL graft was probed and believed to be lax. At the time of presentation for cartilage restoration, he complained of persistent medial-sided knee pain, repeated giving-way, and activity-related effusions.

PHYSICAL EXAMINATION

Height, 5 ft, 10 in.; weight, 145 lb. The patient walks with a nonantalgic gait. He stands in neutral alignment. His range of motion is symmetric to the contralateral knee without any prone heel height difference. He has a trace effusion. He has significant tenderness along the medial joint line. The Lachman examination is grade II with firm endpoints, and he has a grade I to II pivot shift. His KT-2000 test reveals an 8-mm side-to-side difference on maximum manual testing. He has no posterior drop-back or sag, and he has no increased external rotation with manual testing. The remainder of his examination is unremarkable.

RADIOGRAPHIC EVALUATION

Plain radiographs including flexion weight-bearing and lateral views of the left knee reveal no evidence of joint space narrowing. The bone tunnels from prior ACL reconstruction are appropriately positioned, and a fixation screw is noted on the tibial side (Figure C24.1A,B). Magnetic resonance imaging (MRI) examination reveals almost complete absence of the medial meniscus, with no subchondral edema and intact articular cartilage (Figure C24.1C).

SURGICAL INTERVENTION

The patient was indicated for simultaneously performed left knee medial meniscus allograft transplantation and revision ACL reconstruction with bone–patellar tendon–bone allograft. The principal indications for this simultaneous procedure included ipsilateral post-meniscectomy pain and recurrent ACL insufficiency. The primary indications for allograft meniscus transplantation included pain and instability, with consideration given to the role of the posterior horn of the medial meniscus as a secondary stabilizer to anterior translation. At the time of surgery, the ACL was lax to probing and believed to be attenuated (Figure C24.2A). Inspection of the medial joint space revealed near absence of the entire medial meniscus with relatively intact articular cartilage (Figure C24.2B).

The medial meniscus allograft was prepared using a double-bone plug technique. A 10-mm-wide bone–patellar tendon–bone allograft was fashioned with two 10 mm by 25 mm bone blocks (Figure C24.2C). The posterior horn tunnel for the medial meniscus was drilled first, followed by the tibial and femoral tunnels, respectively, for the ACL. The medial meniscus was introduced and secured with vertical mattress sutures and seating of the posterior bone plug into its recipient tunnel. The anterior horn was fixed into a blind tunnel at the anatomic insertion of the native meniscus insertion site. Finally, the ACL was passed and secured with a staple on the tibia and a ligament button on the femur due to slight graft mismatch and partial compromise of the posterior cortex of the femur (Figure C24.2D,E). Postoperative rehabilitation was guided primarily by the ACL protocol except for restriction of weight bearing beyond 90 degrees of knee flexion for the first 6 weeks. Return to unrestricted activities was permitted at 6 months.

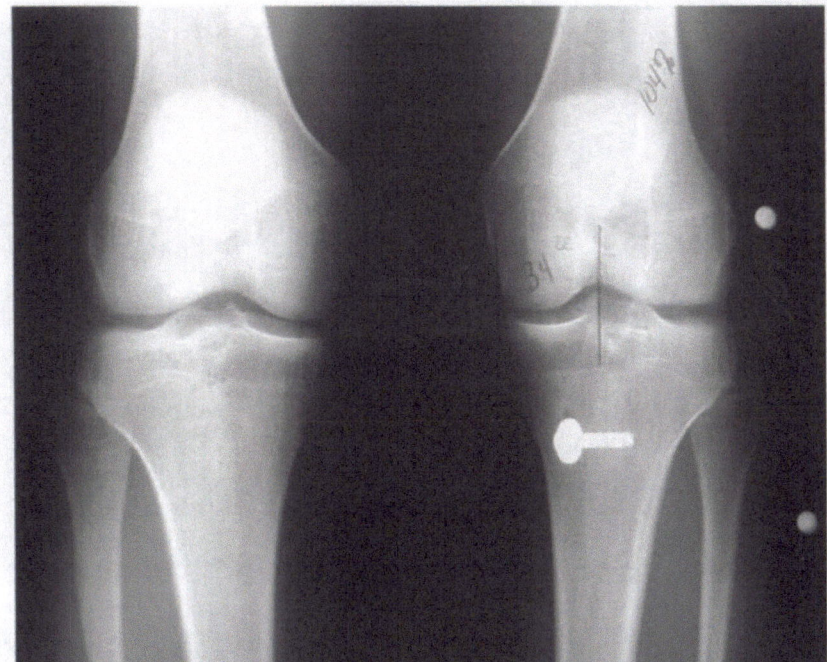
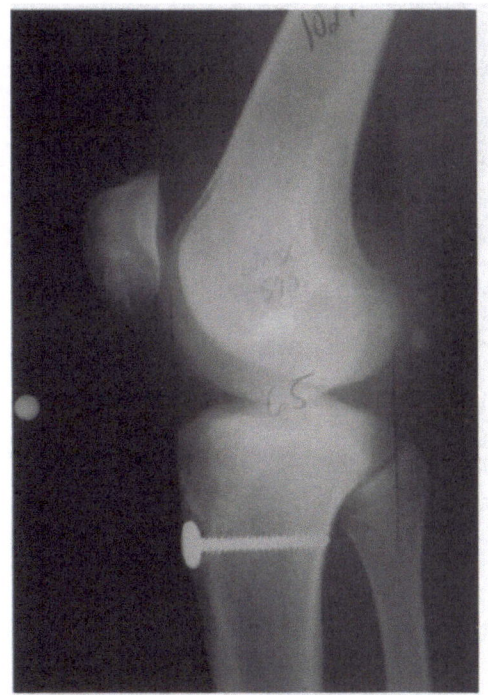

FIGURE C24.1 Sizing X-rays obtained to plan for meniscal allograft reconstruction. Weight-bearing anteroposterior (**A**) and lateral (**B**) radiographs of the left knee demonstrate preservation of the joint space as well as prior anterior cruciate ligament (ACL) fixation in good position. (**C**) MRI reveals almost complete absence of the medial meniscus.

FOLLOW-UP

At 18 months, the patient had full range of motion, denied any medial-sided knee pain, and had no complaints of instability. He had a grade I Lachman examination with a firm endpoint and a negligible pivot shift. Radiographs demonstrated excellent positioning of the ACL graft and proper seating of the meniscus transplant bone plugs. No evidence of joint space narrowing was present (Figure C24.3). Repeat KT-2000 evaluation revealed a 2-mm side-to-side difference on maximum manual testing. The patient recently returned to participating in competitive soccer.

DECISION-MAKING FACTORS

1. Young, high-demand patient with ipsilateral symptoms related to a prior subtotal meniscectomy with a chief complaint of pain and instability.
2. Loss of the primary (ACL) and secondary (posterior horn of the medial meniscus) restraints to anterior translation of the left knee.
3. Intact articular cartilage.
4. A relative contraindication to performing an isolated medial meniscus transplant without ACL reconstruction. Similarly, revision ACL reconstruction without improving the secondary restraints for anterior tibial translation may place the newly reconstructed ACL at continued risk for premature failure.

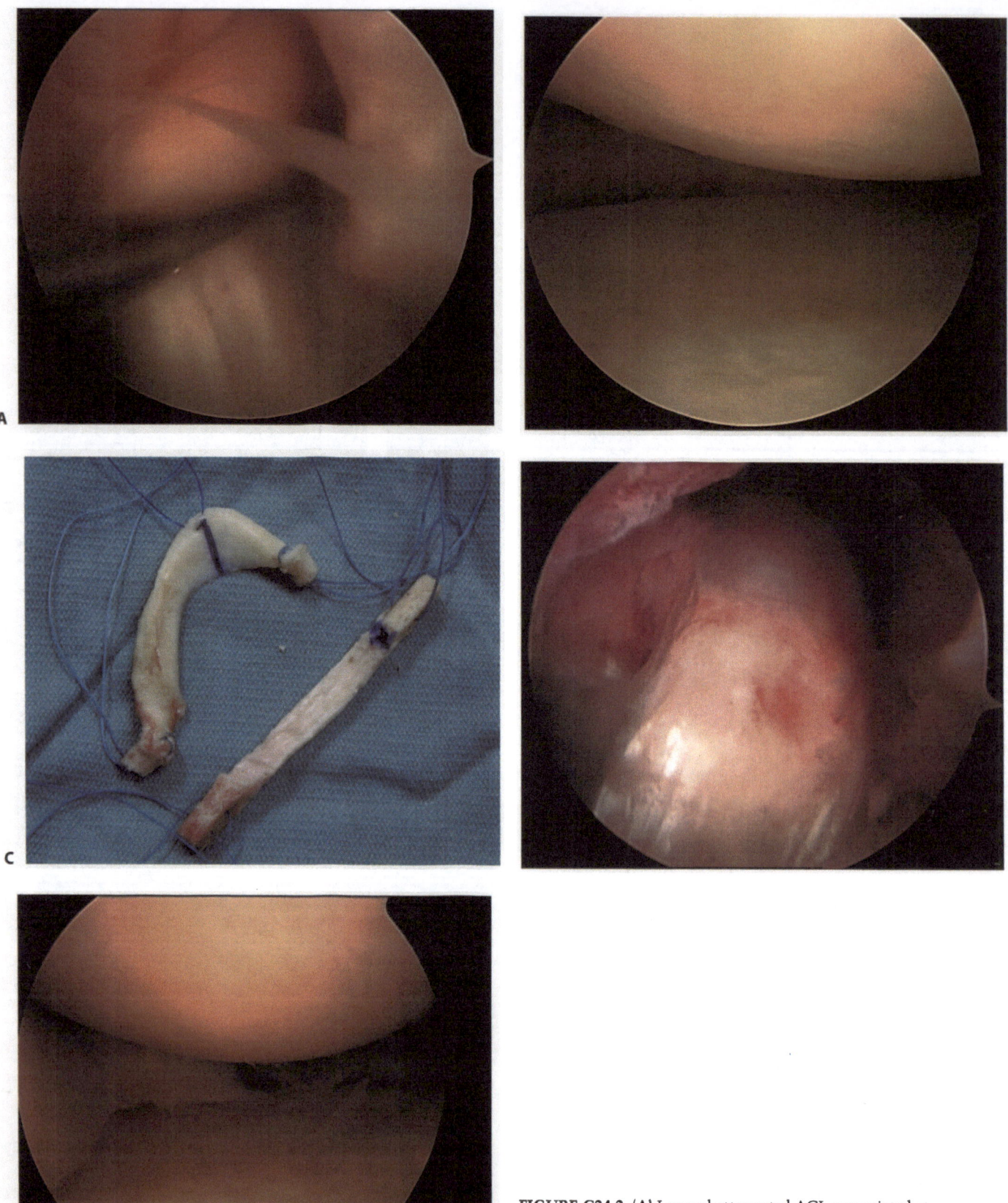

FIGURE C24.2 **(A)** Lax and attenuated ACL appreciated at arthroscopy. **(B)** Arthroscopy of the medial compartment reveals nearly complete absence of the medial meniscus with intact articular cartilage. **(C)** Medial meniscus allograft and ACL allograft terminally prepared before implantation. **(D)** ACL allograft in position. **E.** Medial meniscal allograft secured in position.

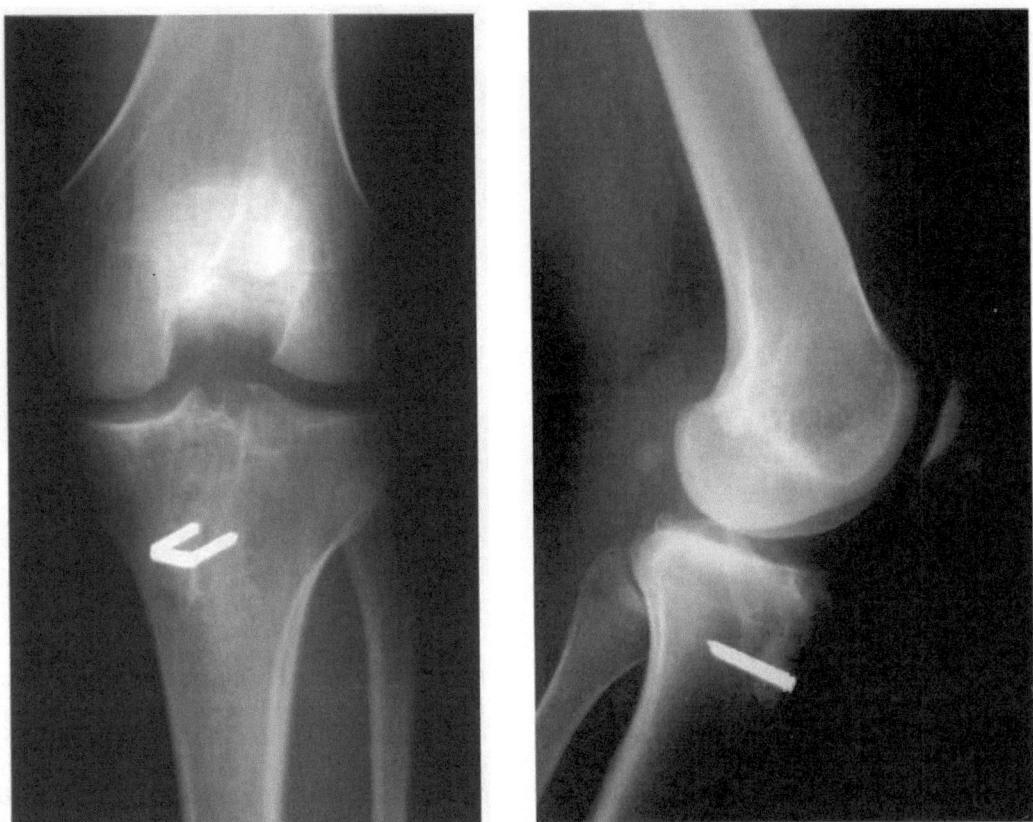

A   B

FIGURE C24.3 Posteroanterior 45-degree flexion weight-bearing (**A**) and lateral (**B**) radiograph obtained 14 months after allograft medial meniscus transplantation and revision ACL reconstruction.

25

PATHOLOGY
Advanced patellofemoral arthritis

TREATMENT
Patellofemoral arthroplasty

SUBMITTED BY
Tom Minas, MD, and Tim Bryant, RN, Cartilage Repair Center, Brigham and Women's Hospital, Chestnut Hill, Massachusetts, USA

CHIEF COMPLAINT AND HISTORY OF PRESENT ILLNESS

The patient is a 41-year-old man with a long-standing history of anterior right knee pain. As a teenager he sustained a patellar dislocation with an osteoarticular fracture. An open VMO quadriceps repair and removal of loose body was performed. Since then, five further arthroscopic debridements have been performed. Presently he complains of chronic right anterior knee pain. He uses antiinflammatories and ice for pain management only. He has pain that awakens him at night when he rolls over in bed. He is able to walk better on level surfaces than on inclines or up and down stairs. Additionally, he must use a handrail one step at a time to ascend or descend the stairs. He has frequent activity-related effusions. He requests a definitive operation that will relieve him of his pain and allow him to rapidly return to work to support his family. His job does not require physical or labor-intensive activities.

PHYSICAL EXAMINATION

Height, 6ft, 1in.; weight, 210lb. Clinical examination demonstrates a relatively fit 41-year-old man with clinically neutral alignment. He walks with an antalgic gait. He must use his hands to get out of a seated position; he is unable to crouch or squat. His range of motion is from 0 to 125 degrees of flexion. Other findings include severe patellofemoral crepitation, a large joint effusion, and a relatively normal quadriceps angle of 15 degrees. His ligament and meniscal examination is unremarkable.

RADIOGRAPHIC EVALUATION

Standing radiographs demonstrate a well-maintained tibiofemoral joint space. Radiographs demonstrate a narrowed patellofemoral joint space (Figure C25.1).

SURGICAL INTERVENTION

At arthrotomy, the tibiofemoral articulations were intact. The patellofemoral joint demonstrated severe erosive grade IV changes to the trochlea and the patella with a convex hypoplastic trochlea (Figure C25.2). A patellofemoral arthroplasty was performed (Figure C25.3). Postoperatively, the patient advanced readily to weight bearing and range of motion as tolerated.

FOLLOW-UP

Within 3 weeks of his patellofemoral prosthesis, the patient was pain free and returned to work. Two years after implantation, he remains satisfied with the result.

DECISION-MAKING FACTORS

1. Advanced, highly symptomatic, isolated patellofemoral arthritis unresponsive to prior efforts at debridement and conservative management.
2. Disease extent poses a highly guarded prognosis for autologous chondrocyte implantation (ACI). Although osteochondral allograft remains a viable treatment option, it also carries a more guarded prognosis, and the patient is unwilling to undergo the prolonged rehabilitation required of this cartilage transplantation procedure.
3. A willingness to maintain relatively reduced activity levels to maximize the longevity of patellofemoral arthroplasty. The patient desires a predictable outcome and has low-demand requirements.
4. Informed consent that should the patellofemoral arthroplasty fail, revision to total knee arthroplasty is unlikely to be compromised.

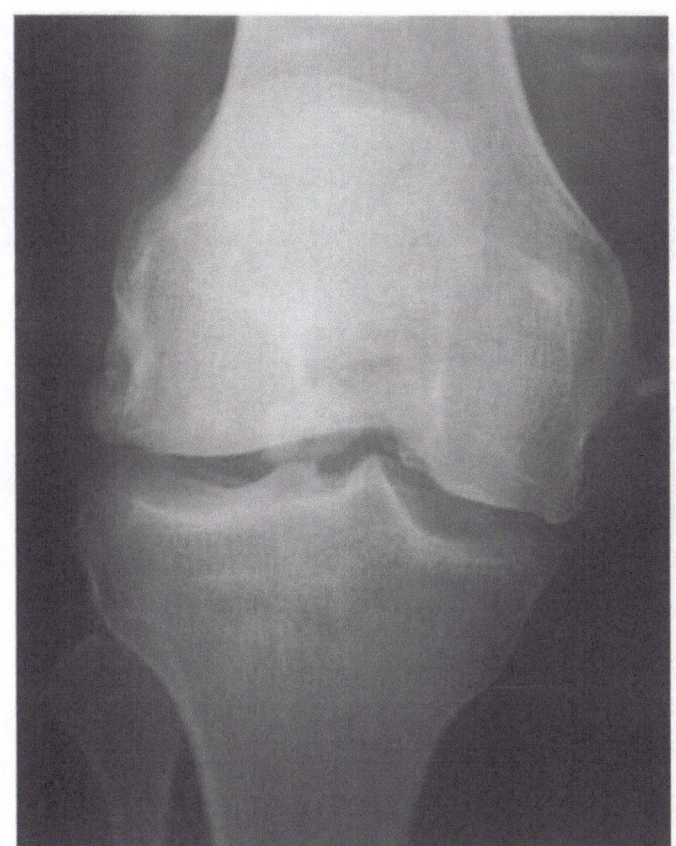
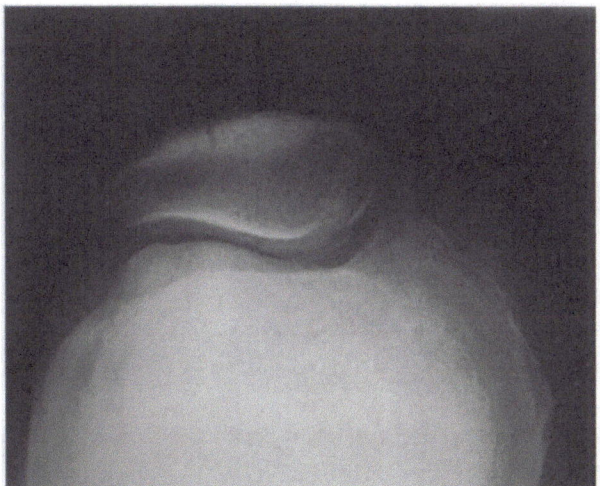

FIGURE C25.1 Preoperative plain standing anteroposterior (**A**) and skyline (**B**) radiographs demonstrate normal tibiofemoral joint space with central and lateral patellofemoral compartment joint space narrowing.

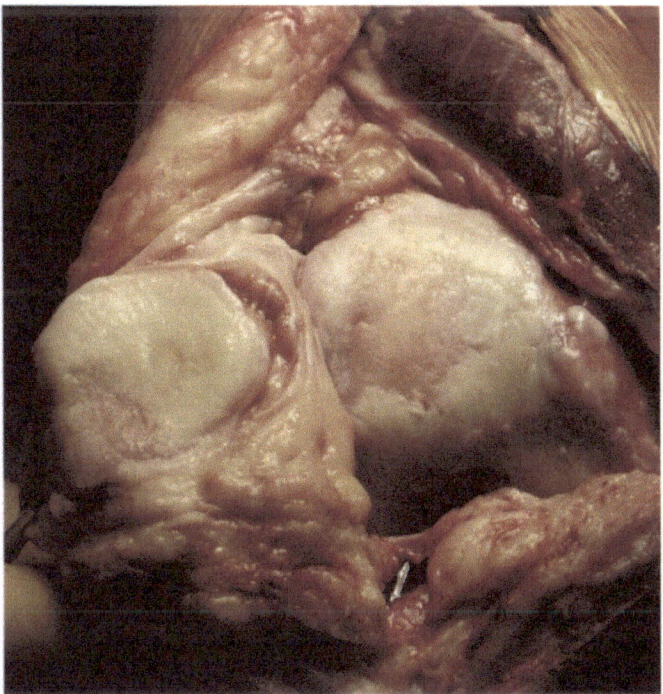

FIGURE C25.2 Appearance at the time of open arthrotomy. The trochlea is convex, hypoplastic, and has severe erosive changes. Similarly, the patella has a large area of exposed bone and has a dysplastic concave appearance.

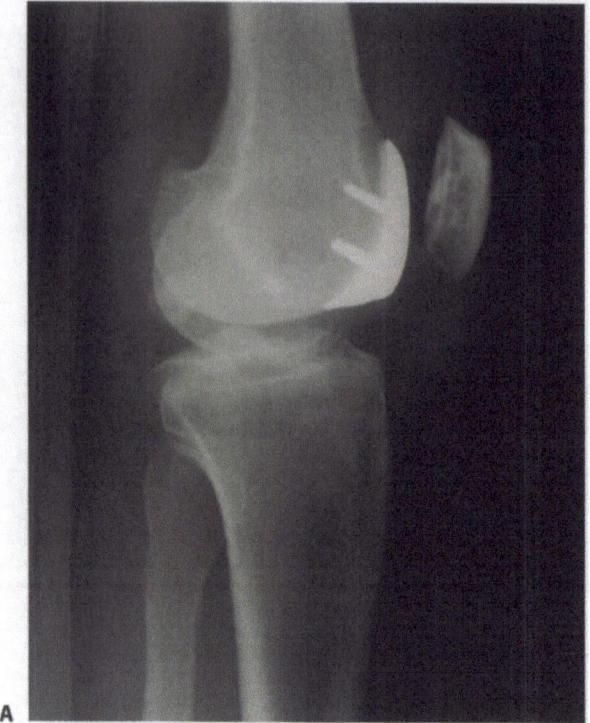

A

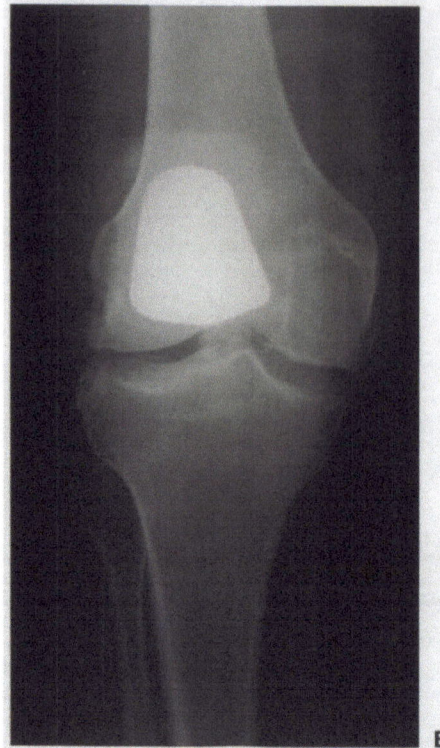

B

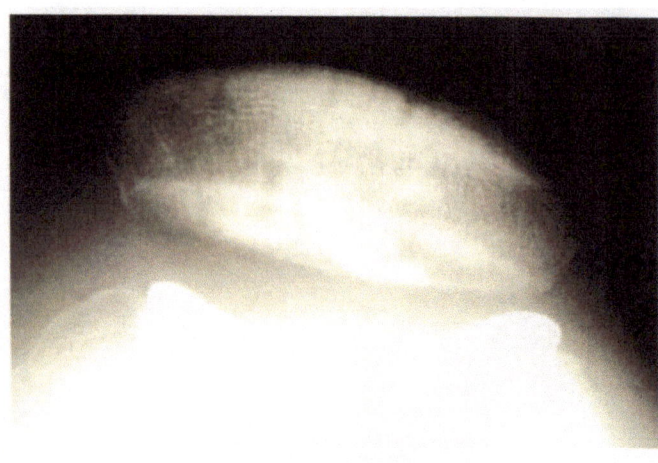

C

FIGURE C25.3 Postoperative plain lateral (**A**), anteroposterior (**B**), and skyline (**C**) radiographs demonstrate inset trochlear cobalt-chrome prosthesis and onset patellar polyethylene prosthesis.

26

PATHOLOGY
Multiple chondral defects

TREATMENT
Autologous chondrocyte implantation of the trochlea and medial and lateral femoral condyles

SUBMITTED BY
Jack Farr, MD, Cartilage Restoration Center of Indiana, OrthoIndy, Indianapolis, Indiana, USA

CHIEF COMPLAINT AND HISTORY OF PRESENT ILLNESS

This patient is a 43-year-old man with a 10-year history of lateral- greater than medial-sided knee pain as well as anterior knee pain. He complains of catching and effusions in his right knee. At the time of evaluation, he provided a history of having undergone arthroscopic treatment previously that provided minimal relief of his symptoms. The patient works as a full-time firefighter and complained of difficulty performing all his duties because of activity-related pain. His desire is to return to higher levels of activity that he previously enjoyed, including jogging and racquetball. At the time of initial presentation, he limited his activities to golf and biking and had gained 40 lb during the previous 2 years.

Review of the operative record indicates that 6 years previously he underwent chondroplasty and drilling of his femoral condyle. A repeat chondroplasty and drilling was performed 1 year before presentation. Despite these treatments, his symptoms recurred.

PHYSICAL EXAMINATION

Height, 5 ft, 9 in.; weight, 228 lb. The patient stands in slight varus alignment compared to neutral on the contralateral limb. He ambulates with a slightly antalgic gait on the right. He has a trace effusion. He has no gross atrophy. His range of motion is 0 to 130 degrees on the right compared to 0 to 135 degrees on the left. His ligament exam is unremarkable. He has marked tenderness on the lateral joint line and, to a lesser degree, at the medial joint line and patellofemoral joint. There are no mechanical signs, and patellar tracking is normal.

RADIOGRAPHIC EVALUATION

Weight-bearing anteroposterior and lateral radiographs show slight medial joint space narrowing and ossification changes in the lateral femoral condyle (due to prior drilling) (Figure C26.1). The Merchant view shows the patella to be centrally located. His long-leg alignment views show only 2 degrees of varus compared to the contralateral side. His magnetic resonance image (MRI) is consistent with a chronic osteochondritis dissecans of the lateral femoral condyle and chondrosis of the medial and patellofemoral compartments.

SURGICAL INTERVENTION

At the time of staging arthroscopy and biopsy for autologous chondrocyte implantation (ACI), grade IV chondrosis was noted at the trochlea (2.0 cm by 3.0 cm), medial (1.5 cm by 2.0 cm), and lateral (1.2 cm by 1.1 cm) femoral condyles (Figure C26.2). These lesions were contained. The opposing articular cartilage was intact. At the time of definitive treatment, ACI was performed for all three lesions (Figure C26.3). No realignment was performed.

Postoperatively, the patient was made protected weight bearing with crutches for 6 weeks and utilized continuous passive motion for 3 weeks initially with restricted motion. The patient slowly advanced to full, unrestricted activities by 18 months.

FOLLOW-UP

The patient had returned to high-level activities including full-time firefighting. Second-look arthroscopy 3 years following the implantation revealed excellent fill and marginal integration of all defects (Figure C26.4).

DECISION-MAKING FACTORS

1. Active patient with multiple focal chondral defects with limited alternatives to ACI, especially because of the concomitant symptomatic trochlear defect.
2. Despite a mild varus deformity, the presence of lateral compartment disease led to the decision to avoid osteotomy.

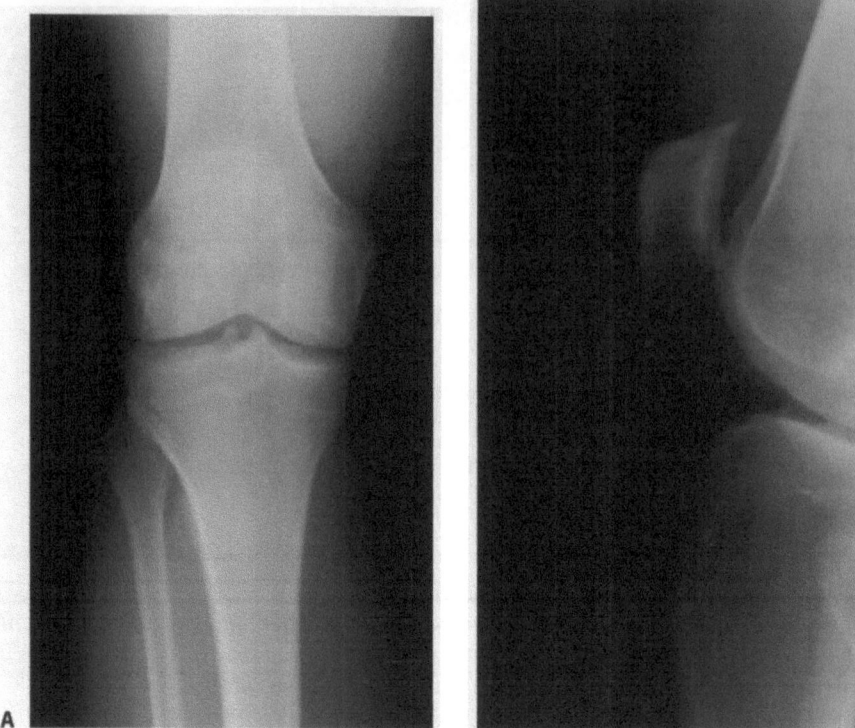

FIGURE C26.1 Anteroposterior (**A**) and lateral (**B**) radiographs demonstrate maintenance of joint spaces.

3. Shallow osteochondral lesion of the lateral femoral condyle amenable to single-stage ACI without bone grafting.

4. Failure of two prior attempts at standard drilling and chondroplasty.

5. Compliant patient willing to tolerate a prolonged rehabilitation period with a desire to return to high-level activities if possible.

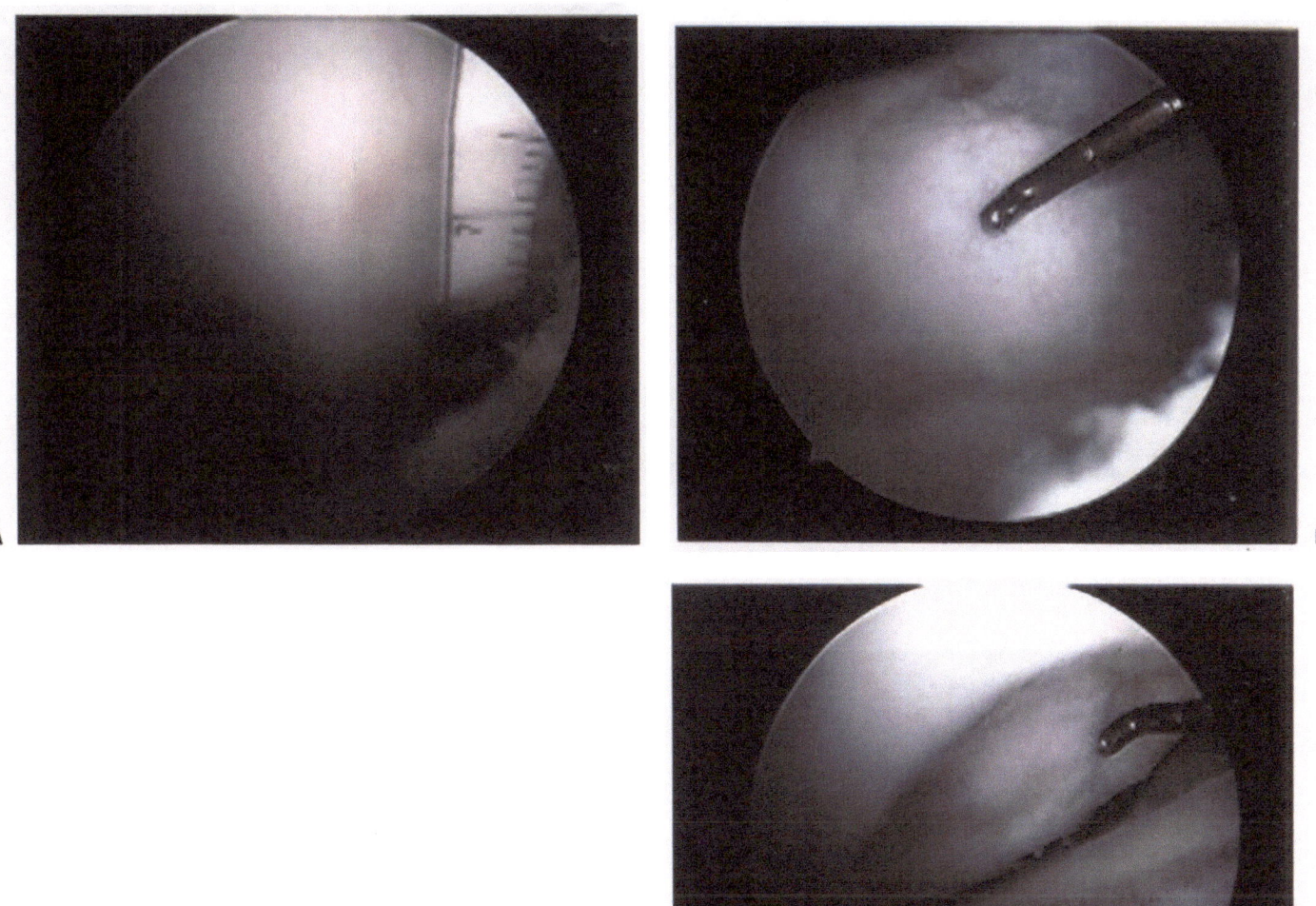

FIGURE C26.2 At index arthroscopy, lesions of the (**A**) medial femoral condyle, (**B**) trochlea, and (**C**) lateral femoral condyle are visualized.

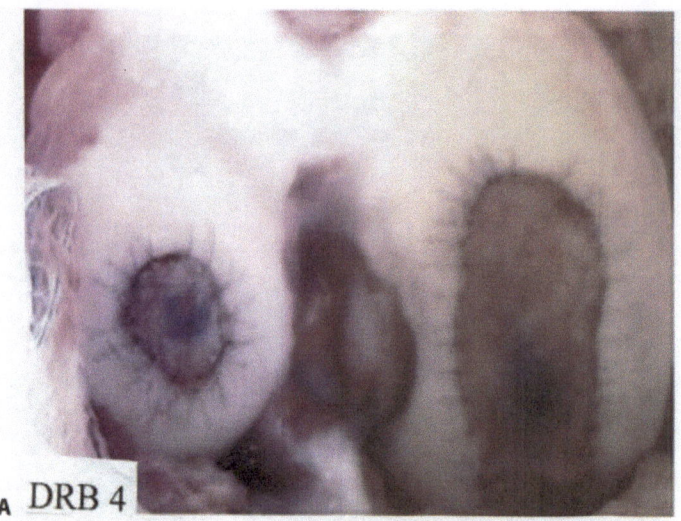

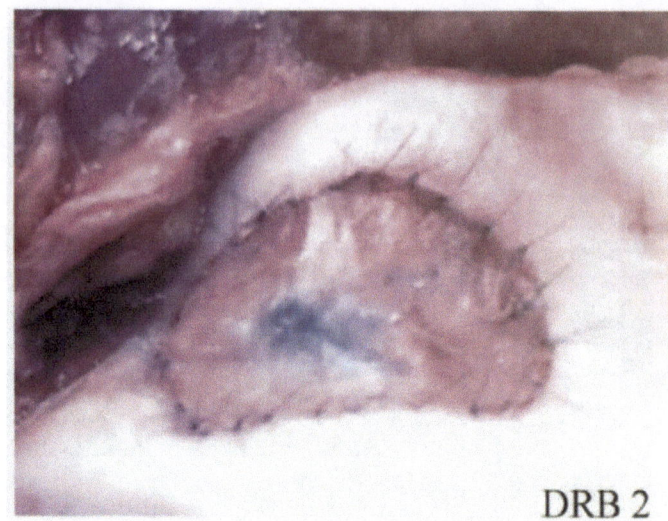

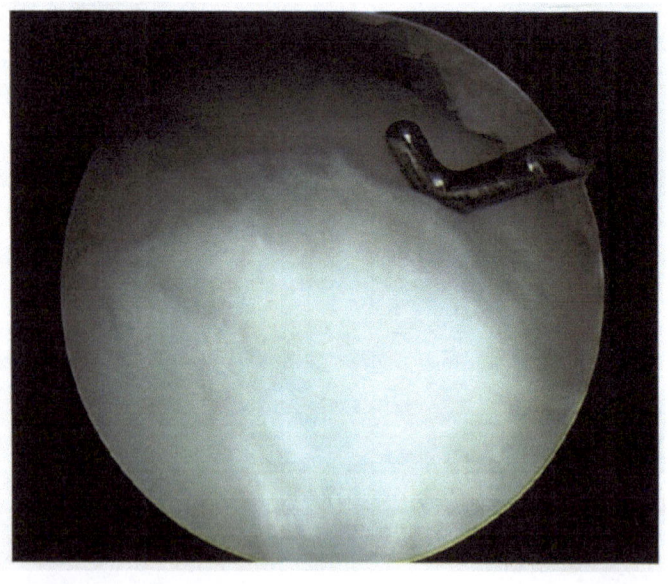

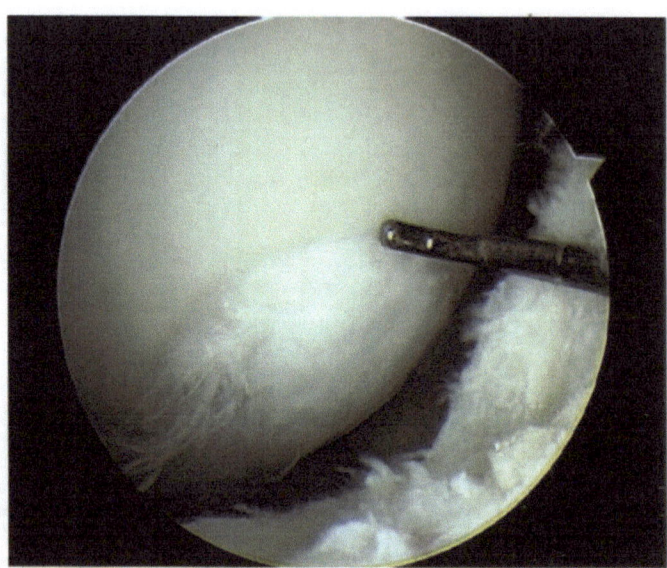

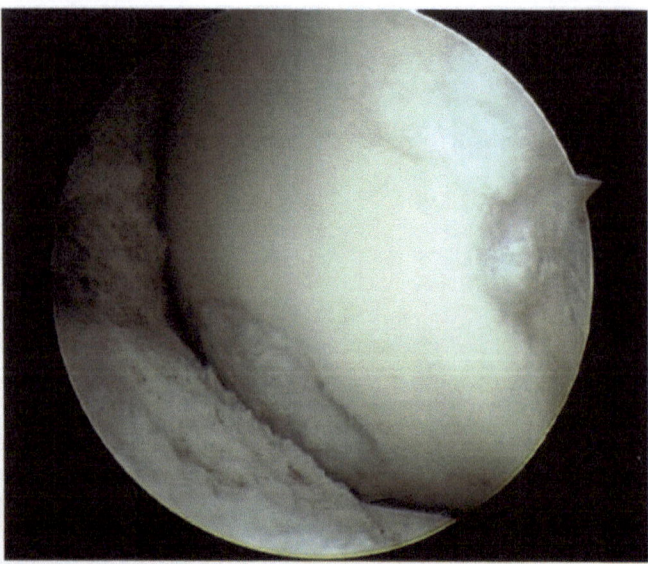

FIGURE C26.4 Second-look arthroscopy demonstrates excellent fill and marginal integration of (**A**) trochlea, (**B**) medial femoral condyle, and (**C**) lateral femoral condyle.

27

PATHOLOGY
Traumatic patellar instability with focal chondral defect of the patella

TREATMENT
Autologous chondrocyte implantation of the patella with distal realignment (Note that the use of ACI for the patella is considered off-label usage, but was indicated and performed with explicit patient and family informed consent and under the guidance of an Institutional Review Board protocol allowing prospective study of this patient at the author's institution.)

SUBMITTED BY
Brian J. Cole, MD, MBA, Rush Cartilage Restoration Center, Rush University Medical Center, Chicago, Illinois, USA

CHIEF COMPLAINT AND HISTORY OF PRESENT ILLNESS

The patient is a 17-year-old female who initially presented with a 3-year history of left knee problems. She first injured her knee while playing basketball when she dislocated her patella. She complains of anterior left knee pain, giving-way, catching of the patellofemoral joint, and residual symptoms consistent with patellar instability. Her symptoms have been getting progressively worse. She rates her overall knee function as being poor and states that before her injury her knee was nearly normal. Previously, she had undergone an arthroscopy during which a small osteochondral lesion of the patella was noted. A 1.5-cm loose body was found and removed. The loose piece was derived from the patella, leaving a full-thickness cartilage lesion of the patella approximately 1.5 cm in diameter with minimal bone loss. At the time of loose body removal, a lateral release was performed. She underwent extensive physical therapy, emphasizing a patellofemoral rehabilitation program. Before this injury, she was a very active adolescent girl participating in multiple sports at her school. At the time of presentation, she was unable to participate in any sports because of her significant knee-related complaints.

PHYSICAL EXAMINATION

Height, 5 ft, 2 in.; weight, 105 lb. The patient ambulates with a nonantalgic gait. She stands in approximately 4 degrees of symmetric mechanical-axis valgus. She has a mild bilateral pronation deformity of both hindfeet. She has a moderate-sized joint effusion. She has significant patellar apprehension with two-quadrant laxity medially and three-quadrant laxity laterally. There is no excessive patellar tilt or subluxation when measured passively. She has a positive J sign and a Q angle of 10 degrees. She has crepitus with active flexion and extension with an audible and palpable catching sensation of the patella at approximately 45 degrees of flexion. The medial and lateral joint lines are not painful. Her ligament examination is within normal limits.

RADIOGRAPHIC EVALUATION

Plain radiographs revealed no significant subchondral sclerosis or joint space narrowing, but did reveal a definite central irregularity of the patella best seen on the lateral view. Merchant views demonstrated the patella to be centered within the trochlea. There was no evidence of trochlear hypoplasia. Magnetic resonance images demonstrate a central patellar chondral defect with slight edema in the subchondral bone in the region of the defect.

SURGICAL INTERVENTION

The patient underwent her second left knee arthroscopy during which a full-thickness chondral defect was noted in the central aspect of the patella measuring approximately 16 mm by 16 mm (Figure C27.1). At the same time, an articular cartilage biopsy was performed with the intention to perform autologous chondrocyte implantation (ACI) of the patella within 3 months of this intervention.

Approximately 10 weeks later, the patient underwent ACI through a lateral arthrotomy centered over the lateral retinaculum (Figure C27.2). A concomitant distal realignment procedure was also performed (Figure C27.3). The patellar defect was essentially central and circular, measuring 16 mm by 16 mm with minimal bony involvement. Postoperatively, she was made heel-touch weight bearing for approximately 6 weeks until radiographs demonstrated evidence of healing of the distal realignment. Although she was allowed to flex her knee daily to 90 degrees, continuous passive motion was restricted to 45 to 60 degrees of flexion during its use for the first 6 postoperative weeks. She advanced

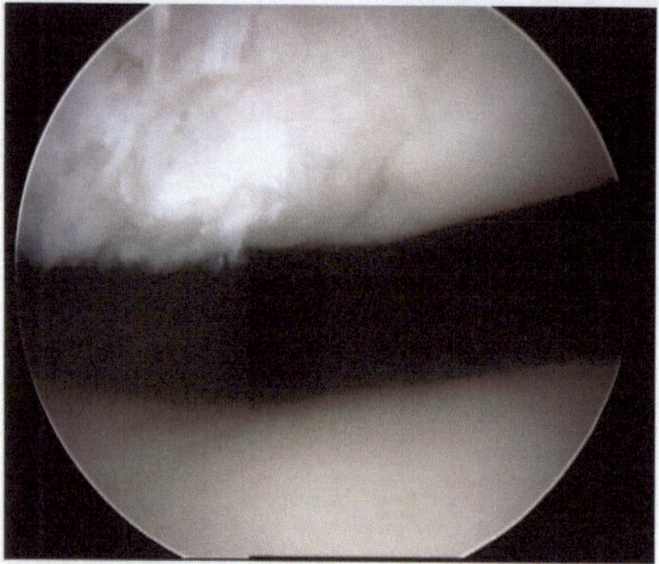

FIGURE C27.1 Arthroscopic photograph reveals full-thickness chondral defect of the patella measuring approximately 16 mm by 16 mm in diameter.

through the traditional rehabilitation protocol for ACI of the patella. She was asked to refrain from any impact or ballistic activities for 18 months.

FOLLOW-UP

Four months following ACI of her patella, with the exception of open-chain kinetic exercise, she remained painfree. Additionally, there was no visible swelling. Her motion was symmetric bilaterally, ranging from 0 degrees of extension to 140 degrees of flexion. The catching sensation she experienced preoperatively was eliminated by 6 months. Because of some discomfort related to the screws placed to secure the distal realignment, she underwent second-look arthroscopy at 12 months (Figure C27.4) and hardware removal. At 2 years postoperatively, she continues to do well with respect to her anterior knee pain and is very satisfied with the results of her surgery. She regularly engages in high-level activities that include running and soccer.

DECISION-MAKING FACTORS

1. Previously failed arthroscopic debridement and aggressive physical therapy program emphasizing proper patellofemoral mechanics.
2. Young, high-demand patient without viable cartilage restoration alternatives.
3. Full-thickness patellar chondral defect causing pain and swelling with mechanical symptoms in addition to patellar instability.
4. Ability and willingness to remain compliant with postoperative rehabilitation.

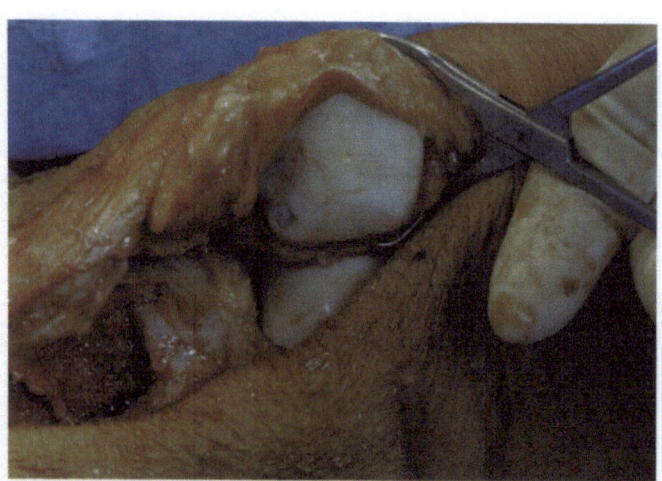
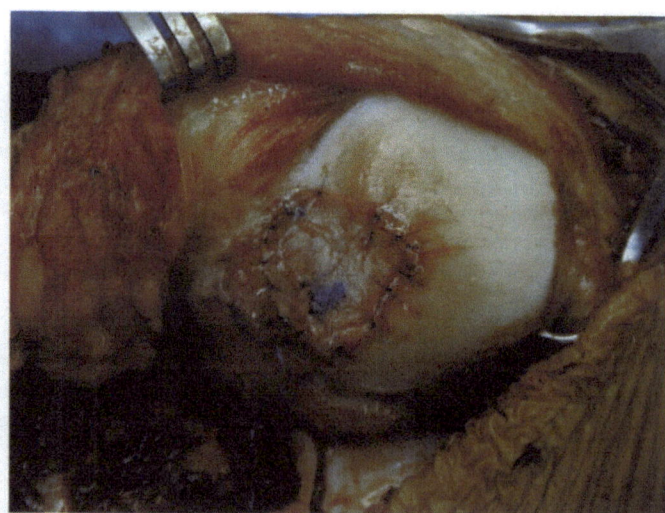

A

FIGURE C27.2 Intraoperative photographs at the time of autologous chondrocyte implantation procedure. Patellar lesion before (**A**) and after (**B**) the periosteal patch is sewn in place.

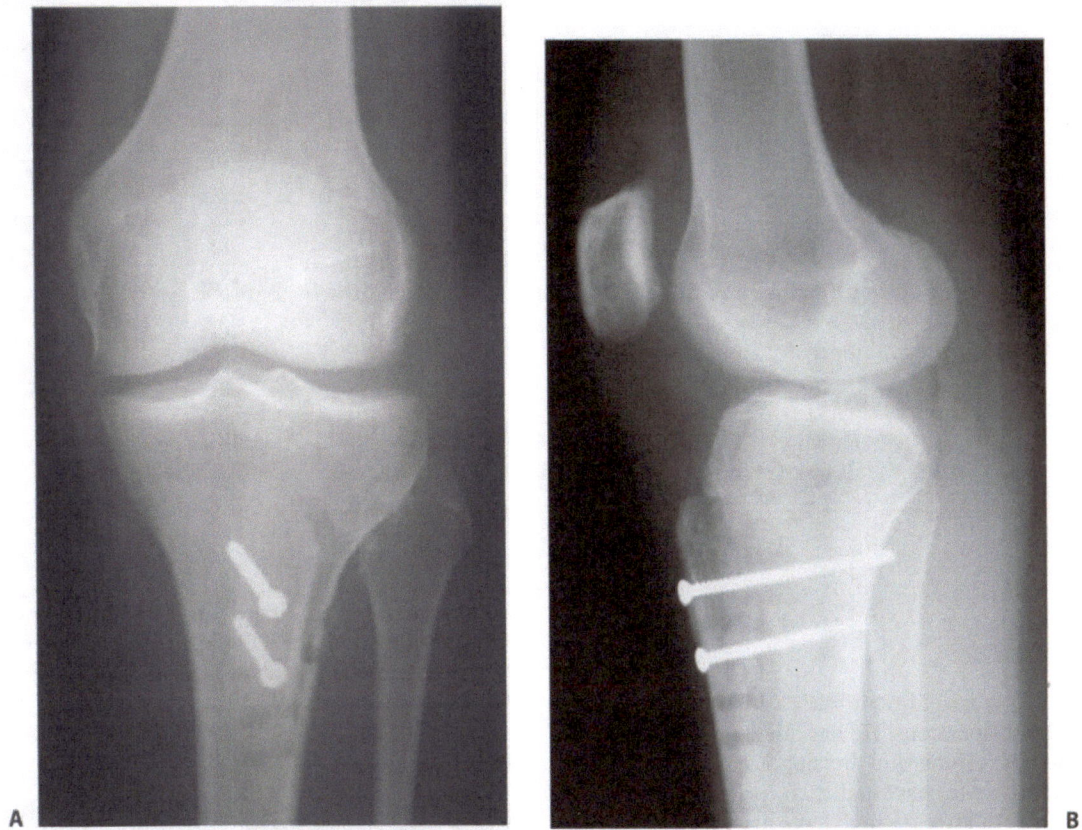

FIGURE C27.3 Postoperative anteroposterior (**A**) and lateral (**B**) radiographs reveal anteromedialization osteotomy of the tibial tubercle.

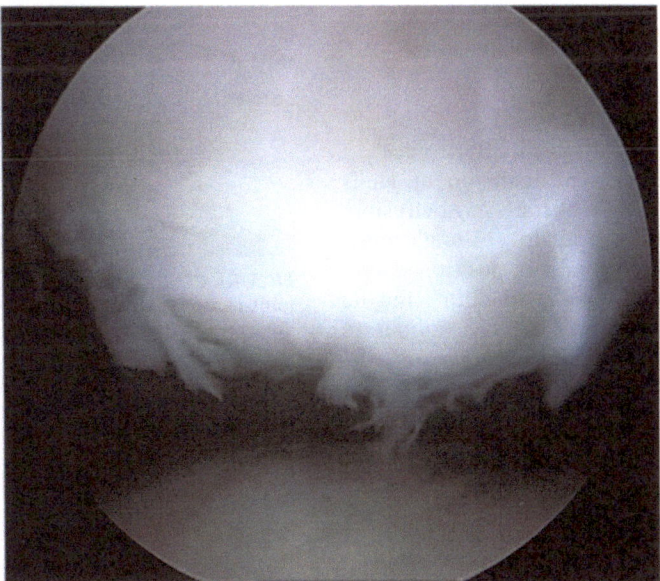

FIGURE C27.4 Second-look arthroscopy at 12 months performed during screw removal from the healed tibial tubercle osteotomy. Defect is filled with firm hyaline-like cartilage with some superficial fibrillation. Integration is good with no areas of exposed bone or delamination.

28

PATHOLOGY
Focal chondral defect patella

TREATMENT
Autologous chondrocyte implantation with distal realignment (Note: The use of ACI for the patella is considered off-label usage. This procedure was performed with explicit patient informed consent.)

SUBMITTED BY
Tom Minas, MD, and Tim Bryant, RN, Cartilage Repair Center, Brigham and Women's Hospital, Chestnut Hill, Massachusetts, USA

CHIEF COMPLAINT AND HISTORY OF PRESENT ILLNESS

The patient is a 24-year-old man with a history of bilateral recurrent patellar dislocations. He has failed physical therapy measures including taping and bracing to maintain patellofemoral tracking. He has had two prior arthroscopic debridements on both knees, which have been ineffective. He has severe right greater than left anterior knee pain which prevents him from participating in any sporting activities. Stair climbing is painful and requires him to use the handrail to ambulate one step at a time.

PHYSICAL EXAMINATION

Height, 6 ft; weight, 175 lb. Clinical examination reveals a physically fit male with symmetric neutral alignment. He is unable to perform a squat. He has a moderate-sized effusion. Range of motion is symmetric. His quadriceps angle measures 25 degrees with the patella in a reduced position. There is lateral subluxation with quadriceps contraction, and he has profound patellar apprehension. He has moderate patellofemoral crepitus. Meniscal compression testing was unremarkable. His ligament examination is normal.

RADIOGRAPHIC EVALUATION

Plain films were within normal limits, demonstrating normal patellofemoral joint space without subluxation or tilt (Figure C28.1).

SURGICAL INTERVENTION

Arthroscopic evaluation demonstrated grade IV chondrosis involving the central and medial patella. There was obvious subluxation and tilt laterally of the patella with the knee in extension. The trochlea articular surface was normal. A cartilage biopsy for future autologous chondrocyte implantation

(ACI) was obtained. Six weeks later, the patient underwent ACI combined with a lateral release, anteromedialization osteotomy (AMZ), and proximal quadriceps advancement. The defect measured 25 mm by 15 mm (Figure C28.2).

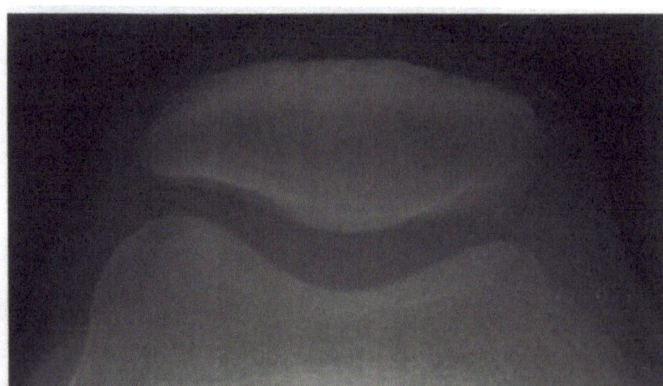

FIGURE C28.1 Preoperative skyline radiograph of the patellofemoral joint demonstrating well-maintained cartilage space.

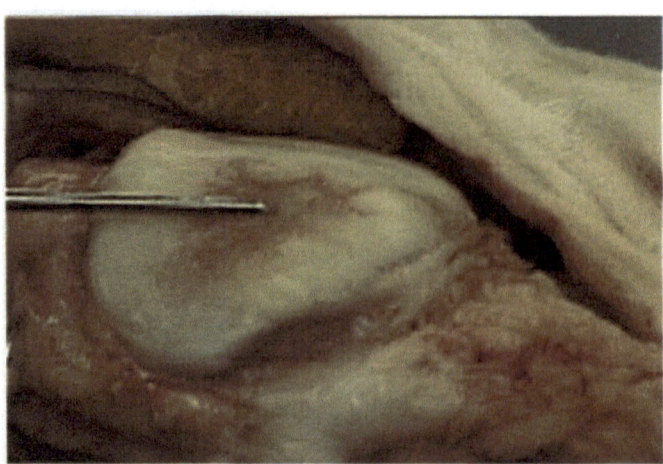

FIGURE C28.2 Appearance of grade IV patellar chondral defect at the time of autologous chondrocyte implantation (ACI).

Postoperatively, the patient was made weight bearing in extension with crutches and began continuous passive motion for 4 to 6 weeks. Activities were gradually advanced as tolerated with impact activities delayed for the first 12 months postoperatively. Radiographs demonstrated healing of his AMZ osteotomy (Figure C28.3).

FOLLOW-UP

One year later, a second-look arthroscopy was performed (Figure C28.4) to remove hardware and to perform a debridement of periosteal overgrowth presenting as retropatellar crepitations with mild discomfort. The patient was painfree afterward, had full range of motion, and ultimately had the other knee reconstructed identically. Four years later he is playing competitive volleyball.

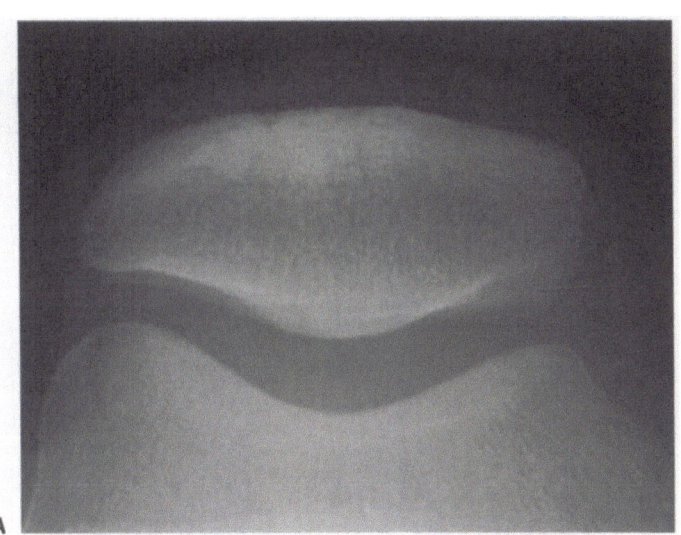

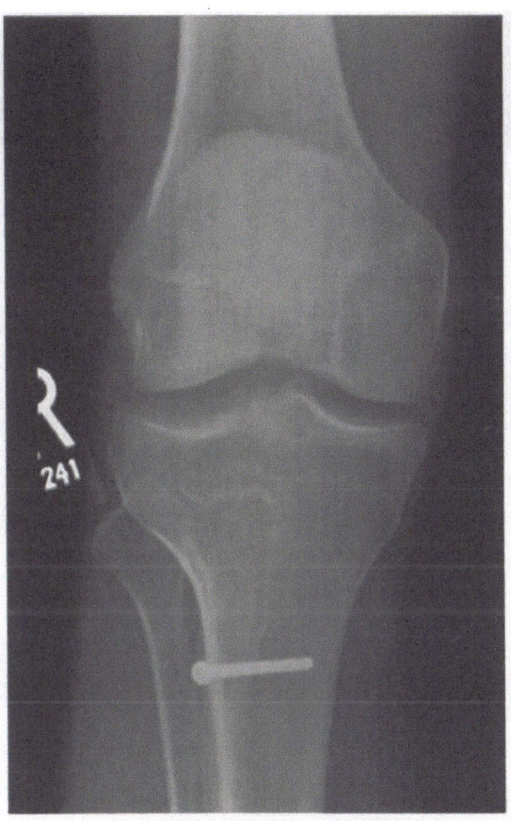

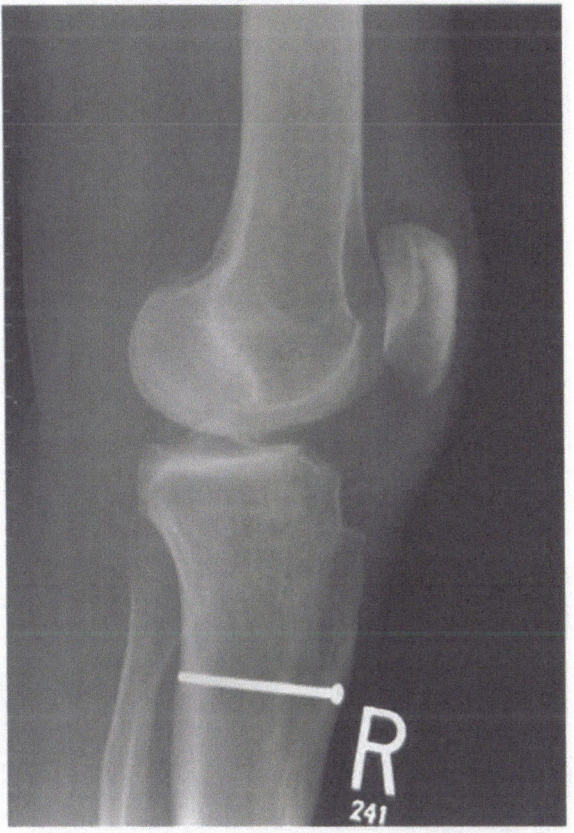

FIGURE C28.3 Postoperative (**A**) skyline, (**B**) anteroposterior, and (**C**) lateral radiographs demonstrate centralized patella and healed anteromedialization osteotomy.

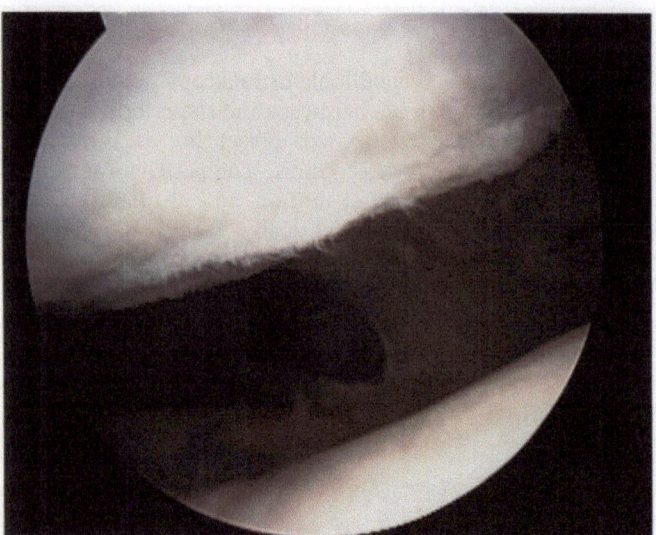

FIGURE C28.4 Arthroscopic appearance of ACI one year after debridement of periosteal overgrowth.

DECISION-MAKING FACTORS

1. Young, active male with symptoms consistent with patellar chondral defect which failed to respond to prior debridements and physical therapy.
2. Contained grade IV defect of the patella of appropriate size for ACI with limited other treatment options other than microfracture (limited goals) and osteochondral allograft (considered not appropriate for a young male with an isolated contained patellar chondral defect).
3. History of patellofemoral instability, increased quadriceps angle, and intraoperative findings of subluxation and tilt leading to decision for AMZ of the tibial tubercle.
4. As apposed to some success in treating inferior and lateral patellar chondral disease with AMZ, it is believed to be less effective when used in isolation for central and medial patellar disease.

CHIEF COMPLAINT AND HISTORY OF PRESENT ILLNESS

The patient is a 36-year-old man who sustained an injury to the medial femoral condyle of his left knee when he fell from a wave runner directly striking his knee. He developed a large effusion, medial joint pain, difficulty walking, and had catching and giving-way type symptoms. Arthroscopy was performed that demonstrated a large grade IV chondral defect of his medial femoral condyle, which was debrided arthroscopically (Figure C29.1). A second arthroscopic abrasion arthroplasty followed by a period of nonweight bearing also failed to improve his symptoms. Biopsy for future autologous chondrocyte implantation (ACI) was then performed. Physical therapy and antiinflammatory medications were also utilized, leading to no improvement in his symptoms.

PHYSICAL EXAMINATION

Height, 6 ft, 1 in.; weight, 210 lb. At presentation, the patient ambulated with a significant antalgic gait using a cane. Clinical evaluation demonstrated mild varus alignment, quadriceps atrophy, and a small joint effusion. Range of motion was symmetric and full. His medial femoral condyle was tender to palpation, as was his joint line. Meniscal compression testing was unremarkable. His ligament examination was within normal limits.

RADIOGRAPHIC EVALUATION

Plain radiographs demonstrate early medial joint space narrowing compared to the contralateral knee. Long-leg alignment radiographs demonstrated early peripheral medial osteophyte formation, minimal joint space narrowing, and mechanical axis falling into the center of the medial compartment (Figure C29.2).

SURGICAL INTERVENTION

ACI of the medial femoral condyle was performed for a grade IV defect measuring 45 mm long by 8 mm wide (Figure C29.3). A closing-wedge valgus-producing high tibial osteotomy (HTO) of 6 degrees angular correction was also performed to slightly overcorrect the mechanical axis to the lateral intercondylar spine (Figure C29.4). Postoperatively, the patient was made nonweight bearing and used continuous passive motion for 6 weeks. Thereafter, he progressed to weight bearing as tolerated. Impact activities were avoided for 12 months postoperatively.

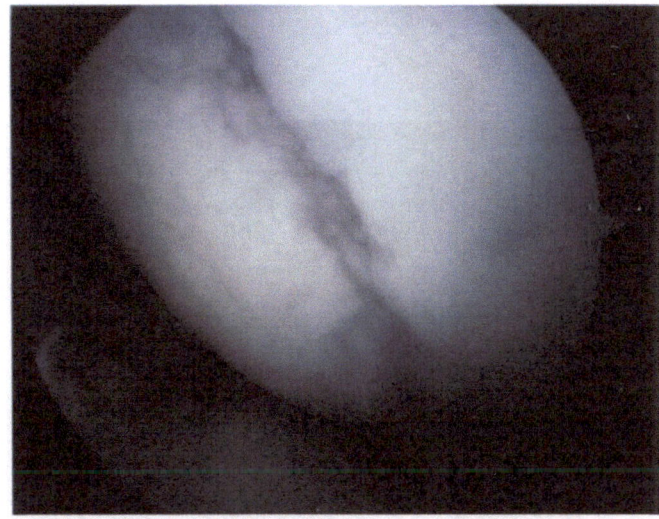

FIGURE C29.1 Arthroscopic appearance of full-thickness chondral defect of medial femoral condyle.

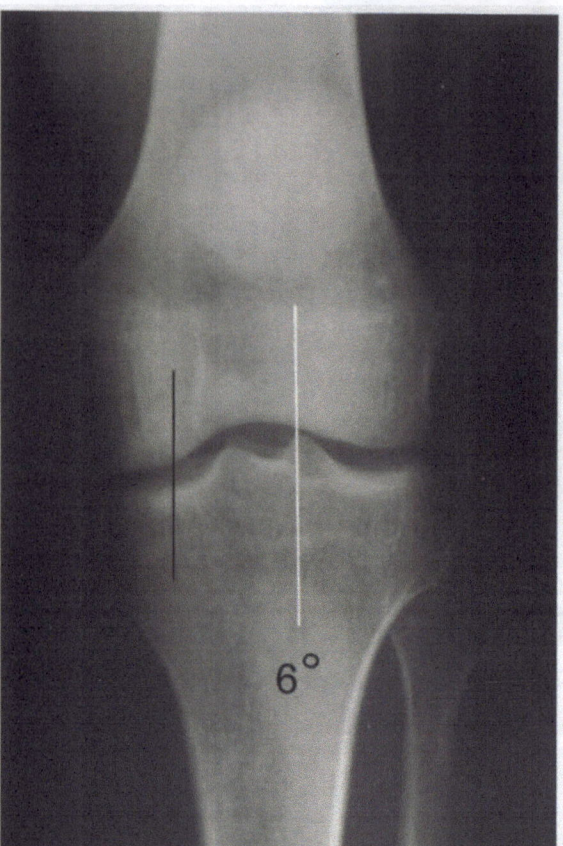

FIGURE C29.2 Cropped standing long-leg alignment radiograph demonstrates the mechanical axis to fall through the center of the medial joint compartment (*black line*) with early medial joint space narrowing compared to the opposite knee (not shown). A planned 6-degree angular correction is drawn (*white line*) to place the mechanical axis through the lateral intercondylar spine in an effort to unload the medial compartment.

FOLLOW-UP

Within 2 years, the patient returned to sporting activities, hiking, and playing with his children without any symptoms. Five years later he remained symptom free with full range of motion (Figure C29.5).

DECISION-MAKING FACTORS

1. Relatively young male with high physical demand level with symptomatic chondral defect unresponsive to prior treatment attempts.
2. Early joint space narrowing with peripheral osteophyte formation on the medial femoral condyle, and the mechanical axis falling through the center of the medial compartment necessitating both cartilage restoration and unloading osteotomy.
3. General indications for osteotomy included medial compartment disease with slight medial joint space narrowing and mild clinical varus deformity and desire to protect the ACI.
4. ACI chosen over other techniques (osteochondral grafting) because of high level of success demonstrated in lesions of this size and location and the avoidance of creating a subchondral defect.

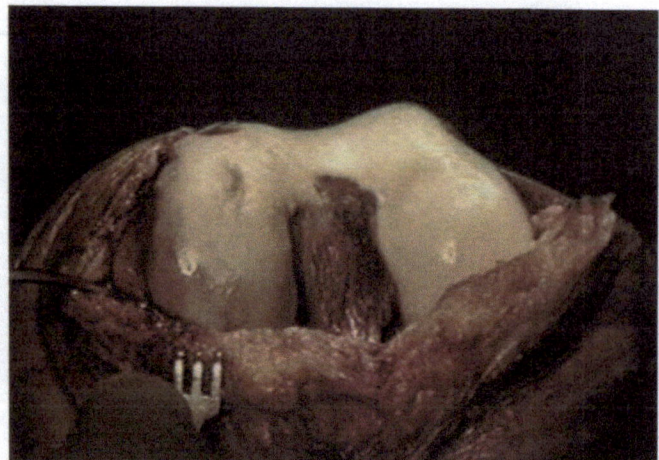

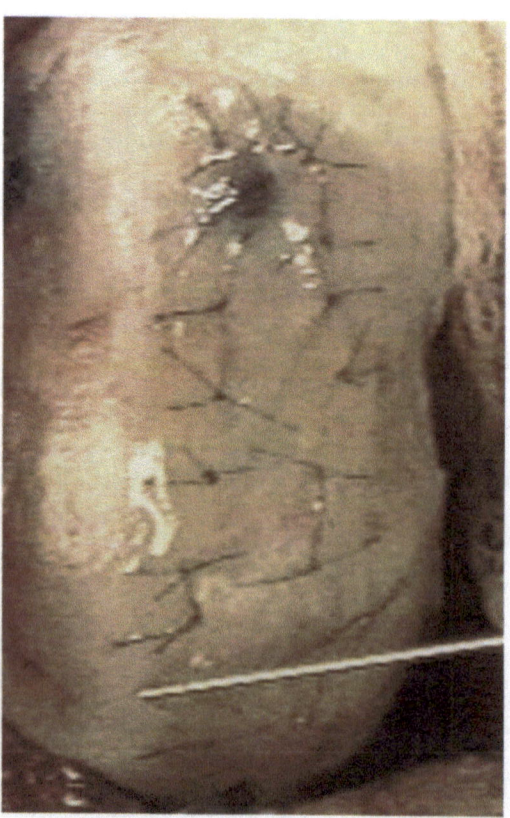

FIGURE C29.3 Clinical photographs of the medial femoral condyle at the time of open arthrotomy for autologous chondrocyte implantation (ACI) (**A**). Note the generalized thinning of the articular cartilage on the medial femoral condyle compared to the lateral femoral condyle and the development of medial peripheral osteophytes compatible with varus alignment and medial compartment overload. These findings were used in part to indicate this patient for simultaneous ACI and high tibial osteotomy (HTO). (**B**) ACI graft being sealed with autologous fibrin glue after injection of autologous cultured chondrocytes.

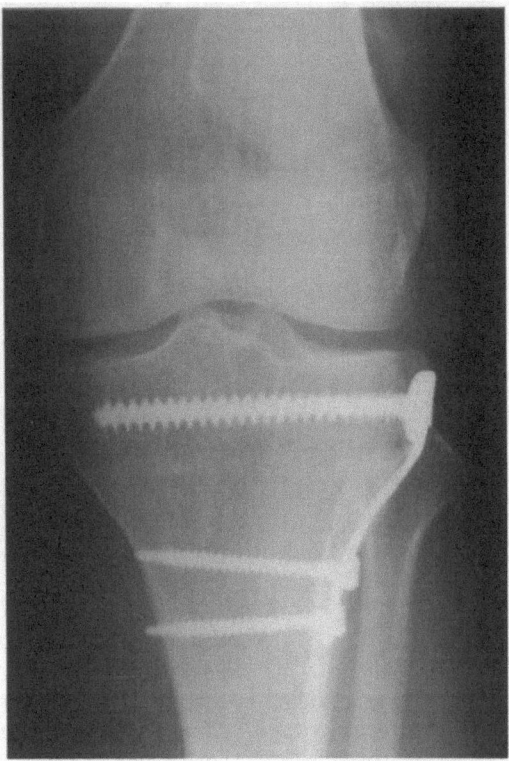

FIGURE C29.4 Standing anteroposterior (AP) radiograph 1 year after reconstructive surgery with restoration of medial joint space.

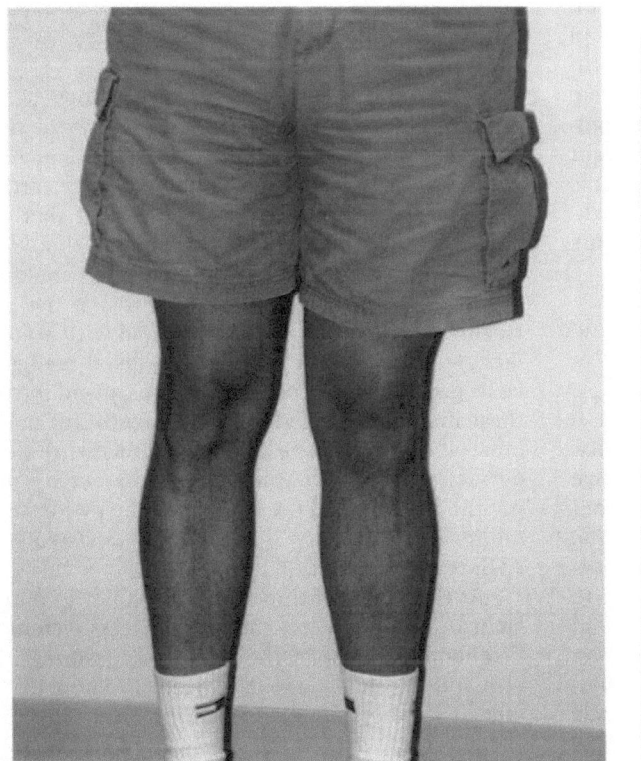

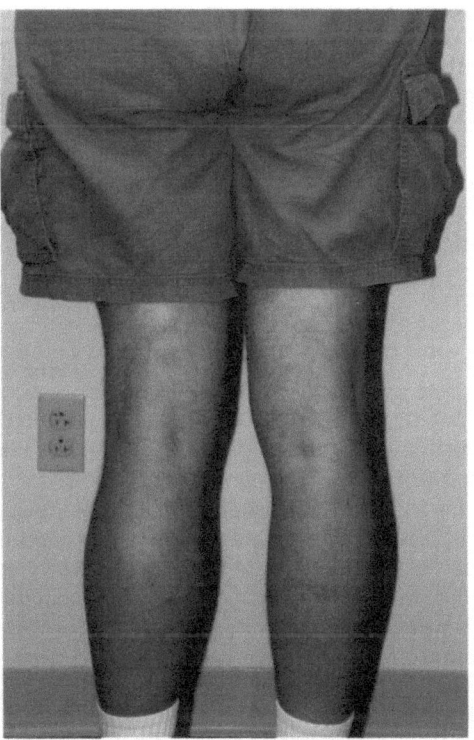

A   B

FIGURE C29.5 Clinical appearance of left knee after ACI and HTO demonstrating slight valgus alignment in the (**A**) frontal and (**B**) posterior views.

30

PATHOLOGY
ACL deficiency with symptomatic trochlear and medial femoral condyle chondral lesions

TREATMENT
ACL reconstruction and autologous chondrocyte implantation

SUBMITTED BY
Brian J. Cole, MD, MBA, Rush Cartilage Restoration Center, Rush University Medical Center, Chicago, Illinois, USA

CHIEF COMPLAINT AND HISTORY OF PRESENT ILLNESS

This patient is a 46-year-old man with complaints of right knee pain, swelling, and giving-way of approximately 2 years duration. He describes a work-related injury occurring 2 years previously when he tripped while carrying a heavy load, sustaining a pop with immediate swelling. Subsequent to that event, he had persistent right knee pain, swelling, and several episodes of his knee giving-way. Following his work-related injury, he underwent right knee arthroscopy, at which time he was diagnosed with at least a partial anterior cruciate ligament (ACL) tear as well as a chondral injury of unclear nature. Chondral debridement was performed without any further treatment. Since that time, he has had severe pain along the medial side of his knee, anterior knee discomfort exacerbated with inclines and declines, recurrent swelling, and giving-way several times a day. Presently, his symptoms are so severe that he is unable to continue working in his present capacity as a manual laborer and presents for evaluation and treatment.

PHYSICAL EXAMINATION

Height, 6 ft, 5 in.; weight, 214 lb. He ambulates with a slightly antalgic gait referable to his right lower extremity. He stands grossly in symmetric neutral alignment. His range of motion is from 0 to 110 degrees as compared to the contralateral side of 0 to 135 degrees. Quadriceps girth on the right side is 2 cm smaller than the contralateral normal side. He has a moderate effusion, and his knee is slightly warm to touch. He has moderate tenderness along the medial femoral condyle as well as the medial joint line. He has moderate patellofemoral crepitus with pain on patellar compression. He has no lateral joint line pain. Ligamentous testing reveals a grade II Lachman's examination with no firm endpoint appreciated. Pivot shift testing was difficult secondary to patient guarding.

RADIOGRAPHIC EVALUATION

Forty-five-degree flexion weight-bearing posteroanterior radiographs are unremarkable (Figure C30.1). Long-leg alignment films demonstrate the weight-bearing line to pass through the center of the knee. Magnetic resonance imaging reveals an articular defect of the medial femoral condyle in the weight-bearing zone as well as some articular thinning of the central trochlea. The ACL appears widened and attenuated on sagittal views.

SURGICAL INTERVENTION

The patient was indicated for arthroscopy to evaluate the articular surfaces as well as the integrity of the ACL. Preoperatively, it was agreed that if the patient had combined pathology of ACL deficiency and articular cartilage disease, that the ACL would be reconstructed at that time using a bone–patellar tendon–bone allograft and, should the articular cartilage disease remain symptomatic, it would be addressed at a later date. It was determined that if the patient had a trochlear lesion that was to be treated with autologous chondrocyte implantation (ACI) then a distal realignment would be be performed concomitantly. Thus, given the magnitude of these individual surgeries and the significant risk for arthrofibrosis if the ACL was initially combined with the ACI, it was decided that the ACL would be reconstructed if indicated during this surgery and the ACI would be performed with a distal realignment only if symptoms persisted following the ACL reconstruction.

At the time of arthroscopy, the ACL was noted to be deficient. Additionally, two articular defects were noted: a grade IV chondral defect of the trochlea measuring 20 mm by 28 mm and a second grade III to grade IV chondral lesion of the medial femoral condyle measuring 25 mm by 15 mm (Figure C30.2). A 200- to 300-mg specimen of articular cartilage was harvested for culturing from the intercondylar notch during the notchplasty for the ACL reconstruction in anticipation

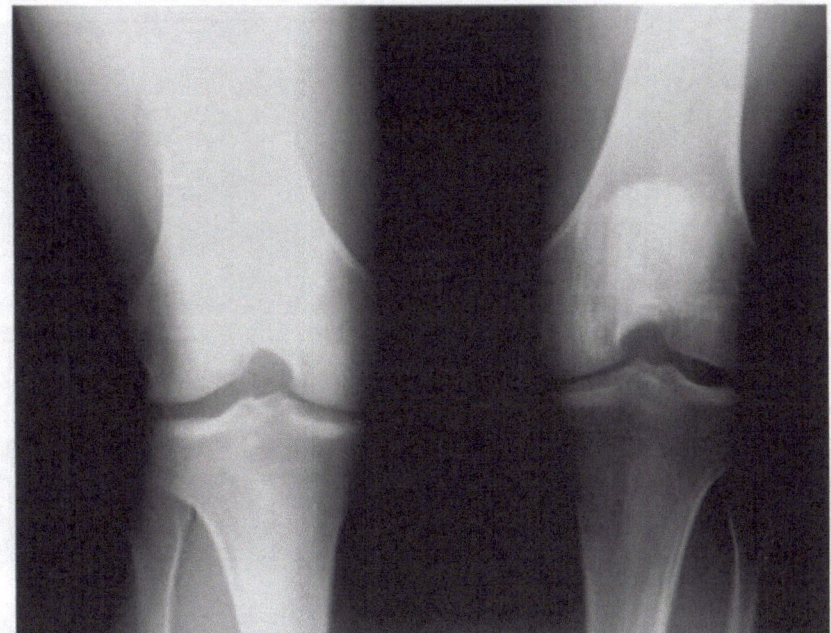 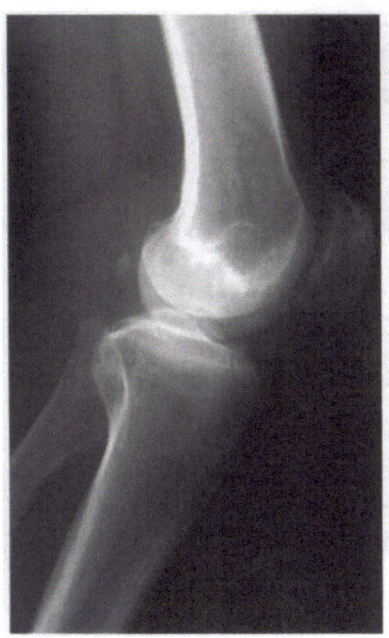

FIGURE C30.1 Forty-five-degree flexion posteroanterior weight-bearing (**A**) and lateral (**B**) radiographs are normal without evidence of joint space narrowing or overt signs of osteoarthritis.

that the ACI would be performed in the future. The ACL was reconstructed without any technical difficulty using the bone–patellar tendon–bone allograft (Figure C30.3). Postoperatively, although the patient did not complain of any further instability, he continued to complain of medial and anterior knee pain with activity-related swelling. At 16 weeks after the ACL reconstruction, the patient underwent ACI of both the trochlear and medial femoral condyle lesions performed in conjunction with a anteromedialization of the tibial tubercle (Figure C30.4). Postoperatively, the patient was initially made nonweight bearing and utilized a continuous passive motion (CPM) machine for approximately 6 weeks. Early in the rehabilitation period, his flexion was limited to 45 to 60 degrees to minimize patellofemoral contact forces on the trochlear healing lesion. Patellar mobilization techniques and flexion to 90 degrees were performed daily to prevent stiffness. He was asked to refrain from any impact or ballistic activities for 18 months.

FOLLOW-UP

The patient is now 24 months following ACI and continues to participate in a home exercise program. His subjective complaints mainly focus on some residual difficulty with kneeling and deep squatting. However, he states that he is significantly improved from his preoperative state and that his medial and anterior knee pain has essentially resolved. He denies any residual instability. His range of motion is from 0 to 125 degrees, and he has minimal quadriceps atrophy. His Lachman examination is a grade I with a firm endpoint with-

out a pivot shift. Radiographs reveal a well-healed distal realignment osteotomy and interference screw placement for the ACL graft in a satisfactory position (Figure C30.5). At 24 months, the patient returned for removal of the screws used to fix the distal realignment and second-look arthroscopy was performed. Both lesions showed excellent fill and integration of hyaline-like cartilage that was minimally fibrillated and relatively firm compared to the surrounding normal articular surfaces (Figure C30.6).

DECISION-MAKING FACTORS

1. Complex problem with ligament deficiency in conjunction with multiple symptomatic articular cartilage defects including a trochlear lesion considered less amenable to fresh osteochondral allograft reconstruction.
2. The need to stage the ACL and ACI because (1) some patients with symptoms believed to be related to chondral injury have reduced symptoms following isolated ACL reconstruction and (2) there is significant risk for arthrofibrosis if all procedures (i.e., ACL, ACI, and distal realignment) are performed concomitantly.
3. Failure of prior attempts at articular cartilage debridement and incomplete symptom relief with isolated ACL reconstruction.
4. High-demand individual with multiple articular cartilage lesions considered most amenable to ACI (i.e., due to size and location) as opposed to other options including fresh osteochondral allograft reconstruction.

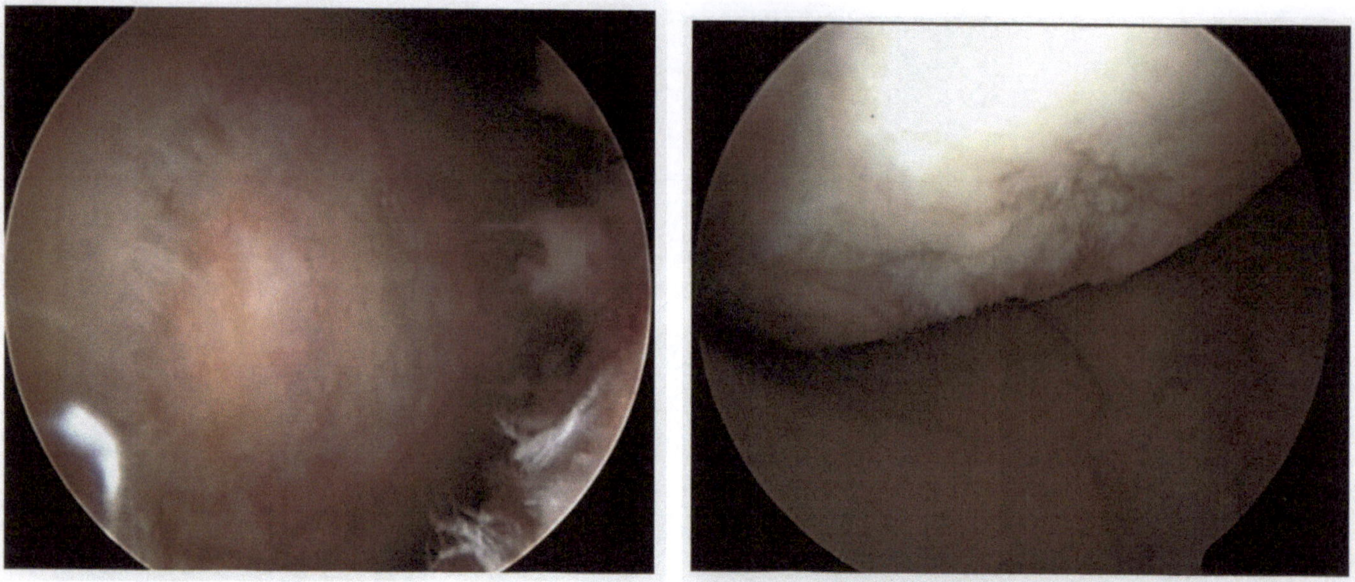

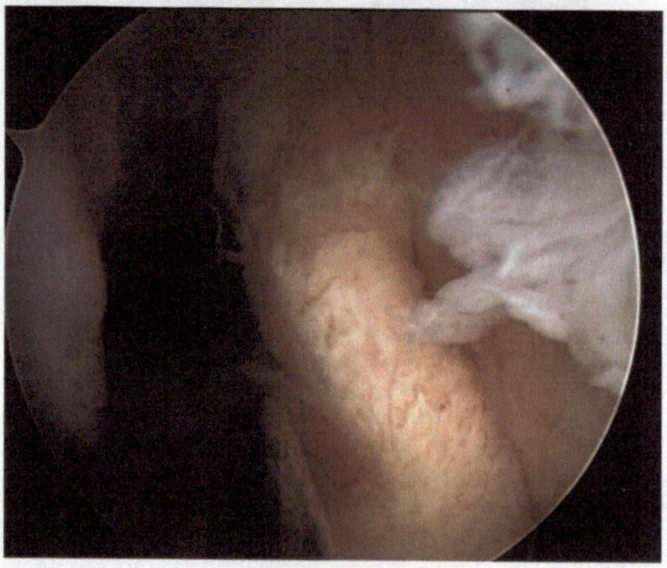

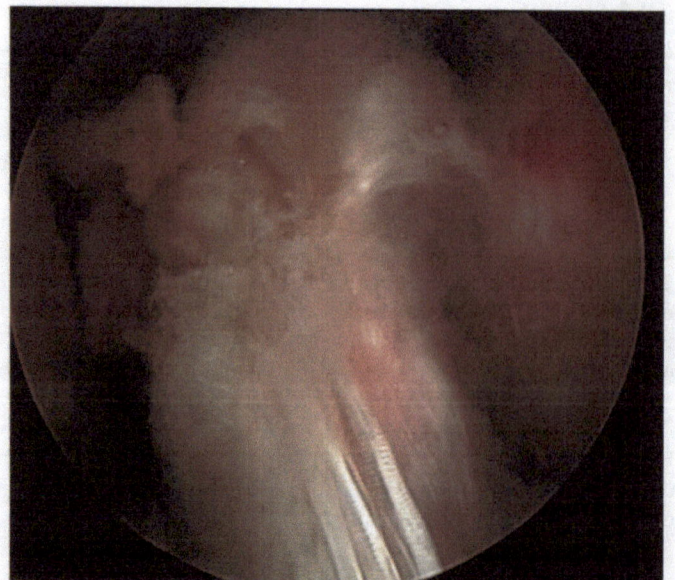

FIGURE C30.2 Arthroscopic photographs obtained at the time of anterior cruciate ligament (ACL) reconstruction and biopsy for staged autologous chondrocyte implantation (ACI). (A) Large grade IV chondral defect of the trochlea. (B) Large medial femoral condyle chondral defect grade III/IV. (C) Deficient ACL with empty lateral-wall sign.

FIGURE C30.3 Arthroscopic photograph of ACL bone–patellar tendon–bone allograft reconstruction secured in place.

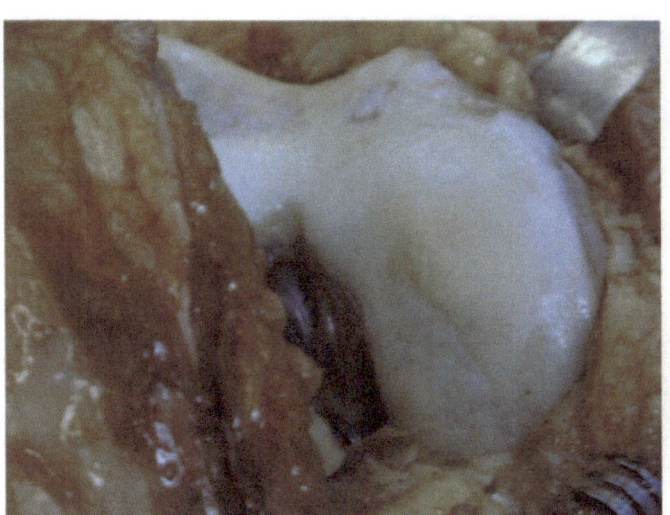
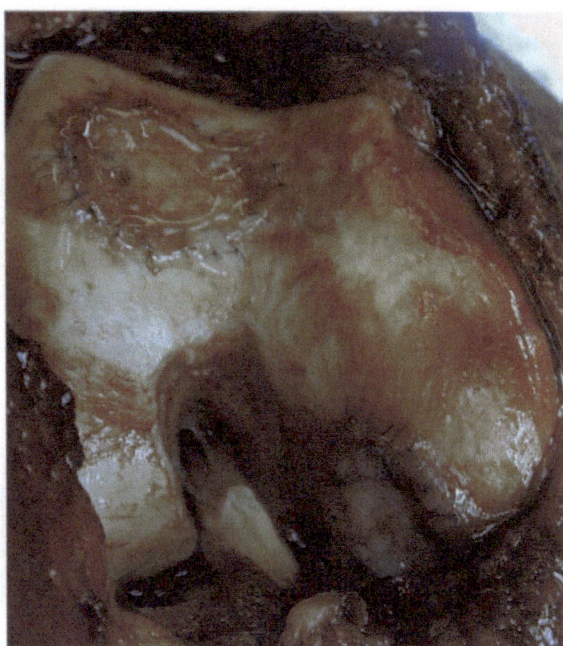

FIGURE C30.4 Intraoperative photographs of (**A**) articular cartilage lesions of the trochlea and medial femoral condyle before preparation and (**B**) the same lesions following periosteal patch and fibrin glue placement.

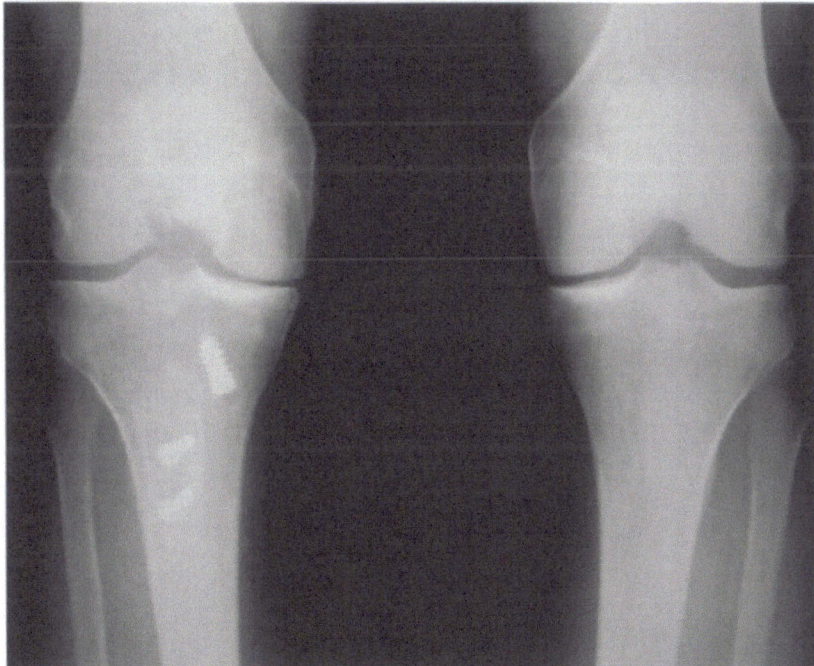
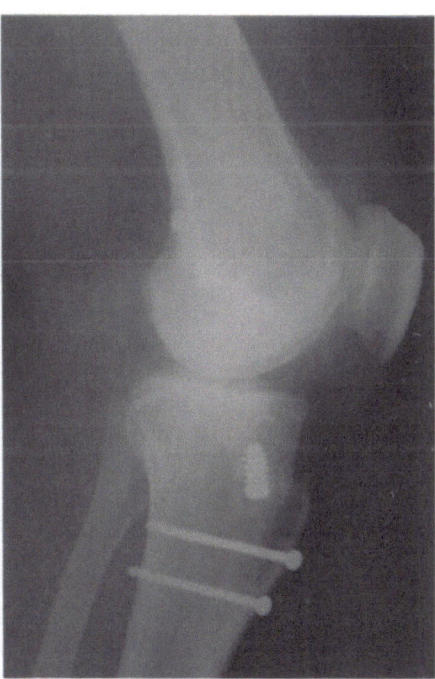

FIGURE C30.5 Twenty-four-month anteroposterior (**A**) and lateral (**B**) radiographs of the right knee reveal ACL reconstruction and distal realignment osteotomy fixation in satisfactory position.

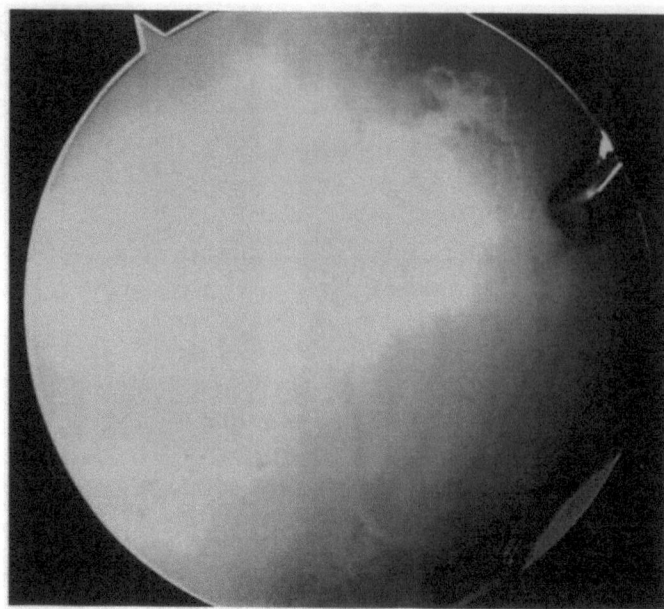

FIGURE C30.6 Twenty-four-month arthroscopic second-look photograph centered on the transition zone between the two defects demonstrates excellent integration and fill following ACI. In this picture, the trochlear defect is visualized almost in its entirety.

31

PATHOLOGY
Focal chondral defect of the medial femoral condyle in a previously meniscectomized knee

TREATMENT
Autologous chondrocyte implantation and concomitant medial meniscus allograft transplantation

SUBMITTED BY
Brian J. Cole, MD, MBA, Rush Cartilage Restoration Center, Rush University Medical Center, Chicago, Illinois, USA

CHIEF COMPLAINT AND HISTORY OF PRESENT ILLNESS

This patient is an 18-year-old girl with a chief complaint of persistent medial-sided left knee pain, predominantly weight bearing in nature, and inability to perform any athletic activities. Her history dates back to the age of 15 years when she underwent a medial meniscectomy. Following initial symptom relief, she developed recurrent medial joint line symptoms and activity-related swelling.

PHYSICAL EXAMINATION

Height, 5 ft, 7 in.; weight, 120 lb. She has a normal gait with slight symmetric valgus alignment. Her knee has a small effusion. Her range of motion is normal and symmetric to the contralateral side. She has pain with palpation of her medial femoral condyle and along her medial joint line. Her ligament examination is within normal limits.

RADIOGRAPHIC EVALUATION

Preoperative radiographs obtained for graft sizing demonstrate no significant joint space narrowing and no femoral condyle or tibiofemoral arthritic change (Figure C31.1).

SURGICAL INTERVENTION

At arthroscopy, in addition to evidence of a prior subtotal medial meniscectomy, she was noted to have a concomitant grade IV focal chondral defect of the weight-bearing zone of her medial temoral condyle measuring approximately 15 mm by 18 mm in size (Figure C31.2). An articular cartilage biopsy was harvested from the intercondylar notch, and the patient was indicated for subsequent concomitant medial meniscus allograft transplantation and autologous chondrocyte implantation. Approximately 8 weeks later, a meniscal allograft transplant with bone plugs was performed using an arthro-scopically assisted approach (Figure C31.3). Following meniscus repair, a limited medial arthrotomy was made to expose the defect and perform an autologous chondrocyte implantation of the focal chondral defect (Figure C31.4).

Postoperatively, the patient was made nonweight bearing for 4 weeks and used continuous passive motion for 6 weeks for 6 to 8 h/day. Thereafter, she was advanced to weight bearing as tolerated. At 12 months, she was permitted to engage in higher-impact activities.

FOLLOW-UP

At 24 months postoperatively, the patient complained of some minor discomfort and activity-related medial joint line pain. A second-look arthroscopy was performed to evaluate the chondral defect and to assess the condition of the medial meniscus (Figure C31.5). The superficial aspect of the autologous chondrocyte implant was gently debrided and the medial meniscus was completely healed to the periphery. At 30 months postoperatively, the patient has returned to all sports with minimal discomfort and denies recurrent effusions or weight-bearing pain.

DECISION-MAKING FACTORS

1. A young, highly active patient with concomitant pathology involving a previous meniscectomy and ipsilateral chondral defect.
2. A relative contraindication to treating either pathology in isolation and the opportunity to treat both abnormalities simultaneously for relative protection of both grafts.
3. Chondral defect size, depth, and location appropriate for autologous chondrocyte implantation with concerns for donor site morbidity and the creation of a subchondral defect if otherwise treated with multiple osteochondral autograft transplants.
4. Rehabilitation tolerant and willingness to be compliant with initial nonweight bearing status.

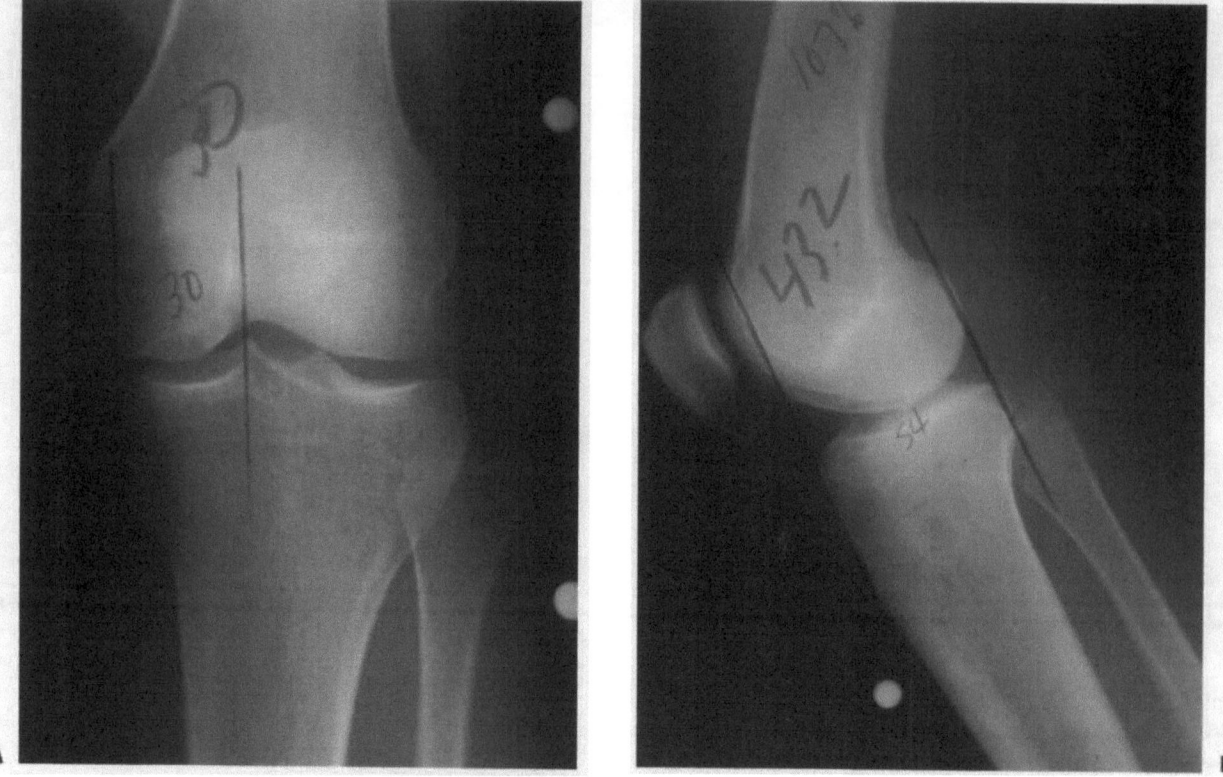

FIGURE C31.1 Anteroposterior (**A**) and lateral (**B**) radiographs demonstrate meniscal sizing with markers in place and no evidence of significant joint space narrowing along the medial tibiofemoral joint.

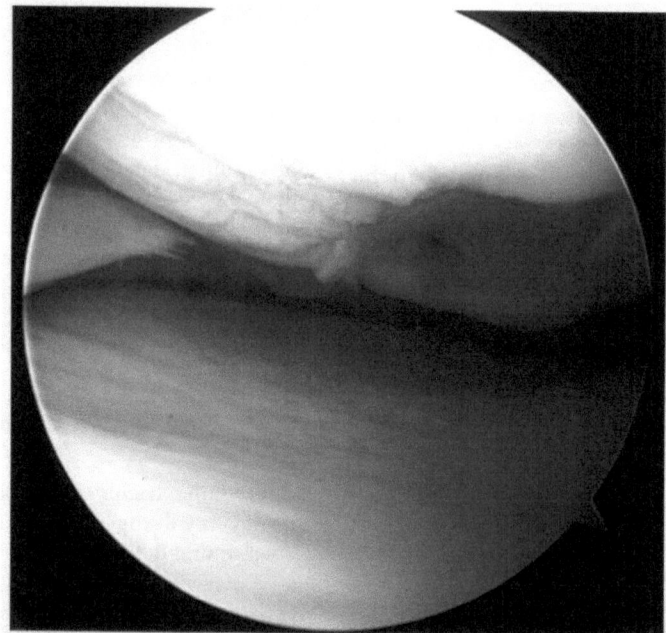

FIGURE C31.2 Arthroscopy demonstrates concomitant pathology of subtotal medial meniscectomy and grade IV focal chondral defect of the medial femoral condyle in the central weight-bearing zone.

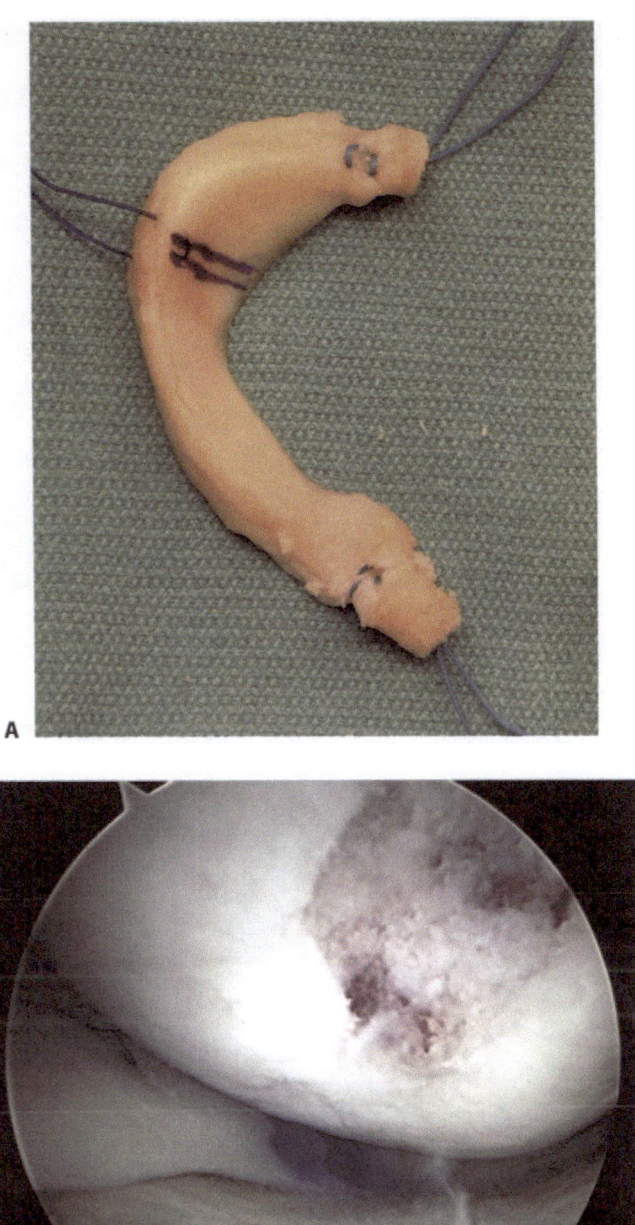

A

B

FIGURE C31.3 (A) Medial meniscus allograft prepared at the time of autologous chondrocyte implantation. (B) Meniscus allograft secured in place before performing the arthrotomy and autologous chondrocyte implantation.

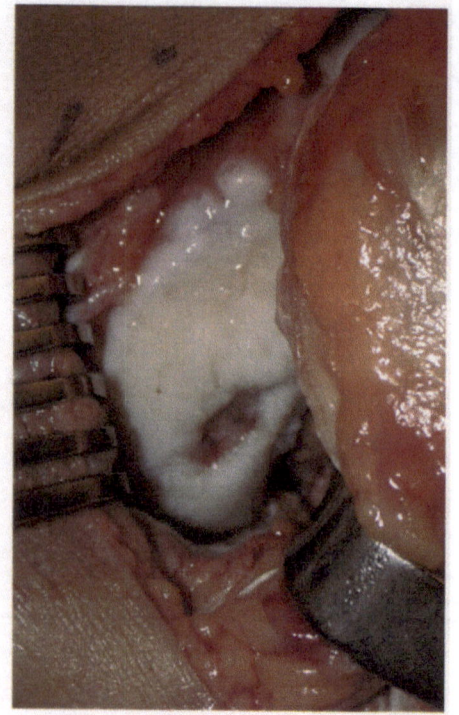

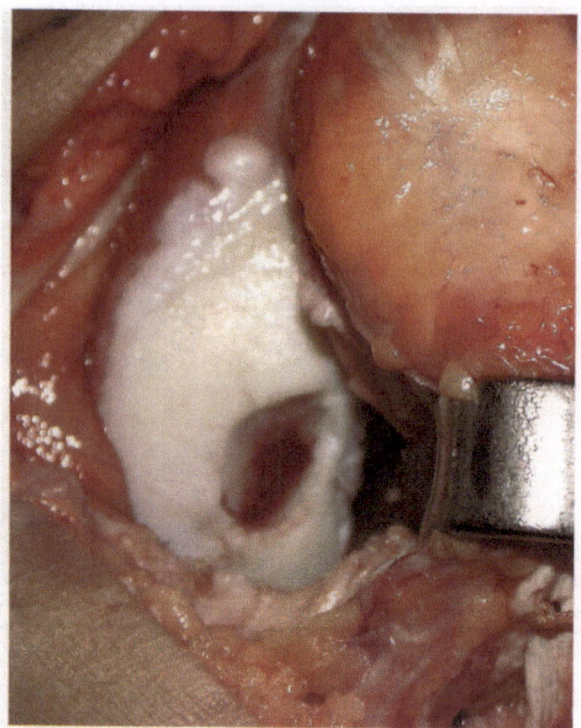

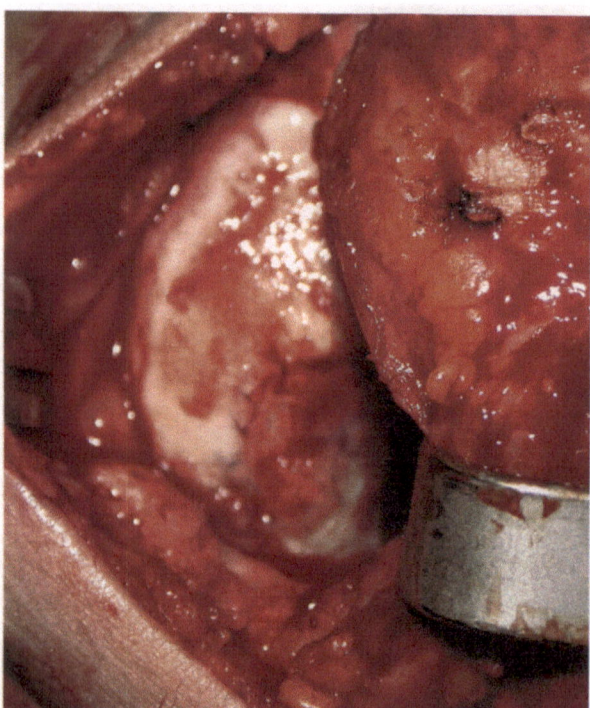

FIGURE C31.4 Medial femoral condyle defect before (**A**) and after (**B**) preparation. (**C**) Defect with periosteal patch in place following application of fibrin glue.

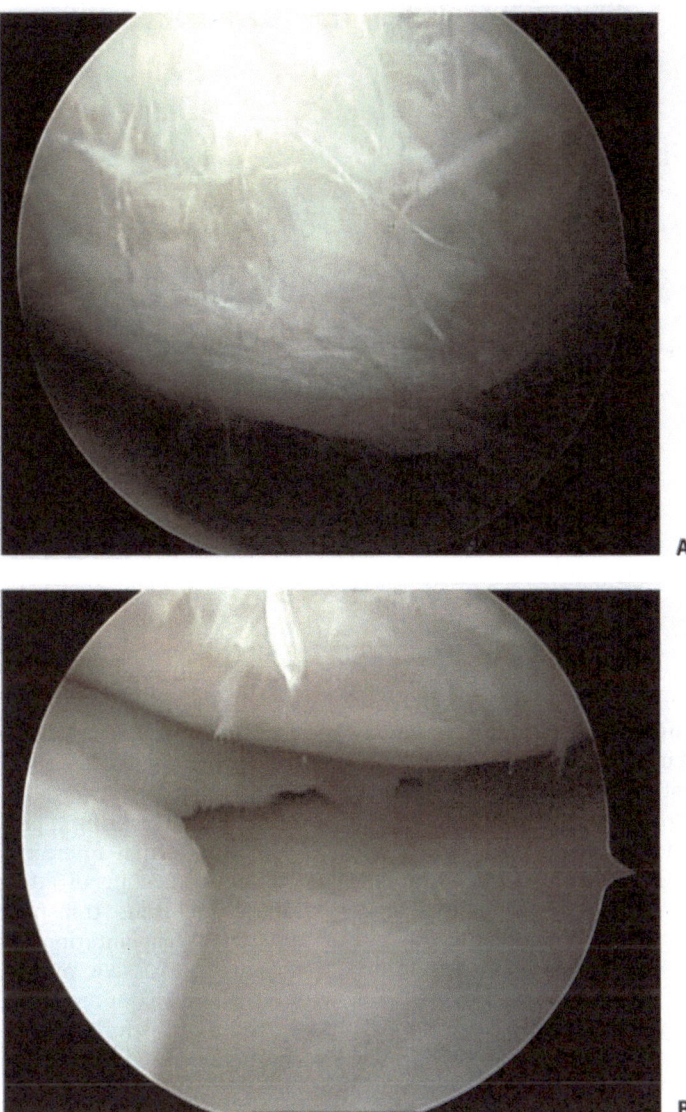

FIGURE C31.5 Twenty-four-month second-look arthroscopy of (**A**) the defect with superficial fibrillation and (**B**) the medial meniscus with complete healing to the periphery and no evidence of shrinkage.

32

> **PATHOLOGY**
> Focal chondral defect lateral femoral condyle, prior lateral meniscectomy, and small focal chondral defect lateral tibial plateau
>
> **TREATMENT**
> Fresh osteochondral allograft transplant lateral femoral condyle, lateral meniscus transplant, and microfracture lateral tibial plateau
>
> **SUBMITTED BY**
> Brian J. Cole, MD, MBA, Rush Cartilage Restoration Center, Rush University Medical Center, Chicago, Illinois, USA

CHIEF COMPLAINT AND HISTORY OF PRESENT ILLNESS

This patient is a 19-year-old college student who was referred with a chief complaint of right knee weight-bearing lateral-sided knee pain, swelling, and inability to participate in high-level sports. Past surgical history is significant for a right knee lateral meniscectomy performed 5 years before his initial evaluation. The patient did well initially, for 2 years, and then underwent a repeat arthroscopy. At that time, he was documented to have grade III to grade IV changes of the lateral femoral condyle and some early tibial plateau changes. This debridement actually led to some symptom relief until his symptoms recurred, and he presented with progression of pain, swelling, and difficulty playing college-level baseball. At this time, he is unable to play baseball and is having some difficulty with other noncompetitive sports and high-level activities of daily living.

PHYSICAL EXAMINATION

Height, 6 ft, 2 in.; weight, 185 lb. He ambulates with a non-antalgic gait. He stands in symmetric and neutral alignment. His range of motion is 0 to 130 degrees. His right knee has a small effusion. He is tender to palpation over the lateral femoral condyle and lateral joint line. Patellofemoral joint demonstrates good tracking with no evidence of crepitus. Ligamentous testing is within normal limits.

RADIOGRAPHIC EVALUATION

Posteroanterior 45-degree flexion weight-bearing radiograph demonstrates signs of femoral condyle flattening, joint space narrowing along the lateral compartment, and early osteophyte formation along the tibial eminences of the right knee (Figure C32.1).

SURGICAL INTERVENTION

The patient was indicated for a diagnostic arthroscopy, at which time he was noted to have an absent lateral meniscus, a grade III to grade IV lesion of the lateral femoral condyle measuring approximately 30 mm by 30 mm, and an area of nearly grade IV cartilage loss in the central region of the tibial plateau measuring approximately 10 mm by 10 mm (Figure C32.2). A formal microfracture of the lateral tibial plateau was performed in an effort to prepare the knee for future lateral meniscus transplantation and fresh osteochondral allograft transplantation (Figure C32.3). The patient utilized continuous passive motion postoperatively and was non-weight bearing for approximately 6 weeks.

Six months following the microfracture, the patient still complained of lateral-sided pain, activity-related swelling, and difficulties with activities of daily living and high-level sports. In consideration of the size of the lateral femoral condyle lesion and the early degenerative changes of the tibia, he was indicated for an osteochondral allograft transplant of the lateral femoral condyle and a simultaneously performed lateral meniscus allograft transplant. Preoperative planning included radiographic sizing images (Figure C32.4). At the time of definitive treatment, the lateral tibial plateau was noted to have excellent fibrocartilage fill of the previously microfractured lesion (Figure C32.5). The patient underwent a fresh osteochondral allograft transplant using a 30 mm by 30 mm fresh osteochondral allograft as well as a concomitant lateral meniscus transplant (Figure C32.6).

FOLLOW-UP

Two years postoperatively, the patient has minimal symptoms and has returned to playing competitive baseball at the collegiate level. Postoperative radiographs demonstrate preservation of the lateral joint space with no progressive joint space loss, as well as incorporation of the osteochondral

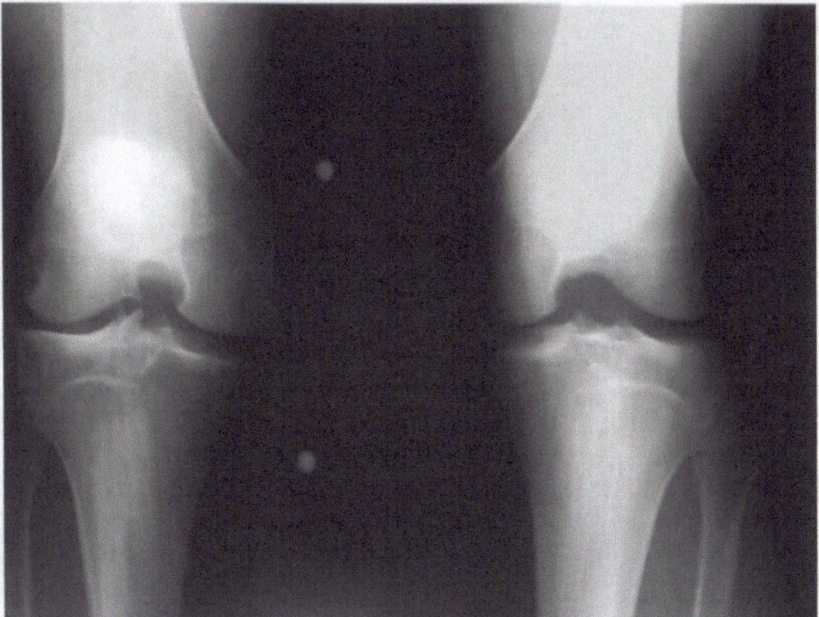

FIGURE C32.1 Forty-five-degree flexion posteroanterior radiograph demonstrates flattening of the right lateral femoral condyle, joint space narrowing, and early degenerative changes along the lateral tibial eminence.

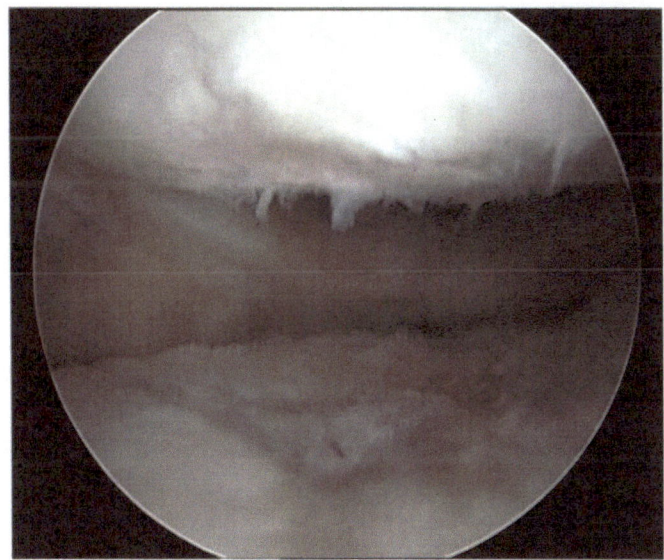

FIGURE C32.2 Index arthroscopy demonstrating diffuse grade IV changes of the lateral femoral condyle, absent lateral meniscus, and a localized area of articular cartilage loss on the lateral tibial plateau measuring approximately 10 mm by 10 mm.

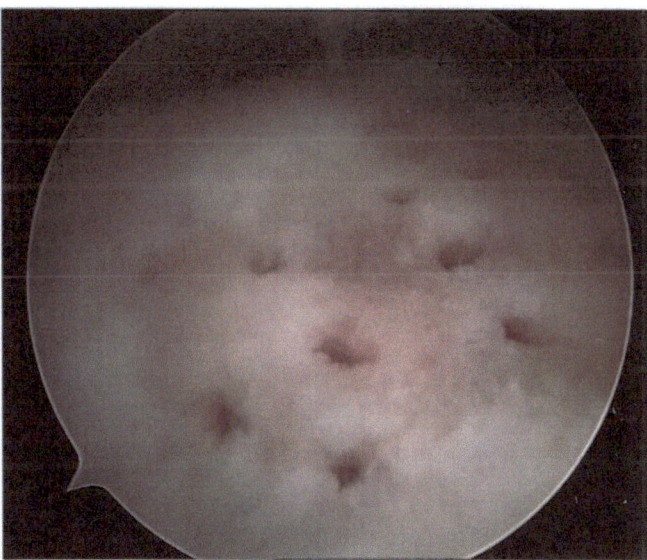

FIGURE C32.3 Focal cartilage defect of the lateral tibial plateau treated with a microfracture technique.

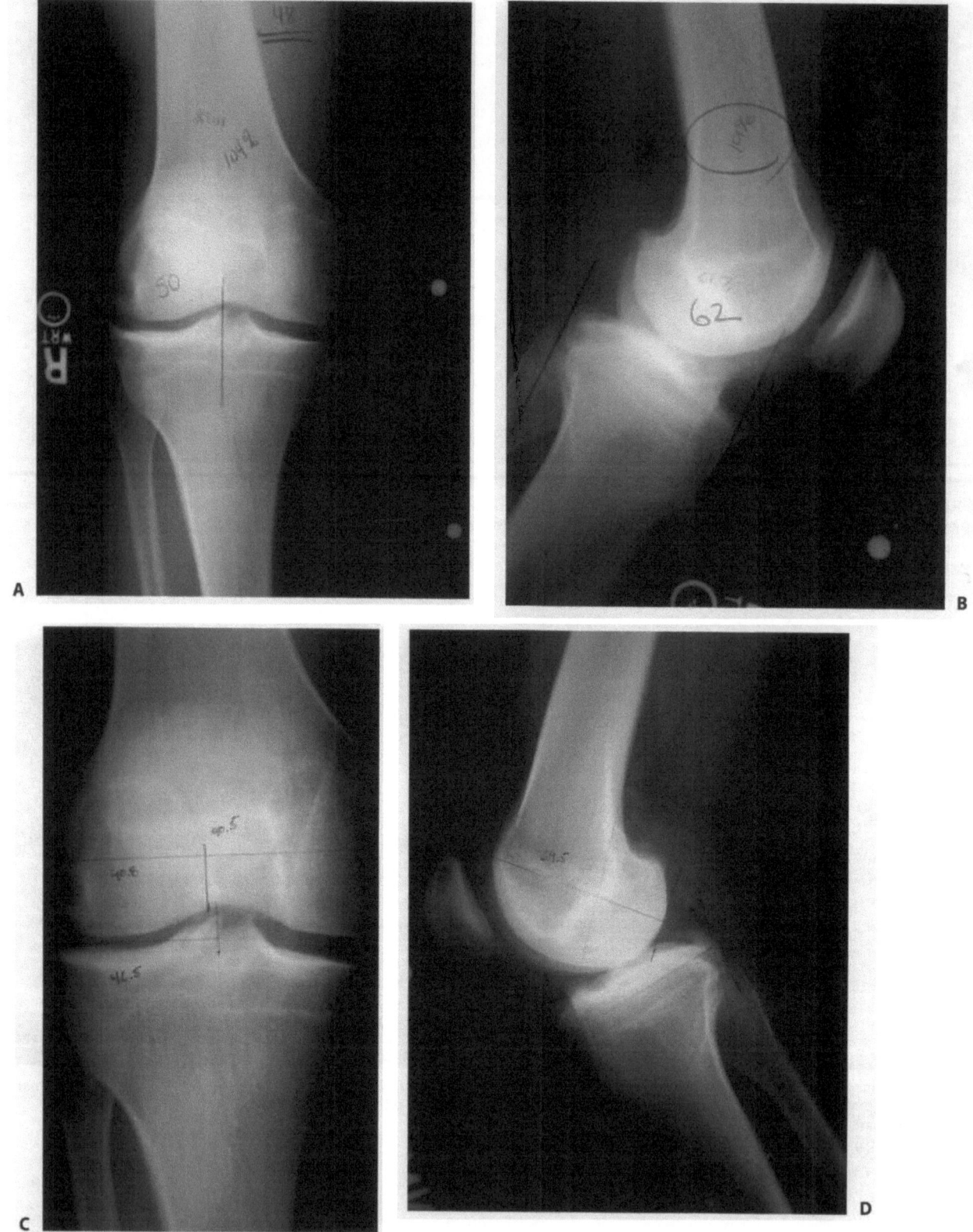

FIGURE C32.4 Anteroposterior (**A**) and lateral (**B**) radiographs with a 100-mm sizing marker in place being utilized for sizing of the allograft meniscus transplant. Anteroposterior (**C**) and lateral (**D**) radi-ographs with magnification markers to calculate the required fresh osteochondral allograft size.

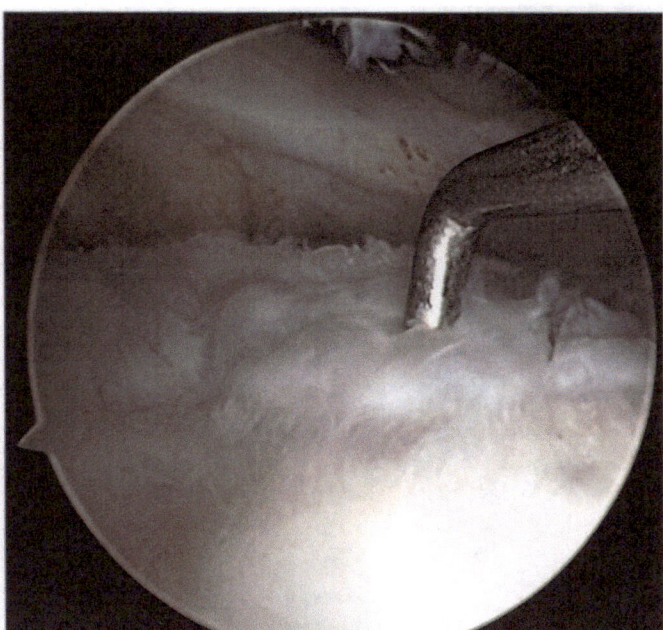

FIGURE C32.5 Six-month second-look arthroscopy following isolated microfracture of the lateral tibial plateau demonstrates fibrocartilage fill of the central tibial plateau defect.

allograft and of the keyhole bone bridge from the lateral meniscus transplant (Figure C32.7).

DECISION-MAKING FACTORS

1. Relatively young and highly active individual with recurrent symptoms following prior lateral meniscectomy and subsequent debridement and microfracture of the tibial plateau.

2. Microfracture of the tibia given the paucity of other acceptable solutions to treat a relatively small area of grade IV chondral change.

3. Lateral joint line and femoral condyle pain with associated ipsilateral meniscal deficiency and articular cartilage disease.

4. Large defect of the femoral condyle with early degenerative change of the opposing tibial plateau considered more tolerant of a fresh osteochondral allograft than autologous chondrocyte implantation.

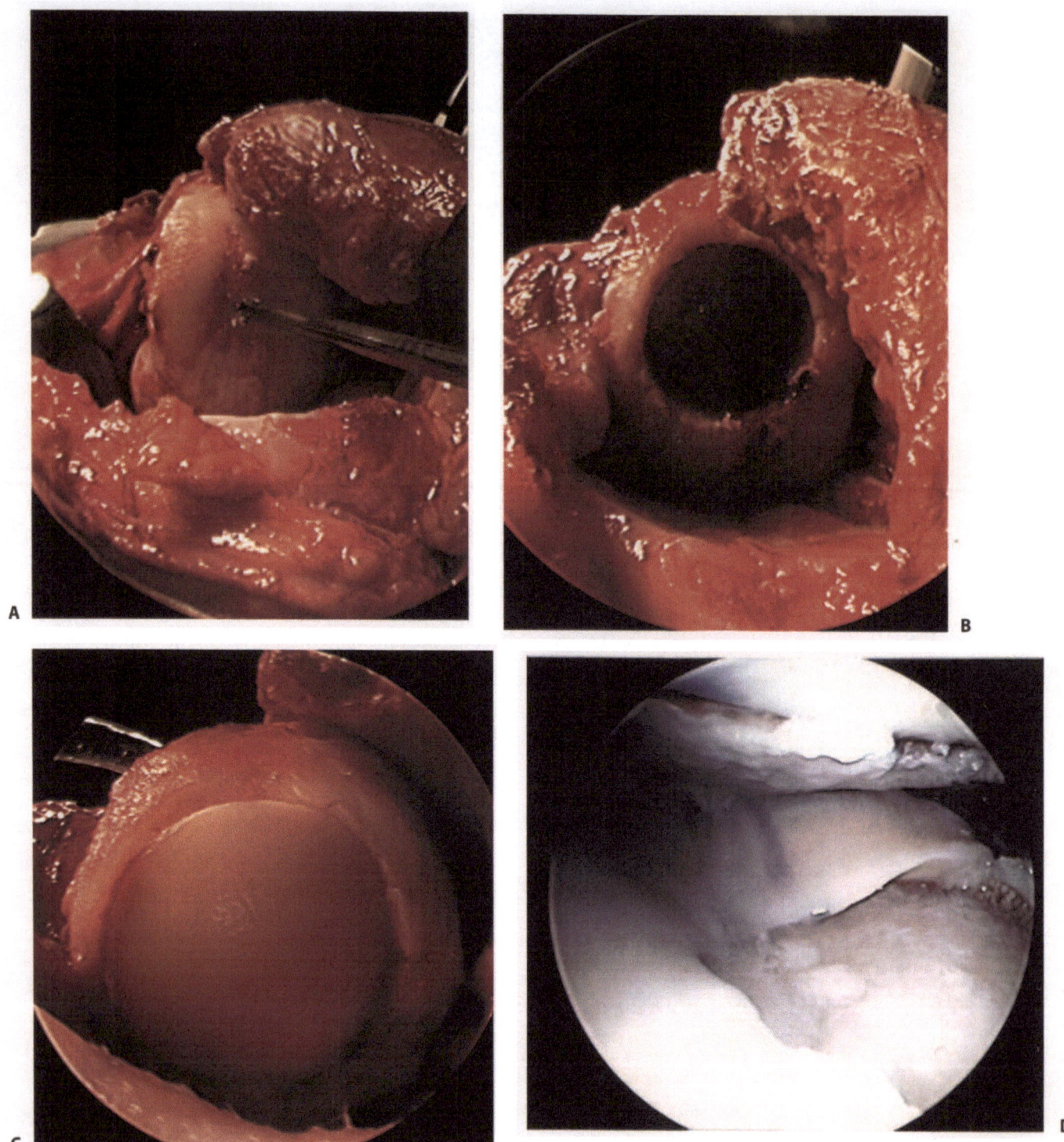

FIGURE C32.6 Intraoperative photograph at the time of arthrotomy of the focal cartilage defect of the lateral femoral condyle (**A**), with preparing the defect (**B**) for a 30 mm by 30 mm fresh osteochondral allograft transplant (**C**). (**D**) Arthroscopic view of lateral meniscus and osteochondral allograft in place.

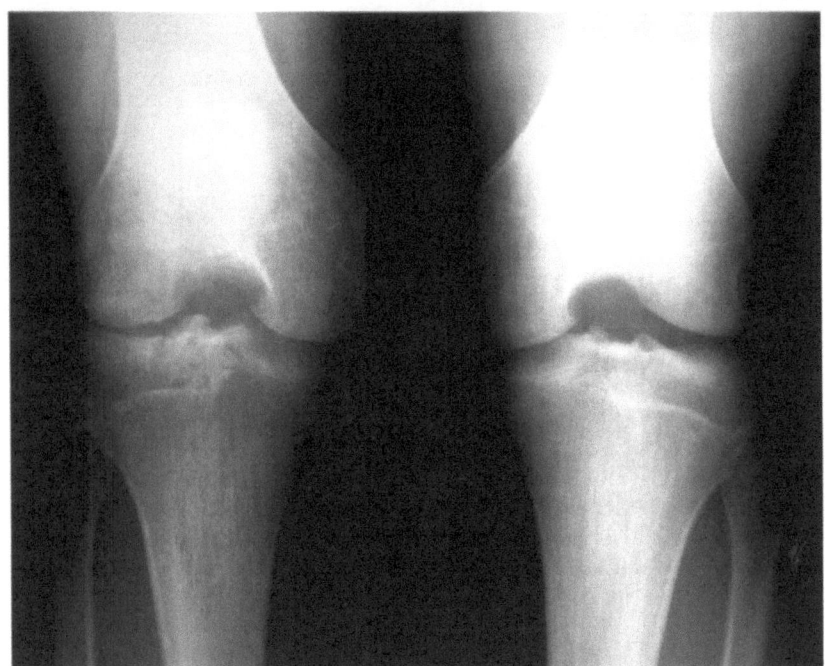

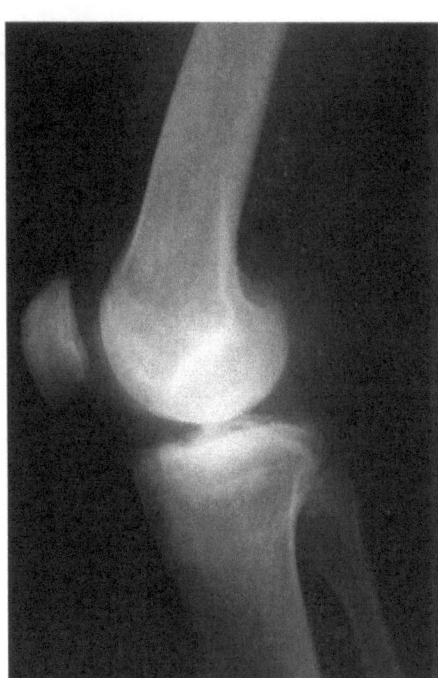

A   B

FIGURE C32.7 Eighteen-month postoperative 45-degree flexion weight-bearing posteroanterior (A) and lateral (B) radiographs demonstrate allograft incorporation, preservation of joint space, incorpora-tion of the lateral meniscus transplant bone bridge, and maintenance of the lateral femoral condyle contour.

33

PATHOLOGY
Bipolar focal chondral defects of the patellofemoral joint with patellar instability

TREATMENT
Autologous chondrocyte implantation of the patella and trochlea with distal realignment (Note that the use of ACI for the patella or for bipolar defects is considered off-label usage, but was indicated and performed with explicit patient and family informed consent and under the guidance of an Institutional Review Board protocol allowing prospective study of this patient at the author's institution.)

SUBMITTED BY
Brian J. Cole, MD, MBA, Rush Cartilage Restoration Center, Rush University Medical Center, Chicago, Illinois, USA

CHIEF COMPLAINT AND HISTORY OF PRESENT ILLNESS

This patient is an 18-year-old female whose chief complaint is that of persistent anterior knee pain, swelling, and recurrent patellar instability. As an adolescent, the patient had persistent anterior knee pain and recurrent subluxation of the patella. She underwent a lateral release at the age of 12, but continued to do poorly until her early teenage years. Subsequent to this, she came to arthroscopy and was diagnosed with a focal chondral defect of the patella and trochlea; the patella was debrided and the trochlea was treated with abrasion arthroplasty. Despite this treatment, the patient continued to have persistent instability and activity-related swelling and anterior knee pain. She was subsequently referred for cartilage restoration 3 years after her last surgery.

PHYSICAL EXAMINATION

Height, 5 ft, 6 in.; weight, 140 lb. The patient ambulates with a nonantalgic gait. She stands in approximately 4 degrees of physiologic valgus bilaterally. Her Q angle measures 10 degrees. Her range of motion is symmetric from 5 degrees of hyperextension to 130 degrees of flexion. She demonstrates some hypermobility of her other joints, including elbow hyperextension and metacarpophalangeal hyperextension. She demonstrates patellofemoral apprehension, a moderate effusion of her left knee, three-quadrant translation laterally, and one-quadrant translation medially of the patella with the knee in extension. She has a palpable clunk at 40 degrees of flexion during active range of motion assessment. Her medial and lateral joint lines are not painful. Her ligament examination is within normal limits.

RADIOGRAPHIC EVALUATION

At presentation, her radiographs demonstrated no evidence of overt patellofemoral arthritis or cystic change. The lateral radiograph demonstrated some evidence of patella alta. The computed tomography (CT) scan demonstrated lateral displacement of the patella relative to the trochlea and mild trochlear hypoplasia. There was no evidence of involvement of the patellar subchondral bone (Figure C33.1).

SURGICAL INTERVENTION

At the time of arthroscopic biopsy for autologous chondrocyte implantation (ACI), a 12 mm by 14 mm grade IV focal chondral defect of the central-to-lateral aspect of the patella and a 12 mm by 14 mm focal chondral defect of the trochlea with fibrocartilaginous fill were identified (Figure C33.2). A biopsy was obtained from the intercondylar notch, and subsequent to this the patient underwent ACI of her bipolar defects of the patella and trochlea about 8 weeks later (Figure C33.3). At the same time, a very oblique anteromedialization of the tibial tubercle was performed. Postoperative radiographs demonstrate elevation and translation of the tibial tubercle (Figure C33.4).

Postoperatively, she was made heel-touch weight bearing for approximately 6 weeks until radiographs demonstrated evidence of healing of the distal realignment. Although she was allowed to flex her knee daily to 90 degrees, continuous passive motion was restricted to 45 to 60 degrees of flexion during its use for the first 6 postoperative weeks. She advanced through the traditional rehabilitation protocol for ACI of the patellofemoral joint. She was asked to refrain from any impact or ballistic activities for 18 months.

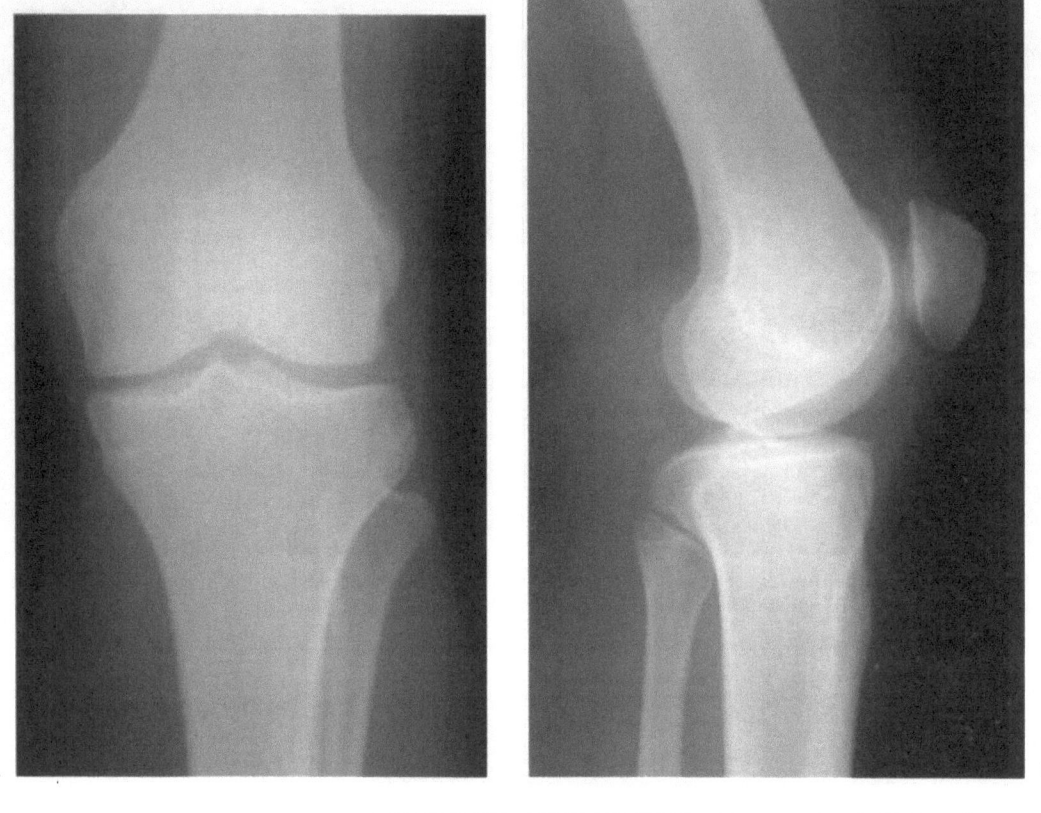

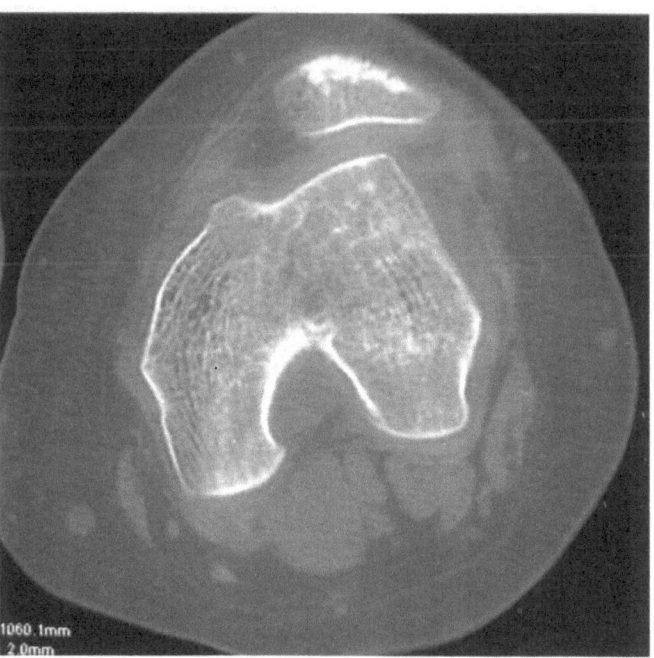

FIGURE C33.1 Anteroposterior (**A**) and lateral (**B**) radiographs demonstrate no evidence of overt patellofemoral arthritis. Lateral radiograph demonstrates patella alta. (**C**) Axial CT scan of the patellofemoral joint demonstrates some lateral displacement of the patella relative to the trochlea and mild trochlear hypoplasia.

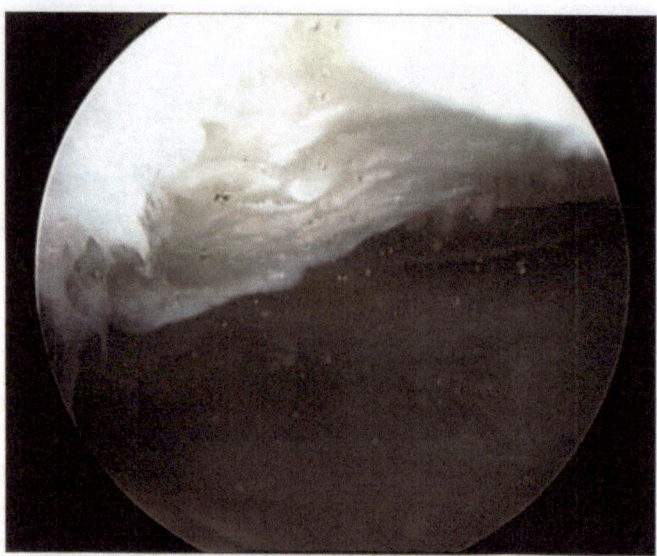
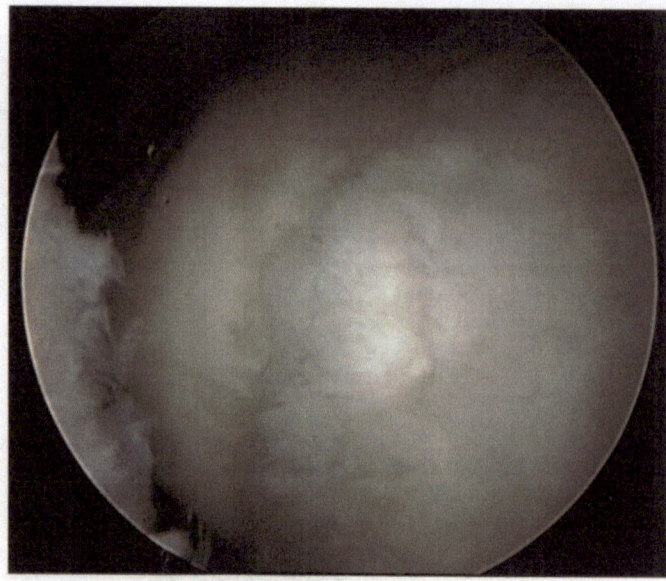

A

FIGURE C33.2 At the time of arthroscopy for biopsy for autologous chondrocyte implantation, a grade IV focal defect of the central-to-lateral aspect of the patella (**A**) and a focal defect of the trochlea with fibrocartilaginous fill (**B**) are identified.

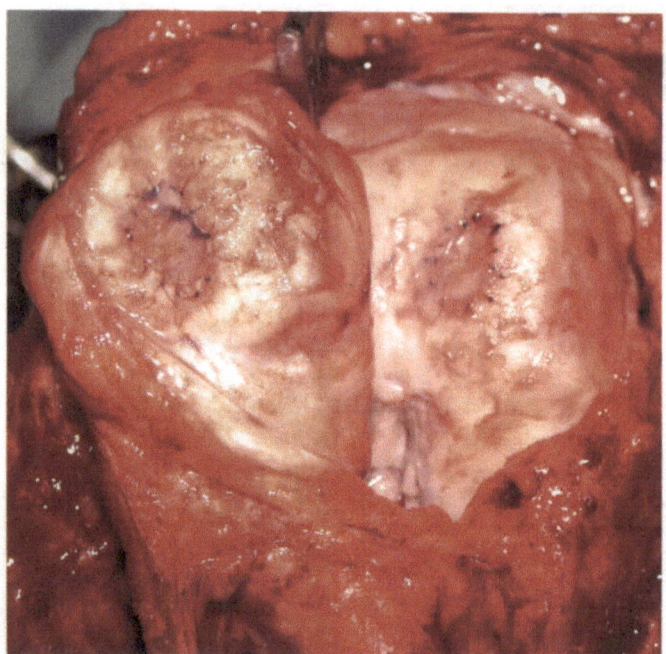

FIGURE C33.3 Intraoperative photograph of autologous chondrocyte implantation for bipolar defects of the patella and trochlea.

FOLLOW-UP

At early follow-up at approximately 18 months, the patient has significantly less pain, no recurrent patellar instability, and she is resuming low levels of activities such as biking, hiking, swimming, and the stair machine for her daily exercise regimen. Postoperative radiographs demonstrate elevation and translation of the tibial tubercle with no evidence of patellofemoral arthritic change (Figure C33.4).

DECISION-MAKING FACTORS

1. Young, highly symptomatic patient with failed primary attempt to achieve cartilage repair tissue of the patellofemoral joint.
2. Bipolar defect of the patellofemoral joint with no other treatment options other than, possibly, osteochondral allograft.
3. Recurrent patellar instability in addition to patellar defect likely to benefit from anteromedialization procedure.
4. Expected additional marginal benefit from concomitant resurfacing procedure in addition to anteromedialization.

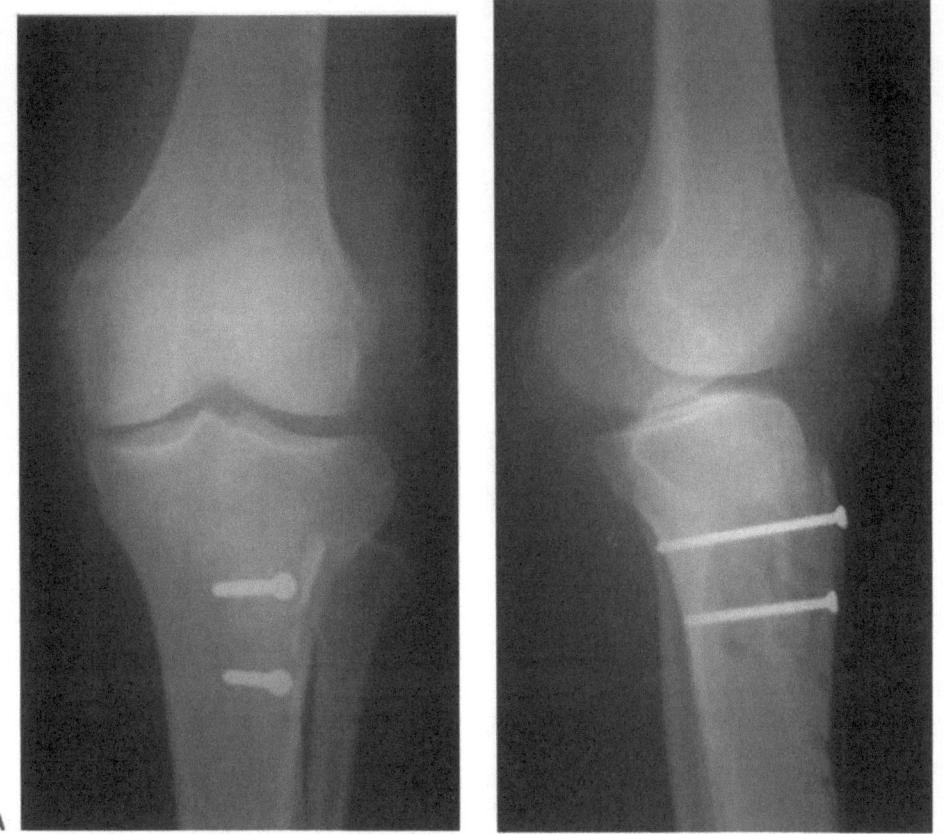

FIGURE C33.4 Postoperative anteroposterior (**A**) and lateral (**B**) radiographs demonstrate elevation and translation of the tibial tubercle.

34

PATHOLOGY
Bipolar focal chondral defects of the patellofemoral joint

TREATMENT
Autologous chondrocyte implantation of the patella and trochlea (Note that the use of ACI for the patella or for bipolar defects is considered off-label usage, but was indicated and performed with explicit patient informed consent.)

SUBMITTED BY
Jack Farr, MD, Cartilage Restoration Center of Indiana, OrthoIndy, Indianapolis, Indiana, USA

CHIEF COMPLAINT AND HISTORY OF PRESENT ILLNESS

The patient is a 28-year-old man who works in his family boiler company as an estimator/troubleshooter. He has a long history of bilateral patellofemoral pain, right worse than left. In his late teens he enjoyed basketball, but had to stop all sports because of severe anterior knee pain and limited his activities to level-ground walking. Review of the operative record reveals that 4 years before presentation, at age 24, he underwent a lateral release and anteromedialization (AMZ) procedure, which was performed with a steep slope osteotomy as malalignment was mild. The articular surfaces at that time were intact, except at the patellofemoral joint where contained grade III chondral defects were noted on the patella and trochlea, each measuring 2 cm by 2 cm. These lesions were treated with mechanical chondroplasty at the time of the AMZ. The patient had minimal symptoms until 2 years later when symptoms similar to his condition 4 years ago developed.

PHYSICAL EXAMINATION

Height, 6 ft, 10 in.; weight, 280 lb. Level-ground gait is normal. Mild symmetric valgus alignment is present. He has a well-healed incision from his prior AMZ. His range of motion is symmetric from 0 to 135 degrees of flexion. His ligament examination is normal. Patellar apprehension is absent. Tenderness is isolated to the patellofemoral joint, where there is 1 cm of medial and lateral displacement. Tilt is reversible to neutral.

RADIOGRAPHIC EVALUATION

Preoperative radiographs of his right knee reveal maintenance of tibiofemoral joint space with near-neutral alignment. Merchant view shows joint space maintenance and a central patella. Evidence of a prior AMZ with internal fixation is present (Figure C34.1).

SURGICAL INTERVENTION

Right knee arthroscopy revealed progression in the size and grade (to grade IV) of the chondral defects of both the patella and trochlea. The trochlea had an intralesional osteophyte treated with impaction (Figure C34.2). Cartilage biopsy was performed. Six weeks later, autologous chondrocyte implantation (ACI) was performed on the patella and trochlear lesions, both of which remained contained, grade IV, and measured 2.5 cm by 3 cm at each site (Figure C34.3).

Although he was allowed to flex his knee daily to 90 degrees, continuous passive motion was restricted to 45 to 60 degrees of flexion during its use for the first 4 postoperative weeks. He advanced through the traditional rehabilitation protocol for ACI of the patellofemoral joint allowing early weight bearing in extension. He was asked to refrain from any impact or ballistic activities for 18 months.

FOLLOW-UP

Postoperatively the patient had progressive diminution of pain. After his pain resolved, he slipped in mud and had acute, new onset medial joint line pain. The medial pain persisted and he was subsequently evaluated arthroscopically. Arthroscopy revealed the areas of ACI were filling with full peripheral integration (Figure C34.4). The medial pain resolved with debridement of impinging scar. At present he is without pain during activities of daily living, and his contralateral patellofemoral pain is now his main concern.

DECISION-MAKING FACTORS

1. Young, highly symptomatic patient with failed primary attempt to unload his patellofemoral joint.
2. Bipolar defect of the patellofemoral joint with no other treatment options other than possibly osteochondral allograft.
3. Bipolar contained lesions treated initially with AMZ in an effort to mechanically unload the defects.
4. Impaction of intralesional osteophyte preceding ACI versus burring at time of ACI in an effort to minimize bleeding.

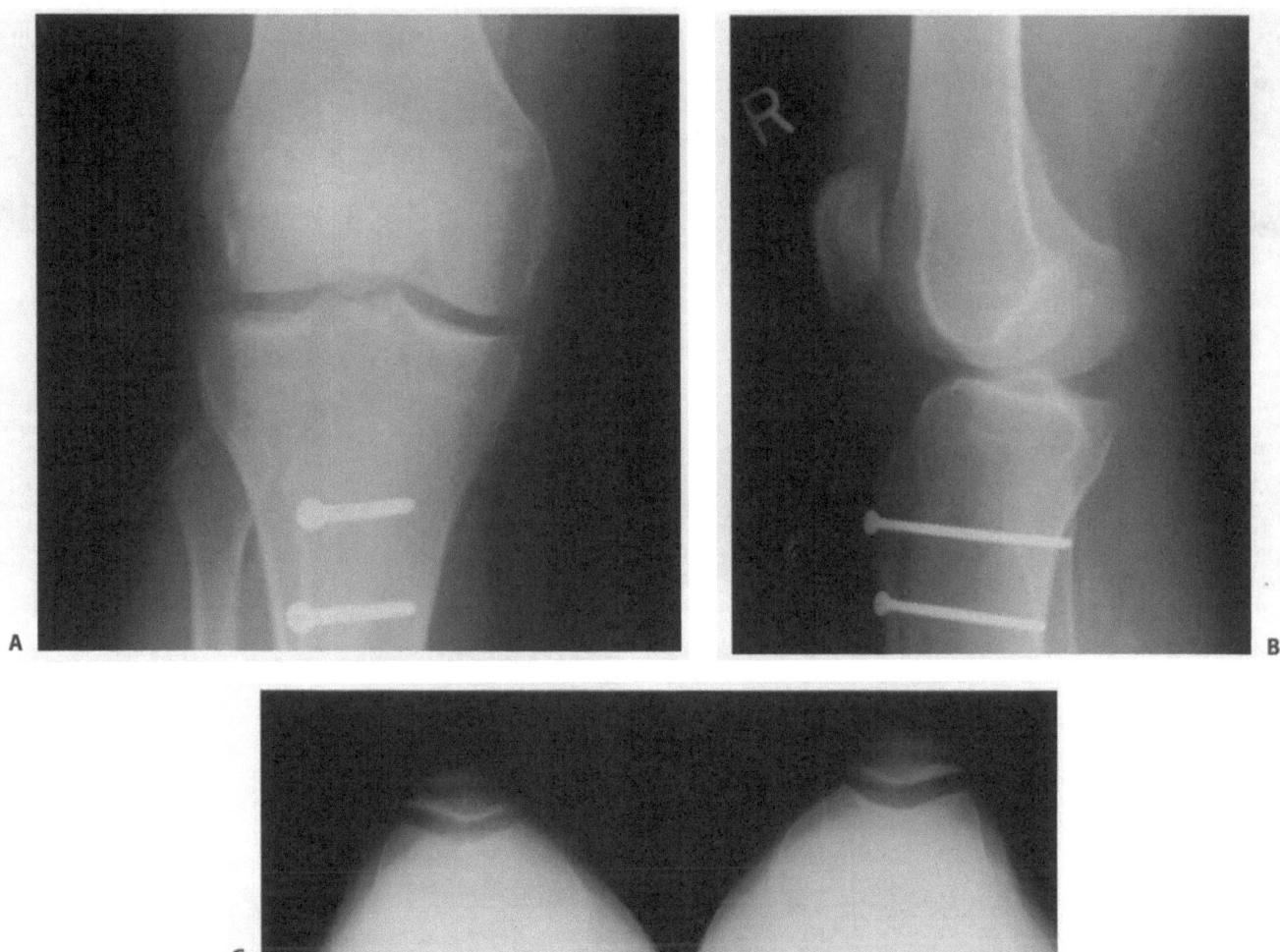

FIGURE C34.1 Radiographs after initial anteromedialization (AMZ) osteotomy. Anteroposterior (**A**), lateral (**B**), and Merchant (**C**) views show maintenance of joint space and central patella.

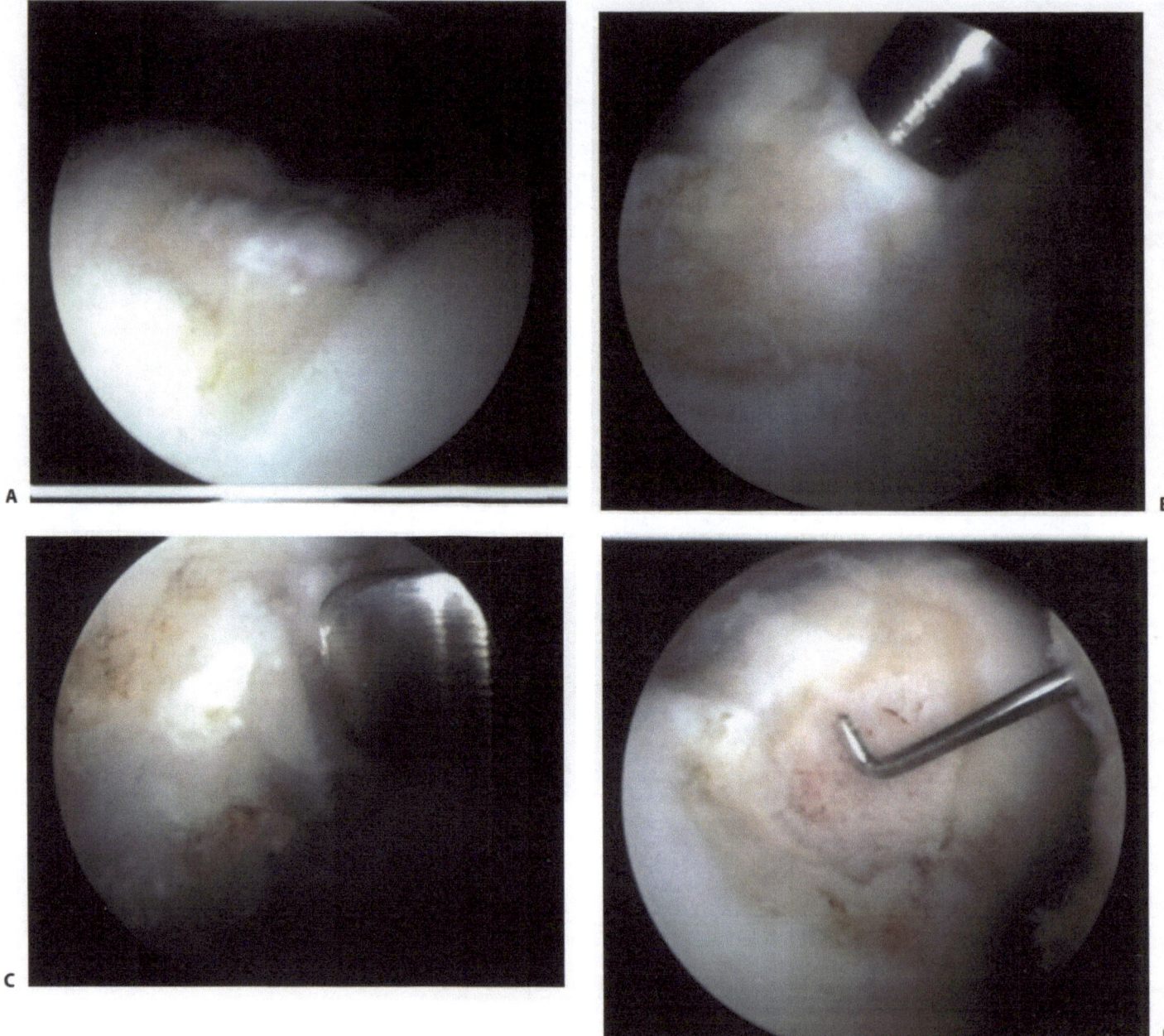

FIGURE C34.2 Intralesional trochlear osteophyte (**A**), raised appearance (**B**), impaction (**C**), and flush area of prior osteophyte (**D**).

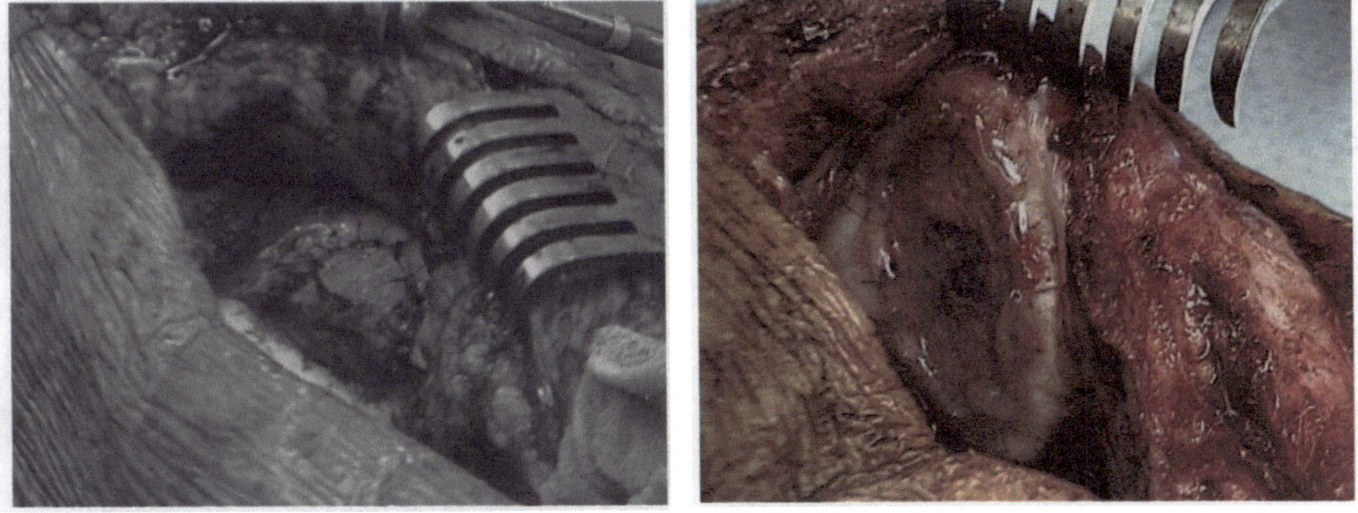

FIGURE C34.3 Intraoperative autologous chondrocyte implantation (ACI) patches in place in the (**A**) trochlea and (**B**) patella.

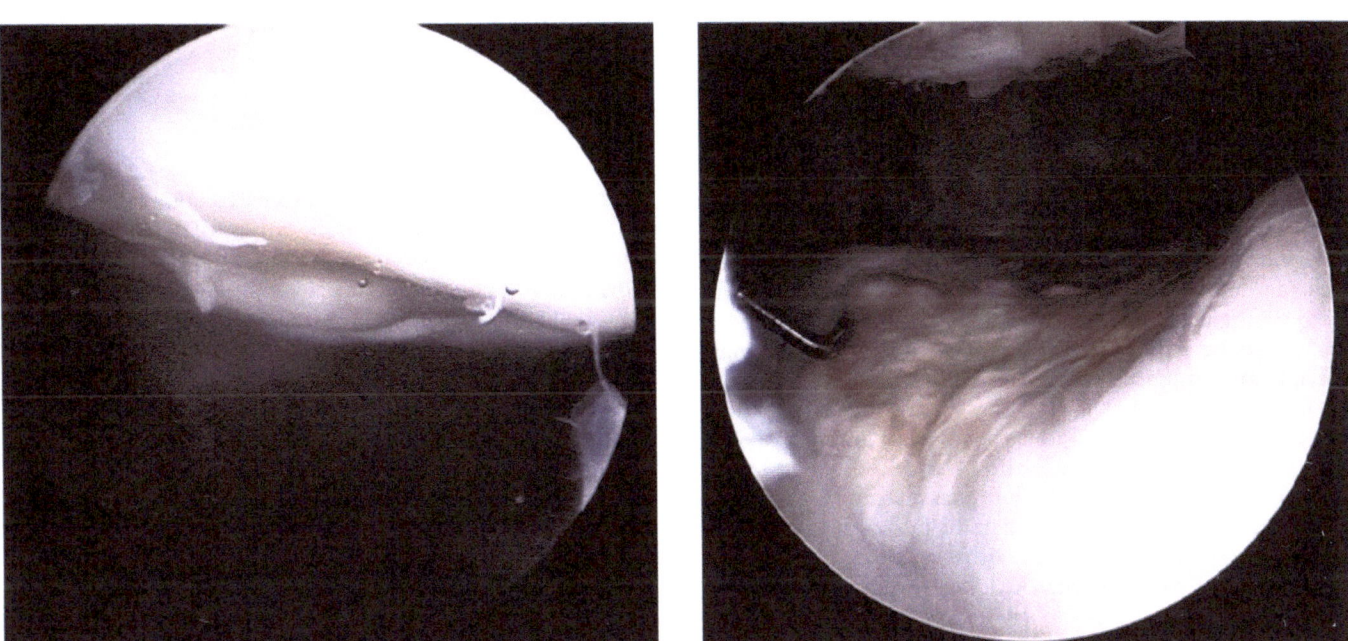

FIGURE C34.4 Second-look arthroscopic view of ACI filling both the (**A**) patellar and (**B**) trochlear defects.

35

PATHOLOGY
Lateral compartment tibiofemoral degenerative arthrosis

TREATMENT
Bipolar fresh osteochondral allograft transplant (At this juncture, the author, as do other surgeons who perform osteochondral allograft transplantation, assigns a significantly guarded prognosis to bipolar biologic resurfacing operations. These surgeons obtain full patient informed consent regarding the guarded prognosis and proceed with surgery only under the auspice that revision to arthroplasty is not knowingly compromised should the allograft fail.)

SUBMITTED BY
Jack Farr, MD, Cartilage Restoration Center of Indiana, OrthoIndy, Indianapolis, Indiana, USA

CHIEF COMPLAINT AND HISTORY OF PRESENT ILLNESS

This patient is a 38-year-old male construction supervisor who is referred for consideration of autologous chondrocyte implantation (ACI) to treat persistently symptomatic chondrosis of the left knee at the site of an old lateral compartment injury. His pain has gradually increased to the point where he can only walk short distances with a cane and an unloader brace. He is on partial disability as he can only perform sitting duties at work. Review of his history revealed a distant sports injury, which was treated with arthroscopic partial lateral meniscectomy. His pain gradually recurred, and he underwent another arthroscopy where a lateral femoral condyle grade IV chondral lesion measuring 2.5 cm by 2.5 cm was treated with abrasion arthroplasty. Additional lateral meniscus was also removed. The tibial plateau was intact at that time. The patient was evaluated for cartilage restoration options and elected to proceed with staging arthroscopy and probable harvest of biopsy for ACI. Insurance appeals delayed staging surgery for 1.5 years.

PHYSICAL EXAMINATION

Height, 5 ft, 10 in.; weight, 165 lb. Gait on the left is severely antalgic even with use of a cane and unloader brace. No effusion is noted. Clinical alignment is in neutral. Range of motion demonstrates 5 degrees of flexion loss compared to the contralateral knee. His ligament examination is normal. Pain is isolated to the lateral joint line without mechanical symptoms. Patellar tracking is normal.

RADIOGRAPHIC EVALUATION

Marked lateral joint space narrowing is noted on 45-degree posteroanterior weight-bearing radiographs. Only mild joint space narrowing is noted on anteroposterior films, and no osteophytes are noted. Alignment is 2 degrees of varus.

SURGICAL INTERVENTION

At arthroscopy, there was new extensive involvement of the tibial plateau with exposed bone without lateral or posterior containment. Evidence of a complete prior lateral meniscectomy was present. The lateral femoral condyle had exposed bone evident with knee flexion past 90 degrees (Figure C35.1). ACI biopsy was not performed in light of the extensive nature of the chondrosis, uncontained lesions, and progression to bipolar status. At the time of definitive treatment, the arthritic regions of the distal femoral condyle and proximal tibial plateau were osteotomized in preparation for fresh osteochondral allograft transplantation. The surgical exposure was facilitated by tibial tubercle osteotomy and osteotomy of the femoral insertion of the lateral collateral ligament and popliteus tendon as well as Gerdy's tubercle (Figure C35.2). Fresh osteochondral shell allografts were prepared and implanted. These grafts included the lateral femoral condyle and lateral tibial plateau with the attached lateral meniscus (Figure C35.3).

Postoperatively, the patient was made nonweight bearing for 8 weeks. Continuous passive motion was used immediately with early efforts to regain full range of motion. Any consideration for high-impact activities was delayed for 18 months.

FOLLOW-UP

Eight-week postoperative radiographs revealed initial graft incorporation and maintenance of joint spaces (Figure C35.4). At 8 months, the patient regained full motion and is ambulating without an aid and without pain.

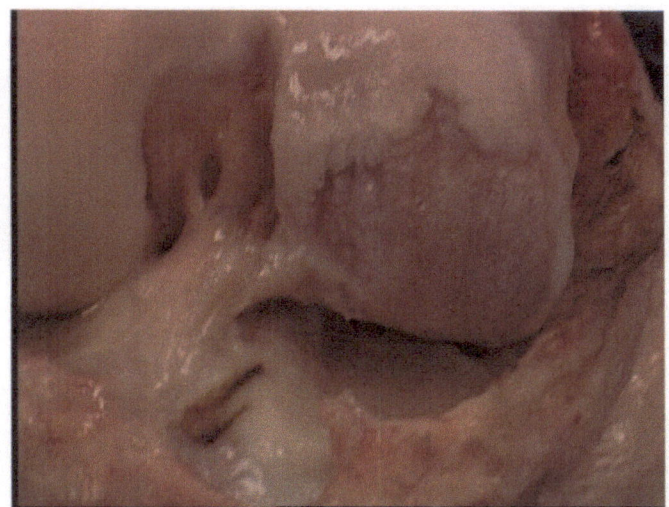

FIGURE C35.1 Intraoperative photograph demonstrates exposed bone of the distal lateral femoral condyle and absent lateral meniscus.

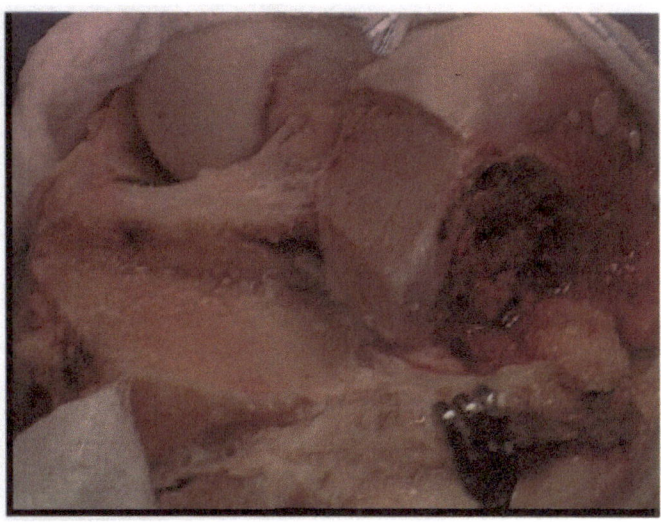

FIGURE C35.2 Host prepared with minimal bone resection of the distal femoral condyle and proximal tibial plateau. Note osteotomized origin of the lateral collateral ligament and popliteus tendon.

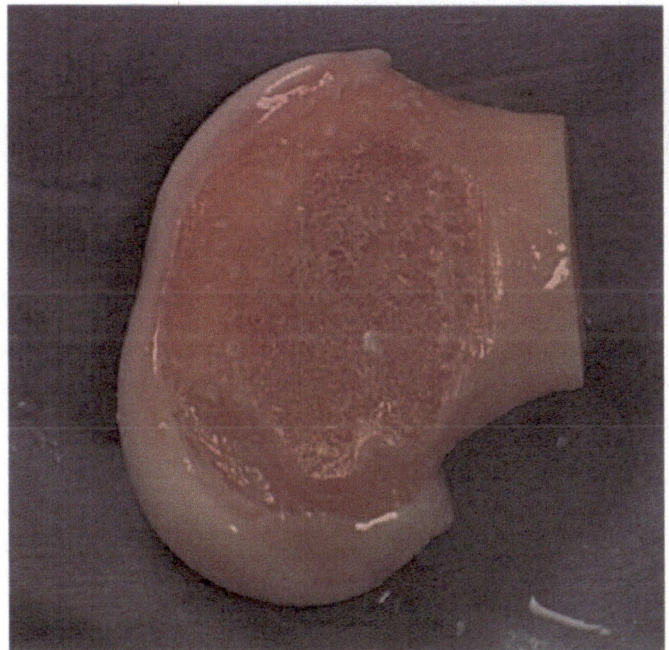

A

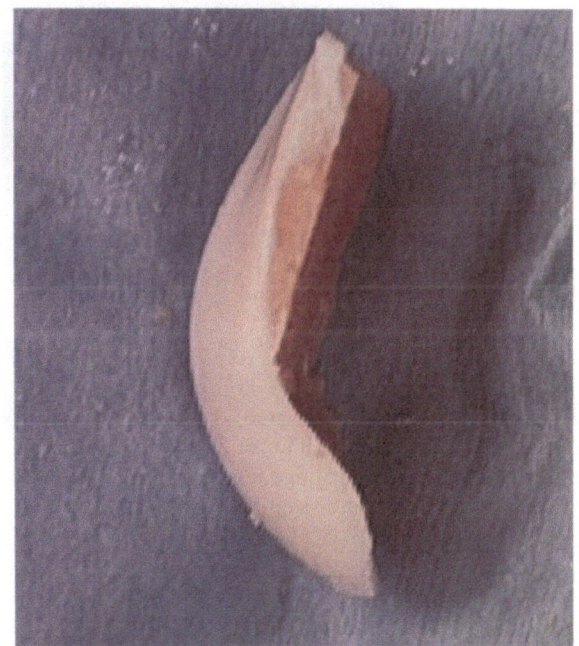

B

FIGURE C35.3 Fresh lateral femoral condyle osteochondral allograft before (**A**) and after (**B**) preparation. (**C**) Distal lateral femoral condyle and composite tibial plateau allograft in place fixed with cortical bone pins.

C

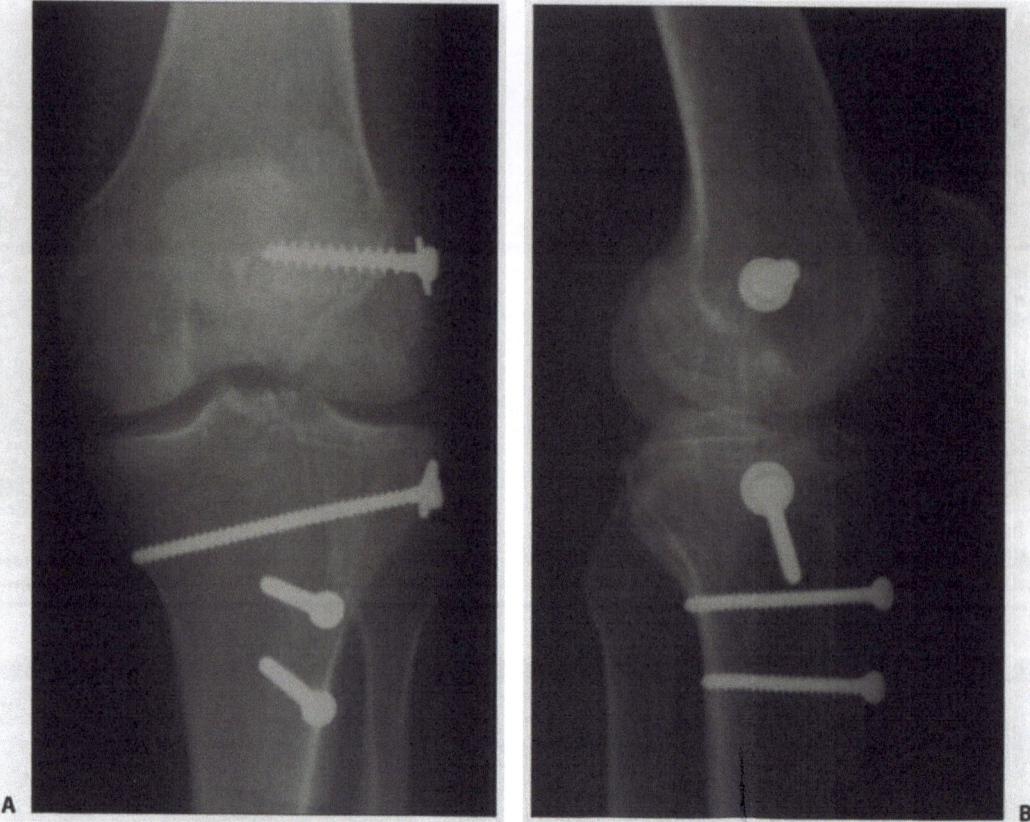

FIGURE C35.4 Postoperative anteroposterior (**A**) and lateral (**B**) radiographs. Note cortical bone pins and fixation of osteotomized lateral epicondyle, Gerdy's tubercle, and tibial tubercle fragment.

DECISION-MAKING FACTORS

1. Relatively young, but severely symptomatic individual with unicompartmental pathology.
2. Young age as a relative contraindication to arthroplasty (i.e., unicompartmental or total knee arthroplasty).
3. Bipolar disease with large uncontained lesions as a relative contraindication to ACI.
4. Neutral to varus alignment eliminating distal femoral osteotomy as a legitimate solution.
5. Absent lateral meniscus in addition to degenerative tibial plateau requiring replacement with composite meniscus and osteoarticular graft.

36

PATHOLOGY
Isolated patellofemoral arthritis

TREATMENT
Bipolar patellofemoral fresh osteochondral allograft with distal realignment (At this juncture, the author, as do other surgeons who perform osteochondral allograft transplantation, assigns a significantly guarded prognosis to bipolar biologic resurfacing operations. These surgeons obtain full patient informed consent regarding the guarded prognosis and proceed with surgery only under the auspice that revision to arthroplasty is not knowingly compromised should the allograft fail.)

SUBMITTED BY
Jack Farr, MD, Cartilage Restoration Center of Indiana, OrthoIndy, Indianapolis, Indiana, USA

CHIEF COMPLAINT AND HISTORY OF PRESENT ILLNESS

This patient is a 37-year-old female nurse who presented with progressive patellofemoral pain of her right knee. She had intermittent pain since a medial arthrotomy was performed 22 years previously to treat a "crushed" patella she sustained from direct impact. Her pain increases with any increase in activity. She experiences marked pain at the end of an 8-hour nursing shift. She is unable to perform squats or climb stairs. Repeated attempts at rehabilitation failed to reduce her symptoms.

PHYSICAL EXAMINATION

Height, 5 ft, 5 in.; weight, 135 lb; body mass index of 23. She ambulates with an antalgic gait. Limb alignment is neutral. She is unable to step up on a 6-in. step secondary to pain. Range of motion is from 5 to 130 degrees of flexion. Pain and crepitus are limited to the patellofemoral joint. She has no patellar apprehension. Her ligament examination is normal. Meniscal findings are absent. Quadriceps bulk is near normal.

RADIOGRAPHIC EVALUATION

Posteroanterior 45-degree flexion weight-bearing radiographs demonstrate neutral alignment with no joint space narrowing. Merchant views demonstrate patellofemoral arthritis in the right knee with no significant subluxation or tilt (Figure C36.1), but there is joint space narrowing at the medial aspect of the patellofemoral articulation.

SURGICAL INTERVENTION

At the staging arthroscopy, the entire trochlea had grade III and IV change and the medial 60% of the patella had grade III–IV change. Both the lesions were diffuse and incompletely contained (Figure C36.2). The tibiofemoral joint was normal. The patient then underwent patellofemoral resurfacing with fresh osteochondral shell allografts (Figure C36.3). Milled cortical allograft bone pins were used for fixation. The exposure was through a steep anteromedialization of the tibial tubercle, which allowed the patella to remain central while the tubercle was elevated in an attempt to potentially decrease the load on the allograft shells.

Postoperatively, the patient was made weight bearing as tolerated with two crutches using a hinged brace set at 0 to 30 degrees for protection. Continuous passive motion was used for 3 weeks, with early full range of motion allowed immediately as tolerated. Return to unrestricted activities was permitted after 6 months.

FOLLOW-UP

The patient is nearly symptom free with maintenance of transplant position and joint space (Figure C36.4). She has minimal patellofemoral crepitus, and range of motion is comparable to her preoperative evaluation.

DECISION-MAKING FACTORS

1. Relatively young, active individual with specific symptoms related to isolated posttraumatic patellofemoral osteoarthritis.

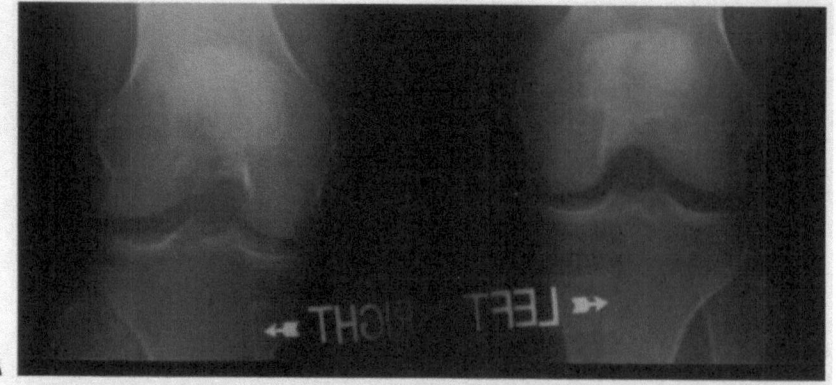

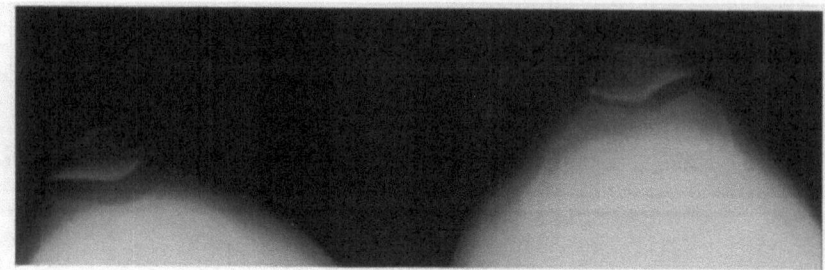

FIGURE C36.1 Preoperative posteroanterior 45-degree flexion weight-bearing (**A**) and Merchant (**B**) radiographs demonstrate isolated patellofemoral arthritis with significant joint space narrowing of the right knee.

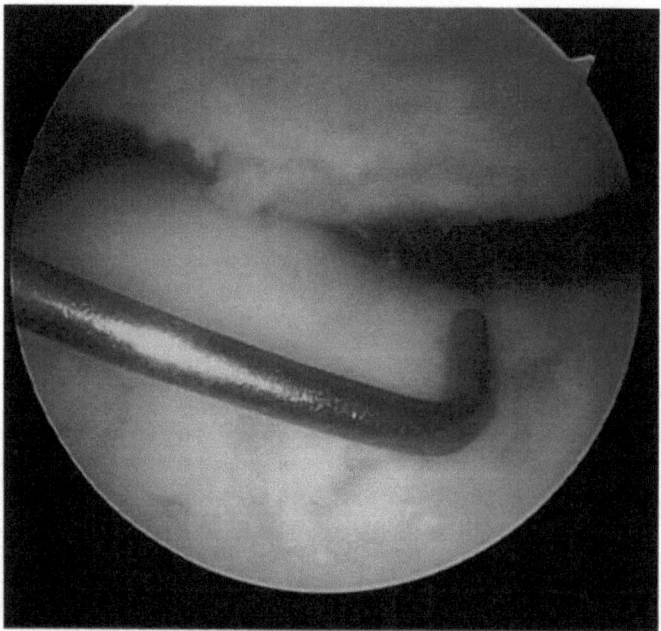

FIGURE C36.2 Staging arthroscopy demonstrates the extensive loss of patellofemoral articular cartilage.

2. Young age as a relative contraindication to arthroplasty (i.e., patellofemoral or total knee arthroplasty).
3. Bipolar defects that are large, diffuse, and incompletely contained, virtually eliminating other cartilage restoration procedures as viable options.
4. Unloading considerations as a part of patellofemoral cartilage restoration include a steep oblique anteromedialization to protect and unload the healing grafts.

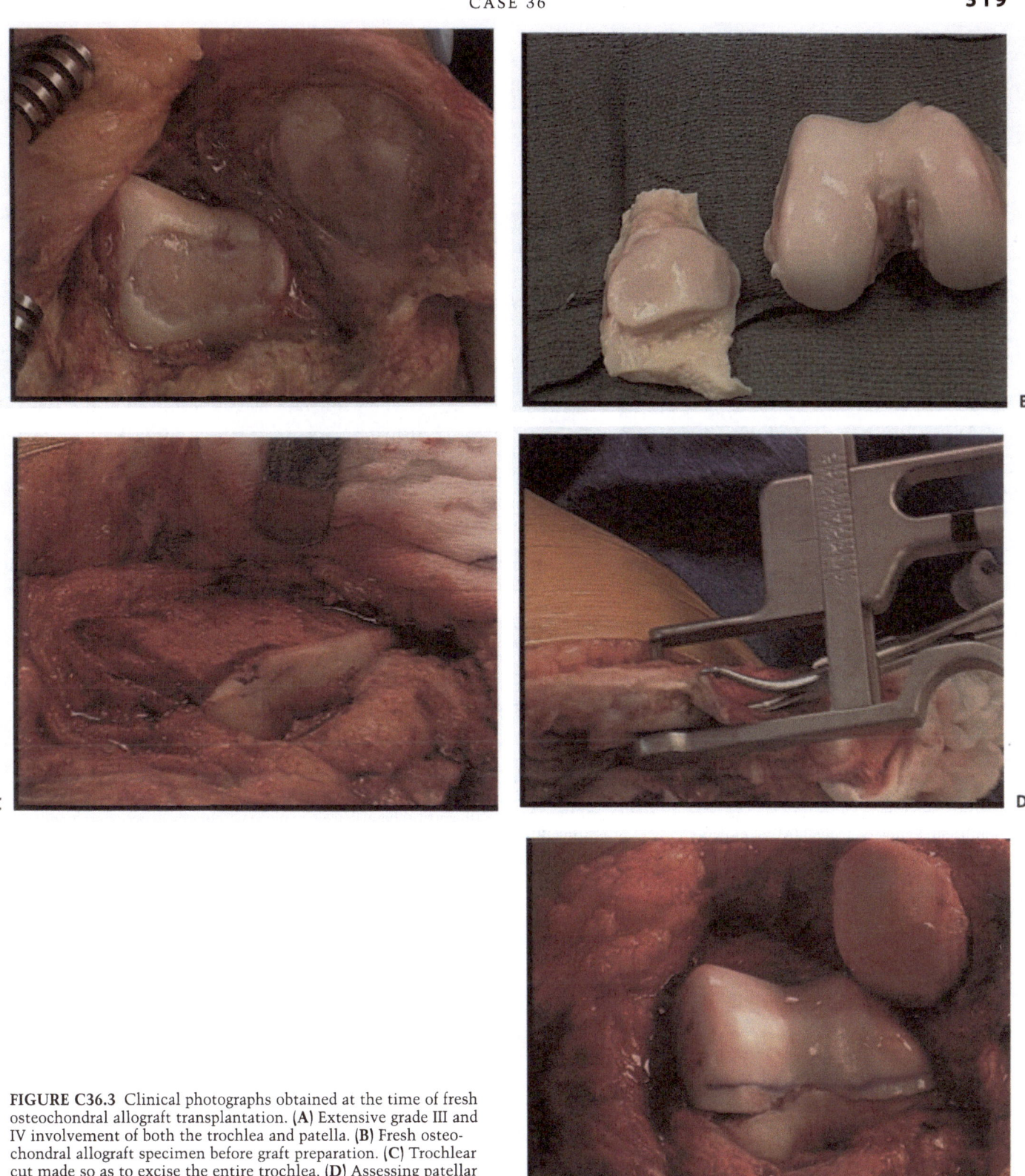

FIGURE C36.3 Clinical photographs obtained at the time of fresh osteochondral allograft transplantation. **(A)** Extensive grade III and IV involvement of both the trochlea and patella. **(B)** Fresh osteochondral allograft specimen before graft preparation. **(C)** Trochlear cut made so as to excise the entire trochlea. **(D)** Assessing patellar thickness to determine osteotomy site. **(E)** Matching osteochondral allografts fashioned and secured to host.

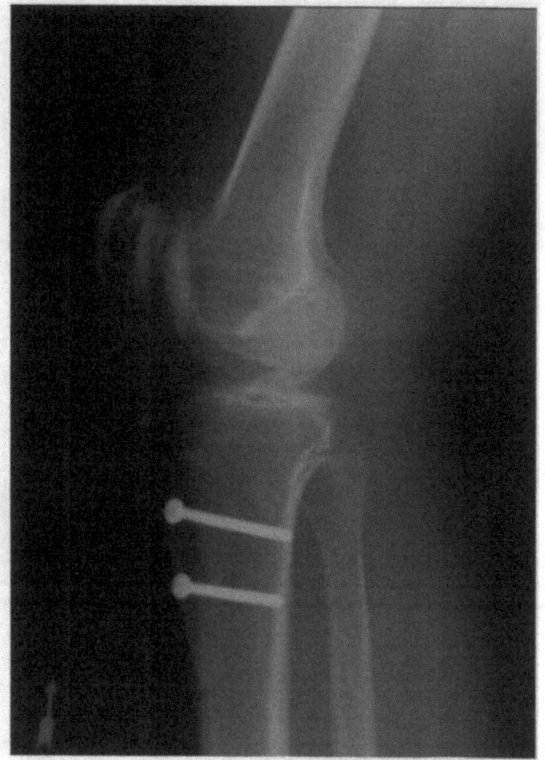

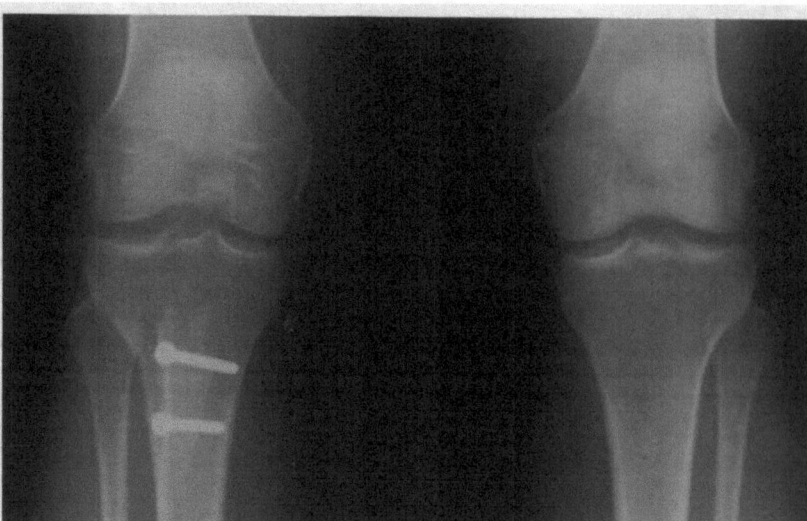

FIGURE C36.4 Postoperative radiographs obtained within the first 3 months after surgery. Lateral (**A**), anteroposterior weight-bearing (**B**), and Merchant (**C**) views demonstrate anatomic placement of the graft with cortical bone dowels in place without evidence of graft collapse or dislodgement.

37

PATHOLOGY
Posttraumatic medial femoral condyle defect, varus instability, and deformity with significant motion loss

TREATMENT
Open release, staged fresh osteochondral allograft transplantation with medial opening-wedge high tibial osteotomy followed by lateral collateral ligament reconstruction

SUBMITTED BY
Brian J. Cole, MD, MBA, Rush Cartilage Restoration Center, Rush University Medical Center, Chicago, Illinois, USA

CHIEF COMPLAINT AND HISTORY OF PRESENT ILLNESS

The patient is a 26-year-old man who sustained a high-energy injury to the lateral aspect of his right knee when a tree trunk struck him while he was working as a tree trimmer. This injury was documented as a lateral-sided ligament injury with an intraarticular fracture of the medial femoral condyle. Initial treatment included open reduction and internal fixation of a medial femoral condyle fracture. Postoperatively, he was made nonweight bearing and his knee was immobilized for several weeks, leading to significant motion loss. At his initial presentation 6 months following this operation, he complained of significant knee stiffness, instability, and medial-sided right knee pain.

PHYSICAL EXAMINATION

Height. 5 ft, 6 in.; weight, 150 lb. Examination of the right knee reveals significant varus alignment with a flexed-knee antalgic gait accompanied by a lateral thrust (e.g., triple varus thrust) (Figure C37.1). His incisions are well healed without any signs of infection. He has a 20-degree flexion contracture and cannot flex past 90 degrees. His patellar mobility is severely limited. He has significant medial joint line and femoral condyle tenderness. On stress testing, he has grade 2 varus instability with an endpoint, and minimal increases in external rotation at 30 and 90 degrees of flexion compared to the contralateral side. His reverse pivot shift and posterior drawer tests are negative. His anterior cruciate ligament (ACL) examination is normal. He is neurovascularly intact distally.

RADIOGRAPHIC EVALUATION

Initial radiographs obtained 6 months following his open reduction demonstrated limited internal fixation of his medial femoral condyle fracture with a significant defect remaining along the central weight-bearing zone (Figure C37.2). Long-leg alignment views obtained following hardware removal and open release of adhesions demonstrated a varus deformity measuring 12 degrees of mechanical axis varus (Figure C37.3).

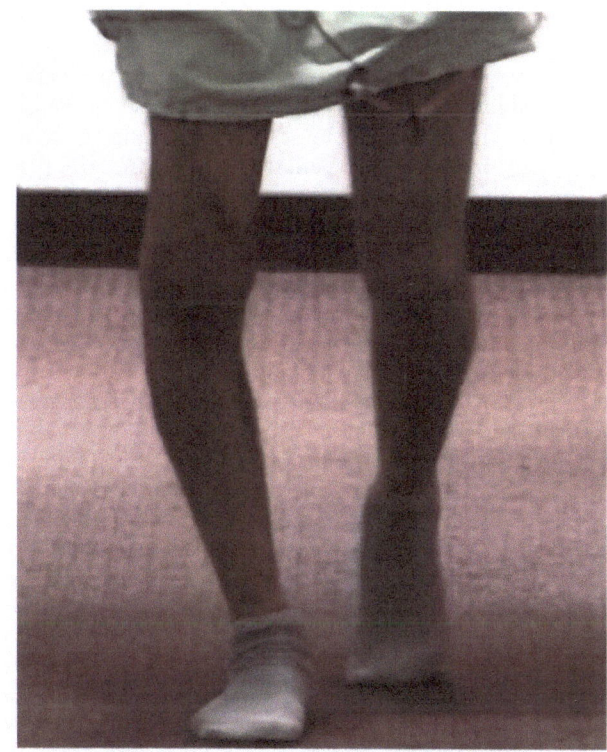

FIGURE C37.1 Clinical photograph obtained during gait demonstrates significant dynamic varus thrust of the patient's right knee due to lateral collateral ligament insufficiency and osteochondral defect of the medial femoral condyle.

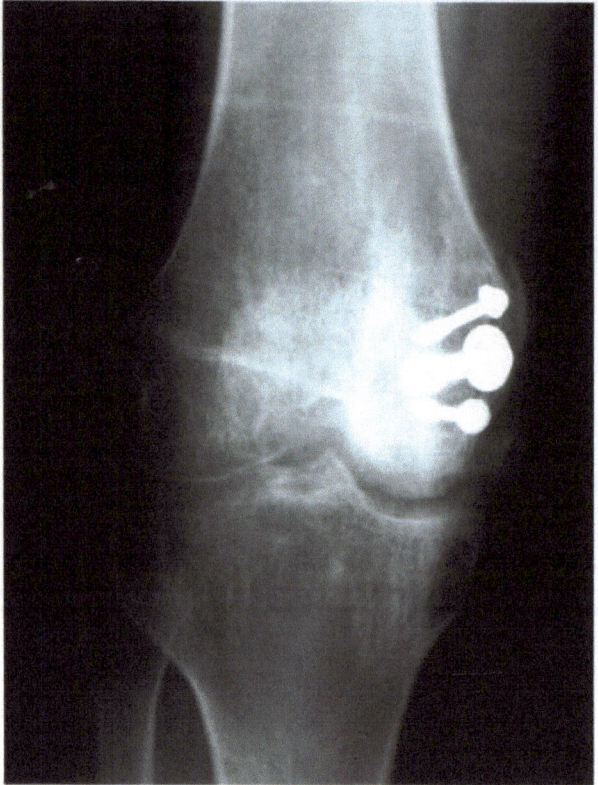 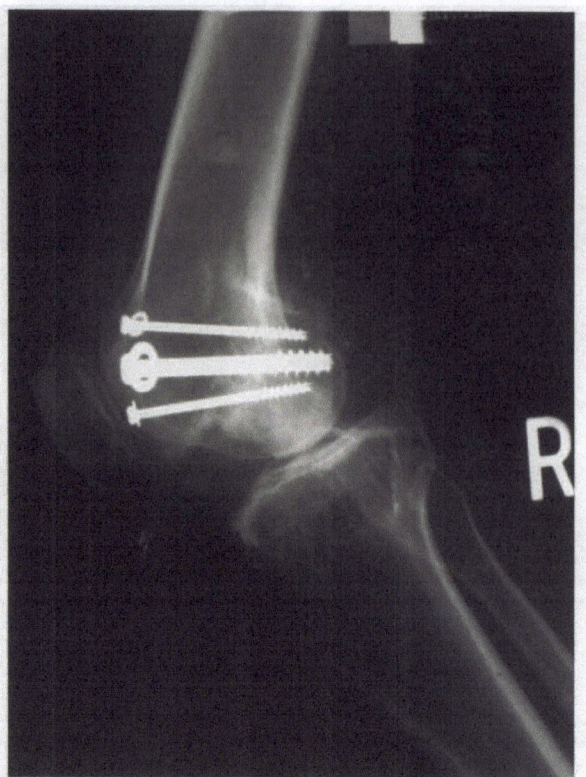

A   B

FIGURE C37.2 Anteroposterior (**A**) and lateral (**B**) radiographs obtained 6 months after open reduction and internal fixation of the medial femoral condyle fracture demonstrate residual osteochondral defect along the weight-bearing aspect of the medial femoral condyle. Also noted is significant osteopenia resulting from a prolonged period of protected weight bearing.

SURGICAL INTERVENTION

Three issues were particularly concerning in this patient: motion loss, varus instability, and a posttraumatic defect of his medial femoral condyle. Initially, the principal focus was on helping the patient regain a functional range of motion. Because of the significant periarticular scarring, the patient underwent his second surgical procedure, which included an arthrotomy, removal of his hardware, extensive intraarticular release, manipulation under anesthesia, and placement in a well-padded long-leg hyperextension cast. Evaluation of his articular surfaces (Figure C37.4) demonstrated a large medial femoral condyle defect measuring 30 mm by 30 mm with more than 10 mm of subchondral bone loss. Following cast removal at 3 days, the patient was placed in an aggressive physical therapy program.

Four months following his open release, his flexion contracture was reduced to 5 degrees and he obtained nearly 120 degrees of flexion. He continued to complain of significant medial knee pain and varus instability. At that time he was indicated for an opening-wedge high tibial osteotomy and fresh osteochondral allograft transplant of his medial femoral condyle. Any attempts to reconstruct his lateral collateral ligament were delayed because of the possibility that the osteotomy might reduce or eliminate his complaints of varus instability and because of the significant risk of recurrent stiffness following the necessary rehabilitation and protection required of this procedure.

Thus, his third surgery, occurring approximately 1 year after his initial injury, included a 15-degree opening-wedge

medial high tibial osteotomy with an iliac crest bone graft and a 30 mm by 30 mm fresh osteochondral shell allograft transplant (Figure C37.5). A headless cannulated compression screw was used to supplement the press-fit fixation of the osteochondral graft.

His knee pain and motion continued to improve over the ensuing 6 months and, despite radiographic evidence of healing at the osteotomy site with valgus alignment (Figure C37.6), he continued to complain of some varus instability, albeit significantly less than his preoperative level of instability. Seven months following the transplant and osteotomy, the patient underwent second-look arthroscopy (Figure C37.7) and a lateral ligament reconstruction using a hamstring allograft fixed at the isometric point of the lateral femoral condyle and passed through the proximal fibula in a figure-of-eight configuration (Figure C37.8). A 1-mm biopsy of the fresh osteochondral allograft was obtained at that time (Figure C37.9). Postoperatively, the patient was made protected weight bearing in an extension brace for the first 6 weeks and progressed to weight bearing and activities as tolerated over the ensuing 6 months.

FOLLOW-UP

At his 18-month follow-up evaluation, he achieved nearly full extension with 120 degrees of flexion. His knee was stable to varus stress in extension and various degrees of flexion. He continues to have a slightly antalgic gait, but complains of no pain along the medial side of his knee. Although he states he

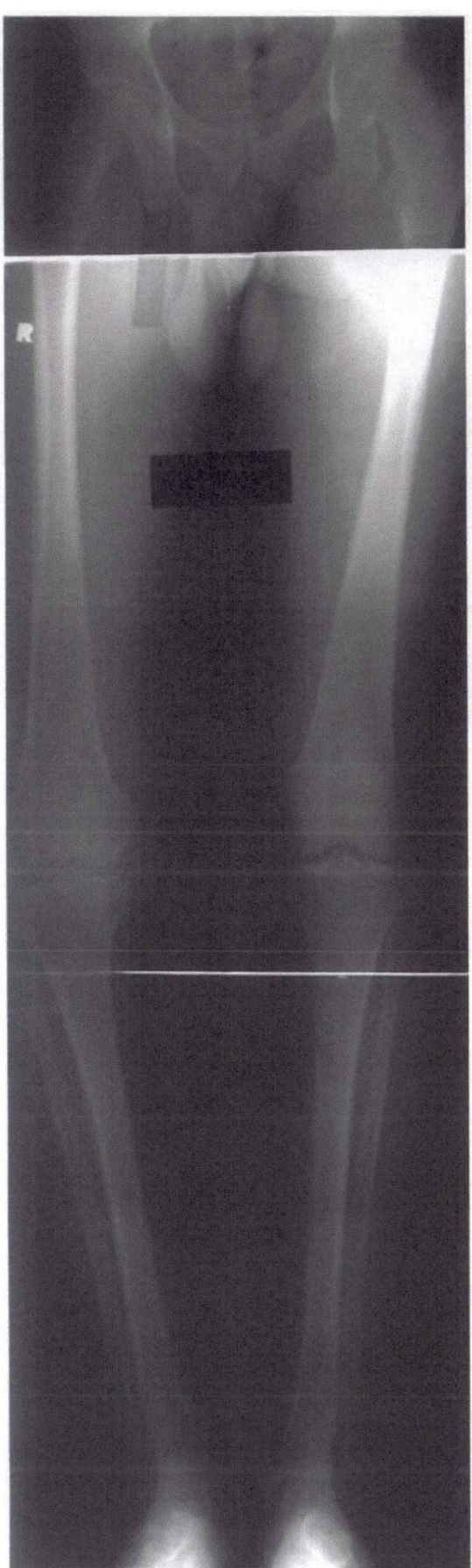

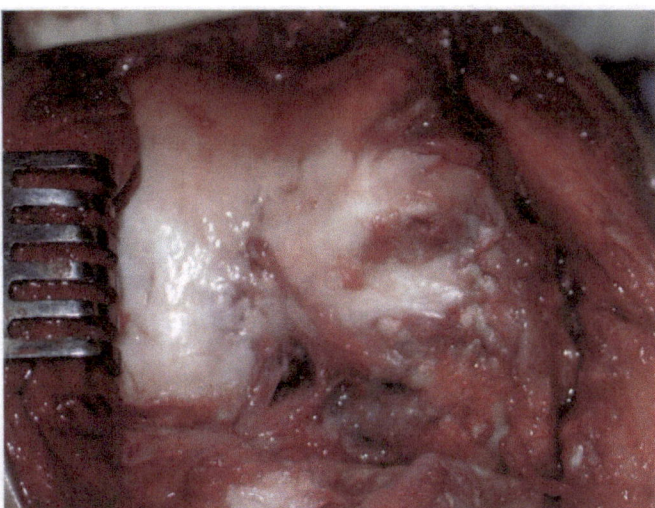

FIGURE C37.4 Intraoperative photograph obtained during the arthrotomy, lysis of adhesions, and hardware removal which was required to regain functional range of motion and prepare for future reconstruction procedures. Note the significant osteochondral defect of the medial femoral condyle measuring approximately 30 mm by 30 mm.

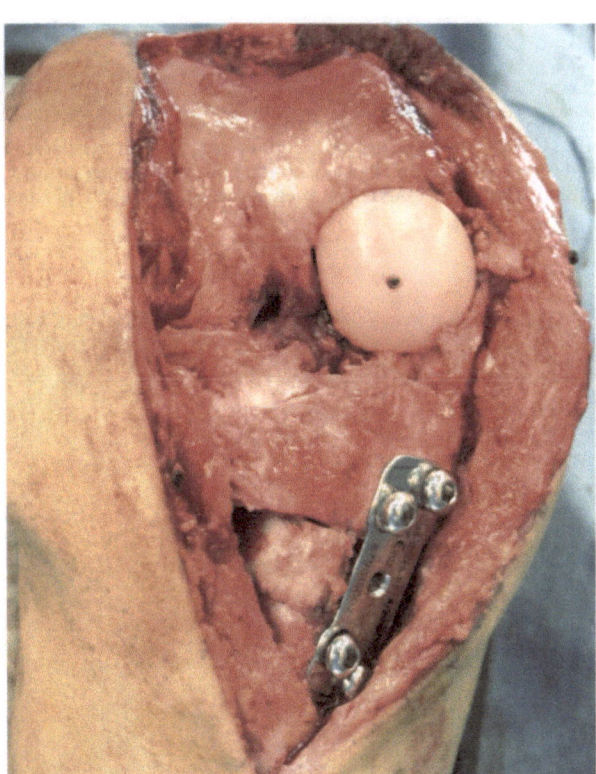

FIGURE C37.5 Intraoperative photograph obtained following placement of the fresh osteochondral allograft and completion of the medial opening-wedge high tibial osteotomy. Note the tricortical iliac crest bone autograft positioned within the osteotomy site.

FIGURE C37.3 Long-leg weight-bearing mechanical axis radiograph obtained following arthrotomy and hardware removal. Note the significant static varus deformity of the right knee due to the lateral collateral ligament insufficiency and osteochondral defect of the medial femoral condyle.

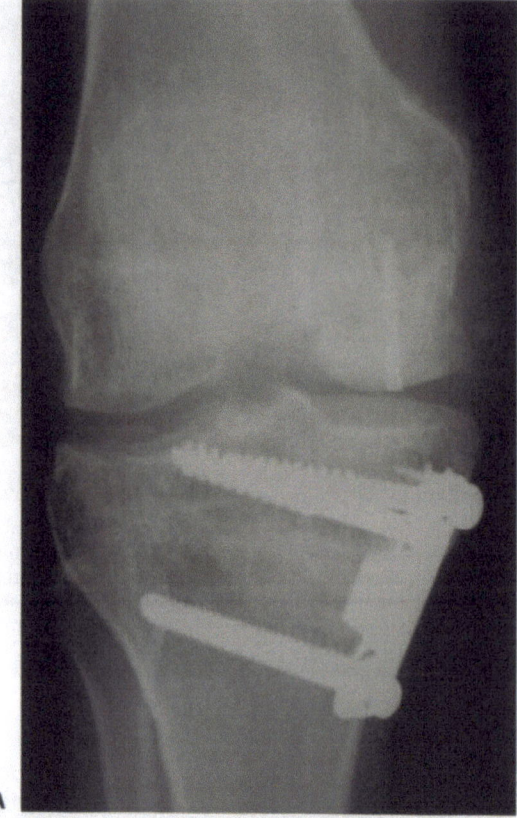
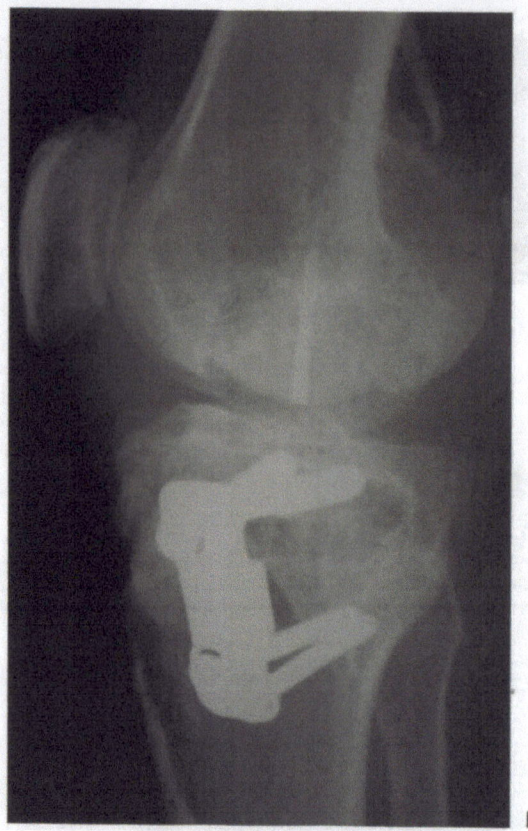

A

B

FIGURE C37.6 Anteroposterior **(A)** and lateral **(B)** radiographs obtained 6 months after fresh osteochondral allograft transplantation of the medial femoral condyle and medial opening-wedge high tibial osteotomy. Note evidence of graft integration without evidence of collapse and bony union at the osteotomy site.

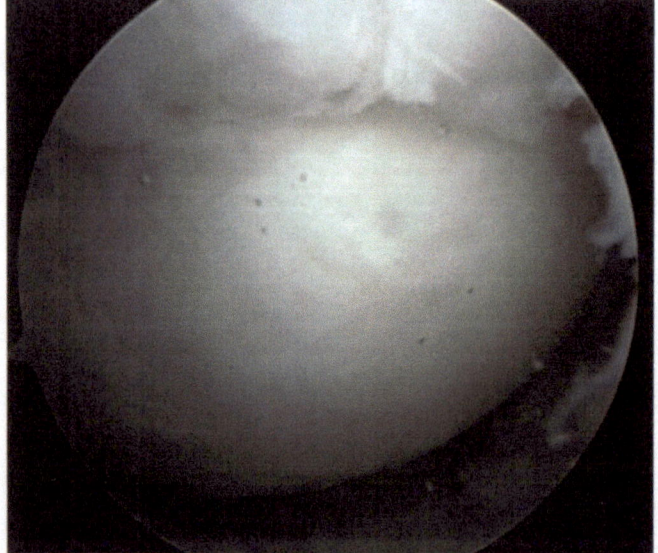

FIGURE C37.7 Arthroscopic view of the medial femoral condyle obtained 7 months following osteochondral allograft transplantation. Note the lack of any articular degeneration of the allograft transplant.

is significantly improved compared to the results following his open reduction and internal fixation, he feels he is not yet able to return to work where climbing and squatting would be required. He continues to participate in an aggressive home exercise program.

DECISION-MAKING FACTORS

1. High-energy injury young, active, male laborer resulting in significant osteochondral defect and varus instability.
2. A requirement to restore motion before articular reconstruction.
3. Large osteochondral defect requiring structural support considered less amenable to other cartilage restoration techniques.
4. Varus alignment requiring medial high tibial osteotomy to correct the deformity, protect the cartilage allograft, and potentially eliminate symptoms of varus instability.
5. Delayed reconstruction of the lateral collateral ligament due to the opposing early-phase rehabilitation compared to the early and full range of motion required following osteochondral allograft transplantation. In addition, the potential for eliminating the need for ligament reconstruction altogether because of the corrective effects of the opening-wedge high tibial osteotomy.

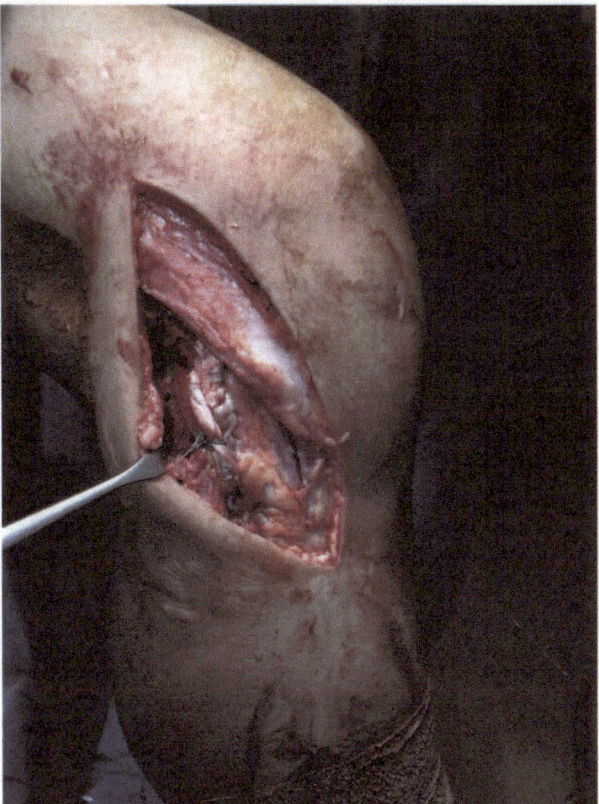

FIGURE C37.8 Intraoperative photograph of the lateral collateral ligament reconstruction using a hamstring allograft. Note graft fixed at isometric point of femur and through a drill hole in the proximal fibula with bioabsorbable screw placed within the fibular tunnel.

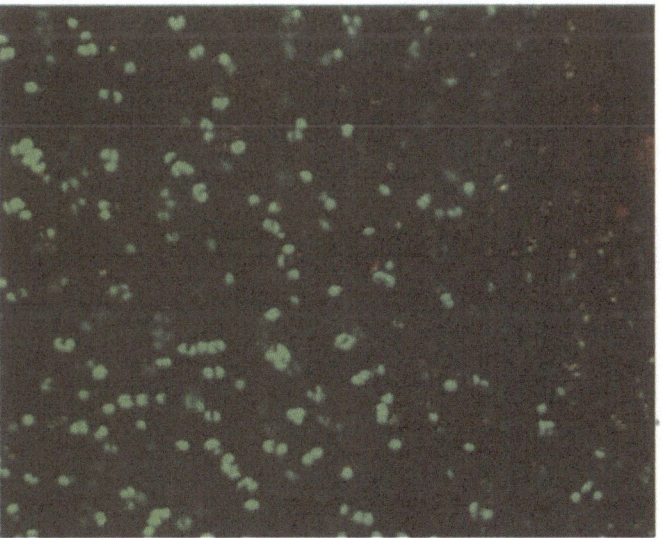

FIGURE C37.9 Biopsy obtained at second-look arthroscopy. Live/dead cell technique analyzed using confocal light microscopy demonstrates a large number of living donor chondrocytes (*green cells*) with minimal evidence of cell death (*red cells*) and maintenance of the cartilage architecture. 10× original magnification. (Courtesy of James M. Williams, PhD, Rush University)

38

PATHOLOGY
Chondral defects with prior medial and lateral meniscectomy and varus alignment

TREATMENT
Staged high tibial osteotomy followed by single-stage autologous chondrocyte implantation and medial and lateral meniscus allograft transplantation

SUBMITTED BY
Jack Farr, MD, Cartilage Restoration Center of Indiana, OrthoIndy, Indianapolis, Indiana, USA

CHIEF COMPLAINT AND HISTORY OF PRESENT ILLNESS

The patient is a 38-year-old medical salesperson who presented with progressive bilateral tibiofemoral joint line pain and activity-related swelling of his right knee. He had a history of medial and lateral meniscectomies performed at the time of anterior cruciate ligament (ACL) reconstruction approximately 8 years earlier. He had no functional instability and initially maintained an active lifestyle including running and basketball, until the gradual onset of medial greater than lateral joint line pain occurred. He has eliminated impact activities and changed to biking and swimming.

PHYSICAL EXAMINATION

Height, 5 ft, 8 in.; weight, 146 lb. Gait of right limb is stiff and mildly antalgic. Clinical alignment is varus with excellent muscle bulk and tone. The knee has a trace effusion. Range of motion is from 5 to 135 degrees of flexion. He has medial and lateral joint line tenderness without patellofemoral findings. His ligament examination is normal. His patellar tracking is normal.

RADIOGRAPHIC EVALUATION

Radiographs demonstrate prior ACL reconstruction with isolated joint space narrowing of the right knee medial compartment (Figure C38.1). Standing hip-to-ankle alignment films show 6 degrees of varus.

SURGICAL INTERVENTION

At staging arthroscopy, focal grade III to IV chondral lesions of the trochlea (1.5 cm by 2.3 cm) and medial femoral condyle

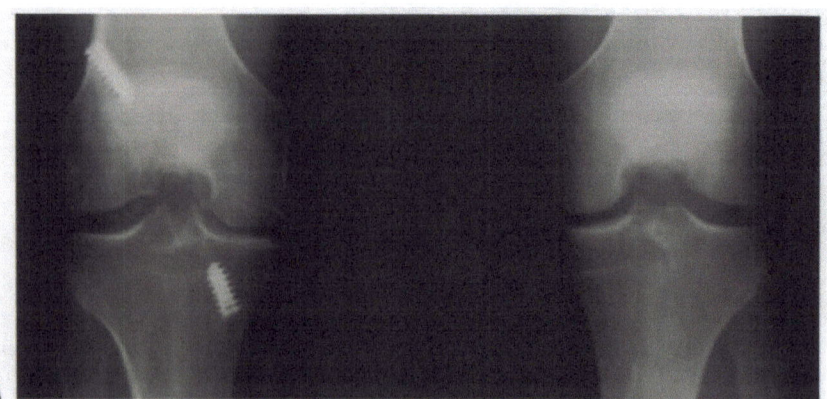

FIGURE C38.1 Preoperative 45-degree flexion weight-bearing posteroanterior (**A**) and Merchant (**B**) views demonstrate prior evidence of anterior cruciate ligament (ACL) reconstruction and minimal medial joint space narrowing.

(1.5 cm by 2.5 cm) were identified. Both menisci were essentially absent. The ACL graft was intact. In light of the varus alignment and medial pathology greater than lateral, the limb was treated at the time of staging arthroscopy with high tibial valgus-producing osteotomy using an opening-wedge hemicallotasis technique with an external fixator. The goal was to correct alignment such that the weight-bearing line would just enter the lateral compartment (Figure C38.2). Cartilage restoration was performed after the osteotomy had healed. Autologous chondrocyte implantation (ACI) was performed on the trochlea and medial femoral condyle defects (Figure C38.3). The medial and lateral meniscal transplants were performed through the same arthrotomy as the ACI, using tibial tubercle osteotomy for exposure and not for realignment (Figure C38.4).

Postoperatively, the patient was made nonweight bearing for 4 weeks and used immediate continuous passive motion during that time for 6 h/day. After 4 weeks, the patient was allowed to progress to weight bearing as tolerated with crutches. Once the patient lost his antalgic gait, the crutches were no longer used.

FOLLOW-UP

Postoperatively, his range of motion reached a plateau of 5 to 115 degrees of flexion. Ten months later, he developed recurrence of his medial pain and underwent arthroscopy. The ACI had largely incorporated, the lateral meniscal transplant had healed and appeared near normal (Figure C38.5), whereas the medial meniscus was torn at the posterior horn attachment. Debridement of the torn meniscus fragment and scar tissue allowed increased flexion to 125 degrees while maintaining extension. The area of incomplete filling by ACI was treated with microfracture. Thereafter, his pain was minimized to significantly less than his initial preoperative condition.

DECISION-MAKING FACTORS

1. Young, active patient with progressive symptoms largely in the medial compartment, but also in the lateral compartment.
2. Staged osteotomy without efforts to overcorrect varus deformity due to bicompartmental nature of the patient's symptoms and disease.
3. Single-stage cartilage restoration procedure to treat both the chondral surfaces and meniscal deficiency such that each procedure provides relative protection against respective graft failure.
4. Minor complaints of anterior knee pain led to a decision to avoid a significant anteromedialization of the tibial tubercle with the tubercle osteotomy performed primarily for surgical exposure.
5. Indications for second look due to pain and motion loss led to management of incomplete ACI fill with microfracture and meniscal tearing with partial meniscectomy.

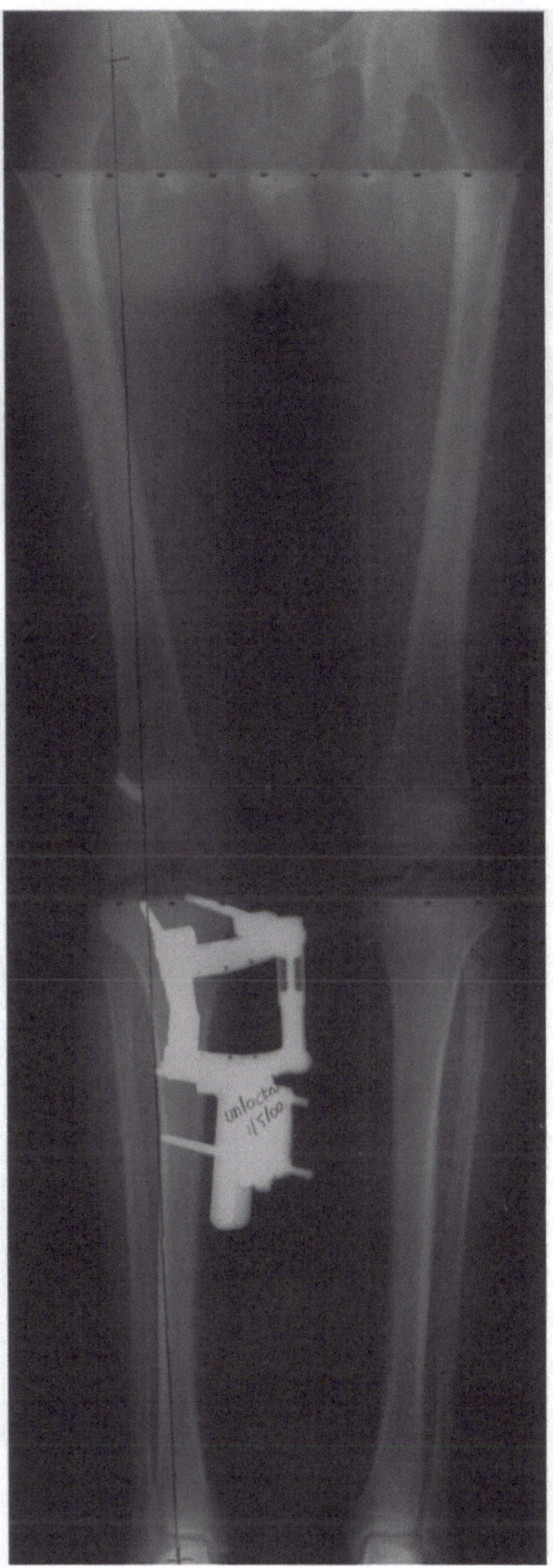

FIGURE C38.2 Postoperative radiograph with external fixator in place, and complete healing of the valgus-producing hemicallotasis high tibial osteotomy (HTO). Note that the weight-bearing line falls into the medial third of the lateral compartment.

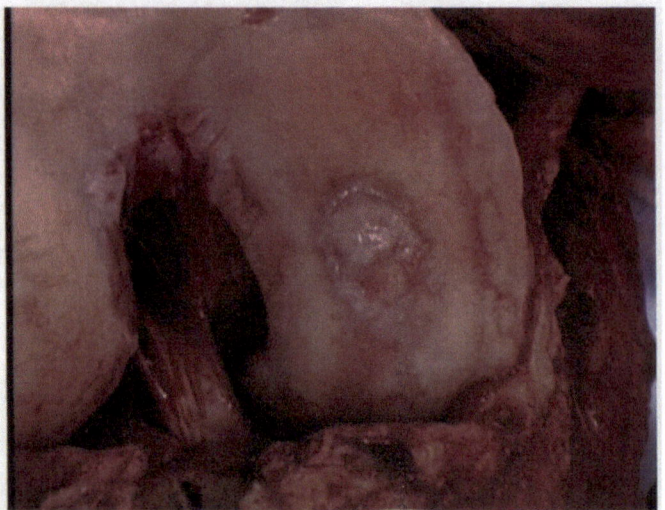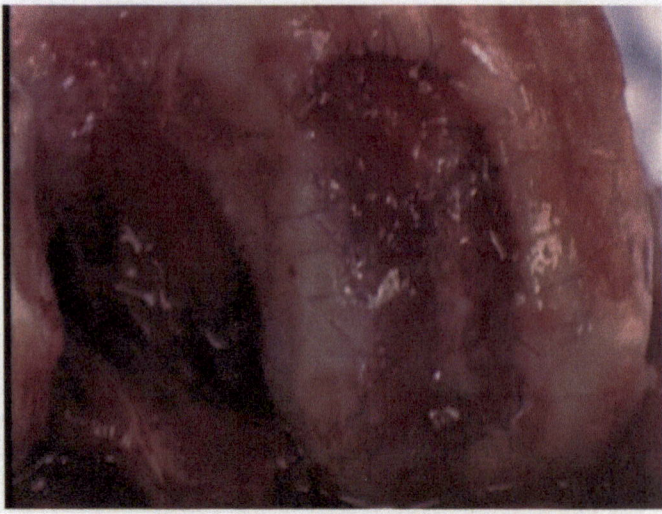

FIGURE C38.3 **(A)** Intraoperative views of the central trochlear and medial femoral condyle lesions (note intact ACL graft). **(B)** Autologous chondrocyte implantation (ACI) periosteal patch in place following preparation of the medial femoral condyle lesion.

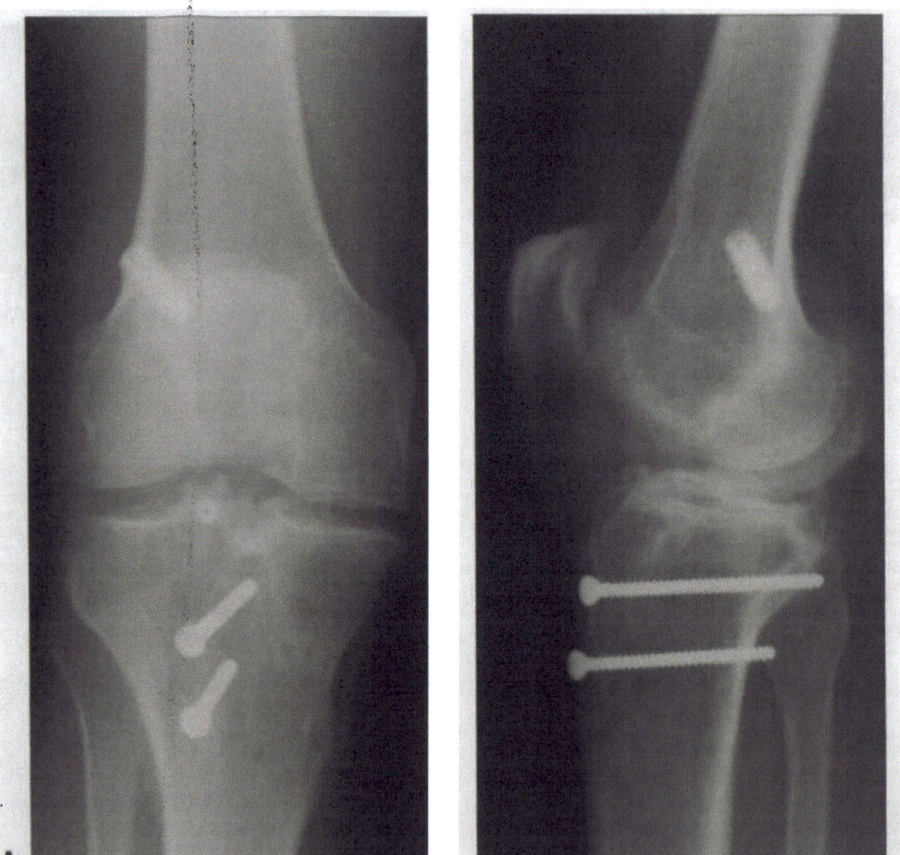

FIGURE C38.4 Postoperative anteroposterior **(A)** and lateral **(B)** films show evidence of medial and lateral bone bridge in slot meniscal transplants and fixation of the tibial tubercle.

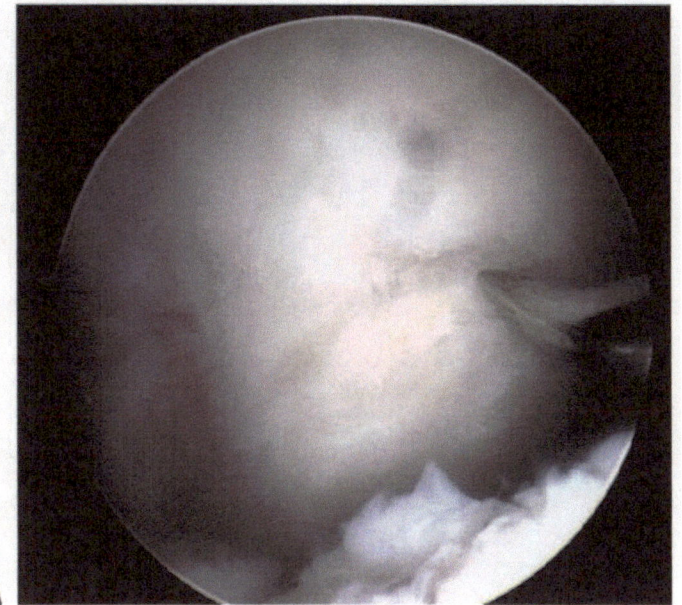
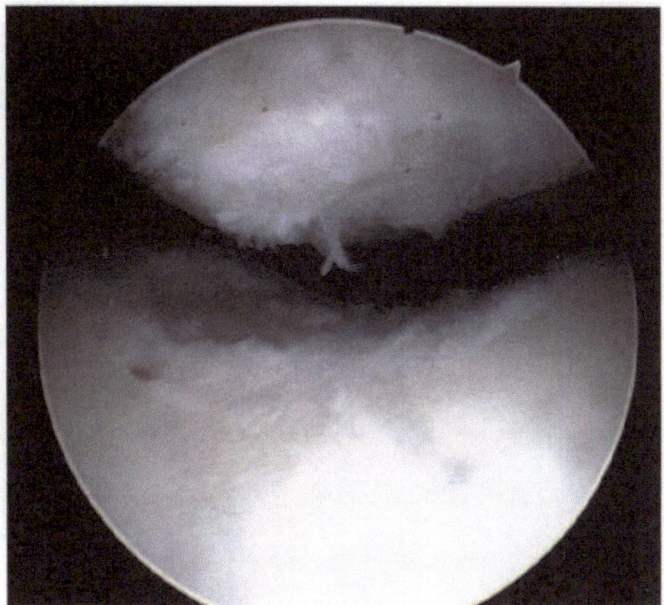
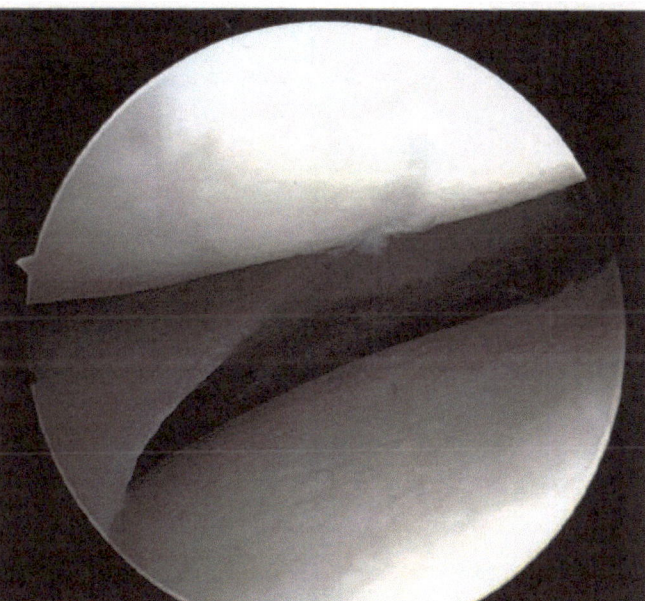

FIGURE C38.5 Ten-month postoperative second-look arthroscopy. (**A**) Treatment of 5 mm by 10 mm area of failed ACI of the medial femoral condyle with microfracture. (**B**) Trochlea shows filling with hyaline-like cartilage. (**C**) Completely healed lateral meniscus allograft.

Index